A PHYSIOLOGICAL HANDBOOK FOR TEACHERS OF YOGASANA

by

Mel Robin

Studio Yoga
P.O. Box 99
Chatham, New Jersey 07928

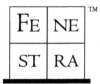

A Physiological Handbook for Teachers of *Yogasana*

Copyright © 2002 Mel Robin

Published by Fenestra Books™
610 East Delano Street, Suite 104
Tucson, Arizona 85705 U.S.A.
www.fenestrabooks.com

ISBN: 1-58736-033-0
LCCN: 2001088499

Book design by Jay Carlis & Atilla Vékony

Printed in the United States of America

Permissions for the following figures have been granted by:
Figures 3.A-1, 5.A-3, 10.A-1; Deane Juhan, *Job's Body: A Handbook for Bodywork,* Station Hill Press, Barrytown, NY, 1998.
Figures 3.A-3, 3.A-7, 6.C-2, 7.A-5, 7.A-6, 7.D-1, 10.D-1, 10.E-3, 16.A-2, 16.C-1, 17.A-1, 17.B-1; L. Heimer, *The Human Brain and Spinal Cord,* Second Ed., Springer-Verlag, NY, 1995.
Figures 3.B-2, 4.A-7; S. Vogel, *Cat's Paw and Catapults,* Norton, NY, 1998.
Figures 4.A-5, 4.E-1, 4.E-2, 4.E-3, 12.A-3; I. A. Kapandji, *The Physiology of the Joints. The Trunk and the Vertebral Column,* Vol. III, Second Ed., Churchill, Livingstone, Edinburgh, 1974.
Figure 4.A-9; B. Calais-Germain, *Anatomy of Movement,* Eastland Press, Seattle, WA, 1993.
Figures 6.E-4, 11.A-4, 11.D-1, 12.B-1, 12.C-1; Himalayan Institute of Yoga Science and Philosophy, Honesdale, PA.
Figure 7.D-2; B. K. S. Iyengar, *Light on Pranayama,* Crossroad Publications, NY, 1999.
Figure 7.A-3, 16.A-1; W. Kapit and L M. Elson, *The Anatomy Coloring Book,* HarperCollins, NY, 1977.
Figure 8.A-3: W. Kapit, R. I. Macey and E. Meisami, *The Physiology Coloring Book,* Addison Wesley, Menlo Park, CA, 1987.
Figures 8.D-4, 8.D-5; I. A. Kapandji, *The Physiology of the Joints. Lower Limb,* Vol. II, Fifth Ed., Churchill, Livingstone, Edinburgh, 1987.

AVIDYA KSETRAMUTTARESAM
PRASUPTATANUVICCHINNO DARANAM
"THE LACK OF KNOWLEDGE IS
THE CAUSE OF ALL PAIN."

YOGA SUTRA 2.4

"THE KNOWN IS LIMITED,
BUT THE UNKNOWN IS VAST.
GO TO THE UNKNOWN MORE AND MORE."

B.K.S. IYENGAR

Contents

PREFACE xiii

ACKNOWLEDGEMENTS xix

CHAPTER 1. EASTERN YOGA AND
             WESTERN MEDICINE 1

Section 1.A. Historical Perspective 1

The Two World Views 2
*Reconciling the Rationality of Medicine with
   the Sublimity of Yoga* 4
*Box 1.A-1: Yogasana, Medicine, and the
   Tomato Effect* 5

Section 1.B. The Goals of *Yogasana* 7

Levels of Consciousness 9

CHAPTER 2. NERVOUS SYSTEMS OF THE
             BODY 13

Section 2.A. Introduction 13

Section 2.B. The Central Nervous System 16

Section 2.C. The Peripheral Nervous System . 17

Connections to the Spinal Cord 17
The Cranial Nerves 17
*Box 2.B-1: Interactions of the Brain's Three
   Systems in the Teaching of
   Virabhadrasana I* 18

CHAPTER 3. THE BRAIN 21

Section 3.A. Structure and Function 21

The Three Broad Areas of the Brain 22
The Cortex: Seat of Conscious Action 24
The Spinal Cord and Brainstem 29
The Reticular Formation 31
The Limbic System 33

Section 3.B. Aspects of Brain Structure and
   Function 35

Blood Flow through the Brain 35
Headaches 37
*Maturation, Aging, and Gender Effects on
   the Brain* 39

Section 3.C. Memory, Learning, and Teaching .42

Memory and Learning 42

Short-Term Memory 43
Box 3.C-1: Learning and Yogasana Practice .44
Consolidation and Long-Term Memory 45
Teaching Yogasana 48

Section 3.D. Cerebral Hemispheric Laterality .49

Bilateral Asymmetry of the Brain 49
*Box 3.D-1: Determining Your Lateral
   Preference for Vision* 52
Cerebral Hemispheric Interactions 53
*Bilateral Asymmetry of the Brain and
   Unilateral Breathing* 53
*Oscillating Dominance of Cerebral
   Hemispheric Laterality* 54
*Using Cerebral Hemispheric Laterality in
   Yoga* 55
*Brain Laterality Can Lead to Body Laterality,
   and Vice Versa* 56

Section 3.E. Brainwaves and the Electroencephalogram (EEG) 57

Characteristics of the EEG 57
*Brainwave Frequencies and Mental
   Functioning* 60

CHAPTER 4. THE SPINE AND ITS
             APPENDAGES 63

Section 4.A. The Spinal Column 63

Structural Components 63
Normal Curvature 68
Box 4.A-1: Ontogeny Recapitulates Philogeny 69
Abnormal Curvature 70
Forward, Backward, and Lateral Bending ...71
Spinal Rotation 75
*Box 4.A-2: Spinal Rotation Can Be Induced
   by Lateral Bending and Vice Versa* 77
Conrotatory and Disrotatory Actions 78
*Misalignment of the Spine and Deterioration
   of the Vertebral Discs* 79
Spinal Muscles, Tendons, and Ligaments ...81
Blood Vessels 81
Keeping the Spine Healthy 82

Section 4.B. The Spinal Cord 83

Structure and Function 84

Neural Connectivity of the Spinal Cord 86

Section 4.C. Intervertebral Discs 87

Structure 87
Function 90
Disc Herniation and Nerve Impingement 90

Section 4.D. Cerebrospinal Fluid 93

Function and Composition 93
Yoga and CSF Pulsations of the Medial
   Suture 94

Section 4.E. The Skull and Pelvis: Axial
   Appendages of the Spine 95

The Skull 95
The Pelvis 96

Section 4.F. *Nadis, Chakras,* and *Prana* 100

Historical Perspective 100
Relation of Chakras to Anatomical
   Features 105

CHAPTER 5. THE NERVES 107

Section 5.A. Types of Nerve Cells 108

Anatomy of Nerve Cells 108
Nerve Function 112
The Motor Unit and Nerve Sensitivity 113
Mental Control of an Individual Motor Unit .113

Section 5.B. Nerve Conduction 114

Generation of an Action Potential 114
Transport of the Action Potential; Conduction
   Velocity 117
Box 5.B-1: What Really Moves When a
   Current Flows through a Nerve? 118

Section 5.C. Nerve Connections; Synapses . .121

Structure 121
Excitation Versus Inhibition 123
Mechanical Effects on Nerves 125

Section 5.D. The Neurotransmitters 128

Acetylcholine 128
The Catecholamines 129
Serotonin 129
Gamma-Aminobutyric Acid 129
Other Neurotransmitters 129
Drug Action in the Synaptic Cleft 130
Endorphins 131

Section 5.E. Transduction of the Stimulus into
   the Sensory Signal 131

In the Retina and Skin 131
The Nature of Neural Information 132

CHAPTER 6. THE AUTONOMIC NERVOUS
         SYSTEM 133

Section 6.A. Introduction to the Autonomic
   Nervous System .133

Origin 133
Homeostatic Control; Feedback and
   Feedforward 133
The Anatomical Center 135
Branches 136

Section 6.B. The Hypothalamus 140

Location and Properties 140
Function 142

Section 6.C. The Sympathetic Nervous
   System 144

Innervation 144
The Effects of Sympathetic Excitation 147
Hormonal Release of the Catecholamines . .147
Cortisol 149
Renin 150

Section 6.D. The Parasympathetic Nervous
   System 150

Innervation 151
The Vagus Nerves 152
The Effects of Parasympathetic Excitation . .152

Section 6.E. Autonomic Balance: Stress and
   Yogasana 153

Stress 153
Yogasana 156
Box 6.E-1: Yogis Can Beat the Lie Detector .160

Section 6.F. The Effects of Emotions and
   Attitudes on Stress 160

Emotions and Stress 160
Physiology Influences Psychology 162
Psychoanatomy .163
The Placebo Effect 164
Box 6.F-1: Examples of the Placebo Effect . .164

CHAPTER 7. THE SKELETAL MUSCLES .167

Section 7.A. Skeletal Muscle; Structure and
   Function 167

Physical Structure 167
Innervation Activates Muscles 176
Vascularization .177
Microscopic Muscle Contraction 178
Muscle Chemistry and Energy 182
Box 7.A-1: Muscular Life After Death 184
Macroscopic Muscle Contraction 185
Types of Muscle Contraction 187
Types of Muscle Fiber 189
Box 7.A-2: What Really Stretches When a
   Muscle Is Stretched, and Why Does It
   Stop Stretching? 190

Box 7.A-3: Muscle Fiber Types in the Poultry World 192

Reciprocal Inhibition and Agonist/Antagonist Pairs 193

Joint Movements in Yogasana 196

Box 7.A-4: The Hands Help Wag the Shoulder Blades in Adho Mukha Svanasana 196

Section 7.B. Muscle Sensors; the Mechano-receptors 198

The Mechanoreceptors in Skeletal Muscle ..198

Structure of Muscle Spindles 199

Function of Muscle Spindles 201

Box 7.B-1: PNF, Contracting in Order to Lengthen 204

Resting Muscle Tone 204

The Golgi Tendon Organs 206

Ruffini Corpuscles 208

Section 7.C. Proprioception 208

Proprioceptors 208

Proprioception and Yogasana 210

Section 7.D. Reflex Actions 211

General Definition of Phasic Reflex 211

The Myotactic Stretch Reflex 212

The Flexional Tonic Reflex 214

Box 7.D-1: Why are Backbends Energizing? 216

A Reflection on the Cervical Flexion Reflex .218

Other Reflex Actions 220

Yoga and the Conscious Control of Reflex Action 222

Box 7.D-2: Conscious Action Pays Off in Yogasana 223

Section 7.E. Resistance to Muscle Stretching .223

When Stretching, Time Matters, and Time Is on Your Side 224

Physical Stretching Can Lead to Mental Stretching 226

Warming Up 227

Stress and Strain 228

Section 7.F. Aspects of Muscle Distress and Injury 230

Muscle Fatigue and Soreness 230

Muscle Cramping and Spasms 231

Paying the Price for Stretching Too Far and/or Too Fast 232

Muscle Memory, Yogasana Detraining, and Over-training 233

CHAPTER 8. THE BONES 235

Section 8.A. Bone Structure, Development, and Mechanics 235

Bone Structure and Development 235

Innervation and Vascularization 238

Bone Mechanics 240

Bone Density 241

Section 8.B. Bone Chemistry 242

Collagen 242

Hormonal Control of Ca^{2+} in the Body Fluids 242

Box 8.B-1: Detoxification 243

Section 8.C. Bone Repair and Remodeling 244

Injury and Repair 244

The Remodeling Response to Mechanical Stress 245

Section 8.D. The Skeletal Appendages 247

The Legs and Feet 247

Box 8.D-1: The Benefits of Rotating the Femurs in Yogasana 249

The Arms, Shoulders, and Shoulder Blades .254

Section 8.E. The Joints 260

The Bones Form the Joints 260

Ligaments and Tendons 262

The Knee Joint as an Example 265

Joint Lubrication and Arthritis 265

Box 8.E-1: A Safe Way to Teach Padmasana 266

Section 8.F. Mechanoreceptors in the Joint Capsules and Ligaments 268

Section 8.G. Osteoporosis 269

Definition, Statistics, and Causes 269

Symptoms and End Results 270

Yogasana, Western Exercise, and Osteoporosis 271

CHAPTER 9. CONNECTIVE AND SUPPORTING TISSUES 273

Section 9.A. Connective Tissues 273

The Body's Glue 273

Collagen 273

Elastin 274

Ground Substance 275

Ligaments and Tendons 275

Myofascia 276

Box 9.A-1. What Price Myofascia? 277

Other Connective-Tissue Types 279

Effects of Age on Connective Tissue 279

Connective-Tissue Injury 279

Section 9.B. Cartilage 280

CHAPTER 10. THE SKIN 283

Section 10.A. Structure of the Skin 283

Section 10.B. Sensory Receptors in the Skin .285

Receptor Adaptation 285
Light Touch 287
Deep Pressure 290
Other Receptors in the Skin 291
The Skin, Emotions, and Touching 291
Yogasana and Touching by the Teacher 291

Section 10.C. Thermal Regulation by Blood
Vessels and Sweat Glands in the Skin 292

Section 10.D. Pain .294

The Physiology of Pain 296
The Psychology of Pain 297
Neural Aspects of Pain 298
*Box 10.D-1: Cultural and Psychological
Factors in Pain* 299
Yoga, Injury, and Pain 301
The Endorphins .303

Section 10.E. Dermatomes and Referred Pain 303

Section 10.F. Glands within the Skin 307

The Sweat Glands 307
The Sebaceous Glands 307
The Tear Glands .308

Section 10.G. Hair and Piloerection 308

CHAPTER 11. THE HEART AND THE
VASCULAR SYSTEM 309

Section 11.A. Structure and Function of the
Heart 310

The Pumping Chambers of the Heart 310
The Valves within the Heart 312
*The Timing of the Cardiac Contractions
and Coordination withValve Positions* . . .313
Cardiac Muscle .314
*Innervation of the Heart: The Cardiac
Pacemaker* 315
*Box 11.A-1: The Cells of the SA Node Share
an Electrical Bond* 316
*Box 11.A-2: Stopping the Heart by Conscious
Control of the Vagus Nerve* 317
The Electrocardiogram 319
*Effects of Western Exercise, Yogasana, and the
Autonomic Nervous System on the Heart* .320

Section 11.B. Blood 322

Chemistry and Function 322
Erythrocytes (Red Blood Cells) 323
Platelets 324
The White Blood Cells 324
The Blood-Brain Barrier 325

Section 11.C. The Vascular System 325

Architecture 325
Mechanics of Blood Flow: Blood Pressure . .330

Venous Flow Against Gravity 332
Thermoregulation 334

Section 11.D. Blood Pressure 334

*Vasoconstriction, Vasodilation, and
Hypertension* .334

Section 11.E. Monitoring Blood Pressure with
the Baroreceptors 339

The Baroreceptor Reflex Arc 341
Other Sensors 342

Section 11.F. Blood Pressure in Inverted
Yogasanas 343

Hydrostatic Pressure 343
*Box 11.F-1: How the Giraffe and the Dinosaur
Gamble When Taking Their First Lunch* . .343
General Effects of Inversion on Circulation .345
Blood Pressure in Semi-Inversion 348
Full-Body Inversions 349
Inversion and Blood Pressure at the Eyes . . .349
*Box 11.F-2: Turning Red During and After
Inversions* 350
Inversions and Hypertension 350
Benefits of Inversions 352
*Box 11.F-3: Inversion (and Laughing) Can
Lead to Urination* 352

Section 11.G. The Lymphatic System 352

Structure and Function 352
Lymph Nodes 353

CHAPTER 12. RESPIRATION 355

Section 12.A. Mechanics of the Breath 355

Journey into the Lungs 356
The Ribs 359
*Using the Diaphragm and the Ribs to
Breathe* 362
*Box 12.A-1. Divers and Yogasana Students
Must Be Aware of the Dead Volume* 365
*Innervation and Control of the Breathing
Centers* 366
*The Effects of Exercise and Emotion on
Respiration* 368
The Function of Hemoglobin 369

Section 12.B. The Three Modes of Breathing 370

Abdominal Breathing 370
Diaphragmatic Breathing 371
Thoracic Breathing 372
Factors Affecting the Breath 373
Rationalizing the Effects of the Breath 374

Section 12.C. Nasal Laterality 374

Internal Structure of the Nose 375
Periodicity of Nasal Laterality 375

*Physiological and Psychological Effects of
  Nasal Laterality* 377
*The Conscious Development and Shift of
  Nasal Laterality* 378
*Relation of Laterality to Other Aspects of
  the Breath* 380
*Connection to Cerebral Hemispheric
  Laterality* 381
Section 12.D. *Pranayama* 381

CHAPTER 13. THE IMMUNE SYSTEM 383

Section 13.A. Lymphocytes and Leucocytes .383
The B Lymphocytes 384
The T Lymphocytes 384
Immunotransmitters 385
Section 13.B. The Autonomic Nervous System
  and Immunity 386
Section 13.C. Malfunctions of the Immune
  System 387
Cancer 387
Allergic Reactions and Autoimmunity 387
Fever 388
AIDS 388
The Brain's Immune System 388
Section 13.D. Yoga, the Immune System, and
  Illness 389

CHAPTER 14. EXTERNAL SECRETIONS . .393

Section 14.A. Saliva and Mucus 393
*Box 14.A-1: Using the Salivary Glands as
  Lie Detectors* 394
Section 14.B. Tears 395
Section 14.C. Sweat 395
Section 14.D. Body Wastes 396
Urination 396
Defecation 397

CHAPTER 15. THE HORMONES 399

Section 15.A. General Features of Hormonal
  Systems 399
Types of Glands and Hormones 401
Rhythmic Release of Hormones 401
Section 15.B. Specific Glands and Their
  Hormones 403
The Hypothalamus 403
The Pituitary Gland 404
The Pineal Gland 404
The Thyroid Gland 405
The Parathyroid Gland 405
The Thymus Gland 405

The Adrenal Glands 405
The Pancreas and Gastrointestinal Glands . .407
The Gonads 408
CHAPTER 16. THE EYES AND VISION 411
Section 16.A. Structure and Function of the
  Eyes 411
External Structure of the Eye 411
Internal Structure of the Eye 413
Vision and Neuroanatomy of the Eye 415
The Ocular-Vestibular Connection 418
Section 16.B. Stress, Vision, and Yoga 419
Stress and Vision 419
Yogic Relaxation for Visual Stress 419
The Eyes Set the Body's Clock 421
Section 16.C. Vision and Cerebral Laterality .422
Crossover of the Optic Nerve 422
The Higher Visual Centers 424
Memory and Visual Laterality 424
Section 16.D. Color Therapy and Yoga 426
Color Therapy 426
Yoga in Colored Lights: A Proposal 428
*Box 16.D-1: The Effects of Colors and the
  Emotions on Muscle Strength* 429
White-Light Starvation 430
CHAPTER 17. SOUND, HEARING, AND
  BALANCE 433
Section 17.A. The Middle Ear 433
The Mechanics of Hearing 433
Yoga and the Middle Ear 435
*Box 17.A-1: Relaxing the Muscles of the
  Middle Ear* 435
Section 17.B. The Vestibular Organs of
  Balance 437
Structure and Function of the Inner Ear 437
Sensors for the Static Position of the Head . .438
*Sensors for the Dynamic Movement of the
  Head* 439
Innervation of the Vestibular Tract 440
CHAPTER 18. THE GASTROINTESTINAL
  ORGANS AND DIGESTION .441
Section 18.A. Structure and Function 441
The Mouth and Esophagus 442
The Stomach 444
*Generation and Containment of Stomach
  Acid* 444
The Small Intestine 445
The Colon 446
Peristalsis 447

Accessory Organs of Digestion 447
The Effects of Stress on the Gastrointestinal
Tract 448
Section 18.B. Digestion and Metabolism 449
Yogasana Practice and the Digestive
Process .449
Metabolism 450
CHAPTER 19. SEXUAL FUNCTION,
GYNECOLOGY, AND
PREGNANCY 453
Section 19.A. Menstruation 453
The Menstrual Cycle 453
Premenstrual Syndromes 454
Inversions at That Time of the Month 455
Section 19.B. Pregnancy 456
The Balance between Estrogen and
Progesterone 456
Muscles, Joints, Ligaments, and Tendons
During Pregnancy 457
Respiratory and Cardiovascular Systems . . .458
The Nervous and Digestive Systems 459
Section 19.C. Menopause 459
Section 19.D. Sexual Function 461
CHAPTER 20. THE EMOTIONS 463
Section 20.A. Depression 464
Symptoms 464
Medicine Versus Depression 464
Yogasana Versus Depression 467
Colored Lights Versus Depression 468
Section 20.B. Mania and Bipolar
Disorder 469
Symptoms 469
Treatment 469
Section 20.C. Anxiety 470
Symptoms 470
Anxiety and Yogasana 471
Other Disorders 471
Section 20.D. Emotion and the Breath 471
CHAPTER 21. TIME AND BODY
RHYTHMS 473
Section 21.A. The Innate Sense of Time 473
Section 21.B. Periodicity of Body Rhythms . .474
Ultradian Rhythms 474
Circadian Rhythms; Physiological Peaks
and Valleys in the 24-Hour Period 476
Ayurvedic Rhythms 483

The Mechanism of the Circadian Clock 484
Yogasana and Chronotherapy 486
The Sleep/Wake Cycle and Relaxation 488
Infradian Rhythms 491
CHAPTER 22. AGING AND LONGEVITY . .493
Section 22. A. Symptoms and Statistics 493
What to Expect 493
Physical Aging 495
Longevity 498
Yoga, Sports, and Aging 499
Section 22.B. Mental and Emotional Effects
of Aging 499
APPENDIX I. *YOGASANA*
ILLUSTRATIONS 503
APPENDIX II. INJURIES INCURRED DURING
IMPROPER *YOGASANA*
PRACTICE 511
Section II.A. Introduction 511
Practicing Yogasanas from a Book, Without
a Teacher .511
Being Too Tired Can Lead to Injury 512
Being Too Ambitious Can Lead to Injury . . .512
Congenital Weaknesses 512
Section II.B. Specific Case Histories 513
Neurological Damage 513
Vascular Damage 515
Muscular Damage 518
APPENDIX III. BODY SYMMETRY 519
Section III.A. Symmetry, Beauty, and Health .519
Section III.B. Symmetry and Yoga 520
Section III.C. The Body's Inherent Lack of
Symmetry .520
Box III.B-1: Preserving the Symmetry of
Tadasana in Trikonasana 521
Section III.D. Handedness 523
APPENDIX IV. BALANCING 525
Section IV.A. Introduction 525
Section IV.B. Mechanical Aspects of
Balancing .526
Balancing a Rigid Block 526
Intelligent Balancing of a Block 527
Section IV.C. Balancing the Body 529
On Becoming a Broomstick 529
Generating a Countertorque 530

Box IV.C-1: How to Use the Floor When Balancing 531

Section IV.D. Other Aids to Balancing in the *Yogasanas* 533

Vision and Balance 533

Box IV.D-1: Using Your Eyes to Balance . . .534

Using the Wall as Support in Balancing Yogasanas 535

Making Your Own Wall for Balancing 536

Redistributing the Mass in the Aid of Balance 537

Box IV.D-2: The Human Balancing Tower . .538

Section IV.E. Balancing in the Standing *Yogasanas* 538

Localizing the Balancing Action in Vrksasana 538

Box IV.E-1: You Have More Sensitivity in Your Big Toe Than You Ever Imagined . . .539

Balancing in the Other Standing Yogasanas .541

Box IV.E-2: Physical Crossover Requires Neural Crossover 543

Section IV.F. Balancing in the Inverted *Yogasanas* 544

Aids to Balancing in the Inverted Yogasanas 544

Box IV.F-1: Resistive Balancing 545

Performing the Inverted Yogasanas 545

Section IV.G. General Points on Keeping Your Balance 551

APPENDIX V. GRAVITY 553

Section V.A. Exerting Pressure on the Floor .553

You Have No Choice 553

Section V.B. The Center of Gravity 554

Section V.C. Gravitational Effects on *Yogasanas* 555

GLOSSARY .557

REFERENCES 575

INDEX .589

PREFACE

I came to yoga from a career as a research scientist with a strong left-brain point of view; once into yoga teaching, my scientific bent innocently led me into assembling two data bases of isolated but interesting facts about *yogasana*-as-it-might-relate-to-medicine and about medicine-as-it-might-relate-to-*yogasana*. These scraps of information were collected in a totally haphazard way, written down as I came across them in the current yoga journals and medical books. Because there was no one book in which such connections could be found, my initial intention was to simply have such files on hand for occasional use in my own classes.

Eventually, the collection grew to two card files encompassing yoga and medicine, with each having about a hundred isolated "facts", but with very few facts connected to anything else in either their own or the other file. At first, these files looked much like a puzzle when all of the pieces are first put on the table. However, as the cards on file accumulated, soon a few new facts could be logically related to others collected earlier, so that small islands of understanding began to emerge. As these islands of coherence grew, they took on the appearance of small essays. At this point, the possibility of writing a handbook connecting the sciences of *yogasana* practice and Western medicine was born in my mind, however, with publication contingent upon the final effort having a coherence that would allow the statement of general principles and an expanded understanding of these two sciences. To this end, I have combed the literatures of *yogasana* and medicine as completely as I can, and lay before you the juxtaposed pictures of the two sciences as I have found them.

Inasmuch as the sciences of *yogasana* and Western medicine evolved independently of one another, it is no surprise that we are trying to assemble a puzzle for which many key pieces are still missing. However, as the pieces of the puzzle connect, with a little imagination one can guess the shape and coloring of the missing pieces with some confidence. I have done this in several places, but have been careful to point out that the "information" is only my best guess for what is going on, and may well be incomplete or even incorrect. Anticipating the future, I also discuss several medical and yogic topics at some length for which there is little or no complementary yogic or medical data; hopefully, these gaps will be filled by more detailed studies in the future. I feel that even with these admitted gaps, there is sufficient correlation of the data in the *yogasana* and medicine cardfiles to warrant placing this admittedly incomplete picture in the hands of interested readers.

Let us take a moment then to define our terms. By "*yogasana*" is meant the scientific practice of the traditional Indian postures, performed with alignment, strength and grace as per the directives of B.K.S. Iyengar [209]. By stabilizing the body through this practice, one can then stabilize and quiet the mind. "Pranayama" is the science of the control of the breath; when the breath is controlled, it is refined, with the result that the mind is again quiet but inwardly alert. By "Western medicine" is meant the scientific study of body systems and their understanding in terms of physiological processes such as heart rate, blood pressure, autonomic stimulation, muscle-spindle response, hormones, *etc* [113].

In this Handbook, I present scientific material of the sort *yogasana* teachers should know and understand, but which committed students might also find interesting. Similarly, the medically inclined will find many yogic aspects of the body mentioned in this Handbook, which have been uncovered over the millennia by the yogis, but not yet investigated by medical science.

Though there are eight limbs to the yoga tree of Patanjali [211], the present work deals almost totally with the third limb, the *yogasanas*, or postures, only tangentially with the fourth limb, *pranayama*, and not at all with the others. This is not to say that they are not all equally important, but it is at the levels of *yogasana* and *pranayama* that the eight limbs of yoga and Western medicine have their largest common ground; hence it is at this level that the integration of *yogasana* and medical understandings makes the most sense.

Similarly, there are many current topics of modern Western medicine that are of tremendous interest and utility, but they too will be ignored, for they do not at present interface with what we know about yoga, just as the higher levels of Patanjali's yoga go far beyond where medical understanding can presently operate. These restrictions will change with time as the two sciences come to recognize one another and their areas of highest sophistication eventually converge on one another.

This Handbook deals with that aspect of yoga that is amenable to rational thought and experiment. Such a mechanistic approach, I feel, is undeniably relevant to *yogasana* practice for beginners. It is equally undeniable that the mechanistic approach is less relevant for the more advanced practitioner, for whom yoga and its effects go far beyond our powers to quantify, measure or understand. Perhaps we can think of the mechanistic approach as equivalent to the use of props, a practice that helps the beginning student in the performance of the *yogasanas*, but is not intended necessarily to be used at higher levels of the yoga tree.

The intended audience for the Handbook consists of yoga teachers with perhaps 5 to 10 years experience (but not necessarily in the Iyengar approach), who have not otherwise been trained in science, but who unavoidably have been exposed to the medical side of yoga without understanding much of that aspect. Perhaps one has wondered about just what is being said by more experienced teachers, but has been hesitant to "look it up" in a medical textbook. Perhaps instead, one is just curious and is in love with the feeling that comes with rationalizing a new idea or sensation based on new understanding. This person will find something new to get excited about in this Handbook, I believe, as will the interested student of *yogasana* who does not yet teach. It is assumed in turn that these teachers are working with beginning students, practicing those *yogasanas* with which beginners most often work.

With the above limitations in mind, the scope of this Handbook in terms of what it is, and what it is not, can be set out in more detail:

What this Handbook is:

1) This Handbook is meant to be a bridge between medicine and *yogasana*, allowing the *yogasana* teacher and the medical researcher to place these two sciences in

relative context, so that each makes the other more interesting and useful.

2) This Handbook is primarily for teachers of *yogasana*. It can be read piecemeal through use of the extensive glossary, so one does not need to study all of the preceding Chapters in order to understand the topic of interest. On the other hand, the Handbook is totally cross-referenced internally, so that one can easily turn to other Chapters to find material related to that under discussion. Of course, some may want to read the entire book, cover to cover: may God bless you.

When the moment comes that you suddenly wonder, "What happens to the blood pressure in *sirsasana?*" or, "Why are backbends energizing?" or, "Why do we turn the leg out in *trikonasana?*" *A Physiological Handbook for Teachers of Yogasana* can be of help to you. Previous to that moment, one's interest level in questions such as these may be less than intense. Nonetheless, it is my hope that using the Handbook will stimulate questions and thoughts in your mind that otherwise might be dormant. Either way, this Handbook will pull you and your students a little deeper into the science of the body and how it works. I believe that medical researchers also will find many yogic gems in this Handbook over which to ponder and possibly put under the microscope of Western medicine.

As one goes deeper into the details of teaching the *yogasanas*, generalizations emerge that allow one to teach, at a certain level, all poses without having to learn the details for each specific pose. And so we hope it also will be with the physiologic effects of the *yogasanas*, where we intend to uncover the generalities of the effects in all poses without having to learn them specifically for each.

3) This Handbook offers discussions of a few scientific topics in Appendices which are somewhat off the main track (for example, Section IV.E, Balancing in the Standing *Yogasanas,* page 538) or otherwise are often confused when used by non-scientist teachers (for example, Appendix V, GRAVITATIONAL EFFECTS ON *YOGASANAS,* page 553). Interesting but tangential discussions of shorter length have been placed in Boxes which may be read or not, without interrupting the flow of the more pertinent text.

4) This Handbook is a what-happens-when-you-do-it text, rather than a how-to-do-it text. It is assumed that the yoga teachers will be familiar with the postures used as examples in the Handbook, and that with the use of the illustrations in Appendix I, medical researchers will be able to follow the yogic text.

5) This Handbook's approach is most strongly focused on the yogic methods of B.K.S. Iyengar [209], as this is the most scientific of the yogas and so is closest to the medical explanations of how the body works. My own practice follows that of Guruji B.K.S. Iyengar.

6) Many beginning students need motivation to practice the *yogasanas*, to return to class, *etc*. Because this Handbook offers rational discussion of the reasons why we work the *yogasanas* as we do, and why we feel as we do while doing them, it can make yoga more interesting to students and so bind them more firmly to their practice.

7) Given that you will be teaching an average cross-section of the adult population, the list below of the seven most popular reasons for adults visiting office-based physicians [114], in large part will reflect the kinds of health problems your students typically will lay at your feet.

1) Hypertension
2) Pregnancy Care
3) Check Up; Wellness Care
4) Upper Respiratory Infections (Colds)
5) Lower Back Pain
6) Depression and Anxiety
7) Diabetes

This Handbook in no way intends to teach therapeutic yoga, however, your teaching will be better if you are familiar with the symptoms of these conditions and at the same time have some understanding of how the relevant body-systems work, and how various *yogasanas* impact on these systems. Most if not all of the items in the list above are at least mentioned in the Handbook, and most are treatable by *yogasana* in the hands of properly trained teachers [209, 306, 379, 421]. If you someday hope to work in the area of therapeutic *yogasana*, you will want a firm understanding of the body and yoga at the level given in this Handbook. In either case, one should be aware that even if a student is in fit condition, performance of the therapeutic poses and sequences can still be of great value, as they act as prophylactics against future conditions not otherwise active at present.

This Handbook is not:

1) This Handbook is not a novel. It is not a continuous, coherent read from one Chapter to the next, but rather, being a Handbook, one can open it in the middle and hope to find information on a particular physiological or *yogasana* item of present interest in compact form and at an understandable yet informative level. In addition to one-stop shopping, the Handbook offers an extensive reference list for those who want to go back to the original sources.

2) Though this Handbook is not a how-to-do-it book on the basic and more advanced *yogasanas*, the Handbook may discuss how a specific posture is performed, so as to illustrate a particular medical or yogic principle.

3) This Handbook is not a complete medical text outlining how the components of the body function. A great deal of detail may be given to medical areas having a direct impact on *yogasanas*, whereas other very important medical areas are not even mentioned due to a lack of yogic relevance at present. A similar statement holds in regard yoga principles which have been ignored because they have no medical basis as yet.

4) This Handbook is not a text on therapeutic *yogasanas*. Though the subject is *yogasana* and medicine, it is not specifically about *yogasana* as therapy, except for a few examples which are given to illustrate specific physical/medical/yogic principles.

5) This Handbook is not a historic description of yoga or of medicine, or their philosophies.

6) This Handbook is not a description of a mature field, though its component parts, *yogasana* and Western medicine, each have long histories and deal with very sophisticated subjects. Because these fields have developed almost completely independently, any overlap uncovered at this late date is more by coincidence than by design. I have tried to include all of the scientifically sound studies dealing with the specific interactions of *yogasanas* and the body-mind.

7) This Handbook is not an easy introduction to the science of the body for non-scientists. It assumes a certain sophistication of *yogasana* practice and understanding, and a willingness to study how the body functions. The medical discussions are relatively high level, and like *yogasana* practice itself, may require the reader to make considerable effort to master the material. Though it has not been my intention, the reader may need other books as well as this one.

My own experience (17 years as student, 12 years as teacher) is that one can more easily keep the experience of *yogasana* practice fresh and full of awareness if one can make the connections between what is being experienced in the *yogasanas* and what one understands of the functions of the body/mind as put forth by Western medicine. I understand that this is over-analyzing something that historically was not meant to be understood in this way, and I know that it is just a reflection of my unthinking tendency to dissect and rationalize everything that comes into view. Nonetheless, I have found this attempt at bringing Western medicine and *yogasana* into some sort of rational relationship to be satisfying to me, and though there are as many loose ends as connections, still the new awareness of the connections has led me to yet more avenues to explore.

Each of the new avenues opened by simultaneously considering Western medicine and *yogasana* has served to refresh and invigorate my practice and my teaching. Each of the hours that I practice and each of the hours that I teach are refreshed by the thought of how these two sciences, which have developed so independently of one another, have come to dovetail as nicely as they do. We can say that the goal in this Handbook is to take the mystery out of Western medicine and out of *yogasana* practice, but not the wonder.

My work on this book has significantly changed my view of yoga. I hope after reading this, you too will find that your sense of self has changed in some significant way, as you come to appreciate more the marvels of your body and mind, their connections, and the ingenuity of the human body/mind in uncovering so many parts of this beautiful mechanism, through both medical practice and *yogasana* practice.

ACKNOWLEDGEMENTS

This Handbook has been road tested on various yoga teachers willing to read the text and give feedback on what needed to be changed. I especially am happy to acknowledge Carol Wipf, Karen Wachsmuth, Eliza Childs, Mary Dalziel, Susan Ahlstrom, and Elaine Patterson, for their valuable help in this important aspect of putting the Handbook together. Special thanks goes to Dr. Arlene Thoma who diligently proofread the Chapter on The Spine. Similarly, I am indebted to Royane Mosely and Nancy Barr for both their skill and patience in regard to drawing and redrawing many of the Figures. Finally, I thank Roger Cole and Fernando Ruiz Pages for several helpful technical discussions, and Jean Fisher for help in searching various databases.

Tom and Susan Parrish of the Quakertown Kungfu Center have been especially helpful in support of this project, and it is a pleasure to acknowledge publicly the time and energy they have volunteered in aid of the completion of this work.

I owe more than I can say to my *yogasana* teachers, Theresa Rowland, Gabriella Giubilaro, Nancy Stechert, and Judy Freedman, each of whom has been an inspiration to me in their depth of knowledge, and their dedication to both their art and their students.

Many of the connections presented in the Handbook between medicine and *yogasana* are not newly discovered by me. Others have considered these two sciences and written briefly on the connections they have found. I have gathered all of their wisdom as best I can into one place, so that the reader can easily find in a Handbook format what they have to say. I hope that I have understood them correctly in reporting their work. In particular, I thank yoga teachers such as Judith Lasater, Arthur Kilmurray, and Roger Cole, who have put so much into the literature on how yoga relates to physiological processes. I have incorporated much of their work into this Handbook, and thank them for all they have explained to me (and you) in regard to how *yogasana* and Western medicine interact.

By necessity, one important reference has been omitted from the reference list, for if I were to specifically acknowledge each item that my day-to-day teacher, Theresa Rowland, has taught me in the past 10 years, it would swell the size of this Handbook to unmanageable proportions. *A Physiological Handbook for Teachers of Yogasana* would never have materialized without the inspiration and understanding I have drawn from her. Of course, eventually all such credit and thanks must be placed at the feet of our guru, B.K.S. Iyengar, whose systematic study of the *yogasanas* forms the basis of any work seeking to tie *yogasana* and medical principles to one another.

Mel Robin
Upper Black Eddy, Pennsylvania 18972
AandMRobin@AOL.com
January 25, 2002.

Chapter 1

EASTERN YOGA AND WESTERN MEDICINE

SECTION 1.A. HISTORICAL PERSPECTIVE

Today's chasm between Western medical science and yoga science is based largely on the differences between Eastern and Western modes of medical experimentation: Western medicine was founded upon the facts learned by dissection of cadavers, in human bodies lacking all energy. On the other hand, dissection of cadavers being forbidden in the Eastern tradition, doctors of that tradition obtained their understanding of the body by observation of living human beings and their patterns of energy [83, 279].

Operating in this way, the yogis intuited the seven major psychic centers of the body, the *chakras*, as listed in Table 1.A-1. Though it was not the original intention to attribute the *chakras* to physical structures, it is amazing to see how closely they correspond to known specific endocrine plexi in the body. The relationship of the *chakras* and their subunits to physical structures in the human body are discussed further in Section 4.F, *Nadis*, *Chakras*, and *Prana*, page 100.

From the Western perspective, the functions of the body have been divided into eleven subsystems: the integumentary system (the external skin), the skeletal system (the bones and joints), the muscular system (skeletal muscles), the nervous system (central and peripheral nervous systems), the endocrine system (hormones), the cardiovascular system (the heart and blood vessels), the lymphatic system, the respiratory system (lungs and breathing), the digestive system, the urinary system, and the reproductive system. The Chapters in this Handbook are based largely on the eleven-part Western scheme of the body.

Though yoga was first mentioned in the ancient Vedic texts of India approximately 3000 years ago, it is thought that it existed

TABLE 1.A-1. RELATION OF THE CHAKRAS TO SPECIFIC ENDOCRINE GLANDS, AND THEIR PSYCHOLOGICAL ATTRIBUTES [279]

Chakra	Endocrine Plexus	Psychological Attribute
Genital	Gonads	Sexuality
Sacral	Adrenal	Fear
Solar Plexus	Pancreas	Power
Heart	Thymus	Love
Throat	Thyroid	Creativity
Brow	Pituitary	Intuition
Crown	Pineal	Bliss

for millennia before that as an oral tradition. Various references to yoga in the ancient texts were drawn together and codified by Patanjali in his work *Yoga Sutra* sometime in the period 200–800 B.C. [113, 306]. In this work, Patanjali laid out the basic philosophy behind the actions one must take in order to bring the mind to a steady, single focus, unwavering, with this then opening the doorway to higher states of consciousness and ultimately to liberation from the pain of ordinary life.

Many variations on the basic theme of Patanjali have taken shape, including the *hatha yoga* approach, which employs the *yogasanas* as focal points for increasing one's strength and sharpening one's concentration. Patanjali says of the postures, that they are to be done in such a way that one is steady, alert, and at ease. The *hatha* form of yoga based upon the *yogasanas* is relatively young, possibly having been introduced as such in the 15th century [432]. Though *Yoga Sutra* mentions no asanas by name, it has survived as the cornerstone of *hatha yoga* practice to the present day.

The *yogasanas* of *hatha yoga* number approximately 700,000, and are performed with the intention of manipulating the body's inherent energy upward through willpower and awareness or downward through relaxation. It is only relatively recently that such yogic exercises have come to be important as therapeutic aids for curing or preventing illness and disease, rather than as points on which to focus one's mental powers in an effort to gain liberation. That is not to say that in the earliest days of yoga, postures were not recognized for their curative values.

It was only in the early 1800's that Western medicine broke away from religion and superstition, leaving behind the influences of the medicine woman, myth, and magic, and adopted instead attitudes based on the medicine man (the physician), science, and experimentation. Since that time, it has succeeded in its own way in inventing, discovering and pushing ahead the frontiers of knowledge about the body and about the mind, albeit, the push has been largely in one direction only (see Subsection 1.A, *Reconciling the Rationality of Medicine with the Sublimity of Yoga*, page 4). In our work, we will try to honor aspects of the traditional *hatha yoga* approach by focusing on the scientifically-documented, objective effects of *yogasana* practice, rather than on the more subjective feelings attendant to this.

The Two World Views

Given the huge number of books on Western medicine at all levels of sophistication, and similarly the huge number of books on *yogasana* (for example [209 and 306]), it is something of a mystery as to why no in-depth book has appeared on the relation between the two. Of course, one also could ask why there is no book relating ballroom dancing to architecture, for example, but clearly in this case there is no reason to expect any overlap of understanding between the two fields, whereas with medicine and *yogasana*, the situation is just the opposite. One can reasonably expect the truths of yoga will stand in one-to-one correspondence with the truths of Western medicine, if indeed they are truths after all.

In regard to this question, perhaps the lack of a book relating *yogasana* to Western medicine may be due to the two world views that pervade human thinking. As shown in Table 1.A-2, there are two world views about most subjects, yoga and Western medicine included. "World View I" has been developed intuitively in the Eastern world, then refined and sharpened by the test of time and out of respect for the sages of the past, whereas "World View II" has been developed in the Western world, and refined by experiment and observation using modern scientific tools and methods. The separate and unquestioned existence of these two World Views implies more or less that they are antithetical: you subscribe to either one of the views or the other. Undoubtedly, the list in Table 1.A-2 could be expanded by adding "Yoga" to the list for World View I, and "Science" to the list for World View II.

Unfortunately, the qualities of the two lists in the Table are so opposite that combining them leads to laughable oxymorons (Intuitive Facts, Subjective Real World, Rational Faith, *etc.*). Among the better oxymorons would be "Yoga Science" or "Scientific Yoga". At best, one might hold the two categories of yoga and science in one's mind sequentially, but not simultaneously, as the dissonance would be too great for that! It is the aim of this Handbook to demonstrate that the fields of yoga and science actually have a much closer and more rational relation than the two World Views would suggest.

Lacking any reconciliation of the apparent conflict between science and yoga, and with the ascendancy of World View II, we have come to a situation in which Western medical doctors, who hold science in the highest regard, hold yoga's understanding of the body in low regard because it has not been "proved" in the accepted Western way. At the same time, yogis hold Western medicine in low regard because it has no precedence historically in the Eastern world in which yoga was born and developed [176].

To see examples of the recent animosity between the two groups, turn to the letters of Seibert [417] and Frawley [145] each arguing one of the two sides of the yoga-*versus*-medicine question, and to the traditional medical view of craniosacral therapy, as mentioned in Subsection 4.D, *Yoga and CSF Pulsations of the Medial Suture*, page 94. A somewhat more optimistic view is

TABLE 1.A-2. COMPARISON OF THE TWO WORLD VIEWS

World View I	World View II
Ancient	Modern
Intuitive	Demonstrative
Subjective	Objective
Irrational	Rational
Faith	Reason
Spiritual	Materialistic
Magical/mystical	Real world
Feeling	Knowing
Sensations	Facts
Right brain	Left brain
Yin	Yang
Soft	Hard
Vague	Specific
Nonlinear	Linear
East	West
Moon	Sun
Feminine	Masculine
Shakti	Shiva

evident in Lipson's review of Western medicine's acceptance of Ornish's work on the efficacy of *yogasana* training in battling cardiovascular disease [284]. It is clear as well that some practitioners of yoga are reluctant to give credit to the substantial improvement in the quality of life that Western medicine has given us through the basic ideas of germs, sanitation, and vaccination.

As Nuernberger [342] has said, Western medicine fails to understand that yoga too is in fact a highly experimental and empirical science, based upon observations of a most discriminating kind and subject to verification by others. It is only with the utmost concentration and effort that yogis are able to perform their amazing physical and mental feats, and the yogic science that has led to these accomplishments should not be belittled or discounted by Westerners.

Ignoring the more esoteric aspects of yogic science, still not everyone agrees as to the possible benefits of yogic stretching. This negative attitude among sports doctors is largely due to the negative consequences of stretching in inappropriate ways, *i.e.*, out of alignment, over-stretching, lack of warm up, *etc.*, as Couch so eloquently points out [94]. Hopefully this attitude will change as more and more of their patients are finally referred to yoga teachers for treatment.

It is the primary aim of this book to bridge the chasm between yoga science and medical science, for each of which I have immense respect, and to discover if possible what each has to offer the other by way of new ideas and/or understanding. That there is reason to think there is common ground between science and yoga is more than just a hope. Looking back at what has been said in the past, consider that "...*When the brain is abnormally moist, of necessity it moves, and when it moves neither sight nor hearing are still, but we see or hear now one thing and now another, and the tongue speaks in accordance with the things seen and heard on any occasion. But all the time the brain is still, a man is intelligent.*" The author of these thoughts is not a disciple of B.K.S. Iyengar and Patanjali, as one might think, but Hippocrates, the father of medicine, who spoke these words in the 5th century B. C. [225].

In a more modern vein, it is said by present-day neuroscientist E. L. Rossi [389] that "*The hypothalamus is thus the major output pathway of the limbic system. It integrates the sensory-perceptual, emotional and cognitive functions of the mind with the biology of the body.*" Is not this statement just that of the yogi defining yoga as the union of body, mind and spirit?

In a different context, Ornstein [346] discusses a dichotomy of attitude much like that presented here as the two World Views. He correlates this separation of attitude with the two cerebral hemispheres of the brain (Section 3.D, Cerebral Hemispheric Laterality, page 49), which are known to favor World-View-I type thinking in the right hemisphere, and World-View-II type thinking in the left hemisphere. As will be discussed further on, there is abundant evidence that, when healthy, our mental processes oscillate between right and left hemispherical dominance once every few hours!

If one has committed one's attitude to one or the other of the two World Views, it can be difficult to accept the other side, as for example in the tomato effect of Western medicine, discussed in Box 1.A-1.

Reconciling The Rationality of Medicine with the Sublimity of Yoga

In 1959, C. P. Snow delivered the much quoted lecture entitled "The Two Cultures", in which he made the point that society has two polarized groups: on one hand, the world of humanism (here called World View I), and on the other, the world of science

BOX 1.A-1: *YOGASANA*, MEDICINE, AND THE TOMATO EFFECT

The Tomato Effect refers to the belief in 18th-century America that tomatoes were poisonous because they are a member of the deadly-nightshade family of plants. However, though they would not eat tomatoes, Americans also knew that in Europe, people already had been eating tomatoes for 200 years without ill effects. Contrary to European experience, American "common-sense" demanded that tomatoes not be eaten! This denial of an experience because it does not correspond with a previously held theory or understanding in spite of strong evidence to the contrary, is known as "The Tomato Effect" in the medical literature [41].

In more recent times, aspirin and gold emulsions were known to relieve the pain of arthritis, however, as more was learned about this disease, the uses of aspirin and gold made less and less sense, until finally, medical students were no longer taught about their use in treating arthritis pain. Though no one had ever challenged the efficacy of the treatments which were admitted by all to be effective, the use of aspirin and gold was discontinued on the basis that their beneficial effects could not be understood. Again, The Tomato Effect, updated to our own time.

Western medicine has made strides in opening its collective mind to alternative therapies, both to its benefit and to that of the patients it treats. This is not to say that there are still no tomatoes hanging on the medical vines. For example, the medical treatment of sciatica as strictly a herniated-intervertebral-disc situation requiring lower-back surgery, ignores the many successes yoga therapy has had with this problem by releasing the compression on the sciatic nerve caused by the tightness of the piriformis muscle within the buttocks. On the other side of the coin, yoga students should understand that a torn meniscus in the knee may require 15 or more years to heal, but that by arthroscopic surgery on an out-patient basis, their knee pain could be cleared up in 10 days!

(here called World View II), and "between the two, a gulf of mutual incomprehension, sometimes (particularly among the young) hostility and dislike, but most of all a lack of understanding." Continuing, he said, "At the heart of thought and creation, we are letting some of our best chances go by default. The clashing point of two subjects, two disciplines, two cultures ought to produce creative chances. In the history of mental activity that has been where some of the breakthroughs come." By not trying to reconcile Western medicine and the science of *yogasana*, we forfeit the chance to experience the clashing point, the chance to make discoveries that will advance both. Hope-

fully, rubbing Western medicine and yoga science against one another will produce not only heat, but light.

From the advantage of hindsight, one can be more specific in defining "Western medicine" in the context of this Handbook. It appears that the largest overlap of *yogasana* practice is with the medical areas of the autonomic nervous system, and its branches, the sympathetic, parasympathetic and enteric nervous systems. Consequently, and in anticipation of newer advances in both medicine and the *yogasanas*, the Handbook mentions all aspects of the autonomic system which are or could be relevant in the future to *yogasana* work. Of course, a full discussion of the autonomic effects with respect to *yogasana* entails descriptions of many other subjects, *i.e.*, muscles, nerves, reflexes, the brain, bones, the breath, vision, *etc.*, and all of these have been included at the proper levels.

As the mind and the body are united in *yogasana*, how can the improvement of the mind through the understanding that Western medicine offers be anything but a further step along the road to yogic awareness? How can the improvement of the mind available through the understanding that *yogasana* awareness offers be anything but an open door to new territories still unexplored by Western medicine? Knowledge of our body and how it functions adds to our bodily awareness, making it more tangible and so more accessible and useful to us. As with everything, we should attempt to come to some balanced (*sattvic*) position on these seemingly opposite points of view on how the body-mind functions.

That the dissonance between Western medicine and yoga seems to be declining at the present moment stems in part from the fact that the nature of medical challenges has changed precipitously in the past few years. Up until the 1970's, the primary concern of medicine was to fight infections caused by outside agents such as small-pox, diphtheria, influenza, tuberculosis, polio, *etc.* Using scientific techniques to identify the disease-causing agent and to then conquer it with drugs or surgery, Western medicine has been so successful that many such scourges are now only of historical interest. The medical community is in love with this scenario, and indeed, it is still very much relevant today in third-world countries. On the other hand, the current medical crises in many other countries now involve chronic degenerative diseases such as cancer, cardiovascular conditions, arthritis, obesity, dietary ailments, drug abuse, *etc.* [163, 331, 335], and less of a threat from pathogenic organisms. As Western medicine slowly takes a turn in the new direction, it will come to consider medical conditions that *yogasana* teachers have been wrestling with for millennia. How fortunate we are that many of these "new" conditions can be ameliorated or avoided by *yogasana* practice! This particular situation is in part responsible for the general public's turning more and more to "alternative medicine" for its ills, one significant part of which is *yogasana*, practiced both for its own sake and practiced as therapy.

Many have spoken of the detachment of the mind that is necessary to reach the highest levels of yogic mental transformation, and I have no reason to doubt what others have said for thousands of years in this regard. With this idea in mind, it would seem fruitless then to try to graft Western medicine and yoga onto one another, for the mind cannot be both engaged in rational analysis and totally detached at the same time. My view is that, because yoga itself is a multilevel structure, it is not unreasonable that the apparent goals of yoga are dependent upon which level is being addressed, and how long a student has been at that level. Furthermore, even at a particular level, there will be many goals, all valid, but with relative priorities depending upon an individual's situation. Therefore, it is neither necessary nor appropriate to have these contrary states operating in the mind simultaneously, but rather they should be present sequentially instead, as discussed below. Approached in this way, the marriage of *yogasana* and Western medicine does make sense.

The eight levels of Patanjali's yoga are hierarchical, so that the Western-style rational analysis that is inappropriate for refining *pratyahara* through *samadhi* may still be of great utility to those working at the levels of *asana* and *pranayama*. This then is the philosophy of this Handbook: at the level of the student working to master the *yogasanas*, there is much to be gained by understanding the physiology that lies behind the manifold effects that *yogasanas* bring into our awareness. However, this rational approach will be less appropriate at the higher levels of *yogasanas* in which the more meditative aspects of yoga are incorporated into the postures.

We take to heart Patel's comments, "...the mind may know, but unless the body experiences, that knowledge will never be converted into understanding...a fundamental reason why the physico-therapeutic sciences as we know them have often failed. Knowledge is being used without understanding" [353]. But this argument cuts both ways, I think. Can it not also be that by ignoring the hard-won knowledge of Western science, yoga teachers who are less than fully experienced in all of the yogic aspects of the body/mind also are operating with understanding that is not supported by knowledge? Would not their understanding be of a higher quality if they had a deeper knowledge of the physiology accompanying the *yogasanas*? What of their students who are necessarily at a lower level of awareness: could they not profit from a rational understanding of *yogasana* even though their teacher might be beyond that point?

Yoga is a scientific system of self-discovery and self-maintenance. Understanding how the body works helps to develop awareness of the body and mind, as is necessary for yogic advancement. Thus, to know and understand the internal workings of the body and mind from both the medical and yogic points of view is a step forward in both yogic mastery and medical science [399].

The close relation between the science of the body as represented by Western medicine and the refined art of yoga as represented by B.K.S. Iyengar in the *yogasanas* is stated repeatedly by him [214]: "Art and science are interrelated and interconnected. Both require study, imagination, discipline and an orderly method. Both depend on technique. All art is science and all science an art. Hence it is hard to compare or differentiate between the two." In this Handbook, we endeavor to forge even stronger links between science and yoga. Hopefully, this will be where *yogasana* and science meet and fall in love.

SECTION 1.B. THE GOALS OF *YOGASANA*

As Patanjali has taught, the chief goal of yoga practice is to still the fluctuations of the mind, and the practice of the *yogasanas* provides an excellent laboratory for developing this ability. Furthermore, within the field of *yogasana*, there are other, lesser goals to be realized. Thus, for example, Juhan [222] states a truth which underlies our practice of the *yogasanas*: "The system of sensorimotor integration is marvelously adaptive, and its simple elements can be manipulated to produce the entire range of complex human skills. Unfortunately, the sense of 'rightness' which comes about through repetition may not necessarily correspond to movements and habits that are 'optimal' in their efficiency. 'Rightness' in this context only means 'familiarity,' *i.e.*, grooves that are well-worn. It is often strongly associated with movements and habits that are merely 'satisfactory' in some limited way, or 'normal' in the sense of 'like before.'

Astonishingly enough, once a sense of normalcy has been established in connection with a way of doing something, perceived inefficiency or even pain are usually not enough to alter our behavior. We will tend to continue to do a thing the way we learned it, the way in which we first established our 'feel' for it, in spite of the fact that subsequent problems develop as a result."

This, in a nutshell, is the way many of us are going through life, trapped in ruts that make every day the same as the one before, and in ways that reduce our responses to life's situations to formulaic, unthinking, mechanical motions. That is, we surrender our awareness and the opportunity to solve a problem in a new and more efficient way to the "old, tried-and-true" methods that seemingly have worked so well for us in the past. As we repeat our actions, our options for response become fewer and fewer, and we become more like the man who has a hammer and sees *everything* as a nail. His perspective may fix a few things, but will leave many more things in ruins.

As discussed so clearly by Desikachar [111], setting our brains on automatic-pilot leads to too many accidents when circumstances change but our methods of handling them do not. We are speaking now in the broadest terms. If we are to navigate successfully through life we must be flexible in every sense, be aware of what is going on around us, and understand what is the optimum rather than the easiest response to each situation. Further, in finding new ways to approach problems, we grow. If our approach is always the same, we have ceased to grow and will therefore stagnate. Stagnation is the enemy of *yogasana*, and attentive *yogasana* practice can be the medicine that banishes stagnation.

Through practice of *yogasana*, we have the tool with which we can raise our level of self awareness, and experiment with new types of strategies for solving life's problems. If we are aware as we work in *yogasana*, we will come to see the common threads of how we approach the solution to all yogic problems, and that a yogic problem is neither more nor less than a metaphor for life's problems in general, and how we go about solving them. If we can, through heightened awareness, find a new way to approach a problem in *yogasana*, and remain aware, then that approach may well be a new and useful strategy in broader life situations.

As we practice *yogasana* with awareness, we can find the unthought-of avenues of attitude, some of which are dead-ends and some of which lead to unexpectedly beautiful and exotic places that we otherwise would never come across if we had remained with the Western scientist's approach.

But the practice of *yogasana* is a two-edged sword; *yogasana* presents its own dangers because it too can be practiced in a rote, mechanical way. If it is practiced in this way, it is just as instructive to the body and mind; it is just that the lesson now acts to reinforce old ideas and ways of reacting, rather than opening up new avenues of behavior. It is from this point of view that we can understand B.K.S. Iyengar's comments on practice that are quoted in Subsection 7.C (*Proprioception and Yogasana*, page 210), where he encourages the student to constantly seek new understanding of the *yogasanas* by observation and questioning of what is being felt, by analyzing the posture and experimenting so as to refine the posture, always being aware of the feeling, and trying today to extend the feeling beyond what it was yesterday.

For those students and teachers for whom *yogasana* practice has become monotonous and consequently whose bodies become dull and unresponsive, it may be that the added dimension of a rational understanding of the physiological effects of the *yogasanas* will brighten their practice again. As I have repeatedly found in my own work, the stimulation that comes from an attempt at understanding the *yogasanas* from a Western perspective can invigorate one and renew one's zest for practice.

Levels of Consciousness

According to Western thought, there are generally agreed to be at least three levels of consciousness in human beings: the conscious, the subconscious, and the unconscious [399]. The highest of these, the conscious, involves the knowing part of the mind, and is active in awareness. However, only a small fraction of the brain is used in conscious thought, and only some of the remainder is involved in subconscious action (as in controlling the autonomic nervous system) and in unconscious modes. Though it is the aim of some people to "use the brain fully", in fact, that state of the brain in which all circuits are simultaneously activated is that of the *grand mal* epileptic siezure! We work in the *yogasanas* to heighten the presence of the bodily sensations at the conscious level, but with no need to use all of its elements simultaneously.

The subconscious is a subtle area, lying just beneath consciousness. One usually has a blurry impression of thoughts lying just below consciousness, but during meditation, such thoughts can be more distinct. The subconscious acts as a buffer area between the conscious level and the forces of the unconscious. The practice of the *yogasanas* can shift many bodily sensations and controlling actions from the subconscious level to that of the conscious. Recent experiments show that subconscious recognition of an external visual stimulus involves a low neural current in the primary visual cortex, whereas the conscious recognition differs only in showing a stronger neural current in the same area [295], and that when the size of the neural current rises above a certain threshold value, the awareness switches from the subconscious to the conscious level. If this finding is true generally, then we see that a practice that strengthens a certain subconscious neural signal will lift the awareness of that sensation into consciousness, and presumably the reverse can happen as well.

Forces originating in the unconscious are extremely powerful. This realm contains the archetypes which are the foundations of our basic drives and instincts. The three areas interact strongly so that the unconscious can indirectly influence the subconscious, so for example, if negativity is preponderant in the unconscious, then this will influence the subconscious in a way that leads to vascular hypertension.

Yogis also recognize a higher level of consciousness, the level of the superconscious. It is the ultimate goal of the yogic practitioner to join the individual consciousness to the universal consciousness and so to reach a blissful state of superconsciousness, that of *samadhi*. The state of *samadhi* is the highest of the eight limbs of yoga, each of which may be considered as a progressively higher state of consciousness than the one preceding it. The eight levels of consciousness in ascending order in the *ashtanga* (eight limbs) scheme are *yama*, *niyama*, *asana*, *pranayama*, *pratyahara*, *dharana*, *dhyana* and *samadhi*. The first four of these are the basis of the yoga of action (*karma*), whereas, *pranayama*, *pratyahara* and *dharana* are the yoga of knowledge (*jnana*), and *dhyana* and *samadhi* are the yoga of devotion and love (*bhakti*) [215].

From the Ayurvedic point of view, the levels of consciousness are represented by the *chakras*, ascending from the *muladhara* at the base of the spine to the *sahasrara* at the crown of the head (Table 4.F-1). The characteristics of these levels are discussed further in Section 4.F, *Nadis, Chakras* and *Prana*, page 100.

The basic qualitative idea of information theory is that the more improbable is an event or observation, the higher is its informational content, *i.e.*, the more likely is it to be a factor in arousing the senses (Subsection 3.A, *The Reticular Formation*, page 31). Thus, when our existence is filled repeatedly with the ordinary and humdrum, the tendency is to lower one's consciousness to the level of the subconscious and put the mind to sleep without a corresponding lifting of subconscious actions into the conscious level. As the consciousness and the mind thrive on information, the "mind is nature's supreme design for receiving, generating and transducing information" [389]. As students of *yogasana*, then, it is incumbent upon us to make each *yogasana* practice interesting and open to new sensations, invention, and creativity, for only in this way can we avoid sinking into the subconscious.

In regard the situation of the levels of consciousness and their interactions in the neophyte student of *yogasana*, consider Fig. 1.B-1. Before a beginner commences *yogasana* practice, the mind is structured as in Fig. 1.B-1a, with sharp divisions between the conscious, subconscious, and unconscious levels of the mind. No mention is made in the Figure of the superconscious level as this is irrelevant to the beginning student. In such a situation in such a student, the straightening of the legs in *paschimottanasana*, for example, will be a deliberate effort of the conscious mind involving the contraction of the quadruceps muscles and, and at the same time, there will be subconscious reflex actions which will change the breathing pattern and also relax the antagonist muscles (the hamstrings, Subsection 7.A, *Reciprocal Inhibition and Agonist/Antagonist Pairs*, page 193) at the back of the legs.

As shown in the Figure, with extended practice of the *yogasanas*, certain of the conscious, deliberate actions of the beginner

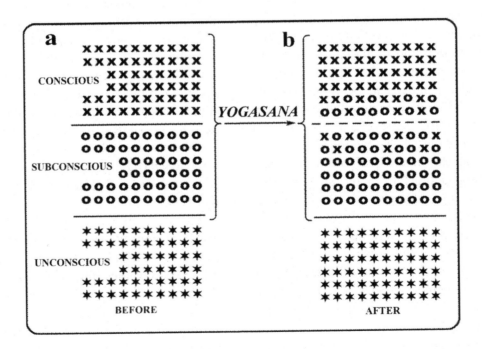

Fig. 1.B-1. (a) Without *yogasana* practice, the human mind is divided neatly into three levels of consciousness. (b) However, once *yogasana* practice has commenced, the boundary between conscious and subconscious levels becomes more indistinct, with practice making some conscious actions become more subconscious (intuitive) and some subconscious actions become more conscious (deliberate).

can become more intuitive/reflexive, *i.e.*, the legs automatically straighten as they should in, say, *ardha chandrasana*, without conscious thought, while on the other hand, the breath is now deliberately moved in a smooth, slow, and rhythmic way. Through the practice of the *yogasanas*, certain subconscious reflexive actions come under the control of the conscious sphere, while at the same time, certain other conscious actions become more reflexive, as if under the control of the subconscious. The result is that the previous sharp line dividing the conscious and subconscious levels is now blurred, Fig. 1.B-1b.

When we practice the *yogasanas* and "turn our awareness inward", we are making a mental effort to blur the line between conscious and subconscious, trying to make the ordinarily subconscious sensations of ordinary awareness surface into the realm of the conscious, much as in Fig. 1.B-1. Neuroanatomically, this means that neural signals that ordinarily ascend only as high as the thalamus are strengthened and elevated instead to the level of the cortex (Subsection 3.A, *The Cortex: Seat of Conscious Action*, page 24).

The work of *yogasana* practice is to bring sensations and the control of subconscious functions (reflexes) into the realm of the conscious and the deliberate, and at the same time, bring deliberate conscious actions, through practice, into the realm of reflex (for example, whenever the feet are set for *trikonasana*, there is an automatic increase in the tone of the quadruceps, *i.e.*, the action becomes reflexive). Thus, by *yogasana* practice, we can forge a link between autonomic and deliberate actions, and this link can be a bridge that can be crossed from either direction. That is to say, the involuntary can be made voluntary, and the voluntary can be made involuntary through practice.

Looked at in another way, as infants, our consciousness is minimal and all of our actions are reflexive, *i.e.*, in the subconscious realm. As we mature, some but not all of the reflexes come more and more under the conscious control of higher brain centers. The goal of *yogasana* practice is to lift the remaining subconscious/reflexive actions into the region of the conscious and to thereby control them through the conscious action of the higher mental centers. At the same time, certain conscious actions are practiced so often that they become more or less reflexive in nature, in that they receive minimal conscious attention, Fig. 1.B-1.

The autonomic responses which yogic exercises bring about are not necessarily *in toto* those sought in yoga, for the body's response to stress is that appropriate to a former way of life which is different than the one we are living today. We must learn in yoga to encourage some of these responses and moderate or reduce others. This is one of the challenges of yoga, for example, not preparing to fight when stressed, or not allowing the blood pressure to rise when frightened. At the same time, the purely physical benefits of *yogasana* practiced as exercise are manifold and well known [209, 216, 306].

Though there are many exercise regimens which offer the participant undreamed-of health benefits, and there are many other relaxation regimens that offer the participant undreamed-of levels of altered consciousness, the practice of the *yogasanas* is unique in offering both. By the study of the *yogasanas*, we come to a state of physical strength and mental tranquility which then allows one to enter into states of meditation; practice of the *yogasanas* prepares the body, the breath and the mind for entering the doorway to meditation [69].

Chapter 2

NERVOUS SYSTEMS OF THE BODY

SECTION 2.A.
INTRODUCTION

For every animate organism, regardless of its size, there exists a sensory system of some sort that allows it to "feel" its environment and a second system that then reacts to that sensation in some way beneficial to the organism. Thus, some one-celled organisms can sense the surrounding temperature and then can move by activation of their cilia in directions that are either hotter or colder, as best serves them thermally. Other bacteria can navigate spatially by sensing the direction of the local magnetic field.

On a much larger scale, even groves of trees can react to their environment. Thus, when evergreen trees within a grove are under insect attack, they are now known to transmit chemical signals diffusively through the air to their neighbors, which neighbors then act in their own time to produce repellent substances in their needles and bark. For mobile organisms the size of trees, the need for speed and accuracy of signaling from one specific site in the organism to another has led to the development of signaling systems that operate instead on bioelectrochemical principles (Section 5.B, Nerve Conduction, page 114) rather than on diffusion. In such systems, a central nerve center is bi-directionally and instantaneously connected with all outlying parts of the organism, both for gathering sensory information about the environment

and for taking physical action in response to what is sensed.

There can be yet another dimension to the signaling/response system. Though signaling systems of the sort mentioned above have been fine-tuned to a high degree in many animals, these responses are largely hardwired in the animal, so that given a particular set of circumstances, the response is always the same. Only in human beings (and possibly other primates [31a]) have there been added the dimensions of volition, imagination, reason, creativity, appreciation of beauty, passion and intellect. The incorporation of these aspects into the neural system of the human being places us at the pinnacle of nervous-system development.

Though the human nervous system is integral and whole, for the purposes of study, it can be artificially divided using two criteria, either on the basis of function or on the basis of structure. Figure 2.A-1 is a hybrid division of the human nervous system in that the primary division into the central nervous system and the peripheral nervous system is based on structure, whereas the peripheral system also has been bisected as well, but in this case, into the autonomic and somatic subsystems on the basis of function.

At the highest level, Fig. 2.A-1, nerves can be assigned as belonging to either a central nervous system concentrated most strongly on the central axis of the body, or alternatively, as radiating from the central axis toward the more distant parts of the body, forming the peripheral nervous

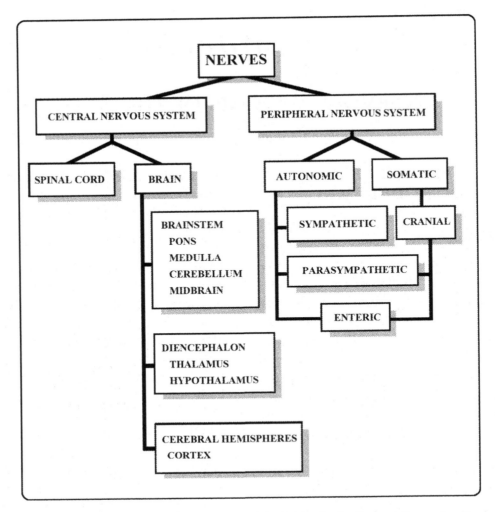

Fig. 2.A-1. Classification scheme for the nerves of the human body. See text for explanations of terms.

system. The central nervous system, consisting of the brain and spinal cord, largely is involved with the coordination and control of body functions such as homeostasis, memory, *etc.*, whereas the peripheral nervous system represents the lines of communication between the central nervous system and the outlying areas. Though the central and peripheral nervous systems are separate anatomically, they are strongly connected functionally through intervening junctions called synapses (Section 5.C, Nerve Connections; Synapses, page 121). In both cases, the nerves that carry sensory information (temperature, pH, blood pressure, muscle tension, *etc.*) from receptors in the peripheral regions to the central region are called afferents, whereas those that carry excitatory neural signals from the central region toward the muscles and glands at the periphery are called efferents.

Each of these two systems can be further subdivided. The central nervous system consists of the brain and the spinal cord, Fig. 2.A-2, and the brain in turn is composed of the brainstem (pons, medulla, cerebellum and midbrain), the diencephalon (the thalamus and the hypothalamus), and the cerebral hemispheres, the covering of which is the cortex. Alternative names are given to

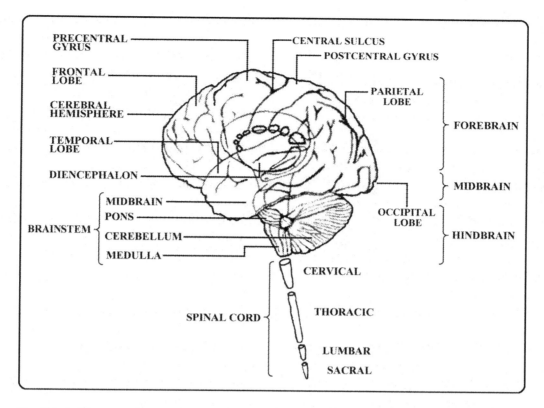

Fig. 2.A-2. The central nervous system and its division into components, taken here as the spinal cord, the brainstem, the diencephalon and the cerebral hemispheres. The covering of each of the hemispheres, the cortex, is divided into four lobes. As shown on the right, an alternative division of the brain yields three regions, the forebrain, the midbrain and the hindbrain.

these areas, *i.e.*, the hindbrain, midbrain and forebrain, respectively.

On the peripheral side, there is the division into the somatic branch and the autonomic branch, the latter of which is further divided into sympathetic, parasympathetic and enteric branches. These autonomic branches are discussed in detail in Chapter 6, THE AUTONOMIC NERVOUS SYSTEM, page 133, and Section 18.A, Structure and Function of the Gastrointestinal Organs, page 441. Not all workers in the field consider the enteric as a separate branch of the autonomic system. Suffice it to say here that the autonomic systems essentially work in an automatic fashion at the subconscious level. Cranial nerves (Subsection 2.C, page 17) are in part parasympathetic.

The somatic branch is concerned with muscles and sensors, and consists of those afferent nerves that carry sensory signals from the muscles, skin and glands via a synapse to the central nervous system, and those efferent nerves that carry excitatory signals via a synapse from the central nervous system to the muscles, skin, and glands.

The definition of the nervous system as shown in Fig. 2.A-1 is deceptive in that each category sits neatly within the borders of its box, whereas in fact, the interaction between systems on the right and those on the left can be so strong that the separateness implied by the boxes simply cannot be supported. Strong interactions are common not only left-to-right, but top-to-bottom as well in this diagram. Though we will use the hierarchy given in Fig. 2.A-1, it is to be understood that the elements shown there are not as independent as the drawing implies.

SECTION 2.B. THE CENTRAL NERVOUS SYSTEM

The central nervous system is composed of the brain, the spinal cord and those structures that stand between them. The structure of the spinal cord within the spinal column is described in detail in Section 4.B, The Spinal Cord, page 83, and so will be described much more briefly here. The bundle of nerves that forms the spinal cord extends from the base of the skull into the region of the lumbar vertebrae, occupying the channel within the bony structure of the spinal column. Indeed, the entire central nervous system is encased within the bone of the skull and spinal column. The spinal cord serves the trunk and the limbs of the body, receiving sensory information from the skin, joints and muscles in these areas, and in turn activating muscles in the same areas via voluntary and reflex mechanisms.

The nerves of the spinal cord are segmented into 31 sectors in registration with the vertebral structure of the spinal column and are divided in the following way:

- Eight cervical branches, serving the diaphragm and the muscles of the neck, arms and hands
- Twelve thoracic branches, serving the trunk and intercostal muscles
- Five lumbar and upper sacral branches, serving the muscles of the abdomen, legs and feet
- Five lower sacral branches, serving the anal and perineal muscles
- One coccygeal branch.

Taken as a unit, the medulla oblongata, pons, cerebellum and midbrain together form the brainstem, an integrated structure which deals with sensory information from the head, neck and face, and in turn controls the muscles in these areas via the cranial nerves. Neural information from the spinal cord also passes through the brainstem on its way upward to higher centers in the brain, and processed information from these higher centers similarly passes downward through the brainstem. Interestingly, there is a mutual neural communication and modulation of the ascending and descending information streams, with selective reinforcement of some signals in both streams, and inhibition of others. The reticular formation passes lengthwise through the brainstem, and is involved in arousal of awareness, among other things. All of these centers (and more) are discussed further in Chapter 3, THE BRAIN, page 21.

Most important in the brain are the cerebral hemispheres, each of which has a covering, called the cortex (Subsection 3.A, *The Cortex: Seat of Conscious Action*, page 24). The cortex is the area of our rational intelligence and the source of our direct and deliberate actions and sensations. The conscious awareness of sensations (temperature, body posture, hunger, *etc.*) are delivered to the sensory cortex in each hemisphere, whereas the motor nerves that consciously drive the muscles have their origins in the somatic or motor cortex.

Though formally not considered to be parts of the central nervous system, it is appropriate here to mention the fibrous sac (the dura mater) in which the central nervous system is contained, and the fluid within the sac in which the central nervous system is suspended (Section 4.D, Cerebrospinal Fluid, page 93). These two non-neural elements are essential to the health, function and maintenance of the central nervous system.

The central nervous system is responsible for the activation of motor nerves that initiate muscle action on both the voluntary and reflex levels (Section 7.D, Reflex Actions, page 211). On the voluntary level, action is possible only if the conscious part of the brain wills the action. That is to say, there must be some part of the brain that serves as a motivational system with input to the somatic motor cortex. Such a motivational system resides within the limbic system of the brain, deep within the cerebral hemispheres [225].

Both the sensory and motor systems of the central nervous system show a peculiar crossing-over of the nerves such that sensory and motor signals appropriate to one side of the body are connected neurally to the cerebral hemisphere on the opposite side of the brain. In some pathways, the crossing occurs at the level of the spinal cord, while in others the crossing is in the brainstem. The side-to-side crossing of the neural pathway is called decussation. A partial decussation of sorts also occurs in the visual and auditory systems in the higher centers of the brain, as discussed in Sections 16.C, Vision and Cerebral Laterality, page 422, and 17.A, The Middle Ear, page 433.

The three major functions of the brain, receiving and weighing sensory input, activating muscles and organs and providing motivation for action, though strongly interacting, are found in distinct areas of the brain and distinct neural pathways are dedicated to their specific functions. Each has subsystems dedicated to more specific tasks, as illustrated in Box 2.B-1.

SECTION 2.C. THE PERIPHERAL NERVOUS SYSTEM

Connections to the Spinal Cord

The length of the peripheral nerve connecting a sensor with the central nervous system can be as short as 1 mm as it is for olfaction, as long as 100 mm for vision, and longer than 1000 mm, as with the mechano-

receptors in the limbs [225]. The somatic part of the peripheral nervous system is activated by centers in the central nervous system at both the conscious (cortex) and subconscious (spinal cord) levels and at points in between (the brainstem and diencephalon). As suggested in Fig. 1.B-1, actions originating at the lower, more unconscious levels can be brought into the higher, more conscious levels through the practice of *yogasanas*.

As its name implies, the autonomic nervous system (Chapter 6, page 133) works normally in an automatic way, silently adjusting the various parameters of the body so as to keep its operating parameters within certain bounds. In doing this, the autonomic system works largely on the internal organs and viscera of the body, adjusting the levels of their functioning to be appropriate for self defense (the sympathetic branch), for relaxation (the parasympathetic branch), or for digestion (the enteric branch). The subconscious actions of the autonomic nervous system are protective in another sense, for were they in the conscious realm, they would flood the consciousness with a mass of data that would make further conscious action impossible. However, as with the somatic branch of the peripheral nervous system, so too can certain of the actions of the autonomic system be brought to the level of consciousness by the practice of the *yogasanas* (Chapter 6, page 133).

The Cranial Nerves

Many of the nerves that serve the head, face, and neck areas of the body are essentially at or above the cervical vertebrae, and so synapse directly with centers in the ventral brain, passing directly through the dura mater at the base of the skull without passing through the spinal cord. However, others go as far south as the lower abdomen, yet they too synapse directly into the brain or brainstem without using the spinal cord.

BOX 2.B-1: INTERACTIONS OF THE BRAIN'S THREE SYSTEMS IN THE TEACHING OF *VIRABHADRASANA I*

Let us see just how the sensory systems, the motor systems and the motivational system of the brain might interact in a student being taught *virabhadrasana I*, Fig. 2.B-1. Beginning with the sensory systems, the various peripheral proprioceptors in the skin, muscles, and joints (Section 7.C, Proprioception, page 208) report on the various joint angles and levels of muscle tension using sensory afferents. From this, the sensory cortex in each hemisphere can synthesize a picture of the current posture on the opposite side of the body, but this will be only partially in the student's consciousness, if at all. At the same time, the teacher's spoken instructions are converted into neural signals that are sent from the ears to the auditory cortex over decussated afferent pathways (Section 17.A, The Middle Ear, page 433). Postural information from the proprioceptors will serve eventually as input to the motor cortex, whereas the spoken information will serve to activate the motivational system in accord with the teacher's instructions.

The outputs of both the sensory and the motivational systems will then serve as inputs to the motor cortex. Using both direct and indirect activation of the relevant muscles, each side of the body is coaxed by the motor cortex in the opposite hemisphere into the position appropriate to *virabhadrasana I*. This will involve the contraction of certain muscles and the relaxation of others. With luck, the end result of these neural interactions will be a pose resembling that in the Figure. As the pose is practiced time after time [345], the muscular actions are smoothed by the basal ganglia and then further refined and coordinated by the cerebellum, Subsection 3.A, *The Brain; Structure and Function*, page 21.

As the pose is practiced repeatedly, a muscular learning process comes into being (Box 3.C-1, *Learning and Yogasana Practice*, page 44), with certain neural pathways being reinforced so that the mechanics of the posture become more intuitive and less deliberate. Note, however, that the Figure accompanying this Box is quite schematic, and ignores many important brain centers that are here only represented by arrows.

Such afferent and efferent nerves are called the cranial nerves [57, 170, 340]. Some of the cranial nerves play a role in the parasympathetic autonomic system, however, all of the components of the sympathetic nervous system have spinal connections rather than cranial connections. Each of the twelve cranial nerves has its origin at the reticular formation within the brainstem, Subsection 3.A, *The Limbic System*, page 33.

There are twelve pairs of such cranial nerves in the body, with each member of a pair serving one side of the body; the names and functions of the cranial nerves are listed below. More information on the roles they play in the body can be found in the relevant Sections in which the various affected organs, sensors and muscles are described.

Cranial Nerve I. The olfactory nerves carry the sensations of odor from the roof of the nasal cavity to the cortex and to the limbic system.

Cranial Nerve II. These are the optic nerves, carrying the sensory signals from the retinas of the two eyes to the occipital lobe at the back of the skull.

Cranial Nerve III. As their name implies, the oculomotor nerves are involved with the extrinsic muscles that move the eyeballs in their sockets and also with the intrinsic mus-

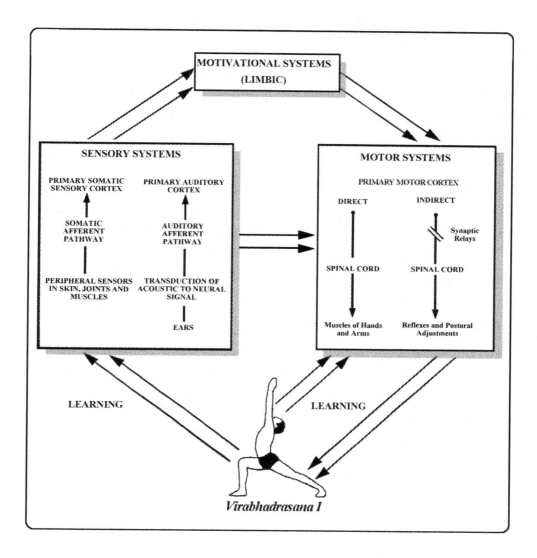

Fig. 2.B-1. The three subsystems of the central nervous system, the sensory, the motor, and the motivational, interact as shown when the student is instructed in *virabhadrasana I*. With practice, learning takes place, with its reinforcing effects on the motor and sensory cortices.

cles that adjust the sizes of the pupils according to the light level. Certain of the fibers in the oculomotor nerve bundle are part of the parasympathetic nervous system as well.

Cranial Nerve IV. The trochlear nerves innervate the extrinsic muscles of the eyes.

Cranial Nerve V. The trigeminal nerves are active in various areas of the face: their afferents originate at the skin of the face, the cornea of the eyes, and from the teeth,

whereas their efferents control the muscles of the jaw when chewing.

Cranial Nerve VI. The abducens nerves are used in the movement of the eyeballs.

Cranial Nerve VII. The facial nerves innervate the muscles of the face and so make the face expressive. Additionally, they are involved with the sense of taste and control saliva production.

Cranial Nerve VIII. The acoustic nerves serve two distinct purposes: they carry acoustic signals from the middle ears to the brain and also connect the balancing apparatus of the inner ears to brain centers.

Cranial Nerve IX. Taste sensations from the back of the tongue, and sensations of pressure and pain in the throat are transmitted to the brain by the glossopharyngeal nerves. Additionally, these nerves activate saliva glands and also help regulate the breathing rate.

Cranial Nerve X. This is the very important vagus nerve, which allows control of many important processes such as breathing, digestion, and heart rate, as well as tension in the vocal cords. More detail on the roles that the parasympathetic vagus nerves play in the body are listed in Section 6.D, The Parasympathetic Nervous System, page 150.

Cranial Nerve XI. The spinal accessory nerves activate the muscles in the neck which turn the head from side to side.

Cranial Nerve XII. The hypoglossal nerves control the muscles of the tongue and throat, and hence are important in the speech process.

As the cranial nerves often synapse to the subconscious centers of the brainstem, they can readily participate in reflex actions such as coughing, vomiting, blinking, swallowing, *etc.* However, as these lower centers are connected within the brain to higher, more conscious centers, their reflexive nature can be controlled in a deliberate way by the conscious brain.

With respect to our practice of the *yogasanas*, the most important of the cranial nerves are the second (optic) which carries the signal sensing our state of balance with respect to the horizon (Appendix IV, BALANCING, page 525), the eighth (vestibular) which again is an important aid in balancing (Section 17.B, The Vestibular Organs of Balance, page 437), and the tenth (vagus) which is extremely important as a regulator of the heart beat and so controls blood pressure, *etc.* (Subsections 11.A, *Innervation of the Heart: The Cardiac Pacemaker*, page 315, and 6.D, *The Vagus Nerves*, page 152).

Chapter 3

THE BRAIN

SECTION 3.A. STRUCTURE AND FUNCTION

That astounding human organ, the brain, is even more so the more we learn of its abilities and the magnitude of the problems it can solve with apparent ease. In this Chapter, we will look at the basic components of the brain, their functions, and how these functions come into play when we practice the *yogasanas*. Needless to say, the subject of the brain, its structure and function, is endlessly complex; in this work we will just scratch the surface, again working to connect the basic elements of brain function to the practice of the *yogasanas*.

The adult human brain weighs 1350 grams (3 pounds) on average, and is thought to contain between 10 and 30 billion nerve cells. By comparison, the blowfly and the ant have brains weighing only 0.084 and 0.00001 grams, respectively, there being only 10 to 20 thousand nerve cells in these cases. Considering then the complex actions that these insects can perform only sets the stage for the amazing feats of a brain a million times larger. Moreover, the human brain with "new" hardware is able to do things that the brains of lower beings can not even dream of doing, even if their brains were magnified a million times.

As if the sheer number of brain cells in the human brain were not enough, realize then that many of these brain cells are connected to up to 60,000 others, averaging about 600 connections per nerve cell. Furthermore, the strengths of these neural connections vary with our experiences. As a consequence, each of us has possible patterns of connection which literally have no limit to their variety. The importance of connectivity cannot be over-stressed, for it is this connectivity and the plasticity of the brain which can change the connectivity patterns on the basis of experience and learning, which has allowed each of us to evolve in our own unique way.

Thanks to the brain's plasticity, neurons which are not used tend eventually to disappear, with their place in the brain replaced by the expansion of other brain functions that are more often used. This use-it-or-lose-it scenario is played out most strongly in the years of early childhood, and is reason enough to engage children in some form of *yogasana* practice at an early age.

Surprisingly, the human brain begins to die as soon as it is born. Our brains contain the maximum number of brain cells that they will ever have at the fourth month *in utero*, and though the brain will increase in size by a factor of three by the time an infant reaches adulthood, brain cells are dying at a rate of up to a million per day, and up to very recently, it was thought that the brain cells do not reproduce themselves once we have reached maturity (however, see Section 22.B, Mental and Emotional Effects of Aging, page 499).

The old idea of the shrinking brain was based on broad investigations of brain size which inadvertently included many subjects who had brain disease of one sort or another. Most recently, repetition of these studies on the brains of healthy subjects has refuted all of these earlier ideas concerning an ongoing brain death as we mature and then age.

It is known that stem cells in the bone marrow mature into red and white corpuscles, and that the skin, liver, gut and perhaps other organs also have stem cells which act to replace worn out cells in their particular organs. Most amazing is the apparent plasticity of stem cells which have been observed to change their character from brain cells to muscle cells, for example, when placed in contact with muscle tissue [470]. At present, the general feeling is that there are few stem cells in the brain, but that the brain is supplied with far too many cells at birth, and that if we stay healthy, the brain does not need replacement cells on a large scale [162]. Many recent experiments in fact suggest that there is some neurogenesis occurring within the brain.

The Three Broad Areas of the Brain

Trying to classify the brain's functions is like trying to classify fruit salad, for there are many ways that each logically can be simplified for understanding. Fruit salad may be described in terms of those fruits that are sweet tasting and those that are tart, or alternatively and just as logically, in terms of those fruits that are red, those that are green and those that are blue. Still again, one could just as logically view the salad as composed of those fruit pieces that are round and those that are thinly sliced. Each of these approaches, while logical in itself, results in categories having different components depending on which criteria were assumed for classification. The same ambiguity arises when trying to group the brain's components into logical units. Looked at one way, two brain functions may seem closely related, but looked at another equally logical way, they are seen to be only distantly related. Alternatively, one might try dividing the brain into geographic regions independent of function. In the end, we have picked one way of defining the brain's subunits, with the understanding that other logical ways exist as well.

At a very broad level, the brain can be divided into three distinct functional-geographic areas, Fig. 2.A-2. The lowest of the three levels, the vegetative/reflexive hindbrain, encompasses the brainstem and works to control various body functions (respiration, digestion, *etc.*) in an automatic way and also to integrate brain reflexes. The effects of the primitive vegetative brain rarely if ever impact on the conscious level, nonetheless, the brainstem is essential for life as it maintains the basic life processes; damage to the brainstem is an immediate threat to life. In fact, the brainstem contains the one intracranial neural structure (the reticular formation) without which our life is impossible [116].

At the highest of the three levels, the cerebral cortex functions as the seat of consciousness as it registers our senses, activates our muscles for motions requiring great finesse, generates and coordinates our thoughts, and is intimately involved in learning and memories. The cortex physically is a layer of folded tissue on the outermost surfaces of the cerebral hemispheres. The evolutionary development of the cerebral cortex is clear in Fig. 3.A-1, where one sees the relative size and convoluted nature of the cortex increases as one ascends this evolutionary series of animals, reaching the apex in man.

Between the levels of the primitive vegetative brain and the sophisticated cortex lies the level of the midbrain limbic system. Physically, the limbic system is found in that part of the brain lying between the brain stem and the cortex, and is itself considered to be a phylogenetically primitive cortex of sorts. The limbic system is the visceral and

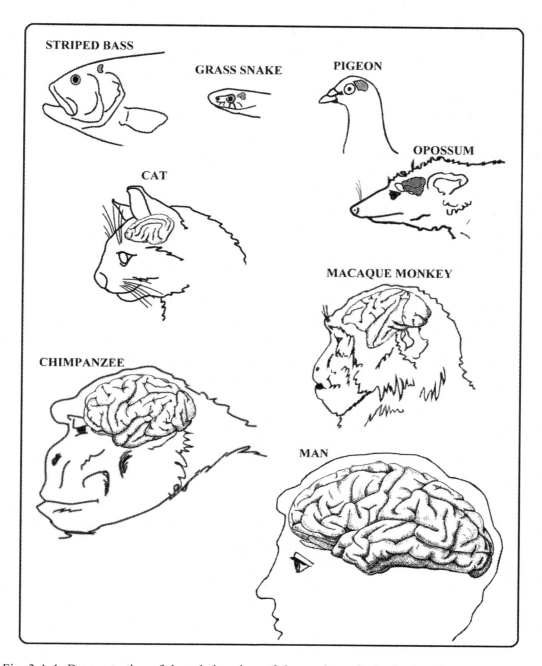

Fig. 3.A-1. Demonstration of the relative sizes of the cerebrum in the brains of water animals (striped bass), land animals that crawl (grass snake), fly (pigeon) or walk (opossum, cat), in the bipeds and in man [222]. Note also the evolutionary development of the forebrain and the increasingly convoluted nature of the cortex.

emotional center of the brain, being involved in behavioral and emotional expression, reproduction and memory, drives and motivations; our senses of pleasure and reward involve stimulation of centers in the limbic system [230]. The limbic system is in continuous contact with the upward-moving sensory signals, and affects the striate muscles, the visceral smooth muscles, and the endocrine glands.

The three levels of the tripartite brain are not as separate as was first believed. It is now known that there is considerable communication between areas of all three levels, and so it has become more difficult than ever to assign a particular function to a particular area of the brain. The various substructures within the three major levels of the brain are discussed more completely below, with the understanding that structures at all levels more-or-less share in the brain's functioning. As Llinas [19] has responded to the question "Where in the brain is the seat of consciousness?" saying "Where in the bicycle is the seat of bicycleness?" so too is it clear that one cannot be too specific about location and function in regard the functional subunits of the brain.

It is interesting to note that 2000 years prior to our own time, Patanjali already had described the brain as consisting of four main sections: the front brain (devoted to analytical thinking), the back brain (devoted to reasoning), the bottom brain (the seat of pleasure and bliss) and the top brain (the seat of creativity and individuality) [211].

The Cortex: Seat of Conscious Action

The cortex, Fig. 3.A-2, is a relatively recent refinement of brain structure, and as such is the crowning achievement of the evolutionary process. The cortex is a thin layer of tissue, heavily folded and creased, covering each of the cerebral hemispheres with a very high density of nerve cells. Six distinct layers of nerve cells have been identified within the cortex, with each layer

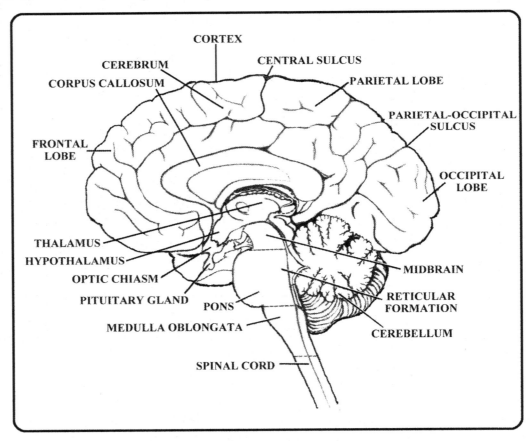

Fig. 3.A-2. Identification of the major components and landmark features in a medial section of the human brain. The temporal lobe is not shown as it does not extend to the midline of the brain.

being responsible for different functions in different parts of the cortex. Being of a gray hue, the outer layer of the cortex is the "gray matter" of which we speak when referring to intellectual powers. Lying within the cerebrum but below the gray matter of the cortex is a thick web of myelinated white matter.

The cortex is such a bulky object that it has to be folded and fissured in order to fit into the skull, especially in those animals in which there is high intelligence and a great need for brain power, Fig. 3.A-1. In human beings, these folds and fissures are constants of the cortex's shape and so serve to divide it into identifiable lobes (see below). Due to its many folds, the cortex has a large area (about 1500 cm^2), with about 3 billion nerve cells in each hemisphere. Much of the brain's work is carried out in the thin layer of the cortex, with the underlying cells serving as point-to-point connections within the brain, or as housekeeper cells with custodial duties. Though filled with nerve tissue, there are no pain receptors in the cortex [116, 291, 434].

With a thickness of only 2–4 millimeters, the cortex and its associated white matter nonetheless are the largest single structure in the brain, accounting for approximately half its volume. This seems at first sight contradictory for an object so thin, but the cortex is so folded and convoluted that only 25% of the brain's cortical area is visible on its surface; the remaining 75% of the cortex's area is hidden in the sulci (grooves) and gyri (convolutions) of the folded sheet [195].

The cortex serves as the conscious reception site for all of the sensory signals in the body, is in control of all of the conscious motor activities of voluntary motion, and is the site for mental activities such as memory, learning, reasoning and language. In performing *virabhadrasana I* (Box 2.B-1, page 18), for example, the cortex will be involved

in positioning the bones of the bent leg, registering the discomfort of the quadruceps of the straight leg, reviewing the pertinent aspects of the pose as remembered from earlier practice, recording, evaluating and storing the new instructions as they are spoken by the teacher and activating/deactivating new muscle groups in response to the teacher's commands. Simultaneously, at a less conscious level, the limbic system is reacting as described in Subsection 3.A, *The Limbic System*, page 33. Virtually all of the signals ascending to and descending from the cortex pass through the brainstem and spinal cord on their way to and from the muscles, sense organs, and glands.

Consciousness as we know it persists even when most of the forebrain has been removed; the essential brain area for consciousness is the thalamus, sitting atop the brainstem (Fig. 3.A-2), and acting as a switching station for neural impulses moving between higher and lower brain centers [369].

Though many functions of the cortex can be pinpointed as occurring in a highly specific area of the cortex, still more so than in the other two brain levels, there also is a delocalization of strongly related brain function over several seemingly unconnected areas. Thus, for example, the related functions of hearing words, seeing words, speaking words and generating words are seen in Fig. 3.A-3 to take place in very different neighborhoods of the cortex [195]. In the same vein, people with aphasia of Broca's area have great difficulty speaking, but can sing with ease and elegance [157].

Taking a somewhat different view of the brain as fruit salad, the cortex can be conveniently divided by its various sulci into four lobes. Such an approach not only divides the cortex geometrically, but also serves to delineate the areas specific to certain brain functions. Each of the lobes separated by

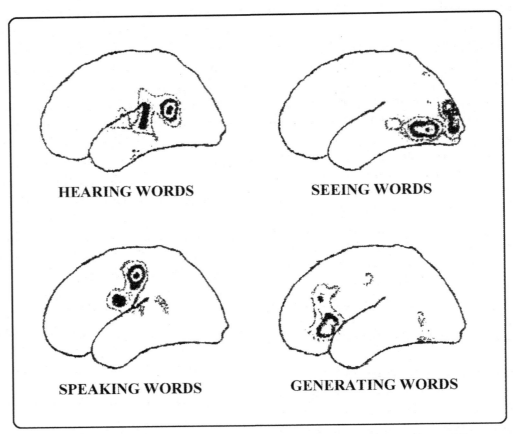

HEARING WORDS   **SEEING WORDS**

SPEAKING WORDS   **GENERATING WORDS**

Fig. 3.A-3. The PET scans of the cerebral blood flow through the left hemisphere of the cortex highlight the functional areas involved in performing various language-related tasks. These scans clearly illustrate how language ability is localized in different areas of the cortex depending upon function, *i.e.*, hearing words (temporal lobe), seeing words (occipital lobe), speaking words (motor cortex) and generating words (frontal lobe).

the longitudinal fissure appears on both the right and left sides of the brain.

The central fissure, also called the central sulcus, Fig. 3.A-4a, is a deep trench in the cortex of each of the cerebral hemispheres, perpendicular to the longitudinal fissure, and serves to separate the frontal lobes from the parietal lobes. Just forward of the central fissure in the frontal lobe is the motor area; all muscles of the body can be activated with neural signals originating here. However, due to a crossing over of the nerve paths (called decussation) in either the spinal cord or the brainstem, activation of the motor centers in one hemisphere contracts muscles on the opposite side of the body.

The frontal lobes, the largest of the four types, are locales for absorbing new information and on this basis planning new strategies; they allow the flexibility lacking in the hardwired brains of lesser creatures. The frontal lobes also deal with language, social behavior and higher mental activities. Note the prominence of the frontal lobe development in Fig. 3.A-1 on going from striped bass to human being.

Just behind the central sulcus in the parietal lobe is the sensory area in which all conscious sensory input is deposited. The parietal lobes are the sites for mathematical calculation, face recognition and most importantly, the ability to integrate experiences. The parietal lobes also deal with language, and have a different physical structure in the two hemispheres.

The sensory cortex within the brain's parietal lobe has been mapped in detail and is found to be laid out in an orderly array, Fig. 3.A-5b, but with the area dedicated to a particular sensory location being in proportion not to the area of that location, but rather proportional to the importance and sensory resolution required of that area. Thus sensations from the tongue, lips and hands are given disproportionately large space in the human sensory cortex, whereas that for the back body and trunk are disproportionately small. It is clear from this what the relative sensory importance of the organs of communication and the organs of posture have come to be in the human body.

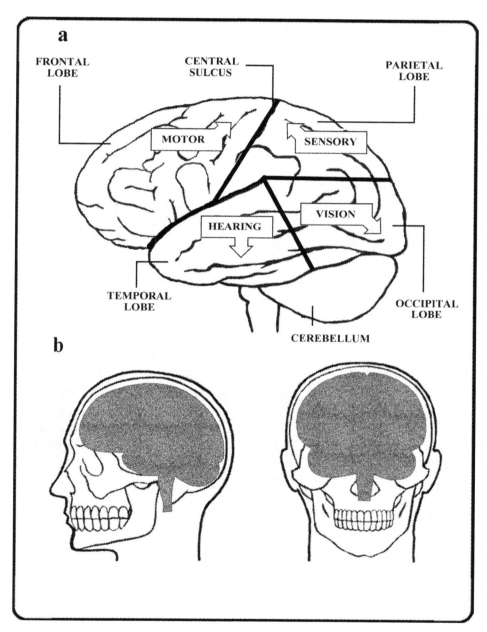

Fig. 3.A-4. (**a**) The surface features of the human brain, showing the lobes, sculpting and areas for motor and sensory functions. (**b**) How the brain rests in the skull as seen from the side and front.

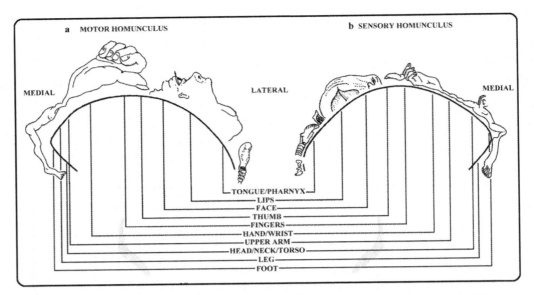

Fig. 3.A-5. (**a**) A map of the motor cortex, showing quantitatively how it is divided with respect to innervation of the appropriate muscles in the body (see also Fig. 3.A-4), and (**b**), a map of the sensory cortex, showing quantitatively how it is divided with respect to sensing tactile information (superficial and deep-pressure) from different areas of the body. The homunculi drawn above the relevant cortical arcs express the relative importance of the various body parts to sensory and motor excitation within the parietal lobes of the cerebral cortices. In both the sensory and motor cortices, the hands and lips of the homunculi require disproportionately large shares of the cortical areas, reflecting our high levels of manual dexterity and language skills.

Interestingly, the kidney, heart and spleen do not have cortical sensory representations, but sensory (pain) signals from them are instead referred to the corresponding skin dermatomes, Section 10.E, Dermatomes and Referred Pain, page 303.

Just in front of the central sulcus in the frontal lobe is a corresponding map of the motor connections which activate the muscles of the body, Fig. 3.A-5a. As might have been expected, the map of motor centers closely matches that of sensory centers, with those body parts having the greatest sensory resolution also having the greatest motor resolution. These distorted homunculi are discussed further in Section 7.A, Skeletal Muscle; Structure and Function, page 167.

The occipital lobes are positioned at the rear of the brain and are concerned exclusively with processing the visual signals from the eyes. Damage to these lobes results in blindness, for the signals sent from the retina are not processed into meaningful images. The temporal lobes are found just above each ear, and receive the auditory signals from the ears, albeit in a largely contralateral way. The temporal cortices are involved in aspects of language communication, in arranging for the storage of learned material in short-term memory and in interpreting olfactory signals.

Brodmann has offered a more detailed sectioning of the brain, dividing the cortical surface into 52 overlapping areas according to function. For example, the visual cortex is found in Brodmann's areas 17, 18 and 19, while areas 4, 6 and 8 correspond to the motor cortex, and areas 41 and 42 are the auditory cortex. As is appropriate for its importance, the primary visual cortex contains twice as many nerve cells as any other Brodmann's area.

However, the Brodmann areas within a cerebral hemisphere are not isolated in any sense. First, there are association fibers that connect one area with another in the same hemisphere. Then there are commissural fibers that connect an area in one hemisphere with another in the other hemisphere. Chief among these is the bundle of intra-hemispheric, myelinated fibers known as the corpus callosum, containing about 300 million distinct fibers. This bundle allows the rapid transfer between hemispheres of information and learning about motor actions and sensations involving all parts of the body, with the exception of the hands and the feet, strangely.

Finally, there are projection fibers in the brain that connect the cortical areas with subcortical areas. For example, the projection fibers carry the heavy neural traffic between the cortex and the thalamus. These fibers should be of great interest to the *yogasana* student as they are the link between the consciousness of the cortex and the subconsciousness of the lower brain centers. The thalamo-cortical neural pathways are discussed further in Subsection 3.E, *Brainwave Frequencies and Mental Functioning*, page 60. As most parts of the body have sensory afferents which project onto the cortex, it is not devoted to a single mode of sense, but integrates all major sensory signals. Projection areas include those for motor, proprioceptive, auditory, and visual sensations as well as speech and interpretation.

On studying the various functions of the major parts of the brain, one is struck by how much overlap of functions there is among the parts. This noncentralization of brain function undoubtedly results in increased mental flexibility allowing many alternate paths to the same result. One such path of a typical sensory signal through the various control centers of the brain and then back to the effector organ is shown sche-

matically in Fig. 3.A-6. In this, the sensory signal from some outlying body part ascends the spinal cord and is then split, with part of the signal ascending as high as the cortex and the other parts going only as high as the fastigial nucleus in the cerebellum. The descending signals from the cortex and the cerebellum then interact in the brainstem before entering the descending tracts of the spinal cord. The final signal activates muscles with a strength that reflects the sum of the influences of many centers in the brain operating at very different levels of consciousness.

Being the most sophisticated neural network, the cortex and its inherent intellectual power is what separates human beings from all other life forms. In an enriched environment offering many experiences, the cortical layers have been found to thicken noticeably with nerve cells. Obviously, the *yogasanas* should be counted among those experiences that enrich the cortex and thereby make it thicker.

A large fraction of the brain's function is inhibitory. In some cases, one can be born with the inhibitions not functioning, and this unleashes the amazing but pathetic performance of the *idiot savant*.

The Spinal Cord and Brainstem

The nerves within the spinal cord control movement of the trunk and limbs, and also receive and process sensory information from the skin, joints, and muscles of the limbs and trunk. See Section 4.B, The Spinal Cord, page 83, and Fig. 4.B-1 for a more detailed discussion of the spinal cord. The vegetative/reflexive hindbrain, also called the brainstem, is continuous with the spinal cord, positioned between the upper end of the spinal cord and the base of the brain, Fig. 2.A-2. The brainstem passes from the skull to the spinal cord through the foramen magnum in the occipital bone of the skull, this being the largest opening into the braincase.

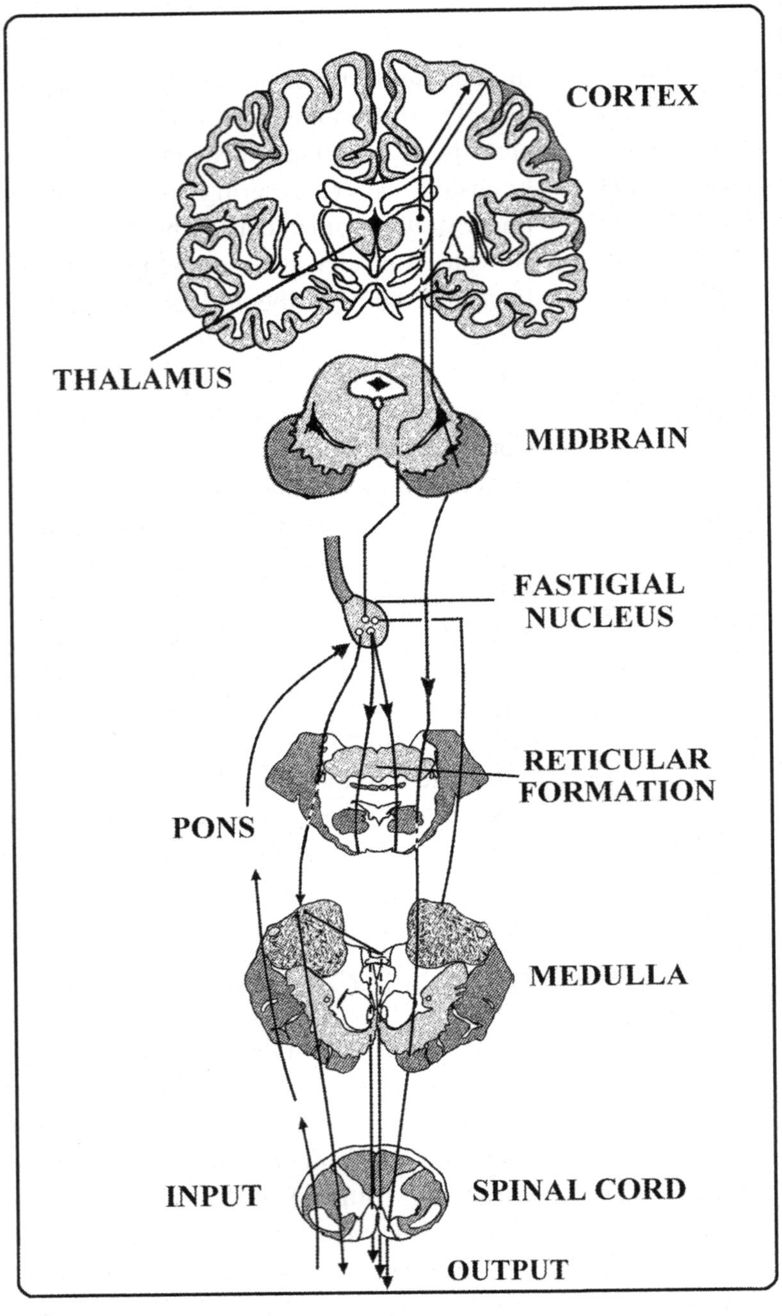

The brainstem consists of four major parts, the medulla oblongata, the pons, the reticular formation and the midbrain, Fig. 3.A-2. The brainstem is a conduit for both ascending and descending information between the brain and the spinal cord, and is also involved in receiving sensory information from the head and controlling muscle action in the face and neck. Containing the reticular formation (see below), the brainstem also regulates the levels of awareness and arousal.

The medulla oblongata, Fig. 3.A-2, is continuous with the spinal cord and is responsible for autonomic functions such as digestion, breathing and heart rate (see Section 11.E, Monitoring Blood Pressure with the Baroreceptors, page 339). It is in this region that the motor fibers for voluntary action connecting the cortex to the spinal cord are decussated, *i.e.*, cross over from left to right and *vice versa* so that muscles on the right-hand side of the body are directed by the left cerebral hemisphere, and *vice versa* [195]. When dreaming during sleep, the medial medulla is inactive so that there is little or no muscle action during the dream.

The pons deals with information about body movement, carrying it from the cerebral hemisphere to the cerebellum. Together with the medulla, the pons regu-

Fig. 3.A-6. Following an ascending sensory signal from a proximal body part (input), the signal bypasses the reticular formation, and may ascend as high as the cerebral cortex; it then returns to the spinal cord (output) via several parallel paths. Note the decussation of the descending signal at the point between the midbrain and the fastigial nucleus.

lates the parameters of blood pressure and respiration. The midbrain controls many sensory and motor functions, including eye movement and coordination of visual and auditory reflexes.

The Reticular Formation

Sensory information from all of the sensory organs (proprioceptive, smell, taste, auditory, visual, *etc.*) enters the reticular formation via the ascending reticular activating system for processing before being sent to the hypothalamus, except for visual information, which bypasses the reticular formation and goes directly to the hypothalamus. Being a column of narrow, vertical sheets in the brainstem, Figs. 2.A-2 and 3.A-7, the reticular formation regulates

motor functions, sleep, consciousness, respiration and vascular functions [195, 230]; it is connected to the gray matter of the spinal cord at one end and to both the hypothalamus and the cortex at the other. Almost all mammals have a reticular formation.

If all of the sensory information sent to the reticular formation were to be forwarded to the higher centers in the brain, there would be an immediate overload. It is the job of the reticular formation to filter this mass of data and to then relay only that part of it that can be of immediate importance. It does this on the basis of change: if signals from sensors or receptors are constant in time, then they safely can be ignored in favor of those few that are changing in time. Any rapid change in the sensory field of the

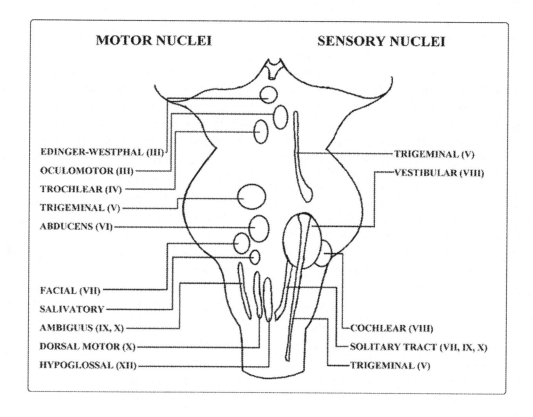

Fig. 3.A-7. Anatomy of the reticular formation showing several of the important brainstem nuclei connected to the cranial nerves in both the afferent and the efferent branches.

organism is immediately forwarded for consideration by the higher faculties. On the other hand, if the reticular formation is damaged or otherwise nonfunctional, the result is eternal sleep (coma), as no arousal is possible [291].

It is generally held that stimulation of any of the sensory organs leads to excitation of the reticular formation and consequently, a state of sympathetic arousal. With this in mind, it is clear why a truly deep state of relaxation in *savasana* requires that the eyes be closed with the room lights off, no external sound, and the body being touched only by the floor. Actually, floor pressure does give a sensible signal for a few minutes, but if it is a comfortable contact, the sensory signal adapts and the sense of pressure fades to zero. Further, any muscular movement beyond that of the breath will be arousing to the reticular formation and so has to be repressed in *savasana*. In contrast, when in the other *yogasanas*, one must constantly make micro-adjustments to the posture in order to keep the proprioceptive map from fading from consciousness.

When one is totally relaxed and there are no external stimuli going to the reticular formation, then the EEG brainwave pattern (Section 3.E, Brainwaves and the Electro-encephalogram, page 57) settles into the low-frequency, high-amplitude alpha mode. On the other hand, any sensory input to the reticular formation brings one into a global, nonspecific state of alertness and preparedness, and the EEG pattern then shifts to that of the high-frequency, low-amplitude beta waves. When teaching *savasana*, one can talk the student toward a state of relaxation, however, in order for the student to achieve this state, the teacher must then be quiet, so that there is no further stimulation of the reticular formation.

Though it is generally assumed that any input signal from peripheral sensors such as eyes, *etc.*, will arouse the reticular forma-

tion as witnessed by the shift away from the alpha brainwave rhythm, and it is generally true, it is also to be noted that in the case of meditating adepts, there is no interruption of the alpha pattern when the eyes are open, in a noisy room, *etc.* One meditator showed no change in alpha pattern when his hand was plunged into ice water and left there for 45 minutes; another maintained a constant, unbroken pattern of alpha waves for 9 hours [201]. According to B.K.S. Iyengar, it is possible to reach such states of inward directedness in the *yogasanas* [210]. The similarities between such deeply meditative states and the hypnotic state have been pointed out repeatedly [104, 107, 201, 380], however, the constancy of the alpha-wave pattern fluctuates when in the presence of distractions in the hypnotic state, whereas this is not the case when in the yogic state [380].

Not only are there ascending somato-sensory and viscero-sensory afferents to the reticular formation, but input as well from forebrain structures and the central nervous system. When functioning properly, there is a high degree of coordination of ascending and descending activities to and from the reticular formation, with ascending activity leading to a change of consciousness from drowsy to attentive. This then leads to somato-motor and autonomic changes on the descending side.

The oculomotor nucleus in the reticular formation (Fig. 3.A-7) is one of over forty such centers in the reticular formation, and is the termination of cranial nerve III. As this nerve and its reticular-formation center are prominently involved with all manner of eye motion [195], such eye motion can be taken as a rough measure of reticular-formation activation, *i.e.*, arousal. The eye movements so often seen in yogic relaxation (*savasana*) suggests that there is residual but random stimulation of the reticular formation in the relaxed state, rather like the beta waves of REM sleep where there is considerable loss of muscle tone, except in the eye muscles [195]. On the other hand, when the eyes are open, there is unavoidable arousal and full relaxation is not possible unless one is in a deeply meditative state.

Activation and deactivation of the reticular formation is readily accomplished with the appropriate drugs. Thus amphetamines stimulate the reticular formation, leading to a hyperalert state of high consciousness and twitching muscles, whereas tranquilizers and depressants lower the level of excitation in the reticular formation, leading to states of relaxation or general anaesthesia, depending upon the dose [222]. *Yogasana* students suffering from depression or low blood pressure should be urged to keep their eyes open in all of the postures intended to energize them, for closing the eyes will allow the reticular formation to relax, followed by a de-energized feeling.

Alcohol and drugs such as marijuana, LSD and heroin have strong effects on the operation of the reticular formation [43], and watching television for 1/2 hour can lull the reticular formation into an alpha-state EEG characteristic of unfocused attention. It is the action of specific cells in the reticular formation that leads to sleep.

The reticular formation receives much sensory information and sends all such relevant inputs to the cortex, thereby alerting it. However, it also acts to filter disturbances when concentrating on an activity. Thus, we tend to hear no other voices when concentrating on the teacher's voice and on the balance when in *ardha chandrasana*, for example, because extraneous input has been filtered out by the reticular formation. The reticular formation is similarly adept at filtering out pain signals or enhancing them as they attempt to gain the attention of the cortex (Section 10.D, Pain, page 294) [186].

The Limbic System

It is most difficult to define the anatomical boundaries of the limbic system because many distant structures are so closely connected neurally to the more obvious limbic centers that it seems logical to include them too. Thus there is no agreement over just what is to be included in the phrase "limbic system" [57, 116, 195, 225]. A simple picture of the brain area generally held to be the site of the limbic system is shown in Fig. 3.A-8. Our text will deal with only a small number of the nuclei within the limbic system, *i.e.*, those relevant to performing the *yogasanas*.

The cerebellum, Figs. 2.A-2 and 3.A-2, has no direct motor function but is the main center for the integration of proprioceptive information, and so is essential for the smooth voluntary actions of the muscles and the learning of motor skills. The cerebellum also coordinates the proprioceptive signals with the signals from the inner ears and from the eyes, and so is a key factor in keeping one's balance. It communicates directly with the cortex in order to guide muscle action and to help maintain posture and balance; it can also inhibit postural reflexes. Emotions have been long associated with the limbic centers, but it is now known [157] that the cortex also contributes to our emotions, moods, *etc.*

Damage to the cerebellum leads directly to a loss of muscle coordination, balance and muscle tone [291, 319, 340]. The cerebellum, like the cerebrum, is divided into lateral hemispheres, is corrugated, and has an outer layer of gray matter covering the white matter within. See Fig. 5.A-2 for a picture of the fan-like Purkinje cell of the cerebellum and the immense web of interconnection that such cells can provide.

The diencephalon (Fig. 2.A-2), yet another part of the limbic system, consists of two parts, the thalamus, which processes much

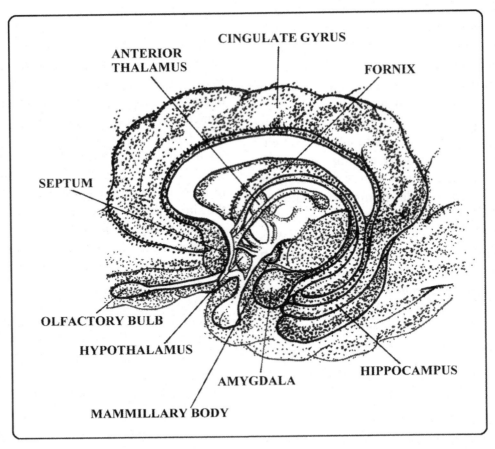

Fig. 3.A-8. Positions of several, but not all of the components of the limbic system within the brain.

of the information traveling up the central nervous system to the cortex, and the hypothalamus, which regulates the autonomic, endocrine and visceral functions, Fig. 2.A-2. Because the hypothalamus has an intimate relationship with both the autonomic nervous system and with the endocrine system, it is a very prominent player in regulating our behaviors [225]. The hypothalamus is of special interest to the *yogasana* student as it is the central organ controlling the reflex actions which we try to bring under more conscious control through practice of the *yogasanas*. The many functions of the hypothalamus and the connections between it and the higher cerebral centers are discussed in Section 6.B, The Hypothalamus, page 140. Though the pituitary gland is formally not a part of the brain, it is connected

to the brain by a stalk, and though it often is referred to as "the master gland", it is in fact controlled by secretions from the hypothalamus.

Lying just above the thalamus in the limbic region are three internal regions: the basal ganglia which regulate motor performance, the hippocampus, involved with memory storage, and the amygdala which coordinates autonomic and endocrine responses with emotional states.

When performing complex actions requiring the proper muscle selection, sequencing, timing, and activation, the basal ganglia are of the greatest importance. Some programs of the basal ganglia are inborn (swallowing), whereas others are learned by practice (the straight-leg lift into *sirsasana*, for example). Three nuclei within the basal ganglia are particularly relevant to our discussion (see below).

All of the information from which the proprioceptive maps of the body position are generated are sent to the substantia nigra, a nucleus within the basal ganglia. Though this mass of information (muscle length, rate-of-change of length, and muscle tension) is handled subconsciously, if the substantia nigra is not working properly, then the fine control of the muscles is lost, movement is jerky and the limbs tremble.

The nucleus called the globus pallidus controls the muscle action when certain body positions are to be held in a fixed position. Also, whenever there is body movement, certain muscles must be braced to support the movement, and this bracing action is under the control of the globus pallidus. As we age, certain holding patterns within the globus pallidus become more comfortable than others, and we tend then to hold these postures to the exclusion of others. This acts to freeze us in the preferred posture so that change becomes nearly impossible. To an extent, the "stiffness" of the aged is in reality a stiffness of the neurological circuits controlling posture, rather than a stiffness of the muscles themselves. However, through the practice of *yogasana* at an early age, the globus pallidus learns how to support a great variety of body postures, and so in this way, one can keep the options for body posture wide open regardless of age.

A third nucleus, the striate body, controls the manner of movement. Again, we tend to fall into stereotypical movements, the patterns of which are stored in the striate body, but through *yogasana* practice, a healthy variety of patterns can be available to us. Diseases of the basal ganglia result in degraded motor control, as for example, the mask-like face and shuffling gait in those with Parkinson's disease.

Returning to the discussion of the student in *virhabdrasana I* first mentioned in Box 2.B-1, page 18, changes are being wrought in the body at the subconscious level as directed by the hypothalamus. In response to the work of the globus palladus in maintaining this pose, the hypothalamus commands the heart rate to increase along with the blood pressure, the blood to leave the gut and go to the working muscles instead, the respiration rate to increase along with the diameters of bronchial vessels, *etc.*, all without any conscious direction from the cortex. At the same time, memories of the action are being stored in the substantia nigra and the hippocampus of the limbic system. Interactions between the hippocampus and the cortex lead to "learning" of the posture, Section 3.C, page 42.

One can only guess that once *virhabdrasana I* has been performed satisfactorily, there is a consequent stimulation of the pleasure center in the hypothalamus that simultaneously activates the muscles of expression (a smile [230]) and reinforces the motivational and physical factors that brought the posture to a satisfying conclusion (Section 6.B, The Hypothalamus, page 140).

SECTION 3.B. ASPECTS OF BRAIN STRUCTURE AND FUNCTION

Blood Flow through the Brain

Physically, the brain is just 2% of an adult's body weight, yet this organ receives 15% of the cardiac output and accounts for 20% of the body's demand for oxygen [225]. The adult brain requires at least 750 milliliters (almost a quart) of freshly oxygenated blood every minute in order to function properly, with a four-fold larger flow of blood through the gray matter of the brain as compared to that through the white matter. Cessation of this flow of fresh blood to the brain for only 5 seconds will induce a change in mental state, 10 seconds will lead to unconsciousness, and cessation for 5 minutes or more will lead to irreversible damage [116]. By comparison, blood flow to the spinal cord can be interrupted for up to 30 minutes without permanent damage. It seems likely that the brain's sensitivity to blood flow lies behind the altered mental states achieved in *padmasana* (Box 8.E-1: *A Safe Way to Teach Padmasana*, page 266) and various inverted *yogasanas* (Section 11.F, Blood Pressure in Inverted *Yogasanas*, page 343).

The huge surface area of the cortex helps in keeping the interior of the brain cool, for the heat load otherwise is quite high (see Table 11.A-2 in regard to O_2 demands by various parts of the body during exercise). This heat load generated by the brain is handled in part by large-area structures within the nose (nasal conchae), which efficiently transfer the heat of the brain into the blood and thence into the inspired and expired air.

Blood carrying oxygen and nutrients (largely the sugar glucose) into the brain moves through two main arteries, the internal carotid and the vertebral, Fig. 3.B-1. The first of these is found on either side of the neck, whereas the other passes through the transverse foramina of the C1 to C6 vertebrae on each side, bypassing C7. The vertebral and carotid arteries supply the Circle of

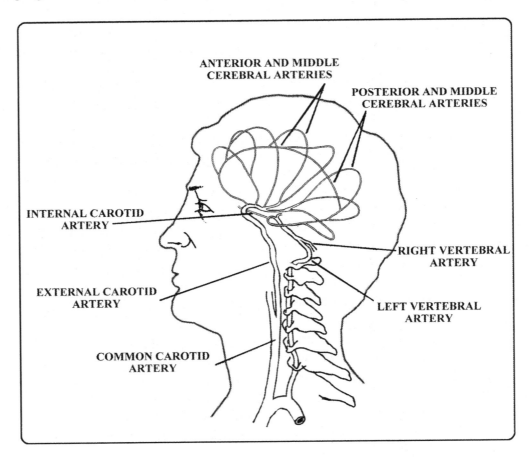

Fig. 3.B-1. Major arteries of the neck and head, showing the left vertebral artery within the foramina on the left sides of the cervical vertebrae. The blood flow is approximately equal through the carotid and vertebral arteries.

Willis, a circular doughnut-shaped structure from which many smaller arteries branch. Once inside the brain, there is further arterial branching in order to serve both exterior and interior structures [116]. Metabolic waste products are carried out of the brain by a complex venous system, converging upon the jugular veins. Blood flow to the brain at age 65 may be as small as 1/3 that at age 25 [141]. Though without proof, one would guess that this diminution of the blood flow to the brain might be slowed by yogic inversions.

That there is sufficient blood pressure to maintain optimum flow through the brain is monitored by the baroreceptor organs (Section 11.E, Monitoring Blood Pressure with the Baroreceptors, page 339), placed within the carotid arteries close to the brain itself. If the neck is squeezed at the carotid arteries, the baroreceptors in that location mistakenly report a high pressure to the brain, which in turn adjusts the heart's action and the associated vascular plumbing such that less blood flows to the brain. As a consequence, the brain is starved for blood and the person faints.

In *yogasana* practice, the throttling of the blood supply to the brain by virtue of the neck posture can have both negative and positive consequences. For example, in the head-forward (flexion) position, as in *sarvangasana, etc.*, the mild throttling of the blood flow through the carotid arteries generally slows the heart as the baroreceptors within the arteries report a high pressure to the hypothalamus. This slowing of the heart beat is welcome as it promotes relaxation (Section 11.F, Blood Pressure in Inverted *Yogasanas*, page 343). On the other hand, when the head is thrown backward as in *ustrasana*, the lack of blood flow through the vertebral arteries can lead to nausea and dizziness, especially if the shoulder blades are not pulled away from the base of the skull.

When the blood flow within the brain is disrupted, the person is said to have had a stroke. The two largest causes of stroke are the presence of a clot that blocks an artery, or an arterial wall that bursts, leading to a hemorrhage. As the formation of clots is favored by a slow flow of blood, strokes from this source are most prevalent about 3 AM when blood pressure is low, whereas at about 8 AM, the blood pressure is rapidly ascending and hemorrhaging then becomes more likely. Should part of the cortex suffer a stroke and so erase sensation or motor control over a part of the body, then nearby areas will eventually move into the vacated cortical space unless a heroic effort is made to hold onto it. Actually, following a stroke, the dead part of the cortex is surrounded by an area that is not dead but is in shock. Through vigorous assisted exercise of the lost function, the shocked part of the cortex can be brought back to functioning, often in the mode of the lost brain cells.

The brain has an immune system which is separate from that of the rest of the body due to the impermeability of the blood-brain barrier; see Subsection 13.C, *The Brain's Immune System*, page 388.

Headaches

Though the brain is a complex web of neurons and records the sensations of pain from all of the other parts of the body, it can feel no pain generated within itself, being devoid of the proper sensors for this. However, pain in the immediate area surrounding the brain often is interpreted as brain pain (headache). That is to say, headache often involves distress in areas surrounding the brain, such as dilation or distension of the blood vessels in the scalp and/or the meninges (the protective covering of the brain), vasoconstriction of the blood vessels, spasms of the muscles of the scalp, neck, shoulders, jaw and face, or a compression of the nerves. There also would appear to be pain receptors in the arteries within the brain. Head pain involves the stimulation of free nerve endings in the head, transmission of the pain signal downward into the spinal cord and then its return up the spinal cord, brainstem, and thalamus to finally register in the cortex [186].

The sensation of headache results when arteries or veins in the brain are pulled, displaced, dilated or disturbed, or when the trigeminal, vagus and glossopharyngeal cranial nerves are pulled, compressed or inflamed [340]. Those headaches that involve the state of tension in the blood vessels are called vascular headaches, whereas those involving muscle tension are called muscle-contraction headaches [117].

The most frequent type of persistent headache is closely associated with on-going depression and anxiety [186]. As discussed in Subsection 20.A, *Medicine Versus Depression*, page 464, depression is largely due to a lack of several neurotransmitters in the brain (mainly epinephrine and serotonin) and this chemical imbalance then can lead to sleep disturbances, *etc.*, Table 20.A-1. When in the throes of depression, the sufferer easily falls asleep, but the depression headache typically begins at 4–5 AM, arousing the sufferer, who then cannot go back to sleep. In contrast, anxiety sufferers have headaches at bedtime and have trouble falling asleep.

The diffuse pain of the depression headache is due to muscular contraction of the band of muscles surrounding the head like a hatband, and strikes most often in the frontal and occipital lobes. The headache type is treated medically with analgesics, antidepressants and muscle relaxants, all of which prompt the sympathetic nervous system to raise the levels of catecholamines in the brain and/or modify the serotonin levels [309]. The increase of the catecholamines can be achieved as well by performing a vigorous set of *yogasanas* emphasizing mo-

tion of the cervical vertebra, followed by an extended relaxation.

As the muscle tension headache is often brought on by tension in the neck, shoulder and cranial areas, the symptomatic posture is one in which the head and shoulders are carried well forward, with the chest collapsed and the thoracic curve exaggerated. *Yogasanas* that work to release tension in these areas can be effective therapy. So, for example, *setu bandhasana*, *viparita karani*, *savasana* and the arm positions for *gomukhasana* and *garudasana*, are effective in reducing the effects of tension headaches [272, 420], as they release tension in these critical areas. As a result of poor cervical posture, nerve compression between C1 and the atlas also can contribute to headache [272]. To the extent that prolotherapy strengthens ligaments that have been pulled into stressed positions by faulty postures, it too has been used successfully to treat muscle-tension headaches [2].

In vascular headaches, the precipitating cause is an over-pressurization of the blood vessels of the brain itself, or of the vessels of the scalp and meninges due to vasodilation. Cluster headaches in which the pain localizes about one eye, and some migraine cases fall into the vascular-headache category. Drug therapy of the vascular headache is centered about regaining a measure of vasoconstriction using alpha agonists, beta blockers, ergotamine and caffeine, all of which act to constrict the smooth muscle of the blood vessels. Certain vascular headaches if not too intense are relieved by drinking a cup of regular caffeinated coffee, but are intensified by drinking a decaffeinated brew. The more effective a cup of coffee is in alleviating headache symptoms, the stronger is the rebound headache when coffee is withheld [384].

Often, the mild vascular headache (but not the migraine) can be eased by the passive performance of a few *yogasanas* in which the forehead is supported on a hard surface, *i.e.*, *adho mukha svanasana* with the head on a block, or *adho mukha virasana* with head on the floor. These postures in which the forehead and/or the orbits of the eyes receive external mechanical pressure stimulate the vagal heart-slowing reflex, and so lower the blood pressure. The acupressure points bladder 2 are also found just above the eyebrows, and are used for headache relief in that type of therapy.

Easing of the distress of migraine headaches through *yogasana* involves passive positions, well supported, with eyes bandaged, minimal movement and minimal external input of sensations, all aimed at minimal activation of the reticular formation and maximal parasympathetic stimulation [378]. It is also felt that disruptions to the regular day-to-day pattern of biorhythms can precipitate headaches.

Maturation, Aging, and Gender Effects on the Brain

In the infant brain, there is considerable rewiring in the first two years, and perhaps less obvious changes for a few years after that. During these early years, there is considerable reorganization as neural paths are developed, unneeded neurons are shed and frequently used circuits are strengthened. As the fetus develops, there is first an invasive innervation of the muscle fibers, with each neuron connected to several muscle fibers, however, with time and use of the muscles, the innervation resolves so that each fiber has only one neuron to stimulate it. Similarly, in the autonomic ganglia, neurons at first have many presynaptic connections, but this later resolves to one per ganglion [225].

Thus one is born with a brain which has the potential to develop in many different directions, but once the pattern is set, then excess baggage is shed. This means that anatomically, the brain of a newborn infant is very much oversized as compared to that of an adult, as can be seen in Fig. 3.B-2, where a five-month old infant has been drawn to the scale of an adult male. In African societies where there is little or no use of calendars, it is decided that a child is ready for school when his body proportions are such that he can reach his hand across the top of his head and hold the opposite ear. Clearly the infant in the Figure has several years to go, whereas the adult would be more than ready for school.

Myelination in the brain continues up to age 7, at which point the learning of language becomes much more difficult. It has only recently been appreciated that significant changes in brain make up and function can continue into the teenage years [302]. Between the ages of 10 and 12, there is a considerable increase in the sizes of the parietal and frontal lobes, and then a shrinking of these up to the early twenties, by which time the brain circuitry has again pared away unneeded neurons and has assumed its final configuration. The parietal and frontal lobes are responsible for such functions as planning, social judgement, and self control.

The effects of aging on the brain are threefold, as there are physical changes, chemical changes and mental changes as we age (see also Chapter 22, AGING AND LONGEVITY, page 493). Chemically, the neurotransmitter dopamine in the brain is very important for movement control and consequently, loss of dopamine leads to Parkinson-like motor problems; in the aging brain, dopamine levels drop by 40%. On the other hand, the level of monoamine oxidase in the brain, a neurotransmitter which helps manage depression, increases with age.

Physically, 70-year-olds have on average 11% smaller brains than 40-year-olds, with the weight of brain tissue decreasing and the ventricular volume increasing. This shrinkage appears to be due to an irreversible loss

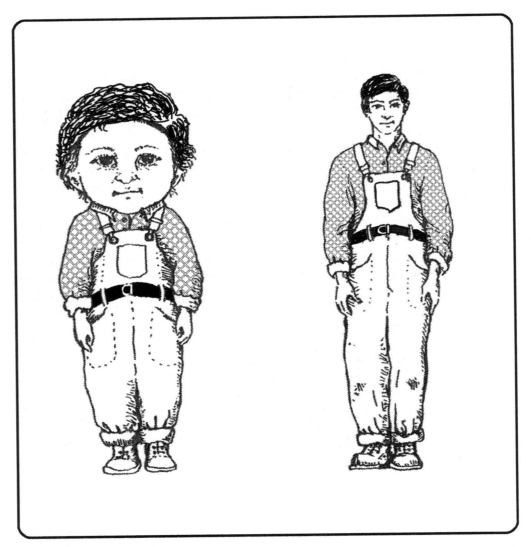

Fig. 3.B-2. Comparison of the relative sizes of body parts in a five-month-old infant drawn to the same height as a grown adult male [472], with both in *tadasana*. Each of the figures is drawn with the proportions appropriate to its age.

of nerve cells. The neurons in the locus ceruleus, sensitive to norepinephrine, decrease in number by 35% in the elderly. The largest changes are in the most important of the brain's regions, the cortex. Here, the number of cells decreases by 40% by age 75, as compared with a 20-year-old. Within the cortex, the largest drop is in the temporal lobe, the site for storage of memories.

There is still discussion of what exactly is going on in the aging brain, for it is argued by some that the shrinkage of the brain is not a decrease of numbers but only of size and form of the neurons. Thus Restak and Mahoney [382] argue that the loss is of neurons not involved in thinking, and that the mature brain is organized differently, has different strengths, and can remodel itself. In the past 20 years it has been realized that the populations studied in the earlier brain work involved significant numbers of people with various illnesses that can affect brain function [187]. Thus, for example, chronic stress can damage the hippocampus and chronically high blood pressure can lead to cognitive decline. On the other hand, in a population of healthy but elderly subjects, there was no neuron loss of any sort, and evidence is becoming stronger that neurogenesis in the brain occurs well into adulthood. In any event, it is agreed that there is a general shrinkage of the dendritic trees connecting a particular neuron to its neighbors and a lowered response to neurotransmitters on aging [153].

Whereas aging seems not to affect the numbers of neurons in the brains of healthy subjects, there is a measurable decrease of the levels of several key neurotransmitters and a decreased affinity for the receptor sites involved in memory and learning. With age, plaques also can form within the axons of the neurons, interfering with the transmission of the action potential, and eventually leading to Alzheimer's disease.

On average, up to 30% of the motor nerves die by the time we are in our later years. Once a motor nerve dies, then its muscle fiber, lacking innervation, also withers and dies, leading to thinner and weaker muscles. This seems to be especially true for muscles of the legs [340]. On the other hand, motor skills of the sort used in *yogasanas* are learned as quickly as in younger people [382].

Despite the obvious outward physical changes in the brain as it ages, its functioning remains relatively unchanged. Thus, the EEG activity (Section 3.E, Brainwaves and the Electroencephalogram, page 57) of the brain decreases only at age 80 years and beyond. What is readily apparent is that with age, the brain slows down more than anything else. With age, memory-recall slows, as do the reaction times for all sorts of mental tests. Still, the aged can often do the job, it is just that they need more time to focus their mental resources on the problem at hand. As one ages, the verbal IQ stays intact as does the knowledge (semantic) memory, while the episodic memory fades. One theory of brain aging has it that the effects are due to stress [382] and the excess cortisol (Subsection 6.C, *Cortisol*, page 149) that it can generate [29], and that yogic relaxation techniques can retard brain aging by lowering cortisol levels in the brain.

One truly significant difference induced by aging is that the aged in general have a problem with accepting new information, unless it is a simple extension of what they already know to be true. As we age, we are less able or willing to try out new ideas and find them acceptable, which is to say, we become mentally inflexible and are discomfited by new thoughts or new ways of doing things. As teachers of aging students, we must be aware of this possible stumbling block to learning and find ways to make the new material seem not so new that learning it is resisted. See Subsection 3.D, *Using Cerebral Hemispheric Laterality in Yoga*, page 55, for a possible way to overcome this situation. Further, since the aging brain finds it harder to stick to a single line of thought and so requires more frequent rest breaks, teaching *yogasana* to seniors should be broken into smaller steps, punctuated by more frequent rest periods [382].

Just as the apparent left-right symmetry of the brain is illusory (Section III.C, The Body's Inherent Lack of Symmetry, page 520), so too is the apparent congruency of the brain functions of men and women. Evidence is now accumulating to show that similar brain functions in men and women can occur in very dissimilar areas. Thus, for example, men use the left side of their hippocampus to find their way out of a virtual maze, whereas women accomplish the same task using the right frontal cortex [326]. Also, it is now known that both of the frontal lobes are used much more by women in the comprehension of language, than by men. Clearly, the division of labor in the male and female brains is not congruent [325].

SECTION 3.C. MEMORY, LEARNING, AND TEACHING

Memory and Learning

The capacity to learn is one of the fundamental activities of man's higher mental functions. Each of us is the individual that we are by virtue of what we have learned and what we remember of that; our experiences shape us, often in important ways of which we are not even conscious. Our personalities are shaped by the knowledge of the world that we have acquired through our senses, our storage of that information in the brain as a memory and the retrieval of that memory. Memory and learning are two sides of the same coin: you cannot learn what you do not store in your memory, and you cannot remember what you have not learned. The scientific study of learning and memory is most difficult and complex, and as might be expected, is changing rapidly.

Each of us has a unique pattern of synaptic connections in the brain, and the expression of these neural patterns is the unique character that each of us has come to be. Certain of these patterns are in-born and hardwired, but others are changeable and allow us to learn (the ability to modify our behavior on the basis of our experience) and to remember (the ability to store and retrieve this modification over time) [224]. That we are who we are largely on the basis of what we have learned and what we remember, is to say that we are who we are largely on the basis of the synaptic patterns of connectedness that we have formed and maintained in the brain. In *yogasana* practice, we will learn and remember important information about ourselves, thus transforming the brain's wiring and so transforming our entire being in the process.

In the broadest sense, there are two types of learning and memory [225]. In the first type, called reflexive memory, the learning accumulates slowly by repetition over many practice sessions, and the memory of the lesson learned has an automatic quality to it, in that it is not dependent on awareness, consciousness, or cognitive properties. Involving perceptual and motor skills, reflexive learning and memory lead to improved performance in many tasks, yet the train of actions necessary for successfully performing a task cannot be articulated. For example, with practice one can learn how to jump into *adho mukha vrksasana* with straight legs and though the sequences of muscle actions are stored in memory in the basal ganglia and cerebellum, yet one is unable to verbally describe what is going on, except at the simplest level. Even certain verbal skills can become reflexive if repeated enough, as when speaking with a regional accent. Much of our practice of the *yogasanas* is reflexive learning.

The second general type of learning and memory is declarative, the type in which one makes a conscious effort to recall learning effects and experiences that can be described verbally. This type of learning/memory depends upon cognitive processes such as evaluation, comparison, inference, *etc*. The declarative memory is being accessed when the teacher of *yogasana* recites to the class the list of points to be attended to when performing *trikonasana*, for example. The acquisition of facts regarding people, places, events, *etc.*, takes place in the hippocampus [105].

It is thought that the two modes of learning and remembering involve different areas of the brain, nonetheless, many learning experiences have both reflexive and declarative elements operating simultaneously, though not necessarily in equal proportions.

There are four generalizations that can be made in regard to learning and the memory of it.

1) Memory has stages in which time is an important factor. Many experiments (and

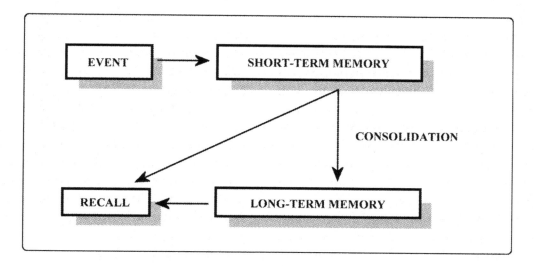

Fig. 3.C-1. The details of an event are stored for about 24 hours in short-term memory and are available for recall during that time. After 24 hours, the details then are consolidated in long-term memory, where they are then available for recall at times as long as several decades later.

accidents) show that memory has a finite lifetime, and within that lifetime, the memory can be disrupted. As shown in Fig. 3.C-1, what we learn from an experience serves as input and is first placed in short-term memory. After being in this place for a time that can last for up to a day, the information in short-term memory is then transferred to long-term memory in a process called consolidation. Information in either the long-term or the short-term memory banks can be searched for, read and outputted: this is what we remember of the stored experience. The physiological and structural characteristics of these two modes of storage are discussed further below. Loss of memory is due either to erasure of the memory or poor performance of the search-and-readout function.

2) Consolidation of a lesson into the long-term memory involves plastic changes in the brain, by which is meant a permanent and detectable alteration of the synaptic circuitry in the central nervous system. By virtue of the different learning experiences we all have had, each of us has a unique synaptic brain structure, and each of us is therefore a unique person.

3) The plastic changes in the brain which occur once something is learned and stored are deposited simultaneously in several different parts of the brain. Furthermore, whereas some lessons are stored in the higher brain centers, others may be stored in the spinal cord (see the discussion on central-pattern generators, Subsection 4.B, *Neural Connectivity of the Spinal Cord*, page 86) and even may be active in a brain-dead person.

4) The reflexive and declarative memories involve different neuronal circuits. Thus the amygdala and cerebellum are active in reflexive memory whereas declarative memory involves the temporal lobe and the diencephalon.

Short-Term Memory

Short-term memory holds fewer than a dozen items, and depending upon the definition of the term "item", some say only three or four items will fit in short-term memory at any one time. Storage time in short-term memory is generally only a few minutes unless the experience is practiced or rehearsed. Given that short-term memory is so limited in capacity, one sees immediately that when teaching the intricacies of a particular *yogasana* to beginners, if one gives more than a few details to the students at one time, their short-term memories will become overloaded and they will abandon the earlier instructions in order to make room for the more recent ones. This is not so much a problem for more experienced students who have laid down permanent memories of the instructions through earlier practices.

Interestingly, information put into short-term storage is easily erased by any sort of trauma or disturbance to the brain. Thus it often happens that in a head-trauma accident, the memories of items far in the past are totally intact, but memories of experiences occurring within a time span of two hours prior to the trauma have been totally forgotten because the short-term memory

has been erased. It is no surprise then, that learned experiences will be most effectively transferred to long-term memory with the greatest fidelity if the brain can be quiet following the exercise, thus allowing for an undisturbed consolidation of the information (see Box 3.C-1 for a further discussion of this and related points on learning). Thus we come to see that the lessons to be learned and remembered through practice of the *yogasanas* will be learned and remembered best if they are followed by a restful period, as with *savasana*!

Physiologically, it appears that "to place an item into short-term memory" means first of all to practice it so that its neural pathway is reinforced. This means the synapses involved in this neural circuit are more conducting of the neural excitation current either because there is a stronger

---

BOX 3.C-1: LEARNING AND *YOGASANA* PRACTICE

From the discussion given in the text, we come to see that one of the physiological benefits of doing *savasana* at the end of *yogasana* practice is that it offers the calm conditions necessary for optimum transfer of the learned neural pattern from short-term memory to the more permanent long-term memory. Though more time consuming, one can then see the sense in doing *savasana* after practicing each *yogasana* as in some forms of *hatha yoga* rather than at the end of the *yogasana* series as suggested by Iyengar [215].

In a situation somewhat parallel to that discussed above, it is known that students will do better on an exam if they will study less and then get a fair night's sleep rather than study for an extended period right up to the time of the exam, for in the latter situation, there has been no time for the learned information to transfer into long-term storage where it might then be available to the student during the test. Though not proven, it seems reasonable to think that consolidation occurs most readily when the mind has shifted from beta-state arousal to alpha-state calm (Section 3.E, Brainwaves and the Electroencephalogram, page 57).

Yet another aspect of learning involves what we might call "the environmental context factor". It has been shown repeatedly that when students study for an examination in the cafeteria, for example, they will do better on the test for that material when tested in the cafeteria, than when tested in the gymnasium. Apparently the learned material is associated in the brain with the environmental context (the cafeteria and not the gym) prevailing at the time it was learned, and is most readily recalled from memory when the environment at the time of testing is congruent with that at the time of learning.

than normal release of neurotransmitter, a heightened sensitivity to the neurotransmitter or a slower degradation of the neurotransmitter in the synaptic cleft (Section 5.D, The Neurotransmitters, page 128). In some way, the learned action in short-term memory is translated into enhanced neural transmission along a specific path, however, the enhancement is fleeting, and if not transferred into long-term memory through the process of consolidation, the memory will be lost forever.

The environmental factor is most obvious in the *yogasanas* when practicing the balancing poses. When these *yogasanas* are learned in a particular setting and the eyes are used to establish the horizon for balancing (Subsection IV.D, *Vision and Balance*, page 533, and Subsection 16.A, *The Ocular-Vestibular Connection*, page 418), then there is a strong mental association of the learning environment as sensed visually with the technical details of the *yogasana*. It is often found then that the balancing is easiest when done while looking at the same environment which was present when the *yogasana* was learned, and that trying to perform the balance in another room or in the same room but facing another view can be more difficult. Needless to say, the *yogasanas* should be practiced with the eyes not holding onto external objects, so that the *yogasanas* can be performed equally well in all environments, and with relaxed eyes.

Finally, though it may seem to be a compliment to the teacher, it is a truism that students will follow their teacher to such an extent that they will come to resemble the teacher in their performance of the *yogasanas*. This means that any weakness of the teacher is transferred to the students to their detriment. It is for this reason (and others as well) that students should be encouraged to work with other teachers who teach the same or related forms of *yogasana*. It often happens that another teacher by

chance will be able to say something in a different way that just makes everything clear to a student who otherwise was not able to get the message, or another teacher will introduce poses to your students that you ignore because you do not do them well or you dislike them for personal reasons, or you are too injured to demonstrate them.

Consolidation and Long-Term Memory

When an activity is practiced so that the memory of it is stored first in short-term memory and then consolidated into long-term memory, it becomes a permanent part of the brain's mode of action. Though all aspects of brain activity can be shut down by deep anaesthesia, by cooling or by lack of oxygen, on recovery, all of the memories in long-term storage are present and available for recall. This strongly suggests that long-term memory involves permanent changes in the brain's morphology, chemistry and/or connectivity.

Noting that chemicals that inhibit protein synthesis have a detrimental effect on long-term memory and that the brain is rich in protein, it was hypothesized and then proven that the deposition of long-term memories in the brain involves site-specific generation of proteins within the brain. On the other hand, the blocking of protein synthesis has no effect on short-term memory.

Furthermore, through the practice of a task, it has been shown repeatedly that the branching patterns of neurons involved in the long-term storage of the experience are changed in number and in type. When a synapse is used often, it may develop more axonal terminals, more dendrites, and more vesicles holding the appropriate neurotransmitters. It also appears that the various motor circuits compete with one another for space within the brain, so that tasks that are practiced tend to expand within the brain (thus allowing for a fine-tuning of the actions in the task), at the expense of those that are not practiced. In this regard, it is interesting to look at the effects of long-term stimulation of an afferent-efferent synapse, as shown in Fig. 3.C-2. As seen there, when the long-term stimulus is somewhat annoying but not noxious, as with the startle response, for example, the synapse tends to change as on going from 3.C-2a to 3.C-2b, *i.e.*, the strength of the synaptic connection decreases. This situation is termed habituation. If on the other hand, the stimulus is truly noxious and warrants avoidance, then the synapse connection becomes sensitized, and takes the strength-ened form shown in Fig. 3.C-2c. In both cases, one has "learned" by a physical adaptation of the neural circuitry.

That experience can change the brain's morphology reflects its plasticity. Like the bones (Subsection 8.C, *The Remodeling Response to Mechanical Stress*, page 245), the brain is undergoing constant modification in response to the environment, to stimuli and to learning and is able to change its architecture in response to these pressures. To learn something, anything, is to permanently change the circuitry within the brain, and without plasticity, nothing can be learned.

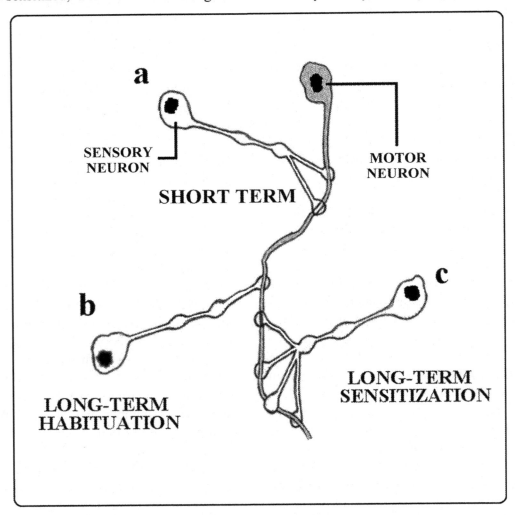

Fig. 3.C-2. (**a**) The short-term afferent/efferent synaptic connections between a sensory neuron and a motor neuron before the action of any long-term stimulus. (**b**) The same neuromuscular connections after long-term habituation, and (**c**) after long-term sensitization.

Unambiguous experiments have shown that, even in cells that last a lifetime, there is a constant replacement of almost all the material in the cell, this continuing for the lifetime of the cell. Thus, in the human being, though a brain cell may exist for 90 years, one half of its protein is regenerated anew every 80 days. The reproduction of the protein is so exact that memories persist clearly for decades even though the proteins that are responsible for them have been reproduced many, many times over [472]. The old idea that the neurons of the brain must not reproduce themselves, for if they did, memories could not be sustained for long periods, is now seen to be fallacious.

Recent research [359] strongly suggests that certain phases of the sleep cycle are intimately involved with the consolidation phase of learning; especially relevant is the REM (rapid eye movement, Subsection 21.B, *The Sleep/Wake Cycle and Relaxation*, page 488) phase, a phase that we go through perhaps a half-dozen times in a night's sleep. This work shows that slow-wave stage-2 sleep and REM sleep both participate in the consolidation process, especially so when the material to be remembered is procedural, *i.e.*, how to do something such as a *yogasana*, rather than a more abstract storage of fact (the square root of 2 is 1.414). Simple skills which are just a refinement of skills learned earlier require stage-2 sleep within 24 hours if they are to be retained, whereas when learning totally new skills, there must be a REM sleep phase within 24 hours if the practiced technique is to be retained. During sleep, there is an active exchange of information back and forth between the hippocampus and the cortex (this also occurs during the day), finally leading to permanent changes of protein structure in the cortex during the hippocampus-to-cortex transfer. The transfer of information between the cortex and the hippocampus occurs during the REM phase of

sleep, whereas the transfer in the opposite direction occurs during the stage-2 phase of the sleep cycle.

The repeated cycling of information back and forth between the hippocampus and the cortex not only transfers the information into long-term memory, but also allows the brain to explore meaning and to integrate the new information with earlier memories, often in creative ways. Learning and remembering the instructions and techniques of *yogasana* practice thus are seen to be a 24-hour job, significant portions of which are completed while we sleep! It is interesting to speculate as to what meaning this has, if any, for the apparent REM-like action of the eyes while relaxing in *savasana*.

Hormones also play a role in memory and learning. The hypothalamus activates the pituitary to release vasopressin, a hormone that not only regulates kidney action and water balance, but also is a vasoconstrictor for regulating blood flow (Subsection 15.B, *The Pituitary Gland*, page 404). In the brain, vasopressin enhances memory and learning. If and when one experiences a frightening situation calling for the activation of the sympathetic branch of the autonomic system (Section 6.C, page 144), the release of vasopressin into the bloodstream will assure that the memory of the event will be retained so that one will act to avoid it in the future [387]. The release of ACTH into the bloodstream during periods of crisis also works to retain the memory of the crisis, and so serves to help avoid it in the future.

The levels of vasopressin in the cerebrospinal fluid show a circadian rhythm (Section 21.B, Periodicity of Body Rhythms, page 474), no doubt correlating with the circadian rhythms of learning and memory abilities that rise and fall during the day [389]. Oxytocin, another pituitary hormone, works to produce short-term amnesia. Its concentration in the body is greatest for women in labor, and can act to make them forget the pain of child birth.

Teaching Yogasana

Learning can take place by mere repetition, but it is faster still and more enjoyable when there is a motivation to learn. An event (lesson) must have meaningfulness for successful learning. The application of this idea to teaching the *yogasanas* is obvious and straight forward. There is a good reason behind the way we do each of the asanas, and there are many good reasons for making yoga work a life-long activity. The teacher at every opportunity should stress why we are doing this work and the physiological and psychological benefits that come from doing it. By doing so, the skeptical student will be won over, and the converted student will find even more reason for dedicated work. Brief comments in this regard show the student immediately that the asanas go far beyond geometry, and will speed their realization of the benefits (see Subsection 6.F, *The Placebo Effect*, page 164).

People tend to repeat behaviors that are rewarded. In the context of *yogasana* teaching, attention or praise from the teacher can act as positive reinforcements, and so can help students learn more quickly and completely.

It is no surprise that most of us learn best by watching with our eyes; almost 90% of our information from outside the body comes to us through the eyes. As a teacher of the *yogasanas*, you should encourage your students to watch you closely as you demonstrate the pose of the moment. In showing the students a new pose, ask them specifically not to try to do it with you as you demonstrate, so that their awareness is totally on what you are doing and not divided between what you do and what they feel at the moment. Not only will the students learn the proper way to perform the asana by watching you as the teacher, but in looking more and more like you, they will come to assume your weaknesses as well as your strengths. For this reason, it will be good for them to be exposed to several teachers both within and outside the particular style that you teach.

For those students who learn better through the auditory channel than through the visual channel, ask the class to "watch closely and listen carefully" as you demonstrate and explain the intricacies of the new pose. When teaching, allow some silent space for reflection and digestion of the previously given information: we all can catch the seven-digit phone number when given the first time if the giver will only stop talking briefly after giving it! [473]

At the neurological level, the repeated excitation of a pathway in the central nervous system (also called "practice") results gradually in an increased ease of transmission of that particular nerve impulse to muscles through that pathway. This is due to the decrease in synaptic resistance, which can arise from more neurotransmitter being released, a longer lifetime for the neurotransmitter and/or more synaptic receptors for the neurotransmitter. This strengthening of the pathway is the basis for the formation of habits and for learning, while explaining the efficacy of practice [106]. Specific pathways for learning are shown in Fig. 7.A-5 and discussed in Section 7.C, Proprioception, page 208.

It seems to be our nature that when left alone, we choose to practice those postures that are least appropriate to our condition [334]. Thus one must be aware that students with low muscle tone, if left to themselves, will prefer to practice relaxation rather than muscle-toning postures, and that depressed students will prefer to practice forward bends rather than backbends, even though their normal posture is rife with forward flexion. Similarly, over-confident people with a prevailing extension in their posture will gravitate toward backbends and shy away from forward bends, if given the choice. In situations such as these, the *yogasana* teacher must emphasize those postures that will bring the student more into balance.

It must be understood that learning and memory do not necessarily function only in the conscious sphere. Thus, through practice, we learn and never forget how to ride a bicycle, how to type a letter or how to walk. In these cases, the neural circuits for such "automatic" muscle actions are developed in the spine rather than in the brain, and once they are activated by higher centers in the brain (consciously or subconsciously), they operate without further control from the higher centers, until turned off by them. Such motor-memory effects are examples of the mixing of conscious and subconscious actions depicted schematically in Fig. 1.B-1. As *yogasana* students become more practiced in the poses, they will find that certain aspects of the poses become more subconsciously attended to, so that the conscious awareness can be turned to more subtle aspects.

SECTION 3.D. CEREBRAL HEMISPHERIC LATERALITY

Bilateral Asymmetry of the Brain

Though the two hemispheres of the brain may seem at first to be identical in appearance and function, there is now abundant evidence that this is not the case. It was first noticed in 1968, that the plenum temporale in the left hemisphere is on average significantly larger than that in the right hemisphere [156], and medical research has expanded upon this to show several other functional aspects of the brain's lack of left-right symmetry. Many anatomical studies as well as experiments in brain function agree unanimously that the two cerebral hemispheres of the brain operate independently and in very different arenas, though remaining in close contact.

It is known topologically that in right-handed people, the brain shows an obvious left-right asymmetry, whereas in left-handed people, the asymmetry is much less pronounced [157]. This may be the reason behind right-handed people being much more strongly committed to their right hands than are left-handed people committed to their left hands. See also Section III.D, Handedness, page 523.

A person's general preference for one hand over the other extends to the other body parts as well: thus nine out of ten people are right handed, eight out of ten are right footed, seven out of ten are right eyed and six out of ten are right eared [90]. Judging from studies of ancient artwork, the 90% proportion of right handers in the human population has been constant for the past 50 centuries, at least. It is the essential differences between the functionalities of the left and right cerebral hemispheres that underlie all of these outward asymmetries of the body.

There is strong evidence that the lifespans of left handers are considerably shorter than those of right handers; though left handers are 15% of the population at age 15 years, this figure drops to less than 1% by age 80 years! Handedness shows only a weak correlation with that of the mother and father, but a rather strong correlation with the presence of birth trauma or stress at the time of birth [90]. This may relate to the fact that the asymmetric development of the brain begins *in utero*, for testosterone temporarily inhibits left-hemisphere development in the fetus [59].

Though language skills appear to be largely localized in the left hemisphere, if this hemisphere is damaged in an infant under two years old, the language skills develop instead in the right hemisphere without any apparent problems. However, if the damage occurs at an age beyond ten years, it cannot be compensated for at all [120]. Because language can be used in so many different ways, it is no surprise that damage to a cerebral area dedicated to a particular language skill can leave other language-skill areas untouched. For example, see Fig. 3.A-3 where different aspects of speech are shown to be located in very different areas of the cortex.

When one is asked an emotional question about oneself, the eyes look to the left consistently, suggesting that the right hemisphere also plays a special role in emotions [120]. It also shows how strongly a purely cerebral process is coupled to motion of the eyes. Further, in cases of depression, it has been found that the intensity of the alpha EEG waves which signal a lack of outer awareness and alertness are very strong in the left prefrontal cortex as compared with that in the right prefrontal cortex, and that procedures that wake up the cortex, switching the activity from alpha to beta waves, is curative [385]. See Table 3.D-1 for a more detailed listing of the differing functions of the right and left cerebral hemispheres.

As Table 3.D-2 shows, there is a strong but imperfect correlation between handedness and the dominant hemisphere for speech. Because 90% of the population is right handed, it is no surprise that 96% of the population is left-hemisphere dominant, as this hemisphere is dominant for motor

TABLE 3.D-1. FUNCTIONS OF THE CEREBRAL HEMISPHERES [225, 230]

Right Hemisphere	Left Hemisphere
Spatial reasoning	Language functions (vocabulary, speech, alphabet)
Face recognition	
Perception of emotions (tone of voice, gestures, attitudes)	Manual control; motor dominance
Feminine (nurture, intuitive, read faces, raise children)	Masculine (hunt, track, chase prey)
	Linear processing (logical, sequential)
Parallel processing (simultaneity)	Analytical
Humorous	Sense of time
Holistic	
Musical	
Proprioception	
Kinaesthesia	

TABLE 3.D-2. LEFT-RIGHT HANDEDNESS (%) VERSUS THE DOMINANT HEMISPHERE FOR SPEECH [225]

	Dominant Hemisphere for Speech		
	Right	Left	Both
Right Handed	4	96	0
Left Handed	15	70	15

control. Right-hemisphere people are less left-handed than left-hemisphere people are right handed (see Table 3.D-2). It also is found that the hearing of speech is in the left hemisphere whereas the hearing of music is confined to the right hemisphere.

Eye movement to the right during thought correlates with left-hemispheric activity and that to the left signals right-hemispheric activity [281, 389]. When thinking logically about a problem, the eyes tend to shift to the right as if transducing information in the left hemisphere, whereas, when thinking analogically, the shift is to the left, as if working in the right hemisphere [389]. Note however that because the optic nerve does not travel through the spinal cord, it cannot decussate in the normal sense so as to send its input to the opposite cerebral hemisphere. A possible mechanism for this visual crossover is given in Subsection 16.C, *Crossover of the Optic Nerve*, page 422.

Results have recently been reported [197] in regard to experiments which clearly show that the strong hemispheric lateralization of alphabetic letter memory (left hemisphere) and of letter location (right hemisphere) in college students occurs in *both* hemispheres simultaneously in people 62–73 years old. Moreover, in certain other mental tasks, the senior people, who were able to use both hemispheres simultaneously, could respond faster than younger students who were limited to using just one side of their brain at a time. It appears that older people can adapt neutral circuitry to accommodate the mental deterioration of aging.

Both vision and hearing are lateral, in the sense that learning or performing nonverbal tasks is better handled through the left eye and ear as expected for right-hemisphere dominance (Table 3.D-1), whereas verbal material is better handled through the right eye and ear, as expected for left-hemisphere dominance [225]. See Box 3.D-1 in order to determine the symmetry of your visual dominance.

Note too that when movie films are viewed through either one eye or the other, the view through the left eye is perceived as more catastrophic and emotional than when viewed through the right eye. This is in line with the thought that the view of the left eye is processed in the visual center of the right hemisphere, where depressive visions reign. In binocular vision, the depressing vision of the right hemisphere is dominated by the joyous vision of the left hemisphere [120], except perhaps in the depressed individual (Section 20.A, Depression, page 464).

The rivalry between the visions of the right and left eyes easily can be demonstrated [285]. Look at a scene with the left eye looking through a long paper tube, and place the open right hand about 3 inches from the right eye, along side the tube. One will see the image of the right hand and the superposed image of the scene seen through the tube, but in the center of the right hand. The two images are seen simultaneously but there is no fusion of the images. After a short time, the dominance will shift so that the tube image will fade and the hole will fill with the image of the missing part of the right hand. A short while later, it will shift back to the original scene.

All mammals have two hemispheres, and in several of these, the separate and independent functions of the two hemispheres have been demonstrated [225]. For example, in birds, the hemispheric laterality allows them to put one half of their brains to sleep and to close the opposite eye, while the other hemisphere and other eye remain alert for predators! [336]. Cats and dogs show a strong paw preference, but it is approximately 50% right and 50% left across each of the populations, unlike that in humans, where handedness is 90% right and 10% left [90].

BOX 3.D-1: DETERMINING YOUR LATERAL PREFERENCE FOR VISION

You no doubt have a strong tendency to write with one hand and not the other, to step up onto a step with one foot and not the other, and to hold the telephone to one ear and not the other. All of these lateral preferences reflect a dominance of one cerebral hemisphere over the other. You can check your vision for hemispherical dominance in the following way [189].

With one arm outstretched, extend the thumb toward the ceiling. Adjust the arm position so that with both eyes open, the thumb is seen to be just below some object in the far field. Now close the right eye and notice if the object shifts with respect to the thumb. With both eyes open, repeat, closing the left eye. Of the people so tested, 54% find that the object does not move when the left eye is closed (Coren [90] reports this figure as 70%), 4% find that it does not move when the right eye is closed and 41% see little or no movement.

If your right eye is the dominant one, then closing the left eye will have no effect on the image since you are seeing it largely with the right eye even with both eyes open, and *vice versa* for the left eye. That is to say, when you are aiming with your dominant eye, the other eye is essentially not functioning. The dominant eye as found here is probably the one that you use when looking through a telescope or keep open when you thread a needle. If there is no shift of the image on closing one or the other eye, then you are ambivisual.

Note that according to Table 3.D-1, if your right eye is dominant, you show a left-hemispheric preference for vision, suggesting that you preferentially view the world in a logical, analytical way, whereas for those who have the left eye dominant, the preferential view is more intuitive and holistic.

All of the above shows clearly that the two hemispheres of the cerebrum have very different functions. In the simplest terms, the left hemisphere of the brain is essentially objective and analytical, dealing best with subjects such as math, the spoken and written word, and critical thought and analytical reasoning of the sort found in the physical sciences. By contrast, the right hemisphere is essentially subjective and intuitive, being most active when dealing with creativity in music and the arts, imagination and insight, as well as the three-dimensional aspects of objects. In contrast to the situation in the left hemisphere, several areas of the right hemisphere can work simultaneously in a parallel manner [346], as is best for integrating visual, kinaesthetic and proprioceptive information as to body posture, body motion, *etc.*

It is interesting as well to note that the characteristics assigned to the functions of the right and left hemispheres in Table 3.D-1 closely match those assigned intuitively in the Introduction (Table 1.A-1) to "World View I" and "World View II", with the former corresponding to dominance of the right hemisphere and the latter to the dominance of the left hemisphere. We see as well that the dominance of the right hemisphere corresponds to parasympathetic excitation of the autonomic nervous system, whereas that of the left hemisphere corresponds to dominance of the sympathetic nervous system, Chapter 6, page 133. Thus the scientific evidence for different functions of the two cerebral hemispheres supports the more intuitive idea of the dual consciousness within each of us [346].

Cerebral Hemispheric Interactions

Though the two cerebral hemispheres have very different and distinct functions, it is not to say that they do not interact, for they do, in two significant ways. In many situations, the distinct functions of the cerebral hemispheres are masked by the significant neural connections between the hemispheres within the corpus callosum, which tends to distribute information and function more evenly between the two hemispheres; in those cases where the corpus callosum has been severed to reduce the severity of epileptic seizures, the inherent differences between the hemispheres are far more obvious. The corpus callosum connects areas of the cortex which are activated by sensors on the midline of the body (the trunk, back and face), but does not connect the extremities (feet or hands).

Though the basic characteristics of the two hemispheres can be neatly set out, in fact, almost all tasks rely on both hemispheres and their interactions. Thus to play the piano well, one must have not only the left-brain technical skills by which the keys and pedals are manipulated in the proper order, but also the feeling and nuance for the fine shading that can come in a personal, intuitive way only from the right hemisphere. With the two hemispheres working together, the result can be beautiful music.

Yogasana practice can be very much like music. In the beginning, we work in a left-brain robotic way, following the detailed instructions of the teacher or the book, without any sense of our own uniqueness. This is not bad, but as we mature in the practice, we should allow room for right-brain input into the process so that, as we experiment and inquire as to what *yogasana* practice is about, each of us will come by our own path to that most exciting discovery: who we really are and what we can become if we choose! In all things done well, we need both the analytical/objective functions of the left brain and the intuitive/subjective functions of the right brain in appropriate proportions.

Pert [357] mentions something that may be of use to yoga students. She finds that she is able to get information flowing readily between the left and right hemispheres by walking with the arms swinging oppositely to the legs, *i.e.*, when the left leg is forward the right arm should have swung forward with it, and similarly with the right leg and the left arm. This simultaneous and deliberate action of the limbs on opposite sides of the body breaks up old patterns of thought/worry and opens the mind/body to new thoughts and points of view. If true, this could be a most useful aid in teaching yoga to older students (Section 3.C, Memory, Learning, and Teaching, page 42).

In addition to the instantaneous communication between the cerebral hemispheres via the corpus callosum, there is a second longer-lasting mode of communication. In this second mode, the character of one of the hemispheres dominates that of the other for a period of a few hours and then the dominance is reversed.

Bilateral Asymmetry of the Brain and Unilateral Breathing

It has been shown [339] that forced unilateral breathing increases spatial memory, but does so equally on the two sides of the cerebrum. However, breathing through the right nostril increases heart rate, systolic blood pressure and consumption of oxygen, as appropriate for stimulation of the sympathetic nervous system [422, 458, 459].

Spatial task performance is enhanced during left-nostril breathing, whereas verbal task performance is enhanced during right-nostril breathing [218]. Left-nostril breathing promotes a higher palmar resistance, indicating less sweating due to parasympathetic increase [458, 459]. Comparison of the entries in Table 3.D-1 with those in Table 12.E-1 suggests that the two types of laterality (hemispheric and nasal) are closely related, and that by choosing which nostril through which to breath, one can dictate which cerebral hemisphere is dominant. This is discussed more fully in Section 12.C, Nasal Laterality, page 374.

Oscillating Dominance of Cerebral Hemispheric Laterality

In addition to the hemispheric lateralities detailed above which are constant in time, *i.e.*, handedness, vision, emotions, *etc.*, there are others which just as clearly oscillate between dominance of the right and left hemispheres, with periods of a few hours. Such oscillating processes in the body are termed "ultradian rhythms". Chief among the ultradian rhythms is the periodic switching of the breath between the two nostrils, this happening every few hours.

The *Swara* yogis have worked with the alternate flow of the breath through the right and left nostrils for over a thousand years, connecting it to many body functions and the general state of health. Hemispheric laterality is implied in the ancient accounts of the *Swara* yogis who envisioned the *ida* and *pingala nadis* as dual and opposing in their effects (Section 4.F, *Nadis, Chakras* and *Prana*, page 100, and Section 12.C, Nasal Laterality, page 374).

The phenomena of nasal and cerebral laterality appear related to a number of other "ultradian" phenomena (Subsection 21.B, *Ultradian Rhythms*, page 474), which are again seemingly under control of the autonomic nervous system (Chapter 6, page 133). This work began in the 1950's, when it was observed that during sleep, there are periodic changes of EEG patterns, heart and respiration rates, eye movement and muscle tone [244]. The period* of these cycles was found to be 3 to 4 hours. It was hypothesized that the physiological oscillation is an expression of a phylogenetically old rest/activity cycle which is ever present, but overlain by other cycles of different periods. The connection was later made to lateralization of the cerebral hemispheres and an oscillating dominance of one hemisphere over the other. Thus ultradian rhythms have been observed for oral behavior, magnitude of the spiral aftereffect, heart rate, vigilance performance, fantasy content of daydreams, and REM/nonREM action during sleep [244].

Now in right-handed people, the left hemisphere specializes in verbal-linguistic, analytical and logical processes and working in a sequential way, whereas the right hemisphere deals with visual-spatial, holistic and nonlogical matters, working here more like a parallel processor, Table 3.D-1. From this, Klein and Armitage [244] argued that performance scores on verbal and spatial matching tests should involve contralateral hemispheres, should rise and fall with a period of about 4 hours, and that the maximum performance of one should fall at the time of minimum performance of the other. These predictions were completely validated by their work.

The suspected connection between nasal and hemispheric oscillations long-ago intuited by the ancient yogis is strongly supported by the work of Werntz [389], who

---

* By "period" is meant the time to go from a maximum in the effect in question, to the minimum and return to the maximum again. Some authors define "period" as the time to go from the maximum to the minimum.

studied nasal lateralization simultaneous with EEG patterns, Section 3.E. She found that when the left nostril was open, there was increased EEG activity in the right hemisphere and when the open nostril was switched either naturally or deliberately from left to right, the EEG-active hemisphere switched from right to left. This is yet another example of how deliberate manipulation of the breath impacts brain function.

Werntz hypothesizes that the nasal and hemispheric oscillations she found were both driven by an oscillation of the relative activities of the sympathetic and parasympathetic branches of the autonomic nervous system (Chapter 6, page 133), via the hypothalamus. Presumably, increased blood flow through the erectile tissue of one nostril is to be associated with increased blood flow through the contralateral hemisphere of the brain! This suggestion is supported by the observations listed in Table 3.D-1, where one sees that all of the effects of having the right nostril open and the left closed are consonant with left-brain sympathetic excitation, while those having the left nostril open and the right closed are consonant with right-brain parasympathetic excitation (see Table 6.A-2).

The seemingly strange fact that sensations from, say, the left side of the body are projected onto the cortex of the right hemisphere is due to decussation, the process in which an ascending fiber enters the medulla on the left side, but by virtue of a lateral synapse to a secondary relay cell, the fiber exits on the right side and travels thence to midbrain, thalamus and cortex on "the wrong side" [230].

The oscillation of the breath between the two nostrils is strongly reminiscent of the recently demonstrated oscillation of mental activity between the two halves of the brain [148]. These experiments show that the proficiency at right-hemisphere verbal tasks waxes and wanes with a period of 90–100 minutes, while the proficiency for left-hemisphere spatial tasks also oscillates with the same period, but is 180° out-of-phase. That is to say, when the right hemisphere is active, the left is quiescent and *vice versa.*

We are now able to cite abundant evidence for the 4-hour periodic shift of mental and physiologic states in the unperturbed body. However, higher brain centers may override this underlying rhythm, as for example, the right hemisphere does control the facial expression showing emotion, however, higher centers can repress this if the emotion is too strong or too embarrassing. In the calm of the *yogasana*, the higher centers again may be significant factors (especially in balancing poses).

Using Cerebral Hemispheric Laterality in Yoga

Note first two things: a) the effects of cerebral and nasal laterality are very subtle, and can easily be missed unless one is very inwardly directed, and b) that the nasal laterality can be directed by pressing the armpit of the opposite side (Chapter 5, THE NERVES, page 107), or by using unilateral forced breathing (Subsection 12.C, *The Conscious Development and Shift of Nasal Laterality*, page 378).

How can we use the effects of hemispheric laterality in our yoga practice? First, following *Swara* yoga, it seems reasonable to spend the first 10 minutes of *savasana* lying first on the left side to warm the body (right nostril open, left hemisphere stimulated along with the sympathetic nervous system) and then on the right (left nostril open, right hemisphere stimulated along with the parasympathetic nervous system) to relax it, provided this is sufficient time to switch nasal laterality, and provided the left-right dominance in the student is strong. The crutch-in-the-armpit reflex (Subsection 12.C, *The Conscious Development and Shift* of *Nasal Laterality*, page 378) would seem to be active in any pose in which one has the *ardha-baddha-padma* grip, *i.e.*, right hand holding the right foot from behind so as to put pressure on the right armpit. This should open the left nostril and promote relaxation, whereas the opposite grip will open the right nostril and promote a lifting of the energy, all other things being equal. Similar effects are to be expected in *pasasana*, *parivrtta parsvakonasana*, *gomukhasana* and *maricy-asana III*. Deliberate shifting of the nasal lateralization is expected especially in *yogadandasana*, but in all of these asanas only after being in the position for 2–5 minutes. On the other hand, in other laterally asymmetric asanas such as *trikonasana*, where there is no direct pressure on the axillae, the lateralization effect will be energizing or calming depending upon which nostril happens to be open at that moment. In any event, the rather subtle shift in the relative activity levels of sympathetic and parasympathetic systems in the course of a *yogasana* practice, may or may not be apparent to the student depending upon their sensitivity to subtle changes in physical, mental and emotional states.

Now B.K.S. Iyengar often states that the learning of the pose on one side can help to teach the other side; perhaps the lateral *yogasanas* such as *trikonasana*, *etc.*, are more easily learned on first going to the right and then this learning is transferred via the corpus callosum to the other hemisphere to help teach the pose to the left side.

To the extent that yoga involves a reconnection of the mind to the body and may be working in part like the placebo response in medicine (Subsection 6.F, *The Placebo Effect*, page 164), it may be relevant to note that the placebo effect is strongest in those with a right-hemisphere dominance, *i.e.*, those who do not overanalyze. The same subclass of people is the most easily hypnotized [389]. As certain aspects of hemi-spheric dominance oscillate, *yogasana* learning may be better at some times (right dominance) than at others (left dominance).

Mood is also lateral, for drugging (de-exciting) the left hemisphere with a barbiturate leads to brief depression, whereas drugging (de-exciting) the right hemisphere leads to temporary elation [225]. From this we see that performing the active *yogasanas* essentially has its effect as a left-brain stimulant, *i.e.*, it is stimulating to the sympathetic nervous system, whereas performing *savasana* is a right-brain stimulant, specifically activating the parasympathetic system.

Coren [90] points out that in gymnasts who are both right handed and right eyed, the center of gravity is moved noticeably to the right in their bodies and that this tends to introduce a twisting motion to their performance. If true, the same effect would be present in the *yogasana* student having a simultaneous preference for the right hand and the right eye, *i.e.*, twisting poses may feel very different on the two sides of the body.

Inasmuch as the turning of the eyes to the right or to the left correlates with accessing either the left or right cerebral hemispheres, respectively, and their attendant moods, one might logically expect that when doing *trikonasana* to the right and looking up toward the left hand, we are accessing the right hemisphere and so visually promote a relaxed feeling, whereas when we do *trikonasana* to the left and look up toward the right, we are exciting the left hemisphere and so visually promote an up-lifting energy.

Brain Laterality Can Lead to Body Laterality, and Vice Versa

It is known that in the general population, there is greater strength, coordination, balance, and proprioceptive awareness on the side of the body corresponding to the dominant hand [5]. Hand grip is stronger, bone density is higher and the muscles larger on the dominant side. One of the tasks then in *yogasana* practice is to work to bring the right and left sides of the body more into balance in regard to the above factors. To the extent that the lateralities of the brain and the body are related, practicing of the *yogasanas* to achieve a more nearly equal balance on the two sides of the body also will work to achieve a similar balance on the two sides of the brain. When the body/brain are strongly lateralized, then such simple actions as interlacing the fingers but changing which index finger is uppermost can have startling effects on the brain as the "wrong" hemisphere becomes involved in the mechanics of the process. The goal in *yogasana* practice is not to force the "wrong" side of the brain to do work it is not meant to do, but to speed the transfer of neural activities between the two hemispheres via the corpus callosum.

The yogic and medical approaches to this subject seem not to be aware of one another, especially in that the yogic approach dwells upon the oscillating character of the hemispheric dominance and the medical approach dwells on the static aspects of the dominance, but neither but rarely mentions the other. Both are discussed in this Section, while the subject of overall body symmetry is discussed in Appendix III, BODY SYMMETRY, page 519. Readers of this Section on cerebral laterality will want to look over Section 12.C on nasal laterality, page 374.

SECTION 3.E. BRAINWAVES AND THE ELECTROENCEPHALOGRAM

Characteristics of the EEG

When the neurons in the cortex are functioning properly, there is a simultaneous electrical activity of large neural populations acting more or less in synchronicity. Such large-scale electrical activity actually can be observed as variations in electrical potential (voltage) on areas of the scalp over the active area of the cortex. The pattern of such voltage changes over short time periods (minutes) is called the "electroencephalogram" (EEG).

The origin of the EEG signals involves the postsynaptic potentials in the pyramidal cells of the cortex and ionic conduction in the extracellular fluid [225]. As the pyramidal cells of the cortex are all oriented in parallel fashion, their synaptic voltages can be summed over a large area to produce a significant net voltage, in contrast to other active cortical cells which are not as well oriented and so have voltage contributions that algebraically sum to a near-zero value.

The EEG patterns, Fig. 3.E-1, are complex and not easily interpretable. In fact, each pattern is a combination of other more basic patterns that are not necessarily obvious in the raw data, but which can be teased out of it using the mathematical technique called Fourier analysis. Using this technique, it is found that there are five general wave patterns corresponding to the preponderance of five different wave frequencies, Table 3.E-1. Furthermore, the spatial patterns of the various basic frequencies may be global or very local with respect to various areas of the scalp. Such electrical data is potentially of great use to those of us studying the relationships between the *yogasanas* and their physiological correlates, because shifts between different EEG levels largely involve changes of levels of excitation in the reticular formation (Subsection 3.A, page 31) within the brainstem. That is to say, the EEG directly indicates the level of mental arousal and awareness.

In the alpha-wave pattern, there is a voltage fluctuation with a frequency of 8–13 Hz, the waves are synchronized, and the waves are prominent when one is relaxed, eyes closed, but awake. Once the eyes open, or one is engaged in intense mental activity

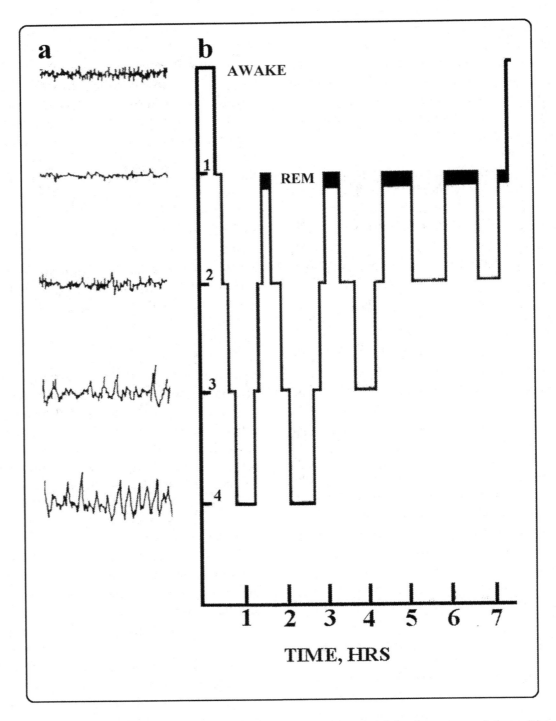

Fig. 3.E-1. (**a**) The EEG traces characteristic of the awake state and the four stages of sleep. (**b**) Typical variation of the duration and sequence of sleep stages in a young adult. REM sleep is represented by the horizontal black bars. As sleep proceeds, the amounts of stage-3 and stage-4 delta sleep drop off and the amounts of stage 1-REM sleep and stage-2 slow-wave sleep correspondingly increase. Note the periodicity of about 90 minutes between sleep stages throughout the night.

or social interactions, the desynchronized beta waves of 13–30 Hz appear, characterizing a state of mental arousal [201]. An EEG state of even higher frequency has recently been reported: the gamma state is synchronized with a characteristic frequency of about 40 Hz, and appears for brief periods while one is integrating visual or other sensory sensations [20, 71]. See Subsection 3.E, *Brainwave Frequencies and Mental Functioning*, page 60, for further discussion of the gamma waves. In contrast to the gamma waves, the delta and theta waves are desynchronized and have relatively low frequencies (Table 3.E-1), and appear in the deeper stages of sleep and meditation.

Cole [78] has observed that placing a student in supported *setu bandhasana* leads to an immediate shift of EEG from beta to theta type, implying a shift from an aroused state to either a deep meditative state or to sleep itself. In other work [79], he discusses how stimulation of the baroreceptors in the carotid sinus and the aortic arch (Section 11.E, Monitoring Blood Pressure with the Baroreceptors, page 339), as when doing wall *padasana*, leads to synchronous alpha waves in the EEG, and contrarily, when one goes from the supine position toward standing, the lessening of the baroreceptor signal promotes a shift of the EEG waveform from alpha relaxation to beta alertness. Among yoga instructors at their practice, it was found that, as the level of cortisol fell, the intensity of the alpha waves in their EEGs increased [223].

In general, the alpha state is attainable only when the eyes are closed as any visual, auditory or tactile stimulation will desynchronize the EEG waveform and raise its frequency into the range of the beta or possibly the gamma states [201, 225, 230]. However, for those who are adept at meditation and yogic discipline [462], there is a more conscious control of the brainwave EEG states, and the above statement does not hold true (See Subsection 3.A, *The Spinal Cord and Brainstem*, page 29). The tranquility of the alpha state also is disturbed by muscle potentials [201], so that students in deeply relaxing poses such as *savasana*, *etc.*, should avoid any muscle excitation (shifting of the weight, scratching, coughing, opening of the eyes, motions of the eyes, swallowing, *etc.*), other than that required for breathing. As the *yogasana* student becomes more adept at meditation, there is a shift of the EEG brainwave pattern from that of beta-wave alertness, to alpha-wave inner awareness, and then to delta and theta states of inward quietude and harmony [462].

TABLE 3.E-1. CHARACTERISTICS OF EEG BRAINWAVES [20, 225, 230, 462]

Name	Frequency, Hz	Amplitude	Synchronicity	Mental State
Alpha	8–13	High	Synchronized	Relaxed wakefulness; tranquility
Beta	13–30	Low	Desynchronized	Mental activity of normal wakefulness
Gamma	ca. 40		Synchronized	Sensory integration
Delta	0.5–4	Very High	Desynchronized	Stage of dreamless sleep
Theta	4–7	Very High	Desynchronized	Dreaming state; reverie

During moderate aerobic exercise the EEG pattern is reported to shift from beta waves to alpha waves, indicating a shift toward a more meditative state [337], and the alpha state persists beyond the cessation of the exercise. It is also reported that the nature of the EEG wave pattern can be changed at will [120]. This ability is related to that in which the yogi is able to defeat the lie detector, Box 6.E-1.

With regard to the EEG waveforms when awake, one can make a rather straight-forward correlation with autonomic excitation by assigning the alpha-wave form to dominance by the parasympathetic nervous system and the beta wave to excitation in the sympathetic nervous system [80]. When in the alpha-wave state, the heart rate and blood pressure decrease, respiration has a decreased rate and becomes more even, while gastrointestinal activity increases. As shown in Table 6.A-2, all of these responses are characteristic of parasympathetic activation.

Interestingly, several of the electrical activities signaled by the EEG waveforms described in Table 3.E-1 are seen as well in various stages of sleep (Subsection 21.B, *The Sleep/Wake Cycle and Relaxation*, page 488). Considering the ease with which babies are rocked to sleep, it is no surprise that an alpha-wave EEG is promoted by mild, low-frequency stimulation of the skin, as by rocking.

Brainwave Frequencies and Mental Functioning

A very new and exciting idea has recently appeared involving EEG waves and a wide variety of serious neurological and psychological disorders [19, 71]. As discussed briefly in Section 3.A, Structure and Function of the Brain, page 29, there is a constant transfer of information back and forth between the conscious levels of the cortex and various lower-level nuclei in the brain. In particular, there are direct neural connections between the thalamus and the cortex, along which the thalamus offers information to the cortex, which decides which elements of the information are truly useful and important, and then sends this back to the thalamus. The thalamus next edits the information received from the cortex and transmits the abbreviated information a second time to the cortex, thereby reinforcing the important aspects of the original message. All of this happens in the space of a few seconds, and involves considerable high-frequency gamma excitation in the EEGs of both the thalamus and the cortex. There are known to be separate and dedicated thalamo-cortical neural pathways for visual information, for auditory information, for touch, *etc.*, all operating in the waking state at the gamma-EEG frequency of 40 Hz. In this process, the thalamus acts as a high-level filter (much like the reticular formation at a lower level), screening out useless sensory signals that otherwise might overload the brain's capacity for decision making.

When we fall asleep, the thalamus blocks almost all of the information flow to the cortex, as the frequency of the thalamic signal drops into the range of the theta EEG waves, 4–7 Hz, and the neural circuits are barely kept simmering.

What is new and exciting here is that in subjects having one of several mental conditions, it has been found that in the waking state, information over one of the ascending thalamo-cortical loops remains at the sleeping theta level, whereas the cortical return signal is at the gamma frequency and increased in intensity. This sort of disrhythmia between the thalamus and the cortex has been found in subjects displaying symptoms as widely disparate as depression, schizophrenia, tinnitus, obsessive-compulsive disorder, Parkinson's, migraine, and epilepsy [47, 385]. In all such conditions, it appears that specific parts of the thalamus have "fallen asleep" in the waking state, leading to a communications mismatch between the thalamus and the cortex for those specific sensory modes. In a variation on the above theme, in psychotic subjects, there is a rapid shifting of the EEG patterns between alpha and beta states [462].

Assuming that the above description holds up to further scrutiny, it has been proposed that the cures for these conditions rest in either pharmacology or electrode implants to reset the thalamic frequencies in rhythm with those of the cortex, much like a cardiac pacemaker. As it is already known that the more relaxing *yogasana* poses such as *savasana*, *setu bandhasana*, and *viparita karani* are effective in switching the brain's

EEG level from beta to theta [78], it may be that through the more arousing *yogasanas* it is possible to raise the "sleeping" EEG of the thalamus from theta to gamma frequency. This possibly is how arousing *yogasanas* such as *urdhva dhanurasana, etc.*, work to overcome depression (Section 20.A, Depression, page 464).

This transfer of information back and forth between higher and lower brain centers in the waking state brings to mind the shuttling of information at gamma-wave frequencies between the cortex and the hippocampus during sleep, leading to consolidation of the information in long-term memory (Subsection 3.C, *Consolidation and Long-Term Memory*, page 45).

Chapter 4

THE SPINE AND ITS APPENDAGES

SECTION 4.A. THE SPINAL COLUMN

Structural Components

The spinal column has the highest priority for our attention in the *yogasanas*, for it is the principal postural axis of the body's skeletal structure, and the spinal cord within it is a conduit for many of the brain's lines of communication to and from the muscles, glands, sensory, and visceral organs.

The spinal column additionally serves as the site for the attachment of many major muscles, including the diaphragm. To the extent that the breath is controlled by the emotions, the emotions impact on that part of the spine closest to the diaphragm, *i.e.*, the middle back, and *vice versa* [7]. In the broadest sense possible, the spinal column and its components are the principal axis of our existence, secondary in importance only to the other half of the central nervous system, the brain (Chapter 2, page 13).

Mechanically, the spine is anchored at its base to the pelvis, a bony structure serving as the point of attachment of the legs to the trunk of the body, as a major joint allowing flexion (forward bending) and extension (backward bending)* of the spine, and as a bowl holding the visceral contents of the abdomen. At the opposite end, the spinal column supports the skull and more indi-rectly, the arms. Whereas the joints in the arms and legs are synovial joints allowing wide ranges of motion, though the joints of the spine and the pelvis also are synovial joints, their main purpose is to bear weight and to act as shock absorbers [476].

The spine is also important in another way, for as it evolved to allow humans an upright posture, it freed the arms and hands for those manual activities that mark us as human. Moreover, once the hand was free to begin to fully develop its abilities, the brain was then stimulated to develop in order to keep pace with the increasing dexterity of the hand [428].

Though one often works in yoga to make the spine more flexible, actually its inherent rigidity is the key to its mechanical stability. The strong spine is both flexible and mechanically well-braced. Considered at the simplest level, the spine consists of a bony yet flexible spinal column which supports the weight of the upper body (Figs. 4.A-1a and 4.A-1b); within this bony structure there is a canal through which the bundle of spinal nerves (the spinal cord, Fig. 4.A-2) passes.

The spinal column is composed of bony building blocks (the vertebrae) set one on top of another, but with offsets front and back, giving the spine its characteristic curvatures. As with the ends of the long bones of the femur and wrist, the vertebrae are composed of cancellous (porous) bone.

---

* In this work, the term "extension" will be taken as the opposite of flexion, and therefore will refer only to backward bending, and not to lengthening of the spine.

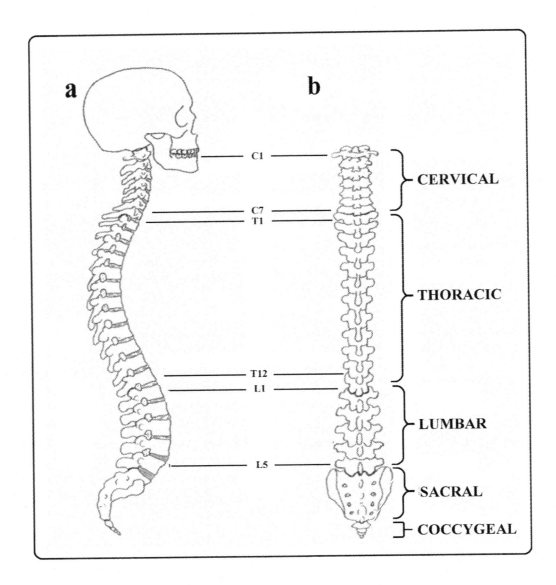

Fig. 4.A-1. (**a**) The vertebrae of the spinal column, showing the cervical, thoracic, lumbar, sacral, and coccygeal members in lateral view. (**b**) Posterior view of the vertebrae of the spinal column.

Because the bone of the vertebrae is cancellous, it can be remodeled when put under a chronic stress, which is to say, it will change its shape to accommodate the stress, Subsection 8.C, *The Remodeling Response to Mechanical Stress*, page 245.

There are seven vertebrae in the cervical region (C1–C7), twelve in the thoracic region (T1–T12), and five in the lumbar region (L1–L5), while in the sacral region,

five vertebrae (S1–S5) are fused into one, and four vertebrae are fused to form the coccyx. The rigid, bony structure of the spine is moderated by the presence of 23 soft, deformable intervertebral discs (Fig. 4.A-3a and Section 4.C, page 87), however, there are no discs between C1 and the base of the skull or between C1 and C2.

The discrete vertebrae in the cervical, thoracic, and lumbar regions have a com-

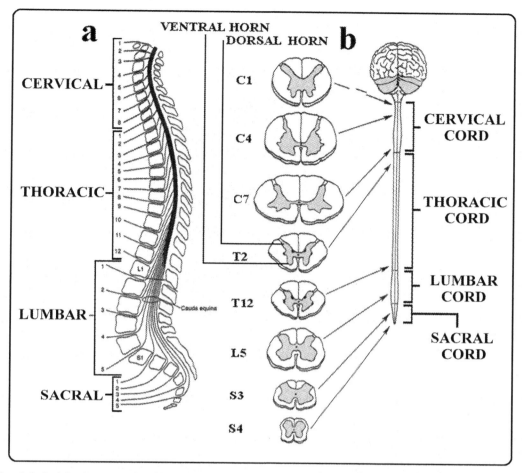

Fig. 4.A-2. (**a**) The spinal cord within the spinal column as viewed with the posterior side to the right, showing the points at which the various spinal nerves exit. Note that the adult spinal cord proper only extends to L1, though nerves exit as low as S5. (**b**) Selected cross sections of the spinal cord taken at the elevations as marked.

mon architecture yet distinctly different shapes (Figs. 4.A-3b and 3c). In each there is anteriorly a heavy, bony vertebral body, which serves for weight bearing, and posteriorly to this, there is an encircling arch of bone which forms the vertebral foramen, the spinal canal. The delicate spinal cord is protected within the canal formed by the vertebral bodies and arches of the vertebral blocks, Fig. 4.A-2a. All of the discrete vertebrae except C1 have a "spinous process" projecting posteriorly (to the right in Fig. 4.A-2a), and it is this aspect of the vertebrae that one feels when palpating the spinal column from behind. The spinous process can be very prominent in the region C7–T1.

Between vertebrae, there also are intervertebral foramina for the entry and exit of local nerve branches. There is a sharp change of vertebral type at each juncture between spinal sections, *i.e.*, at C7–T1, T12–L1, and at L5–S1, Fig. 4.A-1.

Each vertebra has as well a pair of transverse processes extending laterally from the vertebral bodies. In each of the cervical vertebrae C1–C6, two anterior foramen in the transverse processes allow the vertebral arteries access to the base of the skull. Additionally, in each vertebra in the spinal column, the upper and lower surfaces of each transverse process have protruding facets, called the superior articular facet and the

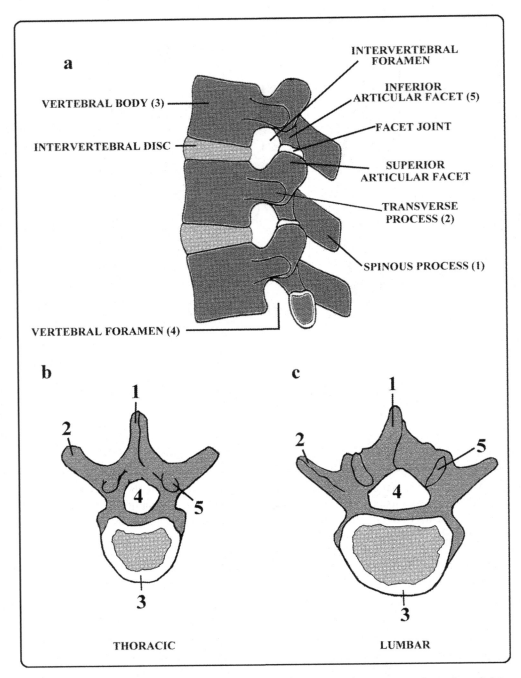

Fig. 4.A-3. (**a**) Stacking of the vertebrae and the intervertebral discs so as to form facet joints as seen with the posterior spine to the right. Numbers in parentheses correspond to those shown in parts (**b**) and (**c**). (**b**) superior view of a vertebra in the thoracic spine, and (**c**) in the lumbar spine. Key: **1**) spinous process, **2**) transverse process, **3**) vertebral body, **4**) vertebral foramen (spinal canal), and **5**) superior articular facet.

inferior articular facet, Fig. 4.A-3. These superior and inferior articular facets on a particular vertebra form synovial joints (Section 8.E, The Joints, page 260) with the articular facets on adjacent vertebrae in order to align and stabilize the spinal column. In particular, the superior articular facets of a given vertebra form facet joints with the inferior articular facets of the vertebra above it, and its inferior articular facets form facet joints with the superior articular facets of the vertebra below it. The attachment of the ribs to the thoracic vertebrae is discussed in Subsection 12.A, *The Ribs*, page 359.

The spine would have little mechanical stability were it not for the facet joints and the vast array of muscles and ligaments (Subsection 4.A, *Spinal Muscles, Tendons, and Ligaments*, page 81) which bind the vertebrae to one another and to the ribs via the transverse and spinous processes [228]. Additionally, the fibrous intervertebral discs (Section 4.C, page 87) act as symphysis joints, holding adjacent vertebrae in their proper positions while allowing limited motion.

Only 4° of rotation can occur about the joint between C1 and the skull (the atlanto-occipital joint), but it does allow head flexion (head bent forward) and head extension (head bent backward), as when shaking the head "yes," however, the largest motion for this movement occurs in the region of C4–C6. Shaking the head "no" involves rotation largely about the C1–C2 joint, especially for angles less than 45° to either side [257]. If the mating surfaces of the atlanto-occipital joint are in some way skewed, then the head is tilted on its axis, and the vestibular organs of balance (Section 17.B, page 437) will generate a constant "off-balance" signal. In response to this, there is a reflexive righting action that can act to produce tension in the neck and possibly result eventually in vision problems and vertigo [260].

The structural gap between the cervical and thoracic vertebrae is filled by the unique structure of C7, with its large spinous process. When C7 is displaced backward and becomes covered with a thick pad of nonfunctional tissue, the stage is set for the development of a dowager's hump [329].

As can be seen in Fig. 4.A-1a, the spinous processes of the vertebrae are inclined about 45–90° with respect to the line of the spinal column itself, looking much like a set of Venetian blinds, whereas the articular facets have angles with respect to the line of the spinal column that change as one moves down the column. The articular facet joints allow movement of the vertebrae, but only by sliding one vertebra upward/forward or backward/downward with respect to its neighbors. For example, when the chin is dropped into the *jalandhara-bandha* position, the cervical vertebrae slide upward and forward, whereas when the head is tipped backward (extension) as in *ustrasana*, the vertebrae slide downward and backward. With facet joints such as these, spinal rotation is achieved by the facet joints on one side of the spine going forward and upward while those on the opposite side go backward and downward.

It is clear from their architecture that the facet joints work best when the motions are simple translations of one transverse process with respect to the next. Note, however, that the articular processes though made of bone nonetheless have a certain flexibility that allows one facet to be pressed against the adjacent one, with a consequent bending of the bone. Working the facet joints in this manner, however, is risking the chance of a broken vertebra, and so should be avoided. Thus, 360° neck rolls are to be discouraged, as this is a motion appropriate to a ball-and-socket joint such as the shoulder, and that is certainly not the case in the cervical spine [271].

The direction and amount of vertebral movement is dictated largely by the interactions among the articular facets of the transverse processes. The interlocking nature of the vertebrae on the one hand stabilizes the spine by limiting its possible motion, but on the other hand, the limited nature of its motion can be a frustration to the *yogasana* student as when backbending or twisting. Note however that the planes of the articular facets face differently in the different spinal regions. For example, for the lumbar vertebrae, the planes of the facets are essentially vertical, allowing easy forward and backward bending (+60° and –35°, Table 4.A-1), whereas spinal rotation drives one lumbar facet into its mate and so is much more difficult in this region (5°, Table 4.A-1).

In these situations, the prescription is to lift the cervical end of the spine away from the sacral end in preparation for either twisting or backbending. This lengthening moves each vertebra away from its neighbors, opens the distance between contacting facets and allows a larger range of motion. Opening of the lumbar spine in preparation for backbending can lessen the discomfort often felt in that region due to lumbar compression of the facet joints. In contrast, when forward bending, the tendency in the spine is for the facet joints to open up, with a stretching of the intervertebral muscles and ligaments.

Normal Curvature

In the newborn infant, the curvature in the upper three regions of the spine is convex as seen from behind, which is to say, the curvature is that of the fetal position, appro-

TABLE 4.A-1. SPINAL DIMENSIONS [228]

	Cervical	Thoracic	Lumbar	Sacral	Coccygeal
Number of vertebrae	7	12	5	5/1[a]	4/1[b]
Curvature as seen posteriorly at given age					
Age					
1 day	Convex	Convex	Convex	Straight	Straight
13 mos.		Convex	Straight	Straight	Straight
3 yrs.		Convex	Concave[c]	Convex[c]	Convex[c]
10 yrs.	Convex	Concave	Convex	Convex	
Adult	Concave	Convex	Concave	Convex	Convex
Forward displacement from posterior, %	33	25	50	Slight	Slight
Kgm weight carried in 100 Kgm man	3	17	37	—	—
Disc thickness, mm	3	5	9	0	0
Thickness/ height[d]	0.4	0.25	0.33	0	0
Nucleus position[e]	5.5	5.5	6.0		
Flexion/extension, deg.	+40/–75	+45/–25	+60/–35	—	—
Lateral flex range, deg.	+/–45	+/–20	+/–20	0	0
Axial rotation, range, deg.	+/–50	+/–35	+/–5	0	0

[a] Five vertebrae fused into one

[b] Four vertebrae fused into one

[c] Very slightly so

[d] Ratio of disc thickness to vertebral height

[e] Relative to 0.0 = front and 10.0 = back

priate to fitting the fetus into the small space of the womb. As the infant first lifts its head and then comes to sit, the cervical and lumbar curves become concave and the otherwise straight sacral and coccygeal sections become convex, Table 4.A-1 and Box 4.A-1. Were the spine to grow into a rigid straight rod, then the process of walking would be impossible, for the jolt of every footstep would be transmitted directly to the brain. However, as the infant matures, the spinal curves develop in a way such that the spine becomes more like a spring, in large part isolating the brain from the mechanical stresses of walking [7]. Additionally, each pair of adjacent vertebrae is separated by a resilient pad of soft tissue, the intervertebral disc. This springiness of the spine due to its unique series of curves is mirrored in the feet, where the arches of the feet act as

springs to absorb the shock to the feet when walking or running; men and women with fallen arches (flat feet) are excused from military service as they cannot march long distances on feet that do not properly absorb the shock of footfall.

If, in the standing adult, one imagines cross sections taken through the neck, chest, and abdomen, one will see where the vertebrae are placed with respect to a line going from the very back of the body at that elevation, to the front of the body at that elevation, Table 4.A-1. In the region of the cervical spine, the vertebrae are seen to be about 35% of the way forward from the back of the neck toward the front of the throat. This position places the cervical vertebrae just under the center of gravity of the head for optimum support. In the thorax, the spine is pushed back so that it is only 25% of the

BOX 4.A-1: ONTOGENY RECAPITULATES PHILOGENY

It is a principle of evolutionary development that "ontogeny recapitulates philogeny", which means that, as an infant matures, it goes through developmental stages that mimic stages in the evolution of its phylum/species. The first noticeable accomplishment of the infant is the lifting of its head, which reverses the cervical curve from convex to concave as seen from the back [231, 249]. With the head and the upper part of its body lifted in this early stage, the infant's pose is reptilian (*bhujangasana*). Later, the infant develops the ability to come onto all fours. With this, the lumbar concavity develops and the stance is quadrupedal (*adho mukha svanasana*; see also Box 8.D-1, *The Benefits of Rotating the Femurs in Yogasana*, page 249). Sitting then follows, representing a simian phase in which the sacrum and coccyx become curved convexly, as in *swastikasana*. Finally, the infant rises to stand (*tadasana*) and move on two feet as befits a bipedal species. Once the spinal curves have developed and the infant stands up and begins to walk, then the hands can be used for more important tasks than just support [43]. All of the *yogasana* practices of the infant are punctuated with deep, intensely restorative sessions of *savasana*.

As pointed out by Kapandji [228], the curvatures of the spine actually strengthen it mechanically by approximately a factor of ten as compared to a straight rod of the same material and dimensions. Similarly, were the spine a straight metal rod, its shock absorbing capacity would be nil, however, when the rod is bent into a helical spring, the same metal "spine" can then be an excellent shock absorber [476]. The various alternating curvatures in the adult spine correspond rather nicely with the five lowest *chakras* as indicated in Table 4.F-1 [7].

way forward along the back-to-chest line. This backward displacement accommodates the large internal organs within the chest cavity. At the waist, the spine is again pulled forward, being situated 50% along the back-to-front line, again the placement being such as to position that portion of the spine just under the torso's center of gravity.

Though the curvatures of the spine are clearly advantageous both from the aspects of mechanical strength, stability, and mobility, there is also a price to be paid: in allowing motion of the spine in many directions, motions also may occur in directions that result in misalignment of the component vertebrae (subluxation) and the woes of "back trouble", Subsection 4.A, *Misalignment of the Spine and Deterioration of the Vertebral Discs*, page 79.

Abnormal Curvature

The most obvious deviations of the spine from the norm involve either the exaggeration or the reversal of the cervical, lumbar, and thoracic curves shown in Fig. 4.A-1a and the deviation of the spine from the strict left-right symmetry shown in Fig. 4.A-1b. As for the lumbar curvature, when standing with the heels, buttocks, shoulder blades and back of the head to the wall, the lumbar vertebra should be no further from the wall than the thickness of the knuckles at the palm of the hand. A similar criterion holds when lying face-up on the floor. Extreme inward curvature of the lumbar spine is called lordosis, or more commonly sway-back, and involves a rotation about the articular facet joints in the lumbar region even in the relaxed position. Though one may sense the occurrence of lordosis in a student with overly large buttocks, the bony part of the back body still may have just the normal curvature. As a person ages normally, the lumbar curve tends to reverse, going from concave inward to convex outward.

The spinal concavity in the cervical and lumbar regions is promoted by intervertebral discs which are thicker anteriorly and thinner posteriorly in these regions. In contrast, if the vertebrae in the thoracic region happen to be wedged oppositely to those in the cervical and lumbar regions, then the result is a kyphotic "dowager's hump", Fig. 4.A-4. Kyphosis, an extreme backward convexity of the thoracic spine, is most often a problem in the elderly suffering from osteoporosis, for in this case the anterior edges of the thoracic vertebrae collapse so as to produce extreme convex curvature. Schatz [412] outlines the postural consequences of having a kyphotic back. In this condition, the neck is thrust forward while the chest collapses leaving little room for the lungs, which instead push downward on the diaphragm and the abdominal organs, forcing the latter to push the abdominal muscles forward, in the process impeding circulation and leading to constipation. Spinal rotation is hindered in an upper back in this collapsed state. Furthermore, when the head is chronically carried in the forward position, there is a possible interference with the blood flow to the thymus gland and possibly a compromised immune system [260].

The kyphosis resulting from a wedging of the thoracic vertebrae is largely irreversible, however, there is also a kyphosis that results from muscle imbalance. For example, young women who are overly self-conscious may try to hide their breasts by assuming a rounded upper back and a collapsed chest. In such a case, yogic opening of the chest and strengthening of the muscles of the upper back as with *urdhva dhanurasana* can reverse the curvature of the spine.

In students with scoliosis (usually female) [312], a section of the thoracic spine is offset from the medial plane to either the right or to the left. As an added complication, the left-right displacement of

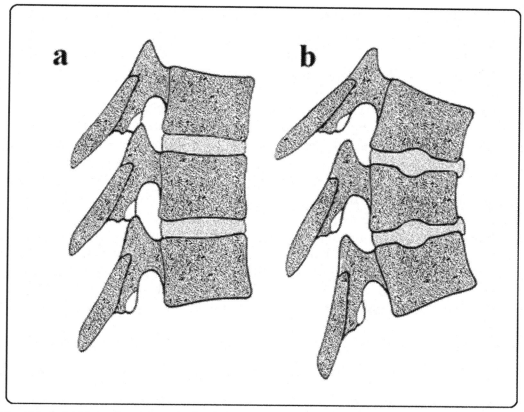

Fig. 4.A-4. (**a**) Normal curvature in the thoracic spine as seen with the posterior to the left, and (**b**) the thoracic kyphosis that results from a wedging of the vertebrae (being thinner on the anterior right-hand edges), leading to a dowager's hump.

scoliosis is often accompanied by a front-to-back asymmetry as well, in which the ribs on one side protrude forward and the ribs on the other side protrude backward (see also Box 4.A-2, *Spinal Rotation Can Be Induced by Lateral Bending and Vice Versa,* page 77). Note too that the data in Table 4.A-1 was assembled from that of "normal" individuals and that yoga students, with their mastery of the spine, may far exceed the values given there (see below), whereas students with spinal problems such as scoliosis may not be able to achieve "the norm" without significant effort.

For students with lordosis or scoliosis, *yogasana* practice can be difficult, for each implies that in the displaced region, the adjacent vertebral facets are already in close contact and so will resist further motion. This would be especially true in backward-bending asanas and in asanas involving spinal twisting. Indeed, as Schatz has pointed out [411], in a student with an abnormal spinal displacement, rotation can be painful in the region of the displacement, or in a more normal region of the spine, the student may over-rotate in an effort to compensate, and so be injured. In either case, one should encourage a more normal alignment and spinal lengthening (Section 8.E, The Joints, page 260) if possible, before trying to rotate fully.

Forward, Backward, and Lateral Bending

As the intervertebral discs (Section 4.C, page 87) act as spinal shock-absorbing cushions, it is no surprise that as one descends the spine and the weight born by a particular vertebra increases, so too does the thickness of the intervertebral disc cushioning it. The ratio of the disc thickness to the thickness of the adjacent vertebrae (Table 4.A-1) is an interesting quantity, in that large ratios reflect large intervertebral separations and therefore high mobility for flexion and extension at that joint. In general, the thicker the disc, the larger the range of motion at that disc [54]. Given this, one sees how important it is to keep the discs healthy as we age, for the alternative is a rigid spine. On this basis, one sees that flexion/extension motions at the cervical vertebrae are most allowed (thickness/height ratio = 0.4), while those in the thorax are even less allowed (ratio = 0.25) than those in the lumbar region (ratio = 0.33), due to the clamping nature of the ribs in the thorax.

Among the joints between thoracic vertebrae, that between T11 and T12 is especially mobile in regard to flexion, extension, lateral bending and rotation. This is so because the lowest two ribs attached to these vertebrae are floating and so are not bound to the sternum. The joint at T11–T12 is the most likely to be stressed when the spine is excessively rotated [54]. The sacrum and coccyx have no mobility to speak of, save for that at the L5–S1 joint and that between the sacrum and the coccyx.

Note that though the cervical and the thoracic vertebrae have nearly the same angular range of motion for flexion (+40º versus +45º), the thoracic region has twice as many joints about which it can bend to achieve this range as compared to the cervical region. Backbending (extension) in the thoracic region is also limited by the pressure of adjacent spinous processes on one another [54, 476].

As seen from the Table, in the average neophyte student attempting *urdhva dhanurasana*, there will be only 60º (25º thoracic plus 35º lumbar) of angular extension available in the thoracic and lumbar regions, meaning that the shoulders and groins will have to supply the remaining 100º or so in order to complete the full backbend. However, as the spine is deliberately lengthened in the *yogasanas*, the disc-to-bone thickness ratio increases, and our spinal mobility increases along with it. Thus *urdhva dhanurasana* becomes possible for the beginner who will work to lengthen the spine.

Kapandji [228] specifies the range of motions observed in the spines of cadavers and states that forward bending (flexion) is largest in the lumbar (+60º), whereas backward bending (extension) is largest in the cervical region (–75º), Table 4.A-1 and Fig. 4.A-5. Though extension also is appreciable in the lumbar region (+35º) [265], 37% of this bending occurs at just one joint, L5-S1 [260, 267]. Lateral bending is largest in the cervical region (+/–45º) and is about equal in the lumbar and thoracic regions (+/–20º). Looking at these numbers, though the disc-thickness/vertebra-thickness ratio as a measure of spinal mobility seems to correlate best with extension, spinal rotation correlates best with lateral flexion. Indeed, Kapandji shows that lateral flexion involves considerable spinal rotation (Subsection 4.A, *Spinal Rotation*, page 75).

It is interesting to compare the range-of-motion values reported by Kapandji (Fig. 4.A-5 and Table 4.A-1) as measured on an "average" population with those attained by accomplished students of *yogasana*. Thus, Kapandji lists the maximal rotation about the cervical vertebrae at +/–50º, whereas students of *yogasana* routinely rotate through 90º at the cervical vertebrae when doing *virabhadrasana II*. According to Kapandji, maximum rotation about the thoracic and lower sections of the spine combined amount to 40º, whereas *yogasana* students rotate by 90º in *maricyasana III*.

As for flexion (forward bending) and extension (backward bending) of the spine, Kapandji reports 45º for movement of the

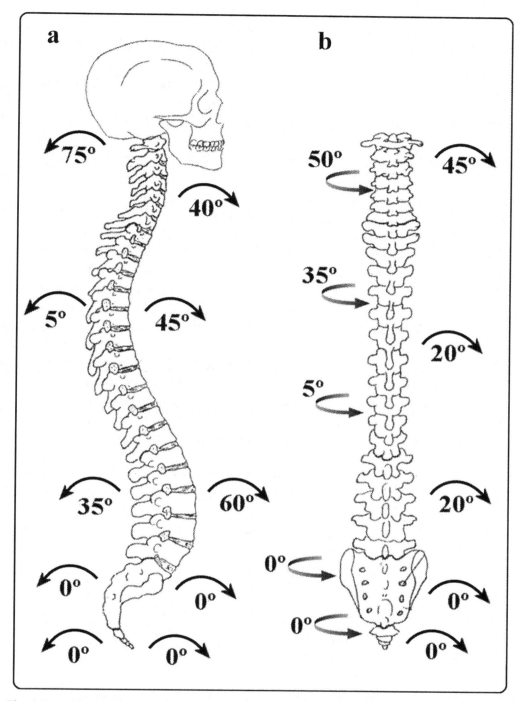

Fig. 4.A-5. (**a**) Maximal angular extension (on the left-hand-side of the Figure) and angular flexion (on the right-hand-side of the Figure) in the five regions of the spine, as measured on a normal population. (**b**) Maximal angles for rotation about the spinal axis (on the left-hand-side) and for lateral bending (on the right-hand side of the Figure) in the five regions of the spine [228].

thoracic vertebrae in forward bends and 25° for the same movement in backbends. Compare this now with the poses shown in Fig. 4.A-6. As a comparative standard, first

consider *tadasana* and measure the angle between the femur of the leg and the average line of the thoracic vertebrae, Fig. 4.A-6a. As these lines are parallel, the angle in question is 0°. For the model (Patricia Walden) in *ruchikasana* (Fig. 4.A-6b), the thoracic vertebrae have an angle of 208° with respect to the femur of the leg in *eka pada sirsasana*, and 174° with respect to the standing leg [482b]! Compare as well Kapandji's backbend "maximum" of 25° for thoracic extension with the 86° apparent in the model's *kapotasana*, Fig. 4.A-6c. It is satisfying to see the large margins by which serious *yogasana* students can exceed the "maxima" of the anatomists. The difference is due in part to the increased flexibility of the *yogasana* student, but also in part to the ability of the student to intelligently work other parts of the body in concert with the stretch or bend coordinates in order to achieve extraordinary lengthening or bending.

The joint between the skull and C1 (the atlas), called the atlanto-occipital joint, is very immobile, allowing only slight forward /backward bending. In flexing the neck in *sarvangasana*, the joint between C4 and C5 is involved primarily, whereas in neck extension as in *salabhasana*, it is the joint between C5 and C6 [260]. Tipping the head back tends to clamp down on the vertebral arteries delivering blood to the brain, as the vertebra slide down on one another in collapse [262]. The joints cited above, other than the atlanto-occipital, are the potential sites of herniated-disc problems in the neck (Section 4.C, page 87). From the point of view of the flexion of the neck, *halasana* will be even more challenging than is *sarvangasana* for the beginner.

As the normal flexion angle at the neck is only 40 to 50° [228, 271], attempts to perform *sarvangasana* with the lines of cervical and thoracic vertebrae perpendicular to one another will induce considerable bending about the higher thoracic vertebrae and the consequent collapse of the upper chest in this *yogasana*. In order to avoid this rounding of the chest, it is much better to

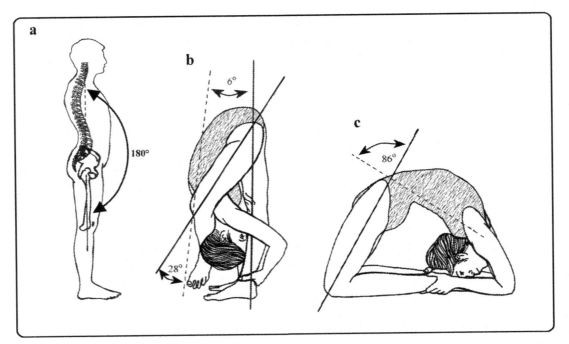

Fig. 4.A-6. Angles formed by the femur bones (full lines) and the thoracic spine (dashed lines) in *tadasana* (**a**), for each of the legs in *ruchikasana* (**b**) and in *kapotasana* (**c**). The model in (**b**) and (**c**) is Patricia Walden.

place blankets under the shoulders and upper arms when in *sarvangasana*; with this, the head can drop back away from the chest, so that the thoracic vertebrae can remain in vertical alignment, and there is a strong vertical lift of the viscera off the diaphragm, lungs and heart [271].

Through articular facets, vertebrae T1–T12 are jointed to twelve pairs of ribs at the costovertebral hinge joints. This, together with the diaphragm, is discussed in Section 12.A, Mechanics of the Breath, page 355.

Kapandji [228] also gives data on how lumbar extension and lumbar lateral bending change with age of the subject, Table 4.A-2. On average, one loses almost 2/3 of one's lumbar range of motion on going from the youngest age group (2–13 years) to the oldest (65–77 years), with the largest part of the decrease coming between the age groups (2–13) and (35–49) years. Fortunately, *yogasana* students are not "average", and so can expect to do much better than average in this regard.

Spinal Rotation

Kilmurray [240] presents an appealing point of view on spinal rotation. He considers the second and fourth *chakras* (the *swadisthana* belly and *anahata* heart centers) as centers which are to be used to drive the rotation, whereas the spine itself acts passively to receive the torsion. In this way, the spine is twisted, but it does not twist itself, as it remains relaxed and is acted upon by the higher and lower *chakras*. Do not create the twist using the head, but instead twist using the belly and ribcage to abet the actions of the lower and higher *chakras*.

When the spine is twisted, there is a tendency for the spine to bend laterally as well; for a twist that will face in a given direction, the direction of the bend is in the same direction, and largely in the lumbar spine [240]. Furthermore, not only does twisting promote lateral bending, but lateral bending promotes twisting. The consequences of this coupling of bending and rotation in two

TABLE 4.A-2. RANGE OF MOTION FOR EXTENSION AND LATERAL BENDING IN THE LUMBAR VERTEBRAE WITH INCREASING AGE [228]

Lumbar Extension	Age, years			
	2–13	35–49	50–64	65–77
L1	6°	4°	2°	
L2	10°	8°	5°	5°
L3	13°	9°	8°	3°
L4	17°	12°	8°	7°
L5	24°	8°	8°	7°
L1–L5 Total	64°	43°	33°	24°
Lumbar Lateral Bending				
L1	12°	5°	6°	4°
L2	12°	8°	7°	7°
L3	16°	8°	8°	6°
L4	15°	8°	7°	5°
L5	7°	2°	1°	0°
L1–L5 Total	62°	31°	29°	22°

yogasanas and in scoliosis are presented in Box 4.A-2.

It is interesting to consider the purely mechanical consequences of twisting the spine. As shown in Fig. 4.A-7, when the opposite ends of a cylinder are rotated with respect to one another, the surface of the cylinder experiences both tension and a shearing force, and the body of the cylinder experiences a radial compression as well. It is this compressional component that squeezes the water out of a wrung-out washcloth while the fibers of the cloth clearly are under tension. Applied to spinal twisting, the compressional force will tend to dehydrate the spinal discs as disc volume and

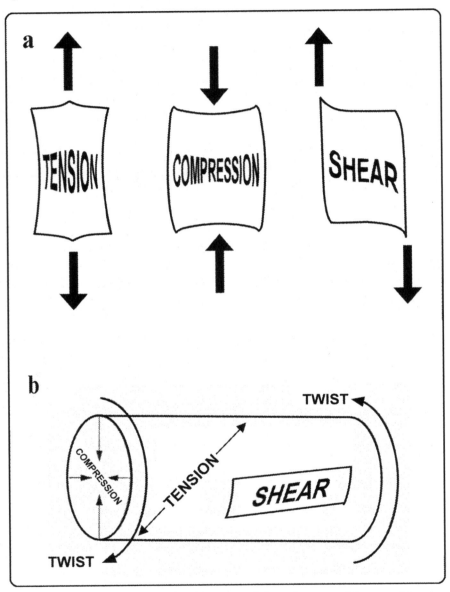

Fig. 4.A-7. (a) A two-dimensional sheet of any material can be stressed in one of three ways: *tension*, when the ends are pulled away from one another, *compression*, when the ends are pushed toward one another, and *shear*, when opposite corners are pulled away from or pushed toward one another. (b) In a three-dimensional object, one adds the stress of twisting the two ends oppositely, which generates tension and shear on the object's surface and radially compresses it at the same time [472].

BOX 4.A-2: SPINAL ROTATION CAN BE INDUCED
BY LATERAL BENDING AND *VICE VERSA*

There is a psychological component to the tendency to bend forward in *trikonasana*: the area in front psychologically represents the known and familiar, whereas the area behind is dark, unknown, and frightening. The beginning student in *trikonasana* must learn to be brave enough to pull the upper body backward so that it is above the triangle of the legs, thus bringing the entire body into two-dimensional alignment.

A second factor, non-psychological in nature, works to align the ribs in *trikonasana*. The lumbar curve results in part because the discs in the lumbar region are wedge shaped, with the thinner aspect of the wedges pointing to the rear [34, 476]. As one bends laterally, the bending is assisted by a rotation of the lumbar wedges so as to place the thinner parts of the wedges to that side on which the intervertebral discs are more compressed, *i.e.*, the side toward which one bends. Correspondingly, the thicker parts of the wedges move toward the opposite side where the vertebral discs are more expanded. The tendency of the thick and thin parts of the discs to change positions when bending laterally results in a twisting of the lumbar vertebrae which ultimately couples spinal rotation to the motion of lateral bending.

This coupling of the lateral bending with twisting is especially synergistic in *trikonasana* and in *parivrtta janu sirsasana*, where the lateral motion in the lumbar spine tends to turn the ribcage to face forward or upward, as the poses require. On the other hand, in *parivrtta trikonasana*, the rotation induced by the bending is in the direction opposite to that demanded by the pose, and so one must overcome this tendency with awareness and practice. The bending-rotation connection described above can be countered by unilateral contraction of the psoas muscle (Subsection 8.D, *The Legs and Feet*, page 247); if the right-hand psoas is contracted, this acts to pull the torso to the right and rotate it to face left, as when doing *parivrtta janu sirsasana*. This bending-twisting action of the contracted psoas is a result of its diagonal orientations in both the left-to-right and front-to-back directions.

The simultaneous occurrence of lateral flexing and rotation of the spinal vertebrae is apparent as well in the spines of those with scoliosis. In this case, the spine is pushed largely to one side and forward when in the neutral position (*tadasana*), with other spinal segments also displaced oppositely in compensation for the primary displacement. The condition of scoliosis is outwardly much like that experienced by beginners in *trikonasana*, except that the rotation-lateral flexion is permanent, and so too are the effects of the misalignment on the internal organs.

When the scoliosis is slight, it is said that its curvature and the discomfort associated with it can be minimized by twisting into the convexity of the displacement, *i.e.*, twisting oppositely to the twist inherent in the scoliosis [316]. Note also that in scoliosis, there often is a partial collapse of the lung on one side of the chest, which spinal twisting and *pranayama* can help to open again. Eighty percent of scoliosis cases are deemed to be idiopathic.

spinal length decrease on twisting, and also will shear the skin of the torso as we twist. It is for this reason that students with "herniated-disc" problems are able to twist without pain only if they consciously lift and lengthen the spine before turning. Lifting the abdomen inward and upward while doing the twist will facilitate the twist and so allow a larger angular rotation to be achieved. On releasing from the twist, the discs and organs will rehydrate with fresh, healthful fluids again.

Conrotatory and Disrotatory Actions

As the spinal column is twisted, there is an unavoidable twisting of the sacral plate in the sacroiliac joint, which tends to misalign it (or align it if misaligned) and loosen the ligaments upon which it is otherwise dependent for stability [270]. When we perform spinal twists such as *bharadvajasana I*, one often finds the pelvis rotating along with the rotation of the ribcage. For the sake of concreteness, imagine the spinal rotation to be toward the right, in which case, the left knee will be thrust forward. To accommodate this unwelcome rotation of the pelvis, one often resets the left femur into the hip joint so that a counter-rotation of the pelvis occurs with respect to that of the ribcage, *i.e.*, a disrotatory motion. In this way, the effect of the twist is amplified by oppositely twisting the two ends of the spine. However, in doing this counter-rotation, one must keep in mind the torque that this produces in the sacroiliac joint, and that the opposite rotation (conrotatory rather than disrotatory) may be better suited to students with lower-back problems.

For safety's sake, in sitting or standing twists where one could actively and forcefully counter-rotate the pelvis with respect to the ribcage (a disrotatory action), the two ends of the spine instead should be rotated in the same direction (a conrotatory action),

as for example, when doing *maricyasana III*. This action will keep the lumbar vertebrae, the sacrum and the ilium bones in alignment, and so will not unduly torque the sacroiliac joint [240, 270]. On the other hand, in twists where the body is lying on the floor (*jathara parivartanasana*, for example) or is inverted (*parsva sirsasana*, for example), the disrotatory twist is more acceptable, but should not be overdone. In right-handed people, twisting to the left is the easier direction in general, as the right arm wraps around the front of the body in this twist as the left arm goes behind the back [5].

For those who wish to rotate the spine with neither conrotatory nor disrotatory motion of the pelvis, the pelvis can be locked in place by twisting with the legs immobilized as when sitting in *vajrasana* or *baddha konasana*.

According to the data of Kapandji [228], the maximum angle of rotation about the vertebral axis decreases in the order cervical (50°), thoracic (35°), lumbar (5°). Although yoga students readily can eclipse these "maximum" ranges of spinal rotation when doing spinal twists such as *maricyasana III*, even in these students, it still seems that the cervical vertebrae rotate about ten times farther than the lumbar. With 14 cervical vertebrae, the owl can turn its head approximately twice as far angularly (270°) as can *yogasana* students with only 7 such vertebrae [473].

Beginning students are susceptible to a second type of spinal twisting, this driven by medial or lateral rotation of the upper arms: when the right arm is below the shoulder and rotated laterally, it tends to take the right shoulder more back than the left shoulder, and *vice versa* when rotating medially [54]. This twisting can be avoided by counter-rotating the thorax, however, such a twist can be advantageous, as in *bharadvajasana I*.

Misalignment of the Spine and Deterioration of the Vertebral Discs

When the vertebrae go out of alignment, a heightened risk of pressure on a nerve in the vicinity of the displacement results. Not surprisingly, there is a clear correlation between the location of the misalignment along the spinal column, the area of the body affected by the misalignment, and the effects that can appear in that area. Tables 4.A-3, 4.A-4, and 4.A-5, list these correlations for misalignment of the cervical, thoracic, and lumbar vertebrae, respectively [351]. Misalignment of the cervical vertebrae also can adversely affect the blood flow through the vertebral arteries to the brain, with consequent neurological problems (see Subsection 4.A, *Blood Vessels*, page 81).

A spinal loading of 600 kilograms (1300 pounds) is sufficient to crush or fracture the anterior portions of the vertebrae and at 800 kilograms (1800 pounds), the entire vertebra is crushed. Unfortunately, at loading far less than this, the osteoporotic spines of the elderly are readily fractured and collapsed. See the Section 8.G, Osteoporosis, page 269, for more discussion of this. When the intervertebral discs have degenerated but not herniated, the vertebrae may come to rub on one another leading to the growth of painful bone spurs and the fusion of adjacent vertebrae. This occurs most often in the cervical region [257]. Poses that challenge the strength or flexibility of the neck or spine must be approached gingerly with students who experience these sorts of problems.

Inasmuch as the spinous and transverse processes are posterior to the vertebral bodies, backbending acts to close the intervertebral joints, forcing bone on bone at the facets. This can be accommodated in part by the flexing of the bony processes. However, one should never rotate about the spine when the column is heavily loaded, as in *urdhva dhanurasana*, as this concentrates the pressure unevenly on the transverse processes and so puts them at risk for frac-

TABLE 4.A-3. EFFECTS OF CERVICAL MISALIGNMENT [351]

Vertebra	Area / Effect
C1	Blood supply to the head, pituitary gland, scalp, bones of the face, brain, inner and middle ear, sympathetic nervous system / Headaches, nervousness, insomnia, head colds, high blood pressure, migraine headaches, nervous breakdown, amnesia, chronic tiredness, dizziness
C2	Eyes, optic nerves, auditory nerves, sinuses, mastoid bones, tongue, forehead / Sinus trouble, allergies, crossed eyes, deafness, eye troubles, earache, fainting, blindness
C3	Cheeks, outer ear, face bones, teeth, trigeminal nerve / Neuralgia, neuritis, acne, pimples, eczema
C4	Nose, lips, mouth, eustachian tube / Hay fever, catarrh, hearing loss, adenoids
C5	Vocal cords, neck glands, pharynx / Laryngitis, hoarseness, sore throat
C6	Neck muscles, shoulder, tonsils / Stiff neck, upper-arm pain, tonsillitis, whooping cough, croup
C7	Thyroid, shoulder bursae, elbow bursae / Bursitis, colds

TABLE 4.A-4. EFFECTS OF THORACIC MISALIGNMENT [351]

Vertebra	Area / Effect
T1	Forearms, hands, wrists, fingers, esophagus, trachea / Asthma, cough, difficult breathing, shortness of breath, pain in lower arms and hands
T2	Heart, heart covering, coronary arteries / Heart conditions, chest conditions
T3	Lungs, bronchial tubes, pleura, chest, breast / Bronchitis, pleurisy, pneumonia, congestion, influenza
T4	Gall bladder, common duct / Gall bladder conditions, jaundice, shingles
T5	Liver, solar plexus, blood / Liver conditions, fevers, low blood pressure, anemia, poor circulation, arthritis
T6	Stomach / Stomach troubles, nervous stomach, indigestion, heartburn, dyspepsia
T7	Pancreas, duodenum / Ulcers, gastritis
T8	Spleen / Lowered immunological resistance
T9	Adrenal and supra-adrenal glands / Allergies, hives
T10	Kidneys / Kidney trouble, hardening of the arteries, chronic tiredness, nephritis, pyelitis
T11	Kidneys, ureters / Acne, pimples, eczema, boils
T12	Small intestines, lymph / Rheumatism, gas pains, sterility

TABLE 4.A-5. EFFECTS OF LUMBAR, SACRAL AND COCCYGEAL MISALIGNMENT [351]

Vertebra	Area / Effect
L1	Colon, inguinal rings / Constipation, colitis, dysentery, diarrhea, hernias
L2	Appendix, abdomen, upper leg / Cramps, difficulty breathing, acidosis, varicose veins
L3	Sex organs, uterus, bladder, knees / Bladder trouble, menstrual troubles, bed wetting, impotency, knee pains
L4	Prostate gland, muscles of lower back, sciatic nerve / sciatica, lumbago, difficult, painful or too frequent urination, backaches
L5	Lower legs, ankles, feet / Poor circulation in legs, swollen ankles, weak ankles and arches, cold feet, weak legs, leg cramps
S1–S5	Hip bones, buttocks / Sacroiliac problems, spinal curvatures
Coccyx	Rectum, anus / Hemorrhoids, pruritis, pain on sitting

ture. Similarly, never allow your students to turn their heads while in *sarvangasana* or *sirsasana*, for the same reason. This means that in the twisting variations of these inversions, the twisting action must take place in the thoracic and lumbar vertebrae, but must not be allowed to extend into the cervical region. For similar reasons, students who are strongly lordotic may experience lower back pain on twisting unless they are careful to first lengthen the spine in order to separate the lumbar vertebrae before twisting about them.

Spinal Muscles, Tendons, and Ligaments

As pointed out by Kilmurray [240], there are three major groups of muscles in the back which attach to the spinal column. The first group, Fig. 4.A-8, has fibers that run almost perpendicular to the spine (latissimus, trapezius, rhomboids, *etc.*), and work to connect the actions of the arms to the spine. Members of the second muscle group, the erector spinae, run parallel to the spine over its entire length, whereas the third group consists of muscles that connect the transverse and spinous processes of each vertebra with those of its neighbors in a criss-cross fashion such that contraction of these muscles can act to rotate the spine about its axis. However, also see Kilmurray's comments in regard keeping the muscles in the third group relaxed during spinal twisting (Subsection 4.A, *Spinal Rotation*, page 75).

The ligamentum nuchae connects all of the spinous processes from C1 to C7; it stabilizes the neck and is stretched in *sarvangasana* [257], and even more so in *halasana*. The anterior longitudinal ligament runs the length of the spinal column on the forward side, and acts to limit the amount of extension possible in backbending [54]. The trapezius muscles are at the back of the neck, being connected to the occiput and to

the shoulder blades (scapulae). Bodily tension accumulates readily in the trapezius, as witnessed by those people who chronically carry their shoulders up around their ears. Students for whom the upper trapezius muscles are chronically short will be at a disadvantage in their *yogasana* work, for they will not be able to lower the scapulae into a position where the scapulae can press the ribcage in order to lift and open it.

The sternomastoid muscles are oriented cross-wise, going from the clavicles to the base of the skull on both sides of the neck, and serve as both neck flexors and neck rotators. Also see Subsection 8.E, page 262, for an extended discussion of the general nature of ligaments and tendons.

Blood Vessels

Approximately half of the blood going to the brain is carried there by the vertebral arteries passing through the vertebral foramina in the cervical vertebrae, Fig. 3.B-1. Almost any head movement imaginable has the potential for interfering with this blood supply to the brain, with resultant dizziness, nausea, or fainting, depending on just how large an oxygen debt is generated in the brain. Occlusion of these arteries is especially likely when the neck is in extension while the trapezius pull the scapulae even more toward the ears. In the elderly, however, occlusion can occur by just rotating the head [39, 480]. The symptoms of occlusion can be eased in a pose such as *ustrasana* by not tipping the head backward and/or by pulling the scapulae away from the cervical vertebrae. Any student experiencing neurological symptoms when the head is tipped backward in extension should immediately change position.

Cautionary tales regarding *sirsasana*, *halasana*, and neck injuries appear in the medical literature [140, 262], and are discussed further in Appendix II, *INJURIES*

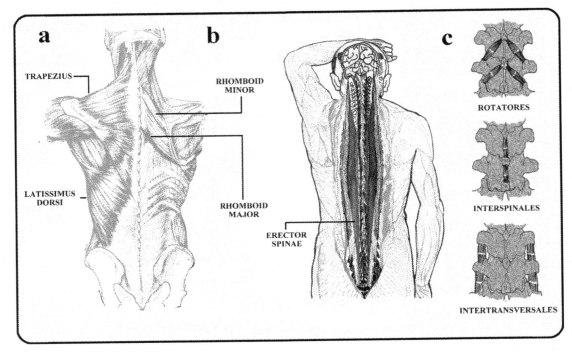

Fig. 4.A-8. (**a**) Posterior views of muscles of the back running almost perpendicular to the spine. (**b**) Muscles of the back running parallel to the spine along its length. (**c**) Posterior views of muscles connecting transverse and spinous processes of neighboring vertebrae.

INCURRED DURING IMPROPER *YOG-ASANA* PRACTICE, page 511.

Keeping the Spine Healthy

It is often said, "A healthy spine characterizes youthfulness of body and mind, and a rigid spine old age and senility" [401]. This truism comes about in part because, as we age, there is a natural shutting down of the vascular system that otherwise nourishes the spinal components. As we age, the nutritional servicing of the spine is less and less by direct delivery of blood via the vascular system, and more and more by the indirect mechanism of diffusion to and from outlying areas.

As the vascularization retreats in the spinal region, the intervertebral discs begin to change. Normally, the nucleus pulposus (Section 4.C, Intervertebral Discs, page 87) of the disc has a tough fibrous covering, however, the inside is soft and jelly-like,

allowing the structure to function as a shock absorber, and also allowing smooth motion between adjacent vertebrae. Over the years, the soft inner part of the disc turns into tough, calcified cartilage, this transformation being complete in some people by the age of sixty [34]. Once calcified, the spine becomes shorter, more rigid and more brittle. The effects of aging on the range of motion of the lumbar spine are shown in Table 4.A-2, where it is seen that the ranges of motion for extension and lateral bending are maximal in the age range 2–13 years, and fall to values much less than half the maximal range by age 65–77 years [228].

Because the spine is deeply involved when forward bending, backward bending and in twisting poses as well, performance of these types of *yogasana* improve the circulation of nutrients into and removal of wastes from the spinal region, and thereby forestall the premature calcification of the spine. The same *yogasanas* that massage the intervertebral discs also massage the internal organs. A healthy spine stays not only supple, but elongates so that the vertebrae do not collapse upon one another, *i.e.*, one's height is maintained on aging. Maintaining a healthy spine involves both exercise *and* rest [7].

Those *yogasanas* that involve flexion and extension of the spine necessarily involve not only the spine proper, but most if not all of the other muscles, organs, and glands within the thorax. Interestingly, the forward bends (flexion) and the backward bends (extension) in many ways have much in common, *i.e.*, both involve compression and stimulation of the internal organs, both improve spinal suppleness and increased spinal length, and both stimulate and release the tension in the associated nerves [404]. The two forms of spinal bending differ however in their effects on the articular facet joints, opening the joints in flexion and closing them in extension, and on the intervertebral muscles and ligaments, where the posterior ones are stretched in flexion and the anterior ones are streched in extension, Fig. 4.A-9. Moreover, the two forms of spinal bending differ in their impact on the autonomic nervous system, with supported forward bends in general resulting in parasympathetic excitation, and unsupported backbends resulting in sympathetic excitation (Chapter 6, THE AUTONOMIC NERVOUS SYSTEM, page 133).

SECTION 4.B. THE SPINAL CORD

Inasmuch as the spinal cord is composed almost totally of nerve tissue, this Section can best be understood by first reading Chapter 5, THE NERVES, page 107, for some of the basic characteristics of such tis-

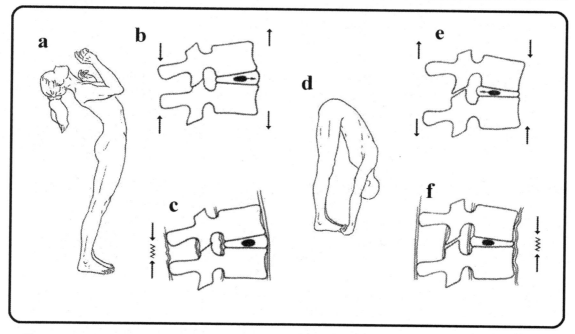

Fig. 4.A-9. (**a**) Extension of the spine, resulting in the pressing of the nucleus pulposus in the forward direction (**b**), with the concomitant stretching of the ligament on the anterior spine and relaxation of the ligaments and muscles on the posterior side of the spine (**c**). (**d**) Flexion of the spine, resulting in the pressing of the nucleus pulposus in the backward direction (**e**), with the concomitant stretching of the ligament and muscles on the posterior side of the spine, and the relaxation of those on the anterior side of the spine (**f**) [54].

sue. Lacking that, several of the possibly obscure terms are defined in the Glossary.

Structure and Function

The spinal cord has three broad functions: (1) it is the pathway for ascending neural impulses from the body's sensors, (2) it is the pathway for the descending neural impulses that drive the body's muscles and organs, and (3) it contains the relatively crude neural circuitry that guides such reflexive actions as vomiting and repetitive actions such as walking [106].

Beginning at the foramen magnum at the base of the skull and passing through the canal of the vertebral column, the spinal cord is a 0.5-meter-long extension of the central nervous system, terminating at the L4 vertebra, though the canal itself extends all the way down to S4, and individual nerves extend all the way to S5 before exiting, Fig. 4.A-2b [195, 225, 229, 230, 313]. The spinal cord is no thicker than one inch at any point and is soft and jellylike, much like the tissue in the brain case [303]. Though some neurons in the spinal cord run its entire length, most are shorter, entering or leaving the cord at intermediate points. The weight of neural tissue in the spinal cord is only 4% that of the weight of the brain [43], however, being tissue with an active metabolism, the spinal cord is well supplied with blood vessels. Surprisingly, nerves within the spinal cord can remain viable for up to thirty minutes without oxygen and/or glucose, whereas after only ten minutes under the same conditions the neurons within the brain irreversibly cease to function [12]. This difference probably relates to the fact that, under normal conditions, the brain has a very high-volume blood throughput, *i.e.*, a strong need for oxygen, whereas that to the spinal cord is quite meager by comparison. The question of the proper oxygenation of nerve tissue is an important one, with many implications for those who practice *yogasana* (see Subsections 5.C, *Mechanical Effects on Nerves*, page 125, and 7.B, *Resting Muscle Tone*, page 204).

The spinal cord is the distal continuation of the central nervous system, and like the brain itself, the spinal cord floats in the surrounding cerebrospinal fluid (Section 4.D, page 93). As seen in cross section, Fig. 4.B-1, the spinal cord shows a central region in the shape of the letter H (this material being called the gray matter) which is surrounded by a field of myelinated white matter (Fig. 4.A-2b). This pattern persists throughout the length of the spinal cord. The white matter of the spinal cord appears so because each of the nerve fibers within it is covered with a coating of fatty substance called myelin. While myelin insures a high velocity of nerve transmission along the fiber, when a myelinated fiber has its coating disrupted, the nerve signal too is blocked at the site of the disruption, rather than being transmitted [303].

The gray matter in the cord is largely involved with the local transfer of neural signals at its particular level in the spinal cord, whereas the neurons of the white matter largely run the full length of the cord. Of course, there are interconnections between the white and gray matter, and there is branching of the white matter at different levels of the cord. Nonetheless, if there were a severe injury to the gray matter at, say, C8, then nerve contact with the fingers and hands would be lost, however, the same injury to the white matter at C8 would mean paralysis not only of the functions particular to C8, but to all functions below that point as well (see Tables 4.A-3, 4.A-4, 4.A-5 and 10.E-1 for listings of the correlation of vertebrae with peripheral body parts).

Nerves that carry sensory information from the periphery to the central nervous system are called afferents, whereas those that carry neural impulses from the central

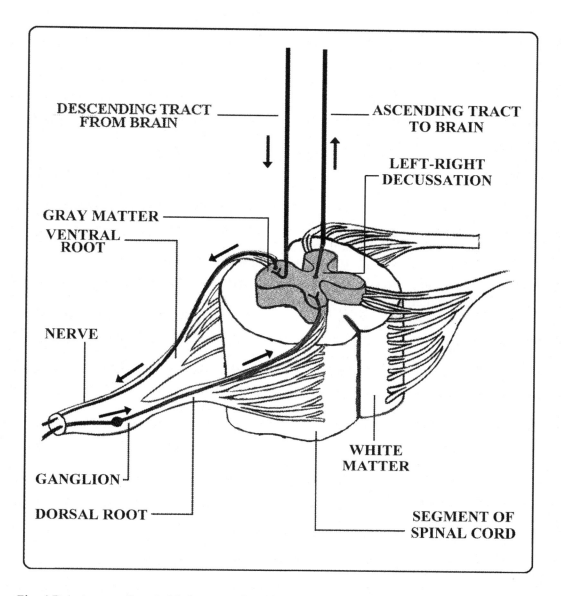

DESCENDING TRACT FROM BRAIN

ASCENDING TRACT TO BRAIN

LEFT-RIGHT DECUSSATION

GRAY MATTER

VENTRAL ROOT

NERVE

GANGLION

DORSAL ROOT

WHITE MATTER

SEGMENT OF SPINAL CORD

Fig. 4.B-1. As seen from behind, connection of the afferent nerves to the white matter of a segment of the spinal cord via the dorsal surface, and connection of the efferent nerves to muscle and organ via the ventral root. White matter also bears ascending and descending tracts of axons to and from the brain, which tracts also synapse to more local neurons. Also shown is possible decussation wherein afferent neurons from the left side of the body synapse across the gray matter to ascend to the brain on the right side.

nervous system to the muscles and viscera are known as efferents. The four prongs of the H-shaped gray matter are the dorsal (posterior, to the rear) and ventral (anterior, to the front) horns, the former of which is a reception point for afferent signals coming from the sensors within the muscles and organs, whereas the latter is the point of departure for efferent motor neurons that eventually will activate the muscles and viscera [195, 303], Fig. 4.B-1.

The white matter of the spinal cord consists of long tracts of afferent nerves transmitting sensory information upward to the higher centers and efferent motor-nerve impulses downward from those higher points to the relevant muscles and organs. Shorter intersegmental tracts connect the longer ascending and descending tracts of the white matter and are used in reflex reactions (see Section 7.D, Reflex Actions, page 211). In both the white matter and the gray, there are many glial cells which help to keep the nerve fibers healthy by performing many housekeeping tasks.

Each spinal nerve will serve a specific body area or part. This segmentation of the nervous system is especially obvious in the dermatome map of the body's skin (see Section 10.E, Dermatomes and Referred Pain, page 303), and can be traced backward in time to the segmentation of the nervous system in an early ancestor of ours, the earthworm! [313]

Afferent and efferent nerves serving a particular peripheral location are bundled together between that location and the spinal cord. However, at the spinal cord, they are separate, with the afferent nerves entering the dorsal surface of the spinal cord, whereas the efferent nerves leave the spine at the ventral side of the spine and then join the nerve bundle, Fig. 4.B-1. Similarly, in the peripheral region, the bundle is again separated into those efferent nerves that will activate the muscles and organs, and the afferent nerves that carry the associated sensory signals.

Each of the vertebra in the spinal column has left and right intervertebral foramina through which nerve bundles pass laterally to the outside, Figs. 4.A-2 and 4.A-3, there being 31 such pairs of bundles (8 cervical, 12 thoracic, 5 lumbar, 5 sacral and 1 coccygeal). Each such bundle has dorsal and ventral components. The nerve roots glide freely through the intervertebral foramina by up to 1/2 inch (12 mm) at L5, unless the sliding is restrained by disc pressure on the root. There are synapsing neural connections of the dorsal and ventral fibers within the gray matter and between axons in the gray and white matter, this going on at a common vertebral level and also between levels. Additionally, there are 12 pairs of nerve bundles that enter and leave the spinal cord at the level of the brainstem above the uppermost vertebra C1; these are cranial nerves I through XII (Subsection 2.C, *The Cranial Nerves*, page 17).

At all levels of the spinal cord, there are both ascending and descending paths involving the autonomic nervous system as well (see Chapter 6, THE AUTONOMIC NERVOUS SYSTEM, page 133). As certain of the sensory fibers ascend and come to synapse in the gray matter of the spinal column, there occurs a decussation, or crossing over, of the fibers such that sensations coming from the left side of the body are sent to the sensory cortex of the right cerebral hemisphere, and *vice versa* (see Section 3.D, Cerebral Hemispheric Laterality, page 49).

Nerve fibers ascending to the brain pass through the reticular formation (see Subsection 3.A, *The Limbic System*, page 33), where they may become relevant factors in the sleep/wake cycle, in arousal and attention, and in the inhibition of pain [230].

Neural Connectivity of the Spinal Cord

One sees that the spinal cord is an active intermediary in the flow of neural traffic signals which flow from all parts of the body to the brain along sensory paths, and from the brain along somatic paths to the muscles (voluntary and involuntary), visceral organs, and glands in all parts of the body as well. However, the function of the spinal cord goes far beyond just being a conduit for two-way nerve traffic, for there is considerable integration of nerve signals and processing of information involving interneurons that goes on within it. Thus, for example, it is known that the neural circuitry that drives certain repetitive but unthinking actions such as breathing, swallowing, chewing, running, walking, and eye movements involve "central-pattern generators" located within the spinal cord itself [172]. Of course, the turning on and off of the central-pattern generators is a task for the higher brain centers, and bringing such repetitive/unthinking actions under more conscious control is a task for the yoga student. Furthermore, as a second example, the descending fibers from the sensory cortex have collateral excitatory and inhibitory synapses with ascending signals from the thalamus in order to fine-tune sensory perceptions [230].

Not all of the sensory fibers synapse at the dorsal horns; only those relaying information about pain, temperature, and crude tactile sensation use this pathway to the thalamus. This is the spinothalamic path; with its slow, unmyelinated type-C fibers (see Table 5.C-2), it is a primitive one and is found in all vertebrates, including man. A second path to higher centers using swift, type-A conductors (Table 5.C-2) is found in humans and primates and carries the information concerning precise localization of touch sensations, pressure, vibration, and proprioception. The fibers of this more modern system run uninterrupted along the length of the spinal cord until they synapse in the medulla oblongata [230]. Of course, sensory and somatic signals from and to the head and neck do not move through the spinal cord.

Unlike broken bones which heal rapidly, and torn ligaments which heal more slowly, badly injured nerves in the spinal cord do not heal and do not regenerate spontaneously [303], however, the more peripheral nerves can repair themselves somewhat more easily than those of the central nervous system.

The largest opening in the skull allowing access to the brain is the foramen magnum in the occipital plate of the skull. It is at the foramen magnum that the brain's pattern of gray matter covering white is reversed, so that in the spinal cord, the white matter covers the gray. However, unlike the gray matter of the brain, that of the spine does not "think", but is used for reflexive subconscious acts instead. It is also at the foramen magnum that many ascending and descending nerves decussate, which is to say, it is at this point that the sensations originating on the left side of the body cross over so as to register in the right cerebral hemisphere, and *vice versa* for those originating on the right. Similarly, the motor nerves from the cortex also decussate at the foramen magnum on their downward paths.

SECTION 4.C.
INTERVERTEBRAL DISCS

Structure

There is a semi-rigid element called the "intervertabral disc," Fig. 4.C-1a, between each adjacent pair of vertebrae in the spine. This disc, composed of a central ball-shaped portion (the nucleus pulposus) which is surrounded by the annulus fibrosus, sits between the relatively flat surfaces of adjacent vertebrae, Fig. 4.C-1b. The nucleus pulposus, a jellylike hydrophilic (water-loving) material consisting of up to 88% water is surrounded by seven annular sheaths made of fibrocartilage having their fibers set at different angles in each of the layers. This arrangement of fibers in the annulus strengthens it, just as it does within the different layers of bone (Section 8.A, Bone Structure, Development and Mechanics, page 235). That the annular sheaths have superior strength with respect to shear thanks to the fibers' mixed orientations is advantageous, for the annulus serves as a casing to keep the nucleus pulposus intact while under pressure.

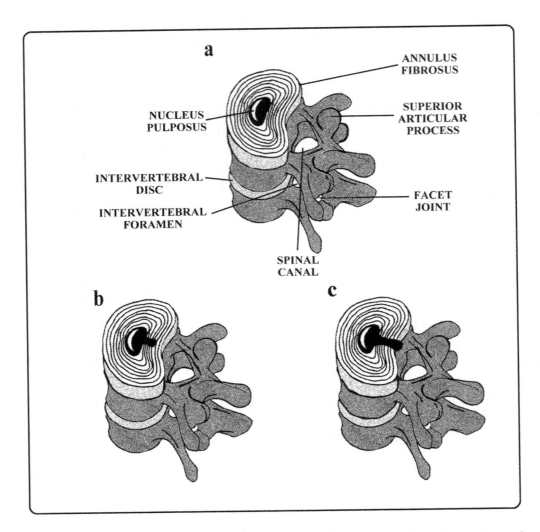

Fig. 4.C-1. (**a**) Superior view of a lumbar vertebra, supporting an intervertebral disc and its nucleus pulposus on its upper surface. (**b**) A bulging but not herniated disc pressing posteriorly toward the spinal canal. (**c**) A herniated disc exudes its nucleus through the torn annulus fibrosus so as to impinge upon the nerve bundle within the spinal canal.

In the adult spine, no blood vessels serve the discs, the vascular system having disappeared by age 20. Instead, the discs are nourished by the diffusion of nutrients and wastes into and out of neighboring tissues [257, 411]. Weight bearing on the spine wrings fluid from around the discs, whereas rest restores the discs by bathing them in fresh fluid. If the discs are not restored, they become thin, brittle and easily damaged [411].

In humans, the intervertebral discs account for approximately 25% of the length of the spine, and so are seen to be a significant structural element in addition to serving as shock absorbers [319], however, the discs lose their elasticity and height as we age. Being somewhat flexible, the intervertebral discs are also important components of the intervertebral joints and the resultant spinal flexibility.

The plateau surfaces of the intervertebral discs are lined with thin layers of cartilage which in turn are perforated by microscopic pores congruent with channels in the cancellous bone of the vertebrae. With axial compression, the pressure drives water from the nucleus pulposus into the pores, and then into the vertebrae and surrounding tissue. As a result of the water loss, the discs thin and consequently, the spinal curves are exaggerated. Due to the pressurized dehydration of the discs, the overall height of a person can decrease by as much as 2.5 cm (one inch) after a day of standing. In the lumbar region, the disc volume decreases by about 20% after a day of standing and sitting [5]. Correspondingly, astronauts measure 5 to 10 cm taller on return to earth from gravity-free space. The effect of gravity on the length of the spine was first raised when it was noted that the vertical spine of a man on horseback shortened after a day's ride, but the horizontal spine of his horse did not.

When lying down at night, the gravitational loading on the discs is relieved (but not the smaller effects of intervertebral muscle tone), and the discs rehydrate so as to assume their larger thickness by morning. When we awake in the morning, the discs are fully hydrated, the vertebrae are pushed apart by the increased thickness of the discs, and the spine has its maximal length. In this case, the various muscles and ligaments that bind each vertebra to its neighbors are pulled taut and consequently, the spine would seem to be at its least flexible in the morning! Conversely, spinal flexibility would seem to be maximal at the end of the day, when the discs are dehydrated, the ligaments and muscles slack, and the spine in a collapsed condition. However, the tautness of the spinal muscles and ligaments are not the only factors determining spinal flexibility. When the discs expand and tighten the spinal musculature, they also lift the bony transverse processes of each vertebra off of and away from that below it (Fig. 4.C-1b), *i.e.*, the facet joints open, and this works to increase spinal flexibility, as was stated in Subsection 4.A, *Forward, Back-*

ward, and Lateral Bending, page 71. It would appear that the pressing of the transverse processes against one another is the more important of the two factors, for it is always best to lengthen the spine before twisting or backbending, even if it tightens the musculature. On the other hand, reversing the above argument leads one to expect that forward bending might be easier late in the day when the spinal muscles and ligaments have relaxed due to collapse of the intervertebral discs, Fig. 4.A-8.

The intervertebral discs show viscoelastic behavior much like that shown by the muscles (Subsection 7.E, *Stress and Strain*, page 228). That is to say, when a disc is loaded and then released quickly, it is compressed and then expanded elastically, so that there is no change in thickness. However, if the loading is large and long lasting, then the disc behaves viscoelastically, losing water during the compression and then regaining its full thickness only after a long-term rest.

Actually, even in zero gravity, there is a strong outward pressure due to water in the discs, and this acts to prestress (preload) them in anticipation of compressive loading from the outside. Because the preloading is most marked in the morning, this is the time when the discs are at their thickest, the spine is at its longest, and the facet joints are most open. (As discussed in Chapter 21, TIME AND BODY RHYTHMS, page 473, there are other physiological markers that suggest that *yogasanas* are best done in the early morning). With increasing age, the discs are less able to achieve the preloaded state and thus they do not inflate well; the result is loss of height, loss of spinal flexibility, and changing spinal curvature in the aged (see Subsection 22.A, *Physical Aging*, page 495, as well); this normal degeneration is speeded along by osteoporosis. Even in a young person, under conditions of constant loading, the discs tend again toward collapse, thus simulating old age. In view of the above, practicing *yogasana* is seen as practicing preventive medicine, thanks to the special attention that the *yogasanas* place on the lengthening of the spine, the release of chronic pressure on the vertebrae, and the stimulation of fluid circulation in their vicinity.

Function

The semirigid nucleus pulposus acts like a swivel ball between the two near-planar surfaces of the relevant vertebrae. As a swivel, it allows relative tilt, rotation, and shearing motion of the two vertebral plates. Though these reorientations may be of small magnitude at one joint, the combined effect along the length of the spine can be substantial (Table 4.A-1). Additionally, the disc acts as a shock absorber, damping out impulsive shocks and spreading its load over a larger area by spreading laterally on compression. Under axial compression, the nucleus pulposus bears 75% of the load, the annulus 25%.

On spinal lengthening, the external loading of the discs is decreased and the internal preloading expands them to a more spherical shape. On spinal compression due to increased loading, the nucleus pulposus flattens and broadens; in a healthy disc, the thickness will decrease by about 1.4 mm for a 100-kilogram (220-pound) load, whereas in a diseased disc the loss of disc height is more like 2.0 mm and recovery will be incomplete on releasing the load. Diseased or not, as the axially-loaded disc broadens, it presses radially on the annulus thereby being transformed from a vertical stress to a horizontal stress.

The loading on the intervertebral discs also may be asymmetric front to back. Thus, for example, the forward slump so common when sitting will act to compress the anterior portions of the intervertebral discs (and to relieve the pressure of one vertebra pressing

on its neighbor), whereas backbending will act to compress the posterior portions of the same discs [265], Fig. 4.A-9. Indeed the discs are said to be wedge shaped front-to-back in the cervical and lumbar regions even when the spine is held vertically. Heavy loading may be sufficient to force one vertebra onto the one below it; however, even the vertebrae themselves have a certain elasticity and can momentarily deform in response to the load [262].

The gravitational loading of the spine in the normal standing posture will act not only to flatten the discs, but due to the inherent curvatures of the thoracic and lumbar spines, these curvatures may increase through the course of a day, and so contribute substantially or even overwhelmingly to the apparent loss of height by nightfall.

Several factors combine to determine the overall mobility of the cervical, thoracic and lumbar spines. Thus, in the cervical region, the orientation of the facet joints, the relatively thick intervertebral discs, and short transverse and spinous processes all combine to infer a large range of motion to the cervical spine. In contrast, motion in the thorax is highly restricted due to the relatively thin discs, the overlapping of the spinous processes and the binding effects of the ribs. In the lumbar region, the facet orientation strongly restricts spinal rotation, but allows large movements in other directions, as does the relatively large thickness of the discs.

Disc Herniation and Nerve Impingement

As the axial compression on the discs increases on going from the cervical to the lumbar vertebrae, Table 4.A-1, the discs at the base of the spine may rupture on loading, especially in the elderly. In this case, the annulus bulges or tears to release the nucleus pulposus into the intervertebral space, and a herniated disc is born, Fig. 4.C-1c. Note that if the herniation is backward as in Fig. 4.C-1d, the nucleus pulposus will press on elements of the spinal cord, whereas if the herniation is forward, there is no direct compression of the spinal cord.

There are many points of view as to the seriousness of the herniation of an intervertebral disc. As there are no nerves serving the discs, there is no direct pain signal to be felt when a disc is injured. However, because of the injury, the load bearing may shift away from the injured site, thereby injuring a nearby site instead which does respond to the secondary injury with pain, tingling, or numbness.

A herniated disc is most often the cause of lower-back pain (lumbago) and/or buttock-leg pain (sciatica). These are often precipitated by a flexion injury, and as flexion is greatest in the lumbar region, Table 4.A-1, herniation (disc prolapse) is most often seen at L4–L5 and L5–S1, whereas cervical herniation is most often seen at C5–C6 and C6–C7 [195]; thoracic herniation occurs most often at T12 [231]. It is said that the disc between L5 and S1 is more or less degenerated in most people by the age of 20 [303]. Nearly 90% of sciatica problems originate either with the rupture of an intervertebral disc and the pressing of this onto the sciatic nerve, Fig. 4.C-1d, or with osteoarthritis of the lumbo-sacral vertebrae [309]. Pain from nerve impingement also may occur when the diameter of the vertebral canal shrinks as with spinal stenosis [323]. The pain of a herniated disc is discussed from the neurological point of view in Section 10.D, Pain, page 294. Moreover, in certain positions requiring pelvic flexion (*supta padangusthasana*, for example), the herniated disc may trap the rootlet to the sciatic nerve so that it does not move through the foramen, and so becomes painfully stretched. Nerve impingement due to a herniated disc can result in pain on the front,

side or rear of the affected leg (corresponding to impingement at L4, L5, or S1), or to numbness at the inner knee, the side of the calf or on the back of the calf, depending again on whether it is the disc from L4, L5, or S1 that is involved [183].

It is still something of an open question as to whether students with lower-back pain should bend forward or backward for relief. A recent study [368] showed that statistically better results were obtained with mild backbending, however, there were a number of subjects who did better with mild forward bending. The backbending result is understandable in terms of a disc that is herniated backward but is pushed forward, away from the spinal cord, by increasing the lordosis, thereby lessening the pain and shortening the time to regain the pain-free range of motion of the spine.

The intervertebral discs also experience an additional compressive force when one rotates about the spine, as in *maricyasana III*, for example [240]. This compression can be avoided if the spinal lengthening is performed as a prelude to the twists. In spinal rotation, some of the sheaths in the annulus are stretched, while others are relaxed, depending on the sense of the twist (clockwise or counterclockwise), and on the fiber orientations within each of the sheaths. Extreme twisting as in *ardha matsyendrasana I* can also lead to tears in the curtains of some of the sheaths, thus weakening the annulus and setting the stage for herniation; this is less likely if the twist is performed in a conrotatory rather than in a disrotatory manner, page 78.

The pain of a herniated disc often follows from the disc contents being forced backward into the spinal canal and impinging on the spinal nerves. Impingement also can be on the nerves serving the pelvis [183], with referred pain then sensed as coming from the groin, rectum, bladder, *etc.* When this is the case, the pain should be relieved by mild backbends such as *setu bandhasana* which force the expelled nucleus forward again [316, 368]. However, such *yogasanas* must be done with deliberate spinal lengthening to be effective pain relievers [60]. Note too that pain is a very subjective sensation, with strong modulation made possible by psychological factors (Section 10.D, Pain, page 294). Many experiments show that our response to pain is a learned behavior, and that through the connection of the spine to the diaphragm and the breathing process, the spine is very strongly involved with problems of a psychological origin [7].

It has been observed that the pressure of a herniated disc on a sensory nerve in the spinal cord sometimes increases the frequency of its action potential and sometimes decreases this frequency, yet both create the sensation of lower-back pain. Further, even removal of the offending disc may not remove the pain if there are other psychological factors at work [153, 402].

The picture of lower-back pain is further complicated by the fact that pressure on the sciatic nerve may originate not with a herniated disc or a subluxation of the vertebrae, but rather with the pressure of the piriformis muscle within the buttocks on the sciatic nerve bundle as it traverses the buttocks region. This is discussed further in Subsection 4.E, *The Pelvis*, page 96.

Sciatic pain is a difficult phenomenon to understand because there is a frequent lack of correlation between pain and hernia. Many people have a disc hernia but report no symptoms, and many others have undergone surgical repair of their herniation without any diminution of the pain, suggesting that mechanisms other than that shown in Fig. 4.C-1 may be at work. For example, if the site of the pressure on the sciatic nerve or one of its components is in the buttocks rather than in the spinal column, the solution then is not vertebral surgery, but stretching the piriformis muscle in the but-

tocks [402]. At the cervical end of the spine, "pinched nerves" may result from the pressure of the trapezius muscles on nerve roots at a distance from the spinal column rather than from the pressure of a herniated cervical disc.

Yet another possible mechanism is advanced by Faber and Walker [132], who argue that the spinal ligaments normally hold the discs in their centered positions between the vertebrae. If and when the intraspinal ligaments become overstretched, their hold on a disc is loosened and the disc is then free to bodily move backward and press on the vulnerable nerves. In this case, one needs joint-proliferant therapy to rebuild ligaments and so strengthen the spine. Sarno [402] also argues that sciatic pain is the result of a high resting-muscle-tone, (Subsection 7.B, page 204) due to psychological tension, and that resolution of the psychological problem will resolve the pain problem.

The facet joints of the spine not only distribute the compressive load on the spine among all of the component joints, but also protect the nucleus pulposus from injury during extreme motions. Were the nucleus pulposus to degenerate or become dehydrated, the facet joints close and so bear more of the weight compressing the spine. When the discs are healthy, 16% of the compressive load of the body weight is carried on the facet joints of the lumbar spine, but this increases to 70% when the discs in the lumbar spine lose their thickness [476]. The increased bone-to-bone contact experienced when the discs collapse can be very painful.

Both the vertebrae and the discs that separate them can be damaged by aging or by overloading them. Thus, the compressional strength of the lumbar vertebrae in 60–70 year olds is only half that in 20–30 year olds, and lumbar herniation is encouraged when stoop lifting with the legs straight, as when recovering from *uttanasana*.

The compressive load on the facet joints of the lumbar vertebrae can be relieved by spinal flexion, whereas extension tends to heighten the forces tending to shear the facets of such joints. This latter can be avoided in backbends by working to keep the lumbar spine extended, pulling the back rim of the pelvis toward the knees.

SECTION 4.D.
CEREBROSPINAL FLUID

Function and Composition

The central nervous system, composed of the brain and the spinal cord, is surrounded by several continuous layers of tissue which hold it as if it were in a sack. The innermost layer of that sack is called the arachnoid [109, 195, 225, 229, 473]. Between the outer layer of the central nervous system and the arachnoid layer is a thin void, the subarachnoid space; the outermost layer of the water-proof sack, called the dura mater or dural membrane, is a tough layer of randomly oriented fibers of great strength. A clear, colorless cerebrospinal fluid (CSF), is generated in the four ventricles of the brain, and fills the subarachnoid space, the spinal canal, and a small channel running down the gray matter of the spinal cord [473] (see also Section 16.A, Structure and Function of the Eyes, page 411).

The CSF acts to cushion the brain and spinal cord from mechanical shocks. Note too that since the brain itself is 80% water and the CSF has a density very nearly that of water, the brain will very nearly float in the CSF. Due to this flotation effect, the average brain of 1400 gm weight in air has a weight of only 50 gm when floating in the

CSF [225].* In addition to mechanically protecting the brain and spinal cord, the CSF also is active in transferring brain metabolites into and out of the deeper recesses of their structures, nourishing the cells in the 2–4 mm outer layer of the brain's surface (Subsection 3.A, *The Cortex: Site of Conscious Action*, page 24) and maintaining a constant environment for the various brain cells. Signals regarding the status of the CSF are sent to the nerve centers in the hypothalamus [389].

The composition of CSF shows it to be somewhat like ultrafiltered blood, *i.e.*, like blood but lacking the red and white corpuscles and virtually all proteinaceous material. In this, it resembles the aqueous humor of the eyeball (Subsection 16.A, *The Internal Structure of the Eye*, page 413) and reinforces the concept of the eye being made of brain-like tissues. However, CSF does differ quantitatively from filtered blood and aqueous humor in the concentrations of certain simple ions [109].

As the ventricles of the brain produce a steady stream of CSF, and the brain and spinal canal are otherwise a closed system, there must be a mechanism for the reabsorption of the CSF, lest the internal pressure of CSF build to dangerous levels. This reabsorption of the CSF is accomplished by small structures in the arachnoid layer called villi, which absorb CSF and empty their burden into the nearby venous blood supply. It requires approximately 125 ml of CSF to fill the subarachnoid and spinal space, and this amount is reabsorbed in about 4 to 6 hours.

The pressure of the CSF within the spinal canal is readily measured by access to this area through lumbar puncture; hydrostatic pressures of only 5 to 15 mm Hg are report-

---

* The near-neutral buoyancy of the brain and spinal cord when floating in the CSF means that upon inversion, there will be little or no tendency for the brain and spinal cord to either rise or fall. It also means that if a particular point on the skull is pressed (as in *sirsasana*), the pressure is transmitted equally to all parts of the brain, not just to that part closest to the point being pressed.

ed [195, 225], corresponding to column heights of water of 70 to 200 mm (3 to 8 inches).

Yoga and CSF Pulsations of the Medial Suture

The dural membrane presses against the medial suture, the front-to-back line in the skull where the parietal bones meet, Fig. 4.D-1. Were the production of CSF to proceed too far, then pressurization of the dural membrane would press to open the medial suture wider. However, the suture contains pressure sensors, such that when over-pressurized, the sensors report the condition to the hypothalamus, which then directs the

production of CSF to slow and the reabsorption of CSF to quicken. Once reabsorption has lowered the pressure at the suture to too-low a value, the sensors then report a contrary condition and the deactivation/activation roles of the production/reabsorption processes are reversed (Fig. 21.B-1).

As a result of the processes described above, the pressure of CSF in the central nervous system oscillates at about ten cycles per minute, and so too does the opening of the medial suture! The monitoring of this CSF pulse is a prime concern of craniosacral therapy [469], the first step of which is to manipulate the bones of the skull so as to release any jamming at the sutures.

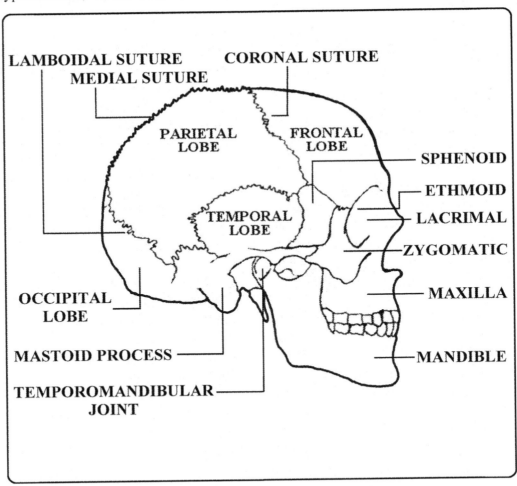

Fig. 4.D-1. The various cranial and facial bones comprising the skull, and the sutures which define the various cranial lobes.

Adjustment of the craniosacral pulse is then possible in the hands of a trained worker, so as to restore good health. Muscle tension can manifest itself as a resistance of the sutures to open and close in response to CSF pulsation [469].

One easily can imagine that the practice of *sirsasana I* and its variations could be a very effective means of keeping the sutures of the skull open, supple and free of calcification. That the sutures of the skull contain blood vessels, innervated pressure receptors, collagen and elastic fibers all suggest that the sutures were meant to be opened, rather than cemented shut.

The stance of the medical establishment in actively denying the existence of the CSF pulse and the movement of the cranial plates about the sutures ("... cranial therapy [is] a quack method of 'manipulating' the bones of the skull. As anyone who has studied anatomy ought to know, the bones of the skull are fused together and cannot be manipulated" [121]) is perhaps another example of the Tomato Effect (Box 1.A-1, *Yogasana, Medicine and the Tomato Effect*, page 5), in operation to this day. If the sutures are indeed closed, one wonders then, "Why is the area in question rife with elastic tissue, pressure and stretch receptors?"

Also within the realm of reason is the idea that the significant rise and fall of the CSF pressure involves a corresponding rise and fall of the CSF level in the subarachnoid space. It is imaginable then, that one could sense the level of CSF in the subarachnoid space by sensing the level of tension in the dural membrane or at the medial suture resulting from the pressurization. Perhaps this is the mechanism whereby B.K.S. Iyengar is able to convert normally subconscious signals into consciousness, thereby sensing the level of CSF in the spinal canal in various *yogasanas*.

Experiments show that the CSF is in motion within its space, especially so when the body is in motion so as to produce different pressures in different parts of the system [109]. Much as energy can be felt to follow a circular path, moving up the front of the chest and down the back in the *yogasanas*, the CSF is known to flow up the anterior side of the spinal cord and down the posterior side [229]. Through this action, the brain and spinal cord are kept bathed in a constantly refreshed pool of CSF, which aids the blood in the maintenance of the brain cells. The health benefits of *yogasanas* in regard keeping the CSF in circulation must be appreciable, especially in *sirsasana I*. However, should this circulation be blocked in some way, then intracranial pools of stagnant CSF are pressurized by the incoming fluid from the ventricles, and should the pressure sensors malfunction at this point, the result is a hydrocephalic condition (also known as "water on the brain"). Dangerously high pressures of CSF can act to extrude the brain through the foramen magnum, the opening in the base of the skull.

SECTION 4.E. THE SKULL AND PELVIS: AXIAL APPENDAGES OF THE SPINE

The skull and pelvis ideally are centered on the axis of the spinal column, and so are known as axial appendages of the spine.

The Skull

As shown in Fig. 4.D-1, the skull is composed of many more bones than one might guess at first, *i.e.*, 8 cranial and 14 facial bones. One might at first opt for only two, the skull and lower jaw, however, this is very much an under-estimation, as the Figure shows. Surprisingly, seven bones must come together to form the eye socket [345].

Each of the various lobes of the brain (Fig. 3.A-1) is protected by a bony plate of the skull. With these plates linked by the appropriate sutures, they add a certain elasticity to the skull, making it a shock absorber, much like the arches of the feet (Fig. 8.D-4) and the vertebral discs of the spine. Flexibility of the sutures of the skull is discussed in Subsection 4.D, *Yoga and CSF Pulsations of the Medial Suture*, page 94.

The lower jaw (the mandible) is held to the skull by synovial joints of the ball-and-socket type, and while gravity encourages the jaw to hang down, the masseter muscles of the jaw keep the lips pursed and the mouth closed. When in a particularly relaxing *yogasana* position, the mouth can be allowed to open somewhat in order to relax the masseters, but the breath should nonetheless continue to move through the nasal passages. Excessive tension in the masseters of the jaw leads to clutching the floor with the toes when standing.

The Pelvis

Because the pelvis has a nonzero height and has joints both to the bones above it (the sacrum) and to bones below it (the femurs), it can be bent at either or both of these places, *i.e.*, at the lumbar spine and/or at the hip joints. If we call these two places for possible motion "the upper hinge" and "the lower hinge", the tendency in beginners is to bend forward, sideward or backward more at the upper hinge; what has to be learned in *yogasana* practice is how to bend more at the lower hinge and less at the upper. That is to say, the upper hinge is to be kept open with the spine straight, and the lower hinge closed at the hip joint(s), either forward, sideward, or backward as the pose demands. It is an open question as to whether the lower hinge should be involved or not in spinal twisting (Subsection 4.A,

Conrotatory and Disrotatory Actions, page 78).

As shown in Fig. 4.E-1, the pelvis consists of eight bony parts and five moveable joints. The bones of the pelvis are the two symmetric ilium bones, which are joined to one another to form a joint anteriorly at the pubic symphysis, to the spinal column through the left and right sides of the sacral plate at the base of the spine, and to each of the legs via the hip joints. The bony plate of the coccyx, joined to the base of the sacral plate, is the eighth bone of the pelvis. Taken together, the pelvic bones form two joints where the sacrum and the ilia meet posteriorly, the pubic symphysis where the ilia join anteriorly, and the two hip joints where the femurs join the pelvis.

Just opposite the joint forming the pubic symphysis, the ilium bones form a wedge-shaped opening in the posterior of the pelvis, and the sacral plate, being a wedge-shaped fusion of five vertebrae as well (Fig. 4.E-1), just fits into this space, forming the sacroiliac joint at each side. The sacroiliac joints are angled at +/–20º from the vertical and are largely synovial joints supported by ligaments.

Both the sacroiliac joints and the pubic symphysis are cartilaginous joints as well. In infants, the mating surfaces of the sacroiliac joint are smooth and allow considerable motion, however, as we age, the surfaces become reshaped so as to have many interlocking hills and valleys which act to strongly restrict motion at this joint; in old age, the joint may become fused and totally immobile. The sacroiliac joint acts as a shock absorber, and should this joint degenerate, then the shock-absorbing task falls more heavily on the intervertebral joints, overloading them and encouraging their degeneration in turn.

The sacrum itself is curved convexly from the rear, just opposite to that of the lumbar spine. Just below the sacrum lies the

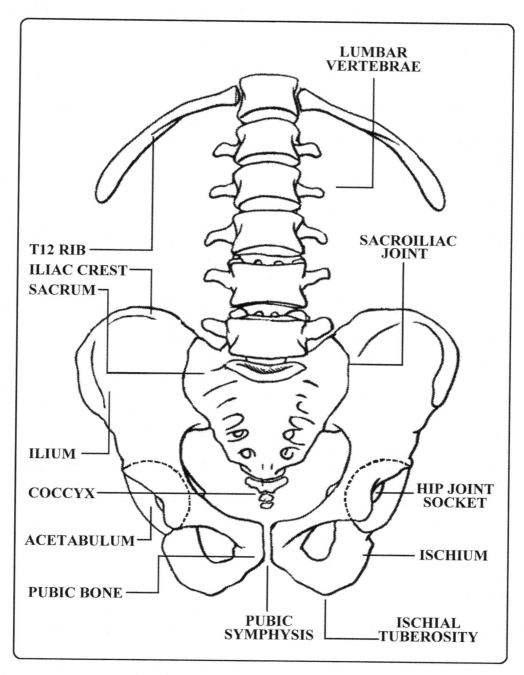

Fig. 4.E-1. Anterior view of the relative orientations of the lowest rib, the lumbar vertebrae and the sacrum with respect to the ilium bones of the pelvis [228].

coccyx, another plate of fused vertebrae, however, it is joined only to the sacrum and not to the pelvis proper [228]. In ancestral animals, the coccyx was responsible for wagging the tail using the muscle joining it to the ischium. The pelvis is supported from below by the femur bones of the upper legs, the connection being made at the socket of the hip joint (acetabulum, Fig. 4.E-1).

In the newborn, the ilium, the ischium and the pubic bones are separate bones which later fuse to form the acetabulum once the legs begin to bear weight [319], whereas the vertebrae of the sacrum maintain their individuality up to about age 25, at which time they too fuse into a single plate [270].

Being essentially a bowl (the word "pelvis" stems from the Latin word for basin), the pelvis has a floor which is a web of muscles designed to control various functions, digestive and sexual. In an upright creature such as man, the pelvis is shaped to carry the organs of digestion, elimination and reproduction. However, the pelvis in the adult male and female are noticeably different, being much broader but shorter in the latter to accommodate childbirth. The joints of the pelvis are important in not only transmitting the forces of the leg bones to the upper body, but also are important in the birthing process. Yet another difference is that in the female pelvis, there are only two segments of the sacrum bound by ligaments to the ilia, whereas for men, the number is three [270].

In adult women, during the latter part of the menstrual cycle, during menopause and during pregnancy, the pubic symphysis and the sacroiliac joints are destabilized by hormones, and so become more flexible. Women in general are more flexible in the pelvic area, whether pregnant or not [5], and because of this, childbirth can misalign the sacroiliac joint [270]. Though the sacroiliac joint is spanned by ligaments, there is only one muscle that spans the joint, the piriformis.

As the sacrum fits nicely into the crevice provided by the ilia and is held in place by relatively few ligaments, Fig. 4.E-2, it is more tightly held when the load on it from above is as large as possible. This means that the sacroiliac joint is most stable when one is standing and is much less so when lying down. For students who are weak in the sacroiliac joint, when twisting in a seated position as in *maricyasana III*, the pelvis should be rotated in the same direction as the chest (a conrotatory motion) in order to keep the lumbar, sacrum and ilia in alignment and so avoid further problems.

The pubic symphysis is a joint within the pelvic girdle, lying opposite the sacroiliac and consisting of two bones which are separated by a thick fibrocartilaginous pad; it is relatively immobile and this rigidity helps to stabilize the sacroiliac joint in turn. However, it occasionally happens that in the course of childbirth, the pubic symphysis separates, allowing the sacrum to move forward. In general, motion about the sacroiliac joints and the pubic symphysis are minimal at best. The joint between the coccyx and the sacrum can undergo flexion and extension only, and only during defecation or childbirth [228].

Front-to-back motion in the pelvis is coupled with side-to-side motion, such that when the top of the sacral plate moves backward (as in *bakasana*, for example), the two pelvic rims move toward one another, whereas the two ischial tuberosities (the sitting bones) laterally move away from one another, Fig. 4.E-3. Because these actions are reciprocal, if one rolls the upper thighs outward as when doing *uttana padasana* [209], the sitting bones move inward and the top of the sacrum is pulled up toward the belly button.

The ischial tuberosities are the bony prominences in each of the buttocks, and bear the weight of the body in a person who is seated. Just how one sits on the ischial tuberosities is of great importance to the student of *yogasana*, for if one sits on the forward edge in *dandasana*, for example, then the pelvis is tipped so that the lumbar spine is pressed forward somewhat, and the proper spinal alignment results, whereas if one sits on the back edge, it is very difficult to pull the lumbar spine into alignment, especially so in related seated poses such as *krounchasana* or *navasana*.

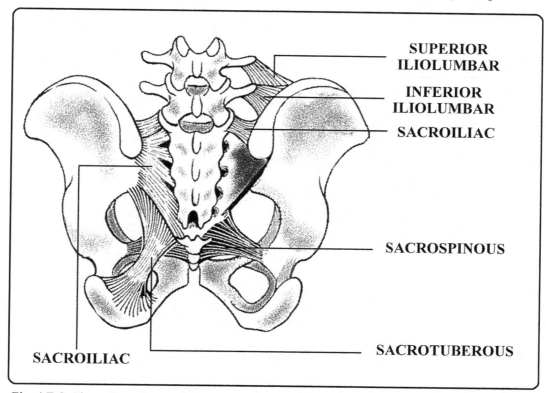

Fig. 4.E-2. The various ligaments of the pelvis, binding the sacrum to the ilium, as seen in a posterior view [228].

Given that the heads of the femur bones are firmly set into the hip joints, and that the strong muscles of the upper legs are attached to the lower rim of the pelvis at several points, it is clear that motion of the pelvis is largely driven by action from the legs (see Section 8.D, The Skeletal Appendages, page 247). Thus lateral opening and closing of the pelvis is dictated by rotation of the legs, and forward-backward tipping of the pelvis is controlled by pressing the thighs backward or forward. Among the more difficult *yogasanas* to perform are those that have one leg positioned so as to encourage the pelvis to tip in one direction and the other leg positioned so as to encourage it to tip in the opposite direction, *e.g.*, *eka pada urdhva dhanurasana* or *hanumanasana*.

One can think of the lower spine, pelvis and upper legs as forming a sort of seesaw in that while standing, for example, if the upper thighs are pressed backward, the lumbar is pushed forward and the spine becomes lordotic (Fig. 4.E-4a), whereas if the lumbar spine is pressed backward and flattened, then the upper thighs are pushed forward (Fig. 4.E-4b). The postures in Fig. 4.E-4 are discussed from the point of view of tonic reflexes in Section 7.D, Reflex Actions, page 211.

It is part of the paradox of yoga that the proper action in most poses is to work both of these seemingly opposite actions simultaneously, *i.e.*, in *tadasana*, one presses the thighs back and at the same time, pulls the navel to the spine, drops the centers of the buttocks toward the heels, and pulls the hamstrings onto the femurs. As a result, the thighs move under the pose to support it and the pelvis tilts to flatten and elongate the lumbar curve, bringing the skeleton into a more vertical alignment. Conversely, if you wish to straighten the legs in *setu bandhasana*, lift the lumbar spine yet higher (but not excessively so) and the thighs will drop

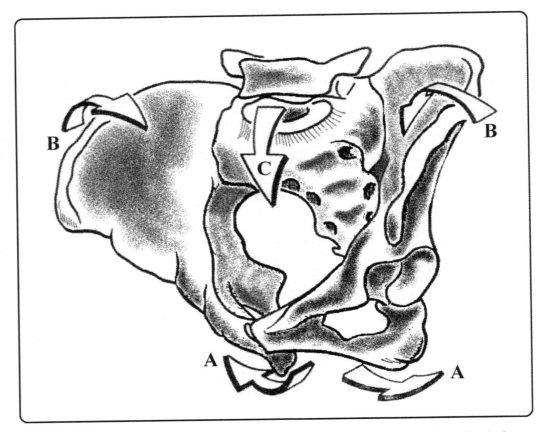

Fig. 4.E-3. A frontal view of the pelvis, showing how an inward rotation of the off-axis femur bones (see Fig. 8.D-1a) increases the distance between the sitting bones (**A**), leading to a decreased distance between the iliac crests (**B**), and a forward thrust of the top of the sacrum (**C**), as in *adho mukha svanasana* [228].

in the direction of the floor and the legs will straighten. Your *padmasana* legs will come to the floor in *matsyasana* if you will lift the lumbar spine higher, as this seesaw action about the pelvis lowers the legs. In *navasana*, the concave lumbar curve will be restored if the thighs of the lifted legs are pressed down, away from the ribs, as this pulls the lumbar spine forward in this *yogasana*.

Note too that the pelvis has its complementary effect on the legs as well. Thus, for example, the tendency of the knees in *tadasana* to be either too close (knock knees) or too far apart (bow legs) reflects misalignment of the femur heads in the hip joints (Section 8.D, The Skeletal Appendages, page 247) [260]. Further, if the psoas

muscles connecting the lumbar spine to the inner/upper femurs are tight, they will roll the thighs out such that one tends to stand on the outer edges of the feet. This is most apparent when beginners perform *urdhva dhanurasana*.

SECTION 4.F. *NADIS, CHAKRAS,* AND *PRANA*

Historical Perspective

Long before the art of dissection was practiced, the ancient yogis were able to deduce certain subtle aspects of human anatomy through close observation of their own bodies [31, 151, 212, 374, 376, 398]. They estimated that within the body there

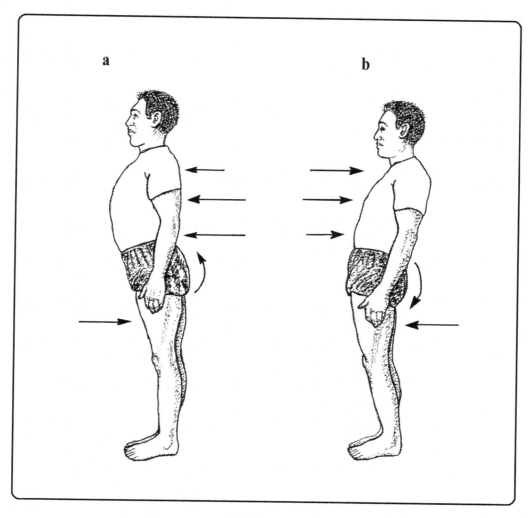

Fig. 4.E-4. (**a**) When the front thighs are pressed backward (and rolled inward) in *tadasana*, the back rim of the pelvis is tipped forward, the spine is pressed forward and the lumbar spine becomes lordotic. (**b**) If instead, the thighs are pressed forward in *tadasana*, the centers of the buttocks descend, the spine is pressed backward and the lumbar region is flattened. Proper alignment of the pelvis and spine in *tadasana* requires the simultaneous application of the actions of both **a** and **b**, *i.e.*, co-contraction of the quadruceps and hamstring muscles.

were between 75,000 and 350,000 channels called *nadis*; the *nadis* are pathways of sensation along which the life force, *prana*, travels. For our purposes, the first of the three most important *nadis* is the *sushumna*, Fig. 4.F-1, located within the *merudanda*, a column extending from the occiput at the base of the skull to the coccyx. The *sushumna* bifurcates at the throat, with branches that ascend both anteriorly and posteriorly,

to rejoin at the *brahmarandra*, a ventricular cavity within the brain.

The two other major *nadis*, *ida* and *pingala*, lie essentially parallel to the *merudanda*, but with each weaving back and forth so as to cross each other and the *merudanda* between 5 and 8 times. The *ida* originates at the right side of the coccyx and terminates at the left nostril, whereas *pingala* originates at the left side of the coccyx and ter-

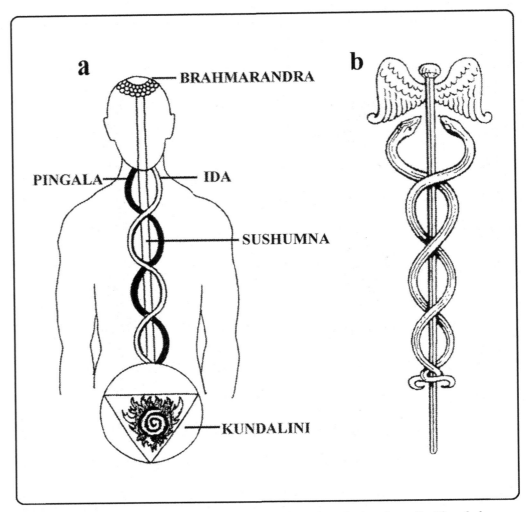

Fig. 4.F-1. (**a**) The vertical *sushumna* and the oscillating *ida* and *pingala nadis*. The *chakras* are those points at which the *sushumna, ida* and *pingala* cross. *Kundalini*, resting at the bottom of the *sushumna*, ascends the *chakras*, finally reaching the crown *chakra* at the top of the skull. (**b**) The ancient caduceus, the medical symbol of the Western world, has a close relation to the symbol (**a**) of the Ayurvedic physicians of the Eastern world.

minates at the right nostril. Those points along the *merudanda* where the *ida, pingala,* and *sushumna nadis* intersect, Fig. 4.F-1, are called *chakras*. The *chakras* are also referred to as wheels, for they are the points from which many other *nadis* radiate.

The seven *chakras* that are generally recognized and their associated properties are listed in Table 4.F-1. When a *chakra* is open to the flow of *prana*, then the characteristics of the *chakra* become manifest in the individual. For example, those people for whom the heart *chakra* (*anahata*) is optimally open are healthy, compassionate, and psychologically stable and centered. The heart *chakra* is associated with the color green and the air element. In contrast, for someone whose highest open *chakra* is the belly *chakra* (*swadisthana*), their personality is friendly and creative, with strong emotional feelings. The color of this *chakra* is orange and the element is water. It must be said that many other interpretations of the *chakras* are available.

TABLE 4.F-1. CHARACTERISTICS OF THE SEVEN *CHAKRAS* [374, 376, 444]

Chakra Name	Position on Spine	Terminal Plexus	Organ/Gland Innervated	Autonomic Association	Color/ Element	Effect on Opening
Crown *Sahasrara*	Crown of head	—	Pituitary, pineal	—	Violet/Electric	Universal love, power, influence, transcendence
Third Eye *Ajna*	C1	Nasociliary	Pituitary, pineal, brain, ears	—	Indigo/Electric	Intuitive, charismatic, knowing, detached
Throat *Vishuddha*	C3	Pharyngeal	Thyroid, parathyroid, throat, eyes	Parasympathetic cranial	Blue/Ether	Communication, creativity, content, nerves centered
Heart *Anahata*	T1	Cardiac	Heart, thymus, lungs, lymph glands	Parasympathetic vagus nerves	Green/Air	Healing, compassion, centered,
Solar Plexus *Manipura*	T8	Celiac	Adrenals, diaphragm, skin	Adrenals T10–T12 sympathetic, vagus nerve	Yellow/Fire	Outgoing, elevation, vitality, psychic awareness
Belly *Svadhisthana*	L1	Hypogastric	Pancreas, ovaries, intestines	Sympathetic from lumbar	Orange/Water	Feelings, friendliness, intuitive
Root *Muladhara*	S4	Sacral	Testes	L1–L3 sympathetic; S2–S4 parasympathetic	Red/ Earth	Healthy, sexual power, passion, confidence

The importance of the *chakras* is understood to be that when they all are open, as through optimum physiological and psychological health, then *prana* can flow unimpeded through *ida* and *pingala* to reach the nostrils. Given this state, a super energy called *kundalini* then can flow up the *sushumna* to the crown *chakra*, resulting in a state of bliss. This sounds at first remarkably like the discussion of nasal laterality, (Section 12.C, page 374), but one must remember that, with respect to *nadis*,

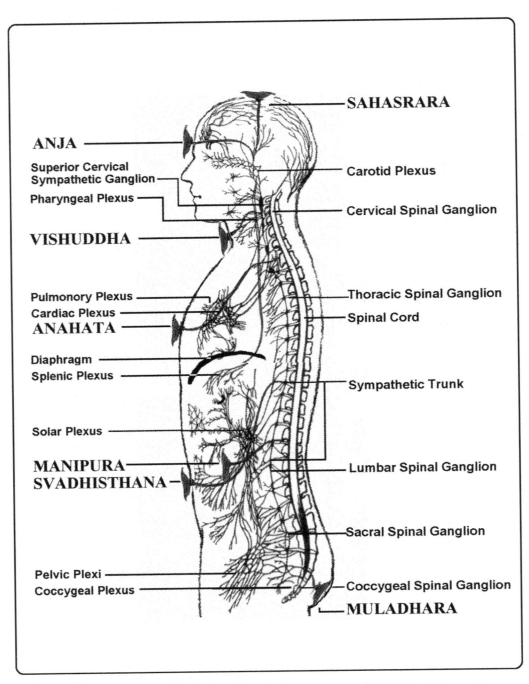

Fig. 4.F-2. Correspondence of the six major *chakras* (upper-case labels) and the various nerve plexi in the body (lower-case labels).

chakras, and *prana*, one is dealing here with structures and/or substances that do not necessarily exist on the physical plane. It is the job of the aspiring student to successively reopen the higher *chakras*. To the extent yoga can influence this flow of nervous energy, *yogasana* and *pranayama* are of use in opening the higher *chakras*. Needless to say, this is but a very brief abstract of a subject that has been studied for thousands of years. For deeper discussions, see for example [130].

Relation of Chakras to Anatomical Features

In trying to set this interesting but inferred topography of *nadis*, *chakras* and *prana* into correspondence with modern anatomical understanding, *ida* and *pingala* may be taken to refer to the parasympathetic and sympathetic nervous systems, respectively, and the *chakras* to the known nerve plexi radiating from the spine. Iyengar [211] further identifies the efferent nerves as the *karma-nadi* (nerves of action) and the afferent nerves as the *jnana nadi* (nerves of knowledge), and states, "Perfect understanding between nerves of action and nerves of knowledge working together in concord, is yoga." With reference to the Chinese system of acupuncture, the yogic concepts of *prana*, *nadi*, *ida* and *pingala* correspond to *chi*, meridians, *yin* and *yang*, respectively.

For the sake of simplicity one, might associate the *nadis* with nerves, the *chakras*

with nerve plexi, and *prana* with nerve impulses. Pushing the analogy further, the *merudanda* is the spinal cord, and *ida* and *pingala* are the two branches of the autonomic nervous system, the sympathetic and parasympathetic (Chapter 6, THE AUTONOMIC NERVOUS SYSTEM, page 133). Indeed, as listed in the Table, except for the crown *chakra*, the other six *chakras* can be put into one-to-one correspondence with known anatomical neural plexi having origins at known levels along the spine and both sympathetic and parasympathetic innervation, Fig. 4.F-2. Each of these plexi (*chakras*) is known to innervate one or more glands and/or visceral organs, just as explained by the ancient yogis. Thus for example, *anahata*, the heart *chakra* of the ancients, can be thought to originate in the vicinity of T1, and to sympathetically innervate the heart, lungs, thymus gland, and the lymph glands. Parasympathetic innervation of the same area involves branches of the vagus nerve originating at cranial nerve X (Subsection 6.D, *The Vagus Nerves*, page 152). On the other hand, the belly *chakra* anatomically has sympathetic innervation at the L1 level, and corresponds to the hypogastric plexus encompassing the pancreas, the intestines, and the ovaries of women.

The possible scientific significance of the colors assigned to the various *chakras* in Table 4.F-1 is discussed further in Subsection 16.D, *Color Therapy*, page 426.

Chapter 5

THE NERVES

All of the sensory organs of the body report the levels of their sensations (signals referring, for example, to pain, temperature, blood pressure, stomach acidity, or the level of oxygen in the blood) to a central site in the body (the central nervous system), where they are evaluated and acted upon. Another set of signals is then sent from the central site to effector organs internal and external (for example, the muscles of the upper arm, nuclei within the hypothalamus, or the blood vessels of the spleen) directing how their states are to be adjusted in order to maintain or change conditions in the body at that moment. The in-coming signals representing the levels of sensation may be either in the conscious realm or in the sub-conscious, with the received information either integrated or not with that from other sensors of the same or different types. Once the totality of the in-coming signal or only a small part of it is held to be a cause for action, the body's response as out-going signals to muscles and organs may be instantaneous or may be drawn out over a lifetime.

All aspects of this sequential information gathering, integration and evaluation, decision-making as to course of action, and setting the course of action in motion is the work of the nervous systems of the body and their component parts, the nerves and the spaces between them. Obviously, there are many decisions that have to be made among an infinity of choices. Were all of the factors that enter into such a decision to be

simultaneously in the conscious realm, we would be overwhelmed.

The nerves of the body are organized into systems and subsystems depending upon function [102, 345]. At the highest level, the nerves of the brain and spinal cord form the central nervous system, Fig. 2.A-1, while those nerves outside the central nervous system (but connected to it) form the peripheral nervous system (Chapter 2, page 13). The central nervous system is the terminus for information coming from the sensory organs, the site of information integration and decision making, and the origin of nerve signals deemed appropriate for activating the effector organs. Those nerves of the peripheral system that radiate from the brain are called cranial nerves (Section 2.C, page 17), whereas those that radiate from the spine are called spinal nerves.

Bundles of nerves having approximately the same origin and destination are called "tracts". There are tracts within the cranial lobes and between lobes, all using the white matter underlying the gray matter of the cerebrum, and tracts that connect the higher brain centers with the lower ones in the spinal cord.

If one imagines the nervous system to be like a railroad, then the nerves are the rails, going from a grand central station out to peripheral ones, the trains are the electric depolarization waves passing along the nerve fibers (see below), some moving rapidly and some much more slowly depending upon the urgency of their cargo. The gaps between communicating nerves, called synapses, are switching centers redirecting or stopping further movement, and the engineer making the decisions as to scheduling, course, speed, *etc.*, is the central nervous system. The ganglia of the nervous system are the large urban centers toward which many rail lines converge and where many passengers change trains. The trip may be one-way or it may be a round-trip, but either way, the train always makes a stop at the central nervous system, except possibly for the enteric nervous system, Chapter 18, THE GASTROINTESTINAL ORGANS AND DIGESTION, page 441.

As passengers on this train, we may view all aspects of the trip with curiosity and take pleasure in what we see, or we may sleep through the entire adventure, unaware of the interesting territory through which we pass. Perhaps we no longer pay attention because we have been there so many times before and we do not make the effort to find what is new about what can be seen from the train.

Our goal in this Chapter is to discuss the nature of the in-coming (afferent) signals from the senses, their transport over a distance of up to 1 meter to the central nervous system, the nature of the out-going (efferent) signals from the central nervous system to the effector organs, and how these signals interact among themselves to prompt a decision for action or inhibition. The latter takes place in the central nervous system, comprised of the brain and spinal cord. Key elements of the discussion define just what is meant by "signal", determine how this "signal" is moved from place to place and how it is turned on and off. In a word, the answer to the understanding of these phenomena lies in the area of *bioelectrochemistry*, an area of science lying at the intersection of the fields of biology, electricity and chemistry.

SECTION 5.A. TYPES OF NERVE CELLS

Anatomy of Nerve Cells

All nerve cells distinguish themselves from the surrounding fluids by a thin but selectively permeable wall known as the cell membrane. As shown in Fig. 5.A-1, the cell membrane has a unique molecular structure, the lipid bilayer. The component molecules of the bilayer each have a polar (electrically charged) head which is strongly attracted to water (it is hydrophilic) and a nonpolar hydrocarbon tail which, by its hydrophobic nature, instead is strongly attracted to other hydrophobic, oily molecules such as itself. Due to these preferences for the types of molecule with which the two ends choose to associate, the bilayer is formed from a tail-to-tail alignment, with the polar heads presented to the aqueous phases on each side of the membrane and the nonpolar tails presented to one another. The bilayer membranes are penetrated by protein channels, which act as gates, allowing or blocking the passage of certain ionic substances, Na^+ for example, from one side of the bilayer to the other. All nerve and muscle-cell membranes are constructed of such lipid bilayers, though the proteins enclosed within the bilayer may be different, as may the protein coats surrounding the bilayers [224, 299].

Being cells that serve as signal-carrying components of a larger system, nerve cells (neurons), receive signals from other neurons via their relatively short but highly branched dendrites (afferents, which conduct signals toward the cell body), and send signals to other neurons, muscles or organs via the axons (efferents, which conduct signals away from the cell body); axons are longer structures up to 1 meter in length. The thicker part of the neuron is the cell body, which is filled with a fluid cytoplasm

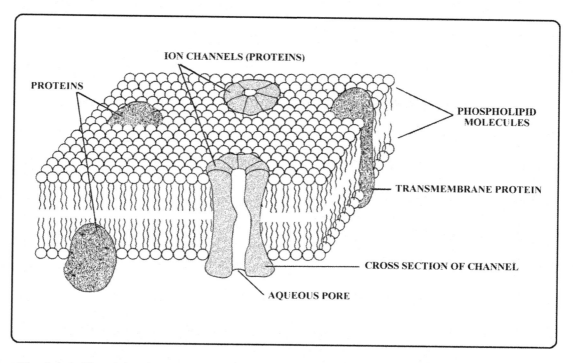

Fig. 5.A-1. The molecular structure of the lipid bilayer membrane, appropriate to all cells in the human body. Shown are the two layers of phospholipid molecules, tail-to-tail, interspersed with various protein molecules, some of which act as ion channels, and some of which only partially penetrate the lipid bilayer.

and several distinctly more solid bodies called organelles. Though the axons of most nerve cells are quite long and thin, containing up to 95% of the fluid content of the neuron, all of the protein synthesis, mitochondria and genetic control functions of the cell lie within the cell body.

The general types of signal-carrying nerve cells are depicted in Fig. 5.A-2. As can be seen there, unipolar cells have a single process appended to the cell body, with the appendage (axon) terminating in dendrites, each of which forms a synaptic connection to neighboring cells, Section 5.C, Nerve Connections; Synapses, page 121. Such unipolar cells are primarily involved in carrying sensory information from the skin to the central nervous system. In a pseudo-unipolar cell, there are two such axonal appendages, each ending in a web of dendrites. One of the two dendritic trees

(the receptor) ends peripherally at skin or muscle, while the other (the transmitter) terminates in the spinal cord. A closely related cell type is the bipolar cell, in which there again are two processes emerging from the cell body, with the receptor process ending in dendrites and the other being a transmitting axon ending with an axonal plate. Bipolar nerve cells are also prominent in the sensory systems, being most often used in the visual, auditory and vestibular systems [57].

Finally, there is the class of multipolar cells in which there is a single axon, but a large and variable number of dendrites, as shown in the Figure; multipolar cells are the most common type of cell in the central nervous system. In the extreme case, the Purkinje cell of the cerebellum has approximately 150,000 dendrites at the receptor end, implying that this cell has 150,000

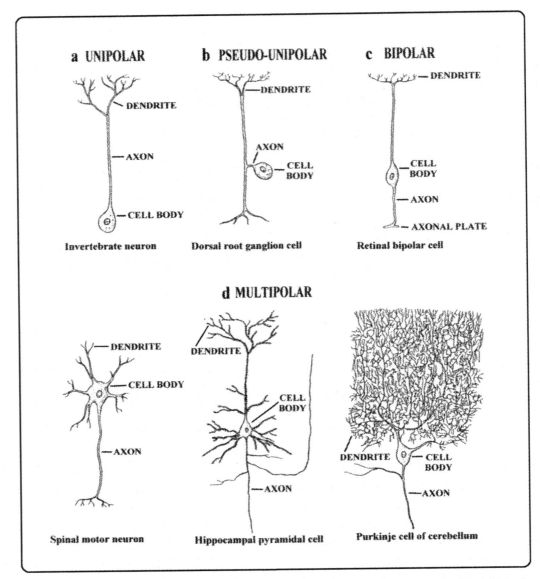

Fig. 5.A-2. Schematic drawings of the branching in (**a**) unipolar, (**b**) pseudo-unipolar, (**c**) bipolar cells and (**d**) three types of multipolar cells. The Purkinje cell is flat and fan-like.

input signals that are summed algebraically and the result sent along the single axon for transmission to an adjacent cell. In addition to the cell types of Fig. 5.A-2 which are actively involved in signal transmission, two other neural cell types called "glial cells" also play important roles.

Nerve cells also may be classified on the basis of their signal-conducting properties rather than on the basis of their shapes. This involves determining their axonal diameter and the velocity of the nerve impulse as it rockets down the axon. This classification scheme is described more fully in Section 5.B, Nerve Conduction, page 114.

As will be seen below, the action of the nerves depends very much on the fact that each cell is wrapped in a membrane which normally is impermeable to certain ions, so that concentration gradients of these ions can be maintained across the membrane, as in Fig. 5.A-3a. The phrase "concentration gradient" refers to the difference in ion concentration at two different points, in this case the inside and the outside of the cell membrane. Because ions are electrically charged, ion gradients imply a net charge separation across the membrane which in turn signifies a voltage difference between the inside and the outside of the membrane.

This is called the transmembrane voltage. When the nerve is stimulated at the receptor end, the permeability of the membrane to specific ions (in this case Na^+, sodium ions) is altered drastically as certain ion channels formed by membrane proteins in the bilayers are opened. The flow of Na^+ ions through the newly opened channels, Fig.

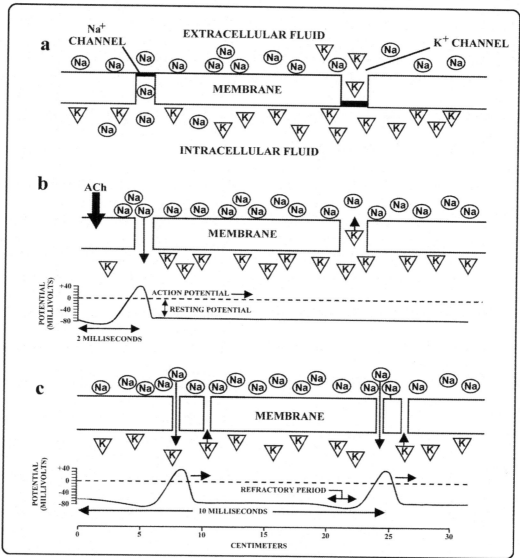

Fig. 5.A-3. (**a**) The neural membrane in the resting state, with the concentration of Na^+ much higher in the extracellular fluid than in the intracellular fluid, and the Na^+ ion channels closed. The reverse situation holds for the K^+ ions, but to a lesser extent. The difference of the Na^+ ion concentrations on the two sides of the membrane results in a transmembrane voltage V of -75 millivolts (mV). (**b**) When the nerve is energized locally by ACh, the ion channels in the membrane open and Na^+ ions flood through them, moving from the outside to the inside of the cell membrane and reducing the transmembrane voltage V to -60 mV or more, *i.e.*, depolarizing it. (**c**) As the channels open sequentially from left to right, one or more depolarization-voltage peaks sweep from left to right on energizing the nerve [222].

5.A-3b, reduces the concentration gradients, and thus the transmembrane voltage. It is this decrease of the induced voltage across the cell's membrane that eventually propagates along the length of the axon as the nerve impulse, or "the signal". The generation and propagation of the nerve impulse is described in more detail in the following Sections.

Not all neurons are simply passive conduits for transmission of a signal from A to B. Were this the case, then it would be hard to see how competing points of view within the brain could be weighed and decided either for or against, or how a compromise ever could be reached. In fact, successful decision making requires the possibility of negative input as well, and this is supplied by cells in the central nervous system called interneurons. The actions of interneurons are always inhibitory, meaning that their action on the transmembrane voltage is to raise it, rather than to lower it as in Fig. 5.A-3b, and thus interneurons act to block transmission of the neural signal. They exert their influence by moderating the interplay between the sensory neurons and the motor neurons, and in doing so, they control our response to the environment. See Section 7.D, Reflex Actions, page 211, for examples of interneurons at work.

Nerve Function

The signal-carrying neurons in our bodies perform three distinct functions. The sensory neurons are afferents, carrying voltage signals from the sensory organs of the body to the spinal cord and brain, and are typically bipolar or pseudo-unipolar, Fig. 5.A-2. Motor neurons are efferents in that they carry signals from the brain and spinal cord to the muscles (skeletal and smooth) and glands, and are generally multipolar. In the brain and in nerve bundles leading thereto and therefrom, many other cell types are found which support the information-carrying role of the neurons, but do not themselves transmit information. These cells, called glial cells, are of two general types. The first of these, the neuroglia, outnumber the neurons by about 50 to 1, and serve to physically support the nerve tissue, acting like collagen (Subsection 9.A, page 273) to glue neighboring units together and so give the brain its large-scale and small-scale shape and structure. Neuroglia also insulate nerves from one another, and aid in the nerve's good health by providing nutrition and by cleaning up debris in the vicinity. They are especially useful in helping to control the ionic concentrations in the extracellular fluid surrounding the nerve cells. The Schwann cells are a second type of glial cell, with a direct impact on nerve conduction. This is discussed further in Section 5.B, Nerve Conduction, page 114.

As is the case with muscles, so too are the nerves a part of the same use-it-or-lose-it game. Thus an often-used neuron can function for a lifetime, and it will have to since neurons do not divide and reproduce once sexual maturity has been reached [313]. On the other hand, unused nerves and nerve circuits eventually wither away in a process called apoptosis. With apoptosis operating in this way, our nervous systems tend to become more highly refined, favoring those circuits used most often (see Section 3.C, Memory, Learning, and Teaching, page 42, for a discussion of how nerves change as they are used repeatedly when practicing *yogasana*, for example), but also becoming more narrow in scope as unused circuits die off as we age [473]. An endless variety of *yogasana* practice will work to keep this scope as broad as possible.

While certain aspects of the nervous system appear fixed, others are capable of reorganization, thanks to the plasticity of the neural circuits in the brain. Thus, by changing the patterns of connection within the nervous systems through their plasticity, we can develop, we can learn, we can grow as individuals in our own unique way. With plasticity, we not only can perform the stereotypical, hard-wired reactions such as walking, but we can also respond advantageously to the trends of the moment, such as riding a unicycle [110]. Not only can we develop new neural patterns, but we can teach them to others. In this context, it is interesting to note that with increasing age there is a shrinkage of mental abilities in general, but at the same time, new connections are made within the brain which can work in beneficial ways to compensate at least in part for losses in other areas [197].

The Motor Unit and Nerve Sensitivity

Though every muscle fiber has a corresponding nerve connected to it for contractile excitation, not every muscle cell receives a unique neural signal, for each motor neuron from the spinal cord branches into between 3 and 300 sub-branches, connecting to between 3 and 300 muscle fibers. Each of the muscle fibers in such a group (called a "motor unit" when considered together with its activating neuron) receives the same excitation signal and at the same time, so that all muscle fibers of a motor unit contract or relax in unison.

The efferent nerves which carry the energizing signal from the spine to the muscles are called the alpha-motor neurons, whereas a second set of efferent nerves, the gamma-motor neurons, adjust the tension within the muscle spindles themselves (Section 7.B, Muscle Sensors; The Mechanoreceptors, page 198).

To put the motor unit in context, those motor units with few muscle fibers connected to the motor nerve offer fine-muscle control as is the case with the muscles controlling the eyes. In contrast, those motor nerves going to several hundred muscle fibers usually innervate muscles used for gross movements such as the postural muscles of the back. Within a large muscle, there will be many independent motor units with little or no coordination of motor-unit firing, for the random contraction and relaxation of multiple motor units provides a smooth muscle action of long duration, whereas the simultaneous firing of all motor units would result in one jerky movement which could be sustained for only a few seconds. Furthermore, by avoiding all of the motor units firing at once, one can achieve a graded response appropriate to the task at hand, *i.e.*, when a large muscle is contracted, the smaller motor units within it are the first to fire, and if that is not sufficient for the task, then other larger and stronger units can be brought into play (Section 7.A, Skeletal Muscle; Structure and Function, page 167).

The various component muscle fibers of a motor unit are not necessarily adjacent to one another but are otherwise in close proximity. The degree of control over the motor unit is apparent when one considers that the motor neuron connected to a hundred or so muscle fibers within a motor unit is itself a part of a web of neurons in the spinal cord totaling approximately 600 nearest neighbors on average, with each of the 600 inputting its excitatory or inhibitory contribution to the transmembrane potential on the motor neuron. These higher-level neurons in turn are connected to approximately 10 billion other neurons within a cerebral hemisphere, all of which again contribute in their own way to the potentials on the intermediate 600! [53] One sees from this that the brain operates by mutual consensus, there being a multitude of inputs competing for expression in the action of the brain.

Mental Control of an Individual Motor Unit

Basmajian and coworkers (summarized in [53]) report on some amazing experimental results, showing that the mind can readily control the firing of a specific motor unit, energizing it and/or other motor units as well, at any chosen time! This series of experiments involved making the motor-unit excitation either visible or audible through suitable electronics, in which case each motor unit has its own characteristic voltage pattern in time when it fires. With a little practice, the subject of the experiment can mentally induce the appearance or disappearance of any one of a number of characteristic motor-unit discharge patterns. This type of biofeedback training requires only about 15 to 20 minutes, after which the control "just happens" without any specific mental effort of the controller beyond thinking of the desired result. After 20 minutes or so of single motor-unit control, the controllers report feeling exhausted, with a stiffness and soreness in the controlled muscles. Note that the learning taking place here is very different from the control of muscles as guided by the proprioceptive signals of tension and position that we normally use when practicing *yogasana* (Section 7.C, Proprioception, page 208). However, that is not to say that one cannot achieve conscious control over single motor units while practicing the *yogasanas*.

The easiest motor units to control are those of the muscles used most often (fingers, arm, *etc.*), while the most difficult to control are those of the muscles used least often, such as those in the back or chest for non-yogis. The degree of difficulty most likely correlates with the relative size of muscles and organs in the somatic motor-cortex homunculus, Fig. 3.A-5. Within a large muscle, the smaller motor units are more easily brought under conscious control.

Some 20% of people cannot learn how to control their motor-unit firing on relaxation. However, if they first contract the corresponding muscle on the other side of the body, then full control of the muscle in question can be achieved. This left-right-symmetry effect probably relates in some obscure way to the inherent left-right asymmetry of the body and the neural cross-talk between them at all neural levels (see Box IV.E-2, *Physical Crossover Requires Neural Crossover*, page 543).

There is a certain resonance between Basmajian's experimental results and Iyengar's statements [211] about bringing every cell of the body under conscious control, of having an awareness at the deepest level of the body. Possibly, without external electronics, Iyengar is able to consciously control individual motor units and sense their levels of excitation in a way parallel to the control shown in Basmajian's experiments!

SECTION 5.B. NERVE CONDUCTION

Generation of an Action Potential

Most neurons, be they sensory, motor, interneuron or neuroendocrine, have in common four local regions which function sequentially in a similar way when the neuron is activated. As a concrete example, consider an afferent sensory neuron in which the sensor is sensitive to the degree of muscle stretch, Fig. 5.B-1. The information flow begins with the input signal from the stretch sensor (called a muscle spindle) at the receptor end of the neuron. Three levels of stretch are shown in the Figure: a brief, gentle stretch (1), a more intense stretch held for the same time (2), and an intense stretch held for a much longer time (3).

The stretching profile (intensity and duration) at the transduction site (the muscle) in each case is transformed from a mechanical stress into an electrical signal called the synaptic potential, A. This transformation is initiated by changes in concentration gradients and in the permeabilities to

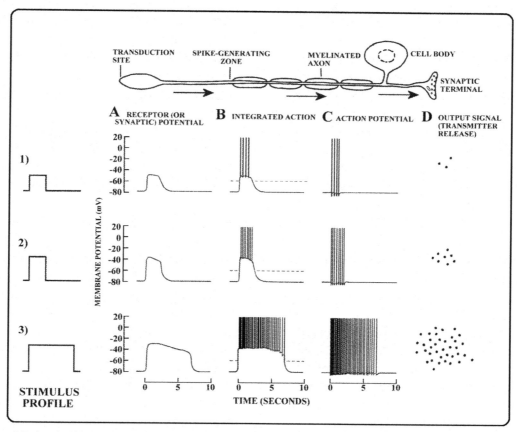

Fig. 5.B-1. The four stages **A** ⟶ **B** ⟶ **C** ⟶ **D** of action, transmitting a signal from the sensory bulb of a muscle spindle (left) to the synaptic terminal (right) along an afferent nerve. Three cases are shown: **1**) A weak stretch (**A**) excites the muscle spindle and generates a receptor potential. This potential is transformed into the frequency realm (**B**) and then becomes the action potential (**C**) that releases a small amount of acetylcholine into the synapse (**D**). **2**) A more intense stretch results in a higher action-potential frequency and consequently more acetylcholine. **3**) A stretch that is both more intense and of a longer duration shows adaptation and a large amount of acetylcholine at the synapse.

certain ions in the cell membranes of the muscle spindles. Further along the axon, the synaptic potential is transformed into an integration signal, B; as shown, this signal contains the profile of the synaptic potential but is also decorated with voltage spikes of constant height but with a frequency* that increases with increasing amplitude of the synaptic potential. It is the spiked part of this voltage profile that becomes the action potential at the far end of the axon, C, with the duration and frequency of the spikes reflecting the duration and intensity, respectively, of the original stimulus in each of our three cases. Finally, the arrival of the action potential at the far end of the neuron acts to release a chemical at the synaptic terminal, D. As shown in the Figure, the amount and

* The " frequency" refers to how many pulse spikes occur in one second, usually given the unit of Hertz (Hz), or equivalently, cycles per second (cps). The shorter the time between pulses, the higher their frequency, and *vice versa*. By way of example, the time between pulse maxima in the alternating-current (AC) house voltage in the US is 0.0167 seconds, therefore its frequency is 1/ 0.0167 = 60 Hz.

duration of this chemical messenger (called a neurotransmitter) is an accurate reflection of the profile of the input stimulus, being stronger and more long lasting in the case of the stronger and longer-held stretch. All four phases of the conduction process are more or less electrochemical in nature, with the second and third serving to shape the electrical character of the signal as it moves down the length of the neuron, while the first is more electromechanical and the fourth phase is more electrochemical in nature.

When there is a constant input signal from a receptor for a long duration as in example 3) of Fig. 5.B-1, the receptor potential tends to fall with time, due to a process called adaptation. This is not due to any fatigue of the sensors involved, but instead reflects the tendency of sensors in the body to respond preferentially to changes in sensory signals rather than to constant sensory intensity (Subsection 10.B, *Receptor Adaptation*, page 285).

But what is it that actually moves down the axon when the neuron is excited? All nerve conduction is based upon the fact that the neural membrane is able to selectively allow charged ions such as Na^+, K^+, Cl^- and CH_3COO^- (acetate ion) to pass in and out of the cell through size-selective channels in the membrane that can be opened by both chemical and electrical means.

In the resting state (no signal at the transduction site), the Na^+ ion concentration is much higher in the extracellular fluid and surrounding glial cells than it is within the neuron, Fig. 5.A-3a, while the opposite is true for K^+. Additionally, in the resting state, the transmembrane permeability for K^+ is much larger than it is for Na^+, and the negatively-charged ions are more numerous within the neuron than outside it. There is thus an imbalance of net charge in the resting state, making the inside of the membrane more negatively charged electrically

than the outside. This difference of net charge across the membrane expresses itself as a transmembrane voltage or potential: typically –70 millivolts (mV) along the entire length of the neuron. As the transmembrane voltage is the same at all points along the length of the neuron in the resting state, no current flows in that direction.

The transmembrane voltage is maintained across the membrane by the expenditure of energy within the nerve cell, for such a nonzero voltage is the result of gradients (differences) in the concentrations of the various ions on the two sides of the membrane which are maintained in spite of the tendency in inanimate situations for such gradients to reduce to zero with time. The energy required to maintain the differences in ion concentration in the resting state of the membrane is supplied by the chemical ATP (Subsection 7.A, *Muscle Chemistry and Energy*, page 182). Actually, the membrane has many channels through which Na^+ ions could flow in order to equilibrate the concentration of Na^+ on the two sides of the membrane, but these channels are more or less closed in the resting state, and therefore the concentration gradient is maintained.

When an appropriate stimulus acts on the input end of the neuron, there is a change in the membrane's permeabilities to Na^+ and K^+, the ion channels open, and with this there is a first-stage flow of ions across the membrane at the transduction site that changes the voltage by +/– 0.1 to 10 mV. The magnitude of the voltage change reflects the magnitude of the impinging stimulus, and the sign of the voltage change (+/–) determines whether the neural impulse will be exciting (+, depolarizing) or inhibiting (–, hyperpolarizing). The formation of a depolarizing potential means that the ion flow acted to reduce the ion gradients, whereas the formation of a hyperpolarizing potential means that the ion flow acted to increase the gradients. The initiating event may be sensory (light, pressure, sound, proprioceptive, *etc.*) or chemical (acetylcholine, norepinephrine, *etc.*); most first-stage voltage changes are depolarizing, but not all of them are so. The first-stage induced voltages in sensory neurons are called "receptor potentials" while those for motor neurons are called "synaptic potentials". The properties of such potentials are summarized in Table 5.B-1.

As can be seen in Table 5.B-1 and Fig. 5.B-1, the time profile of the initial potential will reflect closely that of the initial stimulus, except for a slight relaxation at longer times. The initial induced-potential change of +/− 0.1 to 10 mV passively extends only 2–3 mm along the neuron before it enters the region of integration, Fig. 5.B-1. In this region, all parts of the initial potential which are more positive than a certain threshold (about −65 mV) are converted into pulses of constant voltage, but with a pulse frequency that reflects the amount of voltage by which the signal at that point exceeds the threshold. If the initial signal is too weak or the receptor potential is hyperpolarizing, all parts of the signal fail to reach threshold (−65 mV), no spikes are generated and the signal transmission stops at this point. The amplification of the receptor potentials at the integration stage occurs when the receptor (or synaptic) voltage reaches a value at

which Na^+ channels open in an avalanche fashion and the inner Na^+ concentration soars until such a high voltage is reached that the Na^+ channels close and the K^+ channels then open to allow K^+ to stream out. This brings the membrane back to the resting potential.

Once launched along the afferent fibers to the brain, all nerve signals are identical, *i.e.*, a series of −65 mV peaks differing only in their frequencies, a reflection of their intensities. If the electrical signals from the eyes could be re-routed to the adjacent auditory areas of the brain, then we could hear colors through our eyes! In fact, there are people who have the gift of "seeing" pure colors when they hear pure acoustic tones.

Transport of the Action Potential; Conduction Velocity

Let us assume that the receptor potential is large and depolarizing. In this case, the initial polarization of the region next to the transduction site shows a refractory period of a few milliseconds, during which time the membrane is insensitive to further excitation. However, the strong polarization voltage does serve as a further source of electrical depolarization for the adjacent down-stream region of the axon, and so the integration signal, now called the action potential, moves in that direction only; it cannot move up-stream since the refractory

TABLE 5.B-1. CHARACTERISTICS OF THE VARIOUS ELECTRICAL POTENTIALS RELEVANT TO NEURAL CONDUCTION [225]

Feature	Sensory Neuron Receptor Potential	Motor Neuron Synaptic Potential	Action Potential
Amplitude	0.1 to 10 mV	0.1 to 10 mV	70 to 110 mV
Duration	5 to 100 msec	5 msec to 20 min	1 to 10 msec
Summation	Graded	Graded	All-or-none
Polarity	Depolarizing or Hyperpolarizing	Depolarizing or Hyperpolarizing	Depolarizing
Propagation	Passive	Passive	Active

period is a roadblock for instantaneous motion in that direction, Fig. 5.A-3b-3d. As the shortest refractory period is about 1 millisecond, the upper limit on the number of action potentials that can be generated in a second is approximately 500–1000 [299].

Not only is the action potential mobile in the direction away from the initial stimulus thanks to the refractory period, but it now consists a series of voltage spikes of constant amplitude. The profile of the spikes *in toto* matches the time profile of the stimulus, but the strength of the stimulus is now expressed in the frequency of the action-potential spikes rather than in their amplitude. Understanding how the neural signal can move in a direction perpendicular to the direction in which the ions move is dealt with in Box 5.B-1.

Once the action potential reaches the far end of the axon, each of its spikes triggers the release of a neurotransmitter into the extracellular fluid surrounding the far end of the neuron. The stronger the intensity of the stimulus at the receptor end, the more frequent the bursts of neurotransmitter at the transmitting end of the neuron.

As discussed more fully in Section 4.F, *Nadis, Chakras* and *Prana*, page 100, there is a very suggestive correlation between the nervous system as modern-day anatomists know it, and the paths of vital-energy flow as intuited by the ancient yogis. To the extent that this apparent one-to-one corre-

---

BOX 5.B-1: WHAT REALLY MOVES WHEN A CURRENT FLOWS THROUGH A NERVE?

Note that though a nerve such as one in the sciatic bundle may conduct the action potential for a distance of 1 meter and though the action potential is initiated by the movement of charged ions through the neural membrane, *the ions themselves do not move along the axon*; only the changing energy of the depolarization moves as a wave along the length of the nerve, Fig. 5.A-3. This is much like the case of a boat in the water. As the wave energy moves from left to right on the water's surface, the boat rises and falls in place in response to the wave's crests and troughs, but it does not itself move from left to right. The wave may originate in San Francisco and travel 2000 miles to Hawaii, but the boat only moves up and down by 5 feet as the energy of the wave passes. Similarly, the nerve impulse (action potential) can travel for a meter, but the ions associated with the wave only travel the microscopic distance across the neural membrane. It is the site of the microscopic transmembrane leakage of ions that moves down the length of the axon. Note as well that the conduction of the ionic current in nerves involves far smaller velocities and far smaller distances than is the case for the conduction of an electronic current through a metallic wire.

Yet another way to think about the neural current is to consider a pair of scissors. The top blade of the scissors moving toward the bottom one is like the ions traversing the membrane of the cell wall, however, as the top blade moves toward the bottom one, it is the point of intersection of the blades that moves from right to left, essentially in a direction perpendicular to the motions of the blades. This motion of the intersection corresponds to the motion of the neural current along the axon as the ions (the blades of the scissors) move perpendicular to the axon [207].

spondence is valid, the neural conduction of the transmembrane potential as described above corresponds to the flow of *prana*, the life force. The medium through which the action potential flows, the neural axon, corresponds to the *nadi* of the yogis.

To recap, transmission of the initial signal through the integration zone results in an action potential which can be propagated beyond a meter in humans, as for example in the sciatic nerve. The action potentials are triggered by structural changes in the neural membrane induced by the initial potential. These changes rapidly increase the permeability of the membrane to Na^+, which floods the neuron from outside to generate the all-or-nothing action potential. The action potential originates within a few mm of the receptor end of the neuron, and thanks to the nonzero refractory period, from that point on, propagates down the axon in one direction only. The duration of the action potential reflects that part of the stimulus that is intense enough to generate spikes. As all of the spikes in the action potential are of the same height (voltage), the strength of the initial stimulus instead is reflected in the frequency of the action-potential spikes. The action potential spikes act to release neurotransmitters into the synaptic gap at the far end of the axon.

The picture for nerve conduction is somewhat different when the nerve fiber is myelinated. The axons of the neurons may be wrapped by Schwann cells in a pattern looking like a string of sausages, Fig. 5.B-2. Each spiral wrap of a Schwann cell protects that portion of the axonal membrane from contact with the extracellular fluids, however, at the nodes between the Schwann cells, there is exposure of the membrane and its unusually high number of Na^+ and K^+ channels. The wrapping of the nerves is with a proteinaceous material called myelin, and nerves wrapped in this way are said to be myelinated. All of the nerves of the periph-

eral nervous system are myelinated by Schwann cells [476].

When the first node of the myelinated neuron is depolarized, the effect is so large that it reaches electrostatically to the next down-stream node about 1 mm away, triggering depolarization there. Rather than propagate uniformly down the axon in a wave-like way as in an unmyelinated fiber, in this case there is a rapid jumping of the depolarization condition from one node to the next, with the motion again only in one direction due to the refractory-time effect. Though described above for a depolarizing signal, the same mechanism holds over a short range for a hyperpolarizing one. Nerve

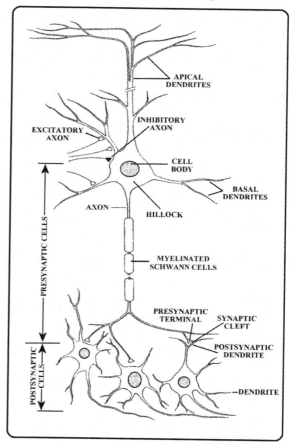

Fig. 5.B-2. The anatomical relationship between the presynaptic neuron (*top*) and the postsynaptic neuron (*bottom*), and the intervening axon myelinated with Schwann cells (*middle*). The neural conduction is from top to bottom.

conduction in myelinated fibers is faster than in the unmyelinated fibers by a factor of more than 100, Table 5.B-2.

As an infant's nervous system is myelinated only in the lower, subcortical regions of the brain, all of its actions are reflexive. With time, myelination proceeds upward toward the cortex, and deliberate muscle action begins as reflexive actions fall away [387].

A general classification scheme will be used here for efferent and afferent nerve fibers based on their diameters and degree of myelination. In general, as the diameter of a nerve fiber increases, so does the conduction velocity, however, fast, large-diameter bundles which would be needed for complex signaling would be too ungainly. A typical motor-nerve bundle in the human body has about 1000 fibers, and were it to be unmyelinated, it would have to have a

diameter of 38 mm in order to have the same conduction velocity that the myelinated fiber has with a diameter of only 1 mm [230]. The smallest diameter motor nerves in the somatic system are myelinated so as to have rapid conduction and a speedy response, whereas the nerves serving the autonomic nervous system are not myelinated and so are not as fast [319]. The afferent neurons in general are slower and are the oldest phylogenetically, whereas the larger and faster fibers (Ia and Ib) are the newer ones. In the autoimmune disease multiple sclerosis, the nerves are demyelinated so that nerve-conduction velocity is very low and muscle control thereby is minimal.

Nerves in class A are somatic and myelinated and are further classified as alpha, beta, or gamma fibers of decreasing diameter [195], Table 5.B-2. The Ia and Ib fibers are sensory fibers (largely in the proprio-

TABLE 5.B-2. CHARACTERISTICS OF EFFERENT AND AFFERENT NERVE-FIBER TYPES [5, 195, 225, 308, 434, 476]

	A_{alpha}	A_{beta}	A_{gamma}	B	C
Efferent					
Diameter (microns)	22	5–15	1–5	3	0.3–1.5
Myelinated	Yes	Yes	Yes		No
Velocity (m/sec)	65–120	40–80	10–50	4–25	0.2–2.0
Refractory period (millisec)	0.4	—	1.0	1.2	2.0
Muscle Type	Fast Twitch	Slow Twitch			
Location		Spindles	Spindles	ANS	ANS

	Ia	Ib	II	III	IV
Afferent					
Sensory Modes					
Sharp pain, thermal			Yes		Yes
Sharp pain, mechanical			Yes		Yes
Slow, dull pain			Yes		Yes
Vibration, skin indentation		Yes	Yes		Yes
Limb proprioception	Yes	Yes	?		
Joint capsule		Yes	Yes		
Golgi organ		Yes			

ceptive systems, Section 7.C, page 208), with conduction velocities of 40–120 m/sec, while the sensory II fibers (sharp pain and slow dull pain) being much thinner, have conduction velocities of only 10–50 m/sec. The C and IV fibers of the somatic and autonomic systems are unmyelinated, and show conduction velocities of only 2.5 m/sec or less. The B fibers are lightly myelinated and are found in the autonomic system. There are other neural classification schemes in the literature, but that of Table 5.B-2 will be used in this work.

Actually, on a macroscopic scale, the strength of response of a neural signal to a stimulus will be reflected not only in the frequency of the action potential from a neural fiber, but also upon the number of fibers so activated in a particular neighborhood. Thus the strength of muscle contraction, for example, will depend upon the frequencies of the action potentials in a particular motor unit, and also upon the number of muscle fibers contained within the motor unit.

The complex action of something like speech involves about 15,000 neuromuscular events per minute of speech, each of which involves many nerves of different lengths and conduction velocities activating dozens of different muscles, yet the brain is able to get all of the timing right so that meaningful sounds result! The same timing is evident in the successful assimilation of the flood of sensory information coming into our brain from various afferent nerves of different length, diameter and velocity.

For example, when we attempt to kick up into *adho mukha vrksasana*, the relevant muscles will be activated and deactivated at the appropriate times by the brain only after it accounts for the different lengths of the nerves involved and their different conduction velocities. That is to say, if two muscles in different motor units are meant to be activated at the same time, but the efferent nerve to one is fast and the other is slow,

even with the nerves of the same length, the initial signal on the slow one must be launched well before that on the fast one if the muscles are to contract simultaneously. The brain handles timing problems of this sort without any sign of conscious effort once the action has been practiced. It is no less a miracle than that of coherent speech that the timing of the muscle action in going up into *adho mukha vrksasana* is handled effortlessly by the brain. The clock that adjusts these timings can be found in the cerebellum and basal ganglia (Chapter 3, THE BRAIN, page 21).

SECTION 5.C. NERVE CONNECTIONS; SYNAPSES

Structure

Given that a sensory organ has successfully transduced its sensation into an action potential which then is transported to the tip of its axon, how does this signal then move through peripheral nerves to the central nervous system? The mechanism for conducting a nerve impulse along the length of a neuron is discussed above (Section 5.B), with the impulse beginning at the receptor sites among the dendrites and propagating to the far end of the axon in the simplest case. In no case does the far end of the axon connect to its eventual destination without interruption. In fact, the nerve paths between the brain and outlying sensors, muscles and organs are frequently interrupted by small gaps called synapses. How such an electrical signal can then move from the axon tip of the transmitter neuron to effector organs or to an adjacent receptor neuron via synapses is the subject of this Section. As will be seen, the synapses will allow the control of propagating action potentials, offering the opportunity to turn them on or off or otherwise amplify or moderate their effects either positively or negatively.

There are two general mechanisms for the transmission of the neural signal across the space (the synapse) that separates two adjacent neurons: the electrical and the chemical. In the electrical synapse, the two adjacent nerve endings are connected by hollow tubes (gap junctions) which are capable of transmitting an ionic current from one neuron to the next, either depolarizing or hyperpolarizing it in the process. Signal conduction through a gap junction can be turned on or off by local changes in the H^+ or Ca^{+2} ion concentrations. The gap synapse is found wherever speed of action and synchronicity of action are important, as in the heart.

In the chemical synapse, there is no structural connective element between adjacent neurons, only a cleft having a width of 200–400 Angstroms (the hydrogen atom is 1.2 Angstroms in diameter), and filled with extracellular fluid, Fig. 5.C-1. When the presynaptic membrane of the transmitter neuron reaches the action potential, it opens channels for the inward transport of Ca^{2+} ions, which in turn stimulate the release at that point of a chemical messenger (neurotransmitter) into the volume of the synaptic cleft. Pending their release, the neurotransmitters are stored in small packets called vesicles located very close to the synaptic cleft, with each vesicle holding about 10,000 molecules of the neurotransmitter [299]; there can be thousands of vesicles in an axonal tip. When called upon to do so, the vesicles move to the very outer surface of the presynaptic neuron and then turn themselves inside out on order to launch their load of neurotransmitter into the synaptic cleft. The stronger the initial stimulus at one end of the nerve, the more fre-

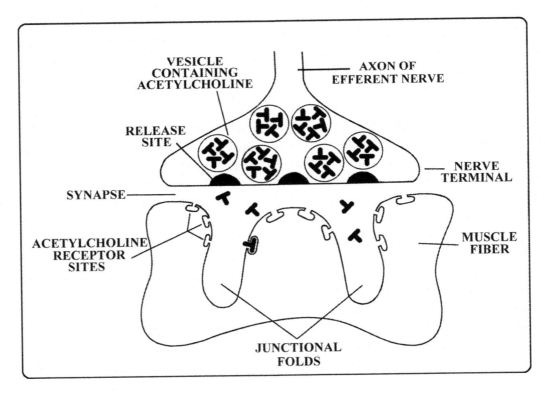

Fig. 5.C-1. Elements of the chemical synapse. In this case, the vesicles within the presynaptic half of the synapse are filled with acetylcholine, and the receptors on the postsynaptic side are shaped to absorb and respond to this neurotransmitter.

quent are the bursts of neurotransmitter released from the vesicles at the opposite end.

The neurotransmitter released on the presynaptic side of the cleft then diffuses across the cleft to the postsynaptic membrane where it is recognized and bound to that membrane. Binding of the neurotransmitter to the postsynaptic membrane then initiates a synaptic potential in that neuron and signal propagation begins all over again, possibly spreading simultaneously to widely separated target organs or brain centers. The chemical synapse works something like glandular secretion, but it is faster and more directed; intermediate cases are known however, in which the cleft spacing is relatively large and the release of neurotransmitter activates many neurons in its locale.

The receptor sites on the postsynaptic membranes are activated by the specific molecule which is released into its synapse, or by ones closely similar in their chemical shapes and reactions. A variety of small molecules and ions (approximately 50) serve as the neurotransmitters in human synapses (see Section 5.D, page 128).

Once having entered the synaptic cleft, the neurotransmitter blocks all further action until it has been cleared from the volume of the cleft and removed from the postsynaptic surface. This involves the reabsorption of the neurotransmitter by the presynaptic membrane, the diffusion of unbound neurotransmitter out of the cleft and the enzymatic degradation of any neurotransmitter within the cleft or on the receptor surface. Clearing of the neurotransmitter signal is very rapid in the case of the small-molecule neurotransmitters (refractory time of less than a millisecond), but can take a very long time in the case of the larger neurotransmitters (refractory times of tens of seconds to several minutes), leading to long-lasting activation of the receptors. In order to get a sustained action at a site with small-molecule neurotransmitters, it is necessary to provide the site with a sustained barrage of action potentials.

Excitation Versus Inhibition

Once bound to the postsynaptic membrane, the neurotransmitter's function is then to open and close ion channels so as to change the electrical-charge state within the membrane. If Na^+ gates are opened, the inner membrane will be flooded with this ion and the membrane will thus be depolarized. If the depolarization effect is large enough, then a depolarization action-potential wave will be propagated, *i.e.*, the signal moves on.

If, on the other hand, the action of the neurotransmitter is to open K^+ and Cl^- channels, letting the first of these out and the second of these into the membrane from outside, then the membrane will be hyperpolarized. In this case, the transmembrane voltage is even more negative and so is discouraged from reaching the more positive threshold necessary for the formation of an action potential; thus this synaptic connection is inhibitory, even if other synaptic connections to the same neuron are excitatory. Depending upon the action and nature of the postsynaptic receptor site, the binding of a particular neurotransmitter can lead to either an excitatory or an inhibitory signal. Thus acetylcholine is an excitatory neurotransmitter in the synapse between motor nerve and skeletal-muscle fiber, but is inhibitory when released in the synapses with cardiac muscle in the heart, where the purpose of the inhibiting action would be to slow the heart rate. If the action of a neuron is to inhibit another from reaching its action potential, then the first neuron is said to be an interneuron. All interneurons are inhibitory. The function of an interneuron releasing the muscular tension in an antagonist muscle (Subsection 7.A, *Reciprocal Inhibition and Agonist/Antagonist Pairs,* page 193) following a sharp pinprick is shown in Fig. 5.C-2.

Moreover, not all synapses are dedicated to a single neurotransmitter and so a single neuron, for example, may have receptors along its length for dozens of very different neurotransmitters, and in turn, it may output many different chemical signals. Thus in Fig. 5.C-2 where a variety of synaptic contacts are shown, one can easily imagine that the various contacts made to the receptor neuron involve different neurotransmitters. Some neurochemicals also play roles as hormones in the body [473].

Nerve fibers either conduct a depolarization wave or they do not, depending in part on the magnitude of the threshold for the action potential. Through experience, this threshold can be raised or lowered to fine-tune the action. Adjustment of the action threshold is more easily accomplished in the chemical synapses. Though somewhat slower than the electrical synapses, the chemical synapses are much more easily modified by experience, and so allow learning to occur through practice. As applied to the *yogasanas*, the reduction of the action potentials through practice means that less nervous energy needs be expended in order to achieve a particular muscular state of contraction. As a consequence, one can stay longer in the pose before nervous exhaustion becomes a factor.

In general, a single motor neuron is able to generate a sufficient action potential at its synaptic junction with a single muscle fiber

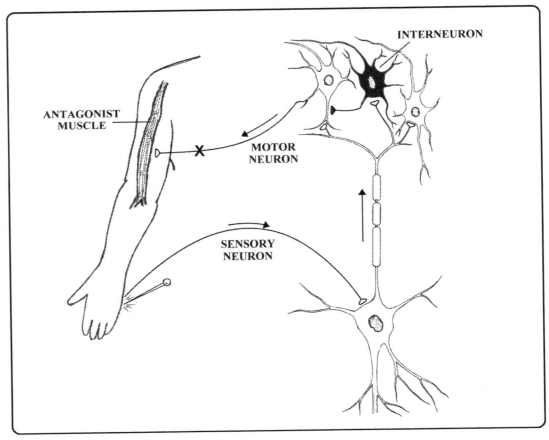

Fig. 5.C-2. A pinprick (*lower left corner*) stimulates a sensory neuron in the skin, however, this afferent neuron synapses with an interneuron in the spine, which then acts to hyperpolarize the motor neuron stimulating the antagonist muscle. Consequently, the antagonist muscle is relaxed through the action of the interneuron.

and so excite the fiber with almost unit certainty. On the other hand, in the central nervous system, the single-neuron receptor potential is far below that necessary for propagation of an action potential. Note however, that on such multipolar receptor neurons there are receptor sites over the entire neuron, and so there can be hundreds of synaptic junctions all in a position to add their signal in a communal way so as to exceed the action-potential threshold, as in Fig. 5.B-2. Often, synapses to the multipolar cell body are inhibitory while those to the dendrites are excitatory and those along the axon are modulatory. The various depolarizing and hyperpolarizing voltages are summed algebraically in both space and time at the hillock where the axon joins the cell body, and depending upon the size of the summated signal, the excitation will prove to be either excitatory and lead to a propagating action potential, or inhibitory due to too negative a net receptor potential. It is in this way that signals from many different organs and sensors from distant points can be integrated and prioritized so as to finally influence a neural action serving the greatest good. In this scheme, learning can occur by changing the relative intensities of the component signals so as to excite or inhibit a potential signal in the receptor neuron.

One can readily see the importance of interneurons in the human body, for in the case of tetanus, the toxin from this bacterial infection acts only on interneurons, blocking their action. As a result, the body loses its muscular inhibitions in the spinal cord, and the body readily goes into muscular spasms, beginning at the jaw (lockjaw) and finally involving the entire body [126]. Once muscular inhibition has been shut down, as when afflicted with tetanus, and the body is subject to muscular spasms when it is touched by something as inconsequential as a small breeze or a soft noise,

then one can fully appreciate the important balancing roles interneurons must otherwise play in our *yogasana* practice. For other examples of the inhibiting effects of interneurons in action, see Subsections 7.A, *Reciprocal Inhibition and Agonist/Antagonist Pairs*, page 193, and 7.D, *The Myotactic Stretch Reflex*, page 212. In a nutshell, the primary action of the higher centers of the brain is inhibitory.

Mechanical Effects on Nerves

External pressure on the body is sensed by several types of sensor organs called mechanoreceptors (Section 7.B, Muscle Sensors; The Mechanoreceptors, page 198), in which the sensor itself is found at the very end of the receptor nerve. The pressure to which these sensors respond may be the result of an external object pressing into the body, or it may be a muscle action which inadvertently presses contracted or swollen muscle tissue, or bone upon a pressure-sensitive mechanoreceptor. However, pressure on the axon of the receptor nerve rather than on the mechanorecptor at the end of the nerve also can result in secondary sensations.

When the axons of afferent nerves are under pressure, the feeling is one of "pins and needles", tingling, radiating pain, or numbness. As nerve fibers are rather fluid and relatively weak mechanically, it is tempting to imagine that the effect of pressure is to throttle the flow of the action potential along the axon, with the "pins and needles" sensation associated with intermittent transmission of the sensory signal, and with numbness resulting when the flow is blocked totally. The situation is worse if both the motor and sensory nerves are affected, if the effect is felt on both sides of the body, or if the disturbance is farther rather than nearer the spine [257]. In yoga work, it can be a good sign to go from numbness to pain, as this signals a release of compression on the nerve in question.

When instead it is an efferent nerve that is under pressure, the secondary effect is one of weakness and tentative action (trembling) of the muscles so innervated, with seemingly low recruitment of motor units. This too is understandable if the action potential which drives muscle contraction is frustrated by the pressure. Remembering that intensity of muscular action depends both upon the frequency of the action potential transmitted along its axon and the number of motor units excited in a muscle, compression can diminish both of these factors, so that the muscular response is weaker [257].

Mechanical injuries to the nerves of the body can result from compression of the nerves as when they are crushed when caught between two bones pressing on one another, from traction which over-stretches and tears them, or from a combination of these situations. Nerves that are injured mechanically are slow to recover their functions, and if the nerve is completely severed, it will die.

Yet another possible mechanism working here to thwart the transmission of the nerve signal is that the compression slows vascular circulation in the compressed area (ischemia), and that, as a consequence of this, the nerve does not receive sufficient oxygen for proper functioning (hypoxia). If there is slight pressure on an afferent nerve, it can suffer ischemia, and this is sensed as pain [260]. As explained in Section 10.D, Pain, page 294, the decrease of oxygen to a nerve or muscle cell results in a release of arachidonic acid, a potent stimulator of pain receptors in the body. Thus in sciatica, pressure on the L4, L5, S1 nerve complex as might be caused by a herniated disc (see Section 4.C, Intervertebral Discs, page 87) can result in symptoms of either pain or even numbness [267].

It is the longer afferent nerves going from the hands and feet to the spine that are most likely to be compressed at some point along their paths, and so tingling or numbness is not unusual in these parts when beginners first do their *yogasanas*. Nerve tissue is almost fluid in character and though it is quite elastic and compressible, too sudden a stretch may over-stretch it and so interfere with nerve conduction, but slow and steady extension is easily accommodated [262].

Many of us experience the secondary effects of pressure on the nerves when going into *virasana* or *supta virasana* and staying there for a few minutes. On coming out of the pose, the legs are tingling and so weak that they can be straightened only with difficulty! The problem here would seem to be that one has a tourniquet effect at the knee, where extreme flexion at the knee and the pressure of the calf against the hamstring muscle both restrict blood circulation and press on the axon of the sciatic nerve. These effects can be avoided by sitting on a block in *virasana* so as to open the angle at the knee, and by rolling the calf muscle out while rolling the thigh in as one sits, so as to avoid pressing one on the other.

The ulnar nerve in the arm offers a good example of what can happen to a nerve when the surrounding musculature and bone are involved in heavy exercise [35]. The ulnar-nerve bundle serves the inner aspect of the hand, traveling up the forearm and passing through a narrow channel (the cubital tunnel) in the elbow on its way to the upper arm [195]. The cubital tunnel is normally circular in cross section and open, however, when the arm is flexed at the elbow, its shape changes to triangular and the channel diameter decreases by more than 50%. Compression of this nerve can result in severely reduced conduction velocities, as well as tingling, numbness, pain and muscle weakness.

Active extension of the arm with the wrists bent as in *adho mukha vrksasana* or *purvottanasana* acts as traction on the ulnar nerve and can extend it by almost 5 mm.* Depending upon the mechanical actions at the elbow, the ulnar nerve in the cubital tunnel is subject to compression, friction and traction with consequent symptoms when poses such as these are practiced. Numbness due to ulnar impingement is occasionally experienced by yoga students when resting in *savasana* with their elbows on the floor at their sides.

Tingling sensations in the arms are possibly due to the compression of nerves or blood vessels as these nerves or vessels pass between the thorax and the arms. Called thoracic outlet syndrome, it may be caused by over-developed muscles or poor posture among other things.

Nerve impingement can occur as well when the vertebrae are misaligned, but with discs not herniated, as discussed in Subsection 4.A, *Misalignment of the Spine and Deterioration of the Vertebral Discs*, page 79. Carpal tunnel syndrome also can be mentioned here [151a], wherein a swelling at the wrist impinges upon the nerves going to the fingers.

The weakened muscular response of a muscle when it is compressed externally is often met in the *yogasanas*, and can be used to one's advantage. This is especially so when the compression is across the direction of the muscle fibers being compressed. Thus the bent leg in *ardha baddha padma paschimottanasana* presses across the quadruceps muscle of the straight leg and so works to relax it in this pose. Similarly, *virasana* done with a pole set between the

hamstrings and the calf muscles on each leg will relax the latter and help them go flat (see also, Subsection 7.D, *Other Reflex Actions*, page 220).

However, one must be careful not to overdo nerve compression, especially by either pressing too hard or by staying too long in a *yogasana* position. For example, when meditators stay for hours in either *padmasana* or *muktasana*, the consequence can be a serious injury to the sciatic nerves in the legs at the points where one leg presses on the other (Subsection II.B, *Neurological Damage*, page 513).

Interestingly, when a peripheral nerve passes through a joint, there is a preferred position within the joint for this. In most cases, the nerve chooses to pass on what is the inside of the joint when the joint is flexed. In this case, the nerve being on the inside will actually experience a lesser tensile stress as compared to the outer path, which would be more stressful to the nerve whether the joint is flexed or extended. The only exceptions to this are the ulnar nerve in the elbow and the sciatic nerve in the hip, both of which follow the outer paths and so become the loci of many neurological problems.

When one moves from *tadasana* to *uttanasana*, not only are the hamstrings stretched, but so too are the peripheral nerves that run along the back of the legs. This extension of the nerves is handled by the body in the following way [5]. As we stand with the back of the legs more or less relaxed in *tadasana*, the nerve bundles in the nerve bed are in a somewhat folded form, accordian style. On elongation of the surrounding muscle, such peripheral nerves

---

* If you fall asleep with your wrist folded either forward or backward, you will wake up with the hand feeling numb from the pressure and traction experienced by the ulnar nerve. Similarly, pressure on the sciatic nerve of the leg due to sitting too long without moving can make the leg "fall asleep".

can lengthen by up to 2 inches (5 cm) by just becoming straighter, with little or no stress being applied. Following this, the inherent elasticity of the nerve fiber will allow another 20% extension, however, when the stress is between 20 and 30% , the extension becomes inelastic and a certain amount of nerve damage is incurred; at 30% extension, the nerve breaks. As the nerve is extended, its diameter decreases and its conduction velocity drops.

As with muscles, a neuron lasts a lifetime if used often, but withers away (through apoptosis) when it is not used at all. In this way, our signaling system tends to become more refined and more narrowed as our skills become more practiced and unused neural circuitry is discarded. This has the effect of making us better and better at less and less [473]. However, the practice of an endless variety of *yogasana* certainly will work to keep the largest possible number of neurons active and healthy.

If the cell body of a neuron is destroyed by injury, then not only does the injured nerve die, but its synaptic neighbors also wither and die afterward. The neural debris is cleared by the glial cells. In the adult, slight damage to axons in the peripheral nerves is self-repairing, but this generally is not so in the central nervous system [225, 303]. However, there is now intriguing evidence that certain of the nerve cells in the hippocampus are capable of regeneration, and that rebirth of these nerve cells is stimulated by exercise [35].

SECTION 5.D. THE NEUROTRANSMITTERS

The message that is sent from the axonal terminal of a neuron to the receptor sites in the neighboring neuron (or muscle cell, or gland) is a chemical one. Within the cell body of the neuron, the particular chemical to be used in transmitting the message is generated in the cell body and packaged in small units called vesicles. Once filled with the appropriate neurotransmitter molecules, the vesicles are then propelled along the full length of the axon via a two-way axonal transport system, to arrive and be stored finally at the very ends of the axons, the axonal terminals. Whenever an action potential travels the length of the axon and arrives at the terminals, this potential triggers the opening of the vesicles and the release of the neurotransmitters contained within them. In turn, the released neurotransmitters flood the synaptic cleft, to be sensed by the receptors on the receiving neuron. The axonal transport system then returns the empty vesicles to the cell body for repair or recycling.

The neurotransmitters injected into the synaptic cleft may be either excitatory or inhibitory. In the former case, they depolarize the postsynaptic membrane thereby initiating a propagating neural signal, or they hyperpolarize this membrane, thereby inhibiting the propagation of a neural signal beyond the synapse.

There are two broad classes of neurotransmitters, the small molecules (usually biogenic amines) and the neuropeptides. Prime among the former are the following.

Acetylcholine

Acetylcholine is the neurotransmitter in all neuromuscular (cholinergic) synapses, in the paravertebral ganglia of the sympathetic trunk, and in the pre- and post-ganglia of the parasympathetic nervous system, Fig. 6.C-1; it is prominent as well in the brain where it influences psychological function [153]. Acetylcholine's action in the neuromuscular case is to depolarize the muscle fiber so that Ca^{2+} channels open and these ions then initiate muscle contraction. Interestingly, the synapse in the adrenal medulla which excretes epinephrine/norepinephrine operates on acetylcholine, for if it were activated by epinephrine or norepinephrine, it would be self-stimulating and out of control.

Acetylcholine is always excitatory at the neuromuscular synapse (where there is no inhibitory signal) and though each acetylcholine release at a neuromuscular synapse results in an action potential, the signal may be either excitatory or inhibitory at the autonomic synapses to the visceral organs. The binding of acetylcholine at a receptor site opens ion channels for only 1 millisecond, after which the acetylcholine is enzymatically degraded or reabsorbed. Given that the ion channels are open for about 1 millisecond, it is theoretically possible then to excite a muscle fiber at up to 500 times per second.

The Catecholamines

The catecholamines epinephrine and norepinephrine circulate in the blood stream after they are released as hormones by the adrenal medulla upon being stimulated by the sympathetic nervous system. Their release is triggered by acetylcholine's action in the neuroendocrine synapse. Because the receptors on the postsynaptic membrane can be of more than one type, the alpha and beta receptors for the catecholamines throughout the body often can be sensitive to both epinephrine and norepinephrine, though some are more sensitive to the former, while others are more sensitive to the latter.

Epinephrine binds to both alpha and beta receptors, but in the case of the small blood vessels, the alpha binding leads to constriction while the beta binding leads to dilation of the vessels. Epinephrine prefers beta receptors such as those found in the heart and gastrointestinal tract where it dilates arterioles.

Norepinephrine is found in high concentrations in the locus ceruleus of the brain, a center which affects levels of attention and arousal [153]. The emotional effects of low levels of the catecholamines in the brain are

discussed in Chapter 20, THE EMOTIONS, page 463. Norepinephrine prefers alpha receptors as found in the vascular smooth muscle, the gut, bladder, spleen and the sphincters.

Serotonin

Though serotonin functions as a neurotransmitter in the enteric nervous system within the gut, it is not found to function in either the sympathetic or parasympathetic branches of the nervous system [155]. See Chapter 20, THE EMOTIONS, page 463, for the consequences of low serotonin levels in the brain. Serotonin exerts inhibitory action by opening K^+ channels which tend to hyperpolarize the postsynaptic membrane. When serotonin is released by the platelets at the site of a wound, it acts as a vasoconstrictor of nearby blood vessels.

Gamma-Aminobutyric Acid

Gamma-aminobutyric acid (GABA) is found largely in the central nervous system, where it acts as neurotransmitter for inhibitory synaptic potentials. It functions by opening channels for Cl^- ions. Its action is opposite to that of glycine, which depresses neural activity in the brain by blocking the Cl^- channels. GABA in the brain influences psychological function [153].

Other Neurotransmitters

Glutamate and aspartate anions are among the most common neurotransmitters in the brain, and work in excitatory synapses. An excess of glutamate in the synapse leads to excessive excitation and nerve death by "excitotoxicity' [155].

Dopamine in the brain is an important neurotransmitter, influencing the control of movement. Loss of dopamine can lead to Parkinson-like motor problems.

Monoamine oxidase in the brain helps manage depression, and actually increases in concentration with increasing age [153].

Neuropeptides which function as neurotransmitters throughout the body number between 50 and 100. As a class, the neuropeptides are relatively short polymers of the various amino acids linked together in a specific order. For example, the neuropeptide oxytocin contains nine amino acids strung together end-to-end in the order cystine - tyrosine - isoleucine - glutamic acid - asparagine - cystine - proline - leucine - glycine, with the two cystine groups joined by a disulfide -S-S- linkage [360], whereas the growth hormone GHRH consists of a chain of 44 such amino acids strung together in a shoestring fashion [225].

The action of a particular neurotransmitter at a particular site is guaranteed by the totally specific nature of the interaction between the transmitter and the receptor site. Because a neuropeptide receptor will only accept that one neuropeptide with the proper ordering of its amino acids, the peptides can range freely over the body via the circulatory system and still activate distant sites with great specificity. For neuropeptides, there are no short-range synapses of the kind ordinarily met with as when acetylcholine is the transmitter.

The dorsal horn of the spinal cord is a locus of neuropeptide receptors, for example, and there are receptors for the neuropeptide angiotensin in both the brain and in the kidneys. Furthermore, the circulating cells of the immune system have receptors for all of the neuropeptide receptors. In a sense, the neuropeptides when coupled with the immune system form a global system of neural consciousness, allowing signals to be sent between any two points in the body [346].

It would be difficult to overstate the importance of the neuropeptides as neurotransmitters. Thus certain short-chain neuropeptides are key players in the body's very successful efforts to erase pain sensations (Subsection 10.D, *The Endorphins*, page 303). Because the neuropeptides were first identified in the brain, it was quite a shock to find so many sources of and receptors for the neuropeptides throughout the body. Consequently, they have come to be viewed as extending the body's intelligence to the furthest points [357]. Once again, there is a certain resonance between such medical discoveries, and Iyengar's repeated dictum to work the *yogasanas* so as to extend one's intelligence to the furthest parts of the body [211].

Drug Action in the Synaptic Cleft

Foreign substances such as mood-altering drugs can strongly influence synaptic chemistry when they have parts or all of their molecular structures similar to those of the natural neurotransmitters. Once within the area of the synapse, a neuroactive drug can act to stimulate a stronger release of neurotransmitter, can compete successfully with the natural substance for a position on the receptor membrane, and/or can block the enzymes that otherwise would destroy the natural transmitter within the synapse. Still others work their effect by blocking the channels otherwise used for transmembrane ion transport. Thus local anaesthetics block the Na^+ channels in the pain axon and so do not allow a depolarization wave to form [473].

Amphetamines both increase the release of norepinephrine into the synaptic cleft and also block the re-uptake of the transmitter. The resulting high concentration of norepinephrine in the cleft then leads to increased arousal, mood, excitability and pleasure. When the concentration of norepinephrine or serotonin is far below normal as in depression (Section 20.A, page 464), then amphetamines can restore normal order and mood by raising neurotransmitter levels.

Norepinephrine and the drug mescaline have closely related molecular structures:

Norepinephrine   Mescaline

It appears that mescaline is tightly bound to the enzyme that otherwise degrades norepinephrine in the synaptic cleft. With this enzyme blocked, the norepinephrine has an unusually long lifetime in the cleft and this leads to hallucinations [434].

A drug such as LSD, which so closely resembles serotonin in chemical structure, can compete successfully with serotonin for receptor sites on the neural membranes and on degrading enzymes and so can drastically alter the synaptic chemistry when ingested [434].

Serotonin   LSD

The acetylcholine receptors also bind nicotine, and are blocked by curare, the paralyzing South American arrow poison. Once the neuromuscular junctions are blocked by curare, no muscle action is possible and either relaxation or suffocation soon follow, depending on whether the application of the drug is local or global.

Endorphins

When the level of exercise brings one to about 90% of $\dot{V}O_{2max}$, beta-endorphins are released into the blood stream from the pituitary [337]. Moreover, receptors for beta-endorphins are found in the hypothalamus and within the limbic system. These neuropeptides act in the synapses of the brain to produce a euphoric feeling, the runner's high. See Section 10.D, Pain, page 294, for a further discussion of the action of the endorphins.

SECTION 5.E. TRANSDUCTION OF THE STIMULUS INTO THE SENSORY SIGNAL

In the Retina and Skin

Having discussed the important aspects of the formation of an action potential and how it might be conducted down the length of an axon, then chemically jump the synapse to the adjacent neuron, we turn briefly to the question of how a sensory organ can initiate such a process, given the wide diversity of sensors in the body. Unfortunately, there are answers to these questions for only a few of the receptor types, and even here, the explanation is sketchy. The best understood of these is the transduction of light at the retina into an action potential along the optic nerve [225].

When light is absorbed by the photopigment in the retina, Section 16.A, Structure and Function of the Eyes, page 411, the pigment molecules first change their geometry in an act called "isomerization". The eventual result of this isomerization is the drastic reduction in the concentration of cyclic guanosine monophosphate (cGMP), a chemical within the retinal cell which effectively holds open the Na^+ channels in the cell's membrane. When the concentration of cGMP drops on exposure of the retina to light, the Na^+ channels close, while at the same time, the K^+ channels remain open to the outward flow of this ion. The net result of the blocking of the inward flow of Na^+ and the unrestricted outward flow of K^+ is the hyperpolarization of the retinal membrane when illuminated.

Remember now that a depolarized excitation wave can propagate for a long distance (over 1 meter), but hyperpolarization cannot (see Section 5.B, Nerve Conduction, page 114). In the retina, the hyperpolarization is able to travel passively for only 2 mm before it connects to intermediate neurons (bipolar and multipolar) and then to the ganglion cells, Fig. 16.B-1. It is not yet clear how the hyperpolarization of the retinal cells eventually is transduced into depolarization of the ganglion cells, but the axons of these latter cells are depolarized and send their signals to higher centers in the brain via the optic nerves.

Transduction in the Pacinian corpuscles, Subsection 10.B, *Other Receptors in the Skin*, page 291, sensitive to deep pressure, is even less clear, involving in some way the mechanical deformation of the sensor bulb, the opening of specific ion channels, and the launching of an action potential.

The Nature of Neural Information

Regardless of the nature of the sensory organ, if its stimulus is strong enough to result in an action potential, then a depolarization wave is launched toward its farther end. Depolarization waves traveling from different sensors are essentially the same:

they are a series of voltage spikes, with frequencies proportional to their intensity of stimulation, but each traveling on its own unique highway, at first. The "signal" in nerve signaling is the depolarization wave (action potential) or its absence. Thus, every neuron in the body at any one moment is either activated or not. The resulting pattern of activations/deactivations across all of the neural space, a pattern of ones and zeros, if you will, is the information of the nervous system. But now to add the aspect of stimulus intensity, one must consider a pattern of zero's, one's, two's, three's, *etc.*, these representing the levels of excitation in a nerve fiber, ranging from none to very intense. As these signals move from the periphery to the central nervous system and back out again, they are repeatedly fused together or separated into multiple branches so that individual neural paths become more and more difficult to define the farther one moves away from the sensory source. Nonetheless, at any one instant, the patterns of zero's, one's, two's, three's, *etc.*, represent a specific state of consciousness, but this is clearly shifting from moment to moment if only because one is breathing, thinking, acting, *etc.*

Chapter 6

THE AUTONOMIC NERVOUS SYSTEM

SECTION 6.A. INTRODUCTION TO THE AUTONOMIC NERVOUS SYSTEM

Origin

As the brain developed and life became more complex, various older brain functions common to insects and reptiles were superceded by newer, more useful ones. Nonetheless, the ancestral reptilian brains remained in the newer animals to perform their functions in less obvious ways. In insects and reptiles, there has never been anything more than this reptilian brain and its associated nervous system; in humans today, the reptilian brain has survived intact as the autonomic nervous system. In addition to this, humans also have the old brain of the limbic system, and the newest addition, the cortex, the function of which is largely inhibitory with respect to the other two [313].

In the first approximation, the autonomic nervous system in humans works without any conscious control, and is inaccessible to conscious inspection. It is able to sense the status of the internal-body apparatus and then signal adjustments to be made so as to keep the body's parameters coordinated and within certain preset bounds. This process is called homeostasis (see below).

When the autonomic nervous system was first uncovered, it was so named because it was believed that its actions were totally automatic and independent of any outside control, in contrast to the central nervous system, Fig. 2.A-1. In agreement with the findings of the yoga masters of the past millennia, medical doctors today know that this supposed independence of the autonomic nervous system is not realistic, for there is possible a strong mixing of the autonomic and central-nervous-system functions.

Homeostatic Control; Feedback and Feedforward

Though the human body can survive under a wide range of conditions, there is a single set of narrowly-defined conditions under which it operates best. Should any of the body's parameters fall outside the optimum range due to either external or internal forces, then the body reacts automatically to regain the optimum value, in a general process called "homeostasis" [225, 313]. For example, the various systems of the body automatically adjust so as to keep the body temperature optimal (98.6° F) regardless of the external weather or internal chemistry. In this case, autonomic adjustment may include shivering, sweating, readjustment of vascular diameters to shift blood flow, *etc.*, all of which work to shift the core temperature in one direction or the other. Other body systems under homeostatic control are the kidneys which regulate the salt content of the body fluids, the circulatory system which concerns itself with the heart rate, blood pressure, and vascular diameters, the respiratory system which is involved with breathing rate and O_2 and CO_2 levels in the blood, and the appetites for water and food intake.

The control of these autonomic functions is by the mechanism called feedback, as illustrated in Fig. 6.A-1. For a particular function, there is an optimum setpoint. A detector for the level of the function in question detects any deviation from the setpoint and so produces an error signal, either positive or negative depending on the sense of the deviation. This error signal is then fed back to the controlling center, thereby either raising or lowering the level of function, until the value of the function is brought back into agreement with the setpoint. For example, sensor cells in the brain monitor the blood supply for the concentrations of O_2 and CO_2 to see that they are within prescribed limits for optimum brain health. If these concentrations are not within the setpoint range, the sensors report an error signal, and the respiratory centers then alter the rate and amplitude of the breath until the concentrations are within the prescribed limits, and homeostasis is achieved. The setpoints for various functions can be reset, as by pyrogens, for example, which induce and maintain fevers. A related setpoint mechanism for system regulation is described in Section 21.B, Periodicity of Body Rhythms, page 474, while yet another type of internal body clock runs on the basis of the transitions between light and darkness as observed visually at sunrise and sunset (Subsection 21.B, *Circadian Rhythms; Physiological Peaks and Valleys in the 24-Hour Period*, page 476).

Alternatively, a homeostatic system may have high and low setpoints as in Fig. 21.B-

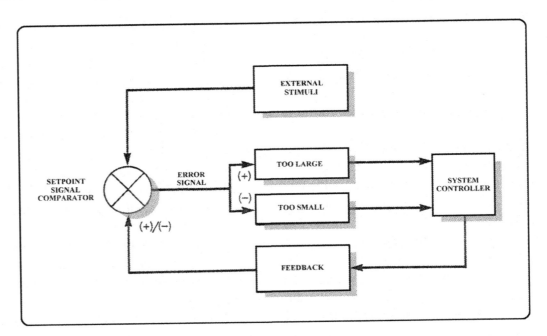

Fig. 6. A-1. A typical feedback circuit for the autonomic nervous system. In this, an external stimulus acts to change a physiological parameter of the system as revealed by comparison of the altered parameter with its setpoint value. This comparison generates an error signal which drives the system controller, which in turn drives the system back toward the setpoint via feedback so as to reduce the error signal to zero. In this way, the setpoint value is maintained subconsciously in spite of external stimuli.

1. In this case, there will be a movement of the system between the two setpoints, and so the system though homeostatic, is never really at a truly constant value, but is always oscillating between the higher and lower limits. In a broader sense, homeostasis consists of a regular oscillation of the level of a controlled function between the high and low setpoints of its comparator.

Elasticity is built into the feedback loops of the body so that every time a limit is exceeded, there is a tendency toward readjustment of the setpoint in the direction of the error. If there is a chronic high or low pressure on a setpoint, *i.e.*, a chronic stress in the body, there will follow a long-term resetting of the setpoint to higher or lower values, respectively. This shift of the setpoint to an extreme value can be unhealthy, for the extreme value will lead to a homeostatic adjustment only when the function being monitored takes an even more extreme value. This is why we need periods of rest and relaxation, which break the tendency of setpoints to be constantly nudged to new, unhealthy values.

On the other hand, through *yogasana* practice, one can deliberately shift the setpoints of otherwise autonomic functions, so that the body maintains homeostasis about a new mean value of the functional variable. This is a mechanistic description of the effect illustrated in Fig. 1.B-1 of the mixing between conscious and subconscious actions through *yogasana* practice.

In a feedforward response, there is again a control loop, but with parameters to be adjusted so as to achieve a goal in the future. For example, in attempting to perform *vrksasana* on the right leg from *tadasana*, feedforward circuits adjust the positions and motions of the limbs in anticipation of raising the left leg.

Most of the centers involved in maintaining the *status quo* (homeostasis) are located in the hypothalamus, the center for auto-nomic action. Nuclei in the hypothalamus receive afferent signals in regard the status of the body's systems, and then via hormonal secretions, neural efferents to target organs, and consciously-directed motivational systems, the internal climate of the body is changed so as to bring it back to optimum functioning. Higher centers in the brain help direct the hypothalamus in its work, interfacing with it through the limbic system.

In the early days, it was thought that the autonomic nervous system was purely vegetative, *i.e.*, that it worked totally at the subconscious level, could not learn new functions, and was closed to conscious intervention. This point of view has come to be radically modified, however, as it is now recognized that, with the appropriate effort, conscious access to the autonomic system is routinely possible. This deliberate, conscious access to autonomic functions can be one of the great practical benefits of *yogasana* practice, especially when the practice is performed with autonomic control in mind.

The Anatomical Center

The main center for autonomic control of body functions is the region of the brain called the hypothalamus, in the diencephalon at the base of the brain, Figs. 2.A-1, 3.A-2. Additionally, input from the hypothalamus impacts on higher brain centers, so, for example, information on drives (sex, hunger, thirst) and emotions, and control of these drives and emotions descends from the limbic system to the hypothalamus, is modified and then returned to the limbic system again. Ascending sensory input to the hypothalamus regarding the status of the internal organs is via the reticular formation (Subsection 3.A, *The Spinal Cord and Brainstem*, page 29), and then out again via the autonomic nervous system. Signals from the hypothalamus also stimulate the pituitary gland to secrete hormones to regulate water, salt, and the metabolic and other hormonal parameters of the body. It is seen from this that the hypothalamus is the primary autonomic control center, weighing input from both above and below, and then directing the autonomic nervous system on this basis. The anatomy and function of the hypothalamus are described in detail in Section 6.B, The Hypothalamus, page 140.

Branches

The autonomic nervous system consists of two main branches, the sympathetic and the parasympathetic; the enteric branch is usually folded in with the latter of these two (Fig. 2.A-1), being considered as just one of the branches of the parasympathetic vagus nerve, however, there is good reason to question this [155]. The first of these, the sympathetic nervous system, is responsible for the "fight-or-flight" response [36]. In this reflexive response, the body and mind shift away from the normal homeostatic condition to one which optimizes the body/mind to either fight to defend itself or to flee from some threat. All of the sympathetic reflexes originate with the fight-or-flight response and so can be understood initially in terms of offering better chances for survival.

In the case of imminent danger, the sympathetic nervous system quickly prepares us to either defend ourselves against the threat, or to run from it. To this end, norepinephrine is released into the neural synapses, making them conductive for a brief moment. Following this, epinephrine and norepinephrine are released from the medulla of the adrenal glands for circulation in the vascular system for several minutes, in support of the initial reaction. When in this state, heart and respiration rates increase so as to furnish oxygen to the muscles, blood is diverted from internal organs to the muscles, mental alertness increases, the pupils

of the eyes dilate, as do the bronchioles of the lungs. And this is only a highly abbreviated list! In our present-day life, some of these responses are no longer logical or necessary, but they are present nonetheless as the "normal" responses to the stresses of modern-day living.

Arousal in the sympathetic nervous system is an all-or-nothing affair in that when the system is activated, *all* of the responses under its control are activated simultaneously, all with one goal, to protect the body from an outside threat. If the threat is in the form of an emotional stress rather than physical, the sympathetic response nonetheless is the same: all systems go. Actually, it now appears that there is some selective excitation possible in the sympathetic nervous system, but not much.

The global arousal of the body's defenses by the sympathetic nervous system is moderated by the responses of the body to the parasympathetic nervous system, Section 6.D, page 150. This system restores calm to the body's internal workings, slowing the heart and lowering the blood pressure, among other things. In general, the two subsystems of the autonomic nervous system are working simultaneously in a cooperative way, balanced as is appropriate to the situation at hand. Through stimulus from the hypothalamus, the relative amounts of sympathetic and parasympathetic excitation can be altered so that one of these becomes more dominant, yet both are functioning. These functions of the two branches of the autonomic nervous system are discussed in more detail below, together with the evidence that in humans the autonomic control of these internal functions can be brought under conscious control, especially through practice of the *yogasanas*.

The enteric nervous system controls the involuntary actions of the digestive system and is often classified as part of the parasympathetic nervous system, however, it has been shown to be able to operate efficiently without any connection to the central nervous system or to the vagus nerve of the parasympathetic nervous system. The enteric system uses serotonin as a neurotransmitter (Subsection 5.D, page 129), a compound not found in either the sympathetic or parasympathetic branches. It thus would seem worthy of recognition as a third branch of the autonomic system [155].

Aspects of the skeletal and the various branches of the autonomic nervous systems are compared in Table 6.A-1. The effects of autonomic action on the functions of the

TABLE 6.A-1. COMPARISON OF THE SKELETAL AND AUTONOMIC NERVOUS SYSTEMS [155]

Nervous system	Final Neurotransmitter	Target Organs
Skeletal	Acetylcholine	Skeletal Muscles
Sympathetic	Norepinephrine	Glands, blood vessels, heart, smooth muscles
Parasympathetic	Acetylcholine	Glands, blood vessels, heart, smooth muscles
Enteric	Acetylcholine, serotonin	Gut

TABLE 6.A-2. INFLUENCES OF THE SYMPATHETIC AND PARASYMPATHETIC NERVOUS SYSTEMS ON BODILY FUNCTIONS[a]

Site/Function	Sym	Parasym	Source/ Target[b]	Reference
Heart				
Rate	+	–		[80, 159, 195, 229, 230]
Contractile force	+	–		[230]
Coronary diameter, alpha receptors	–	+	T1–T4/CN X	[230]
Coronary diameter, beta receptors	+	+	T1–T4/CN X	[230]
Vascular resistance	+	–		[80]
Stroke Volume	+	–	CN X	[195]
Blood				
Clotting	+			[159, 343]
Blood pressure	+	–	T1–T4/CN X	[80, 159, 195, 343]
O_2 concentration	+			[343]
Red cell count	+			[319]
Core temperature	–	+		
Intestinal circulation	–	+		[473]
Brain				
Left hemisphere	+	–		[80]
Right hemisphere	–	+		[80]
Reticular formation	+	–		[80]
Posterior hypothalamus	+	–		[80]

Site/Function	Sym	Parasym	Source/ Target[b]	Reference
Anterior hypothalamus	−	+		[80]
Basal forebrain	−	+		[80]
Solitary tract	−	+		[80]
Alertness	+	−		[343]
Preoptic hypothalamus	−	+		[80]
EEG				
High frequency beta wave	+	−		[80]
Low frequency alpha wave	−	+		[80]
Habituation	−	+		[80]
Synchronicity	−	+		[80]
Sleep, stage 1	−	+		[462]
Sleep, stage 2	+	−		[462]
Sleep, stage 3	−	+		[462]
Sleep, stage 4	−	+		[462]
Sleep, REM	+			[225]
Eyes				
Lens curvature	−	+		
Pupil diameter	+	−	CN III	[159, 195, 230, 319]
Ciliary tone	−	+	CN III	[195, 229, 230]
Blink rate	+			[154]
Lachrimal output	+			[229]
Eyelid elevation	+	−		[80]
Intraocular pressure	+	−		
Sphincter pupillae	0	+		
Dilator sphincter	+	0		
Gastrointestinal Tract				
Peristalsis	−	+		[195]
Lumen sphincter tone	+	−		[230]
Gall bladder tone	−	+		[230]
Bile duct tone	−	+		[230]
Secretions	−	+		[159, 195]
Nutrient absorption	−	+		[473]
Anal sphincter	−	+		[473]
Metabolism				
Glucose	+	0	Liver	[159, 230, 319]
Fat	+			[159, 343]
Basal	+	−		[80, 230]
Glycogen synthesis	+	0	Liver	[230]
Skeletal Muscles				
Tone	+	−		[80, 159, 343]
O_2 consumption	+			
Vasoconstriction, alpha arteries	+	0		[195, 229, 230]
Vasodilation, beta arteries	+	0		[230]

Site/Function	Sym	Parasym	Source/ Target[b]	Reference
Lactate production	+	−		[80]
Coordinated excitation	+	+		
Smooth Muscles				
Vasoconstriction, arteries	+	0		[155, 229, 230]
Respiration/Lungs				
Rate	+	−		[80, 159, 229]
Blood vessel diameter	−	?		[195, 230]
O_2 consumption	+	−		[80]
Glandular secretions	+			[195]
Bronchiole diameter	+	−		[229, 230]
Nasal erection	+	0		[26, 374]
Nasal laterality, R open/L closed	+	−		[80, 374]
Nasal laterality, L open/R closed	−	+		[80, 374]
Glandular Secretions				
Nasal mucus	−	+		[229, 319]
Salivation	+	+ +	CN VII, CN IX	[225, 229, 319]
Lacrimal	0	+		
Gastric	−	+		[159, 343]
Adrenal medulla, adrenal cortex	+ +	0	T10–T12	[343]
Pineal gland	+			[195]
Chemical Release				
Insulin	−	+	Pancreas	[318, 343, 425]
Thyroxine	+			[343]
Epinephrine	+	0	Adrenal medulla	[80, 195, 343]
Norepinephrine	+	0	Adrenal medulla	[80, 195, 343]
Cortisol	+	−	Adrenal cortex	[80]
Glucose	+	−		[225, 230]
ACTH	+			
Aldosterone	+			
CRF	+			
Lactic acid	+	0		[80]
Glycogen	0	+		[230]
Beta Endorphin	+	0		[230]
Thyroid hormone	+	−		[80]
Oxytocin	+			[195]
Vasopressin	+			[195, 225]
Fatty acids	+	0	Adrenal cortex	[159, 195, 230]
Glucagon	+			[343]
Skin				
Raises finger tempurature	0	+		[80]
Lowers finger tempurature	+	0		[80, 159]
Sweating	+ +	0	T1–L3	[159, 195, 229, 230, 319]

Site/Function	Sym	Parasym	Source/ Target[b]	Reference
Piloerection	+	0	T1–L3	[230]
Vasoconstriction	+	0	T1–L3	[159, 195, 229, 319]
Shivering	−			[343]
Kidney, Bladder, Genitalia				
Urinary output	−	0		[230]
Urinary sphincter release	0	+		[319, 473]
Rectal bladder release	0	+		[319]
Detrussor tone	0	+		[230]
Trigone tone	+	0		[230]
Penile/clitoral erection	0	+		[229, 230, 473]
Ejaculation	+	0		[195, 230, 473]
Other				
Immunity	+/−	+		[80]

----

[a] Lists the effect of activation of either the sympathetic or parasympathetic nervous system on the site, function, process, or event as either enhancing/increasing (+), no effect (0), or inhibiting/decreasing (−).

[b] Lists the neuronal paths used in the activation and the target organ if there is one. "CN" is cranial nerve (Subsection 2.C, *The Cranial Nerves*, page 17).

body are manifold, and many if not all of these are within the reach of the *yogasana* practitioner. The results of an extended search of the literature in this regard are presented in Table 6.A-2. For a more detailed account of the interaction between mind and body *vis-a-vis* the autonomic nervous system, see Section 6.F, The Effects of Emotions and Attitudes on Stress, page 160.

The roles of the sympathetic and parasympathetic nervous systems have been interpreted by Iyengar [211] using the classical Indian concepts of the *nadis* (Section 4.F, page 100), with the sympathetic nervous system corresponding to the *ida* and parasympathetic to the *pingala nadis*, respectively. When, through *yogasana* practice, the energies in these two *nadis* become "fused", they then generate energy which is available to all parts of the body through the *sushumna nadi*, the central nervous system. Anatomically, sympathetic dominance is associated with increased electrical activity of the beta waves in the EEG of the left cerebral hemisphere and parasympathetic dominance is associated with increased activity of alpha waves in the EEG of the right cerebral hemisphere (Section 3.E, Brainwaves and the Electroencephalogram, page 57). The many aspects of cerebral laterality, mood, the breath, and autonomic dominance are discussed in Sections 3.D, Cerebral Hemispheric Laterality, page 49, and 12.C, Nasal Laterality, page 374.

The huge number of autonomic functions that are being monitored continuously for deviations from their setpoint values suggests why this function is normally assigned to the subconscious. If all of this information were to appear in the conscious realm, the knowing/thinking mind would be so swamped with setpoint information as to be rendered nonfunctional in regard to making other conscious decisions.

SECTION 6.B. THE HYPOTHALAMUS

Location and Properties

Neurologically, the hypothalamus is the head ganglion of the autonomic system. As such, it is responsible for an amazingly large number of regulatory functions, all aimed at homeostasis and carried out largely in the subconscious so that we are hardly aware of their occurrence until something goes wrong. A list of the hypothalamus's responsibilities would include regulation of the body's temperature, water balance, energy resources, feeding behavior, and rates of heart action and breathing. Speaking geographically, the anterior part of the hypothalamus is reserved for the control of the parasympathetic system, whereas the posterior part is reserved for control of the sympathetic system [342].

The hypothalamus is a rather poorly defined organ lying at the base of the forebrain, Fig. 2.A-2, within the diencephalon of the limbic system. Rossi [389] states, "One seeks in vain for clarity regarding the basic anatomy and functions of the hypothalamus." It is composed of a poorly organized mass of subregions; its nuclei (Fig. 6.B-1), all of which communicate with one another, are used for regulation of the autonomic, neuropeptide, endocrine and immune systems, all of which communicate again with one another. Its small size (being the size of a pea, and weighing only a few grams, it occupies less than 1% of the

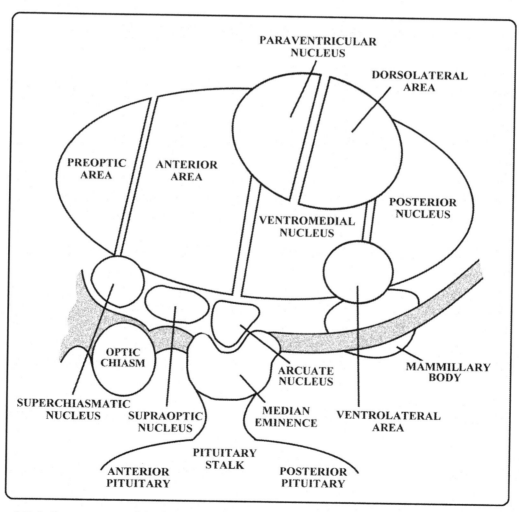

Fig. 6.B-1. Component nuclei of the hypothalamus within the brain and their relation to the pituitary gland, as seen from the left side; the entire organ weighs only 4 grams. See Table 6.B-1 for descriptions of these nuclei.

human brain's volume) belies its importance to the body's well being, for, on a volume-to-volume basis, no other part of the brain receives as much blood as is pumped through the hypothalamus, and Swanson [455] states, "It may very well be that gram for gram the hypothalamus is the most important piece of tissue in any organism." In lower creatures such as insects and reptiles, the hypothalamus is the highest brain center in the nervous system.

In addition to its effects on the purely physical parameters of the body, the hypothalamus also can affect the emotional climate, for it is intimately connected to the limbic system. The early experiments on hypothalamic stimulation strongly suggested that this complex is involved with the expression of emotional states as well as the more obvious somatic, endocrine and autonomic roles [225]. In humans, the hypothalamus controls the emotions of anger, fear, pleasure, contentment and placidity, the sex drive, *etc.*, but with an overlying control by the forebrain so as to make the expression of the emotions acceptable and appropriate. The hypothalamus integrates emotional and visceral response to emotional stress.

As discussed in Subsection 21.B, *Circadian Rhythms; Physiological Peaks and Valleys in the 24-Hour Period*, page 476, hormonal levels in the body rise and fall in patterns that are keyed to the light/dark cycles of the Sun. This timing is accomplished by neurological signals from the eyes that go directly to the hypothalamus, which then is able to turn hormone levels on and off at the proper times by reference to sunrise and sunset. The pineal gland (Section 15.B, page 404) is also involved in this timing scheme. In a well-regulated body, the hormonal levels are optimum for

yogasana practice between the hours of 4:00 to 6:00 in the morning.

As discussed above, the hypothalamus has a hormonal connection to the pituitary gland within the brain and is directly responsible for autonomic functions such as blood pressure, heart rate, breathing rate, metabolism, muscle tone, *etc.* It also has neural connections to the limbic system (which deals with emotions) and through the limbic system, with the prefrontal cortex (which deals with thoughts). It is through this web of interconnections that bodily reactions, thoughts, emotions, and behaviors all come together to influence one another in nonlinear ways. For example, with this map, it is easy to trace the connection between fears hidden within the limbic system, the flexional reflex, and the sympathetic response of the autonomic nervous system that results when doing *urdhva dhanurasana* (Section 7.D, Reflex Actions, page 211).

Function

As there are both ascending and descending nerve fibers both leaving and entering the hypothalamus, it is the central information agency of the entire body. Being the major output pathway of the limbic system, the hypothalamus integrates the sensory-perceptual, emotional and cognitive signals of the mind with the biology of the body* [389]. But not all of the hypothalamic nuclei are connected to the autonomic nervous system, for some are involved only with the endocrine, neuropeptide, somatic or with the immune systems, in non-autonomic ways.

Interestingly, the information flowing into the hypothalamus is of two sorts, neural impulses flowing through the body's network of nerves, and chemical hormones cir-

---

* Note how closely this matches the aim of yoga, phrased as the union of the body, the mind and the emotions/spirit! As we shall see, the hypothalamic control of the autonomic nervous system is indeed a very important factor in understanding how yoga affects the body/mind, and *vice versa*.

culating through the body's fluids. Similarly, the output of the hypothalamus involves both neural impulses and the release of hormones and neuropeptides into the body fluids. There are then four possible modes of action involving the hypothalamus: neural input/neural output, neural input/hormonal output, hormonal input/hormonal output, and hormonal input/neural output. All four of these modes in fact, are used by the hypothalamus.

Hormonally, the pituitary is the master gland controlling the body's growth, reproductive capabilities, metabolism and response to trauma and stress, by controlling the hormone levels in the body. However, even the pituitary is under the control of the hypothalamus. Thus the hypothalamus releases hormones that act specifically upon the pituitary to either stimulate or inhibit its secondary release of hormones into the blood stream. In particular, the hypothalamus dictates the pituitary's control over growth hormone, follicular stimulating hormone (FSH), luteinizing hormone (LH), adrenocorticotropic hormone (ACTH), thyroid stimulating hormone (TSH), prolactin, antidiuretic hormone (ADH, vasopressin), and oxytocin (Chapter 15, THE HORMONES, page 399). In its only inhibitory action, the hypothalamus inhibits the pituitary from releasing prolactin, which otherwise stimulates the flow of breast milk [340].

The hypothalamus exerts an effect not only on the pituitary, but on other brain centers to which it is neurally connected. Note then its connections to the amygdala (emotions), and the hippocampus (memory). In turn, the hypothalamus is influenced by direct connection to the olfactory nerve (emotional memory of odors), and to the eyes (where it dilates the pupils and sets the internal clock according to the light/dark sensations of the eyes). Centers within the hypothalamus regulate the feeding reflex (generating hunger and satiety sensations to

promote and inhibit eating), adjust the levels of sugar in the blood (mobilizing the release of sugar into the blood from storage sites), control the water balance in the body via control of the release of hormones from the kidneys (creating a thirst sensation when short on water, increasing urination when overloaded with water), raise and lower the blood pressure, and initiate shivering in order to raise the body's muscle tone and thereby generate heat, but initiating sweating in order to cool the body. Hypothalamic centers can decrease the heart rate, inhibit the thyroid, maintain the sex organs, promote the secondary sexual characteristics, promote breast feeding and uterine contractions, and regulate the menstrual cycle. The hypothalamus regulates metabolism via the thyroid gland, the sensations of hunger and satiety, and the general level of digestive action at any one time. All of this in an organ the size of a pea!

With neuronal connection to centers both higher and lower than itself, a chain of command can be drawn up for the hypothalamus: it is controlled from above by the amygdala and the thalamus, which in turn are controlled by the cortex, whereas the hypothalamus is in control of the autonomic nervous system.

Certain nuclei or hypothalamic areas (Fig. 6.B-1) have been identified with certain functional responses, as listed in Table 6.B-1. This Table lists in a clear way the multitude of functions for which specific nuclei or nuclear areas of the hypothalamus are responsible. Note however, that some autonomic functions are governed by subcortical structures connected to but outside the hypothalamus.

Operant conditioning is not limited to the skeletal-motor system. Responses mediated by the autonomic nervous system, such as blood pressure and heart rate can be modified by appropriate reinforcements [225]. The great and well-documented successes

TABLE 6.B-1. LOCALE AND FUNCTIONS OF CENTERS WITHIN THE HYPOTHALAMUS [195, 230, 389]

Center	Function
Lateral hypothalamus	Triggers increased heart rate and blood pressure, peripheral vasoconstriction, skeletal muscle vasodilation, general sympathetic activity
Posterior hypothalamus	Cutaneous vasoconstriction; piloerection; promotes secretion of epinephrine and thyroxine; increase of metabolic rate; generates and conserves body heat
Dorsolateral hypothalamus	Adjusts salt concentrations in fluids
Anterior hypothalamus	Activates heat-loss centers; reduces heart rate and blood pressure; increases GI secretions; initiates sweating; inhibits thyroid
Preoptic	Controls sexual, maternal behavior; causes body to cool; sleep/wake cycle
Supraoptic	Secretes hormones
Paraventricular	Controls water, salt and thirst; secretes hormones; promotes eating of carbohydrates
Suprachiasmatic nucleus	Drives circadian rhythms; vision
Median eminence	Excretes hormones to pituitary
Solitary nucleus	Receives information from viscera

of biofeedback in controlling what are otherwise automatic body functions are testimony to one's ability to willfully intercede in the workings of such systems.

SECTION 6.C. THE SYMPATHETIC NERVOUS SYSTEM

It is understandable that the hypothalamus is more concerned with excitations in the sympathetic nervous system than with excitations in the parasympathetic because sympathetic excitations can save one's life in an emergency. And though the sympathetic alarm response does have its place in emergency situations, it can also lead to problems if it is continued for a long period. On the other hand, one can exist without activation of the sympathetic nervous system, however, without it, one cannot do strenuous work, cannot fend for one's self and cannot survive in a harsh environment.

Innervation

The efferent fibers of the sympathetic nervous system originate in the spinal cord at levels between T1 and L3. Exiting through the lateral horns of the cord, they immediately synapse in chain structures which parallel the spinal column, forming the paravertebral ganglia of the sympathetic trunk, Fig. 6.C-1a. Fibers entering the paravertebral trunk may continue through without synapse, may enter at one level and leave at another, or may enter, synapse and leave at the same level. It is a characteristic of the sympathetic nervous system that there is a synapse close to the vertebrae, followed by a long axon to the effector organ. Neural components of the parasympathetic nervous system also have a synapse between the vertebral column and the effector organ, but in this case, the synapse is much closer to the organ than to the vertebrae, Fig. 6.C-1b.

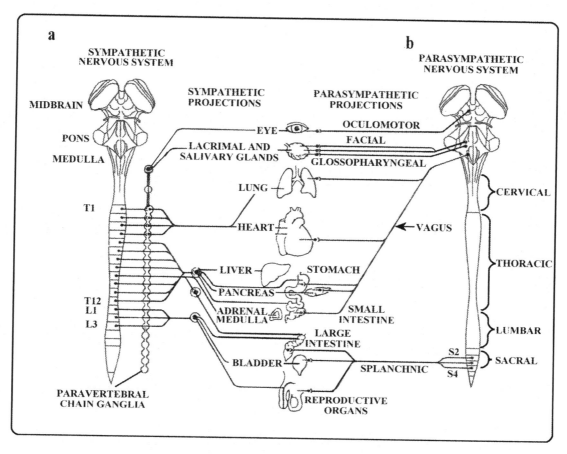

Fig. 6.C-1. The sympathetic (**a**) and parasympathetic (**b**) divisions of the autonomic nervous system. Note that several organs are innervated by both systems, and that the two subsystems use very different points of entry and exit on the spinal cord. Only a small number of the organs and muscles innervated by the autonomic nervous system are shown.

All synapses in the paravertebral trunk use acetylcholine as the neurotransmitter. There are a few ganglia which are not bundled with the other spinal nerves, namely, the nerves to the pupil of the eye, the salivary glands and the blood vessels of the head, heart and bronchi, Fig. 6.C-1.

Fibers leaving the paravertebral trunk then travel along with arteries to a second ganglion complex (plexus), this one still removed from the effector organ and activated by the catecholamines (except in the sweat glands and in the vascular system of the muscles, where acetylcholine again is the neurotransmitter), Fig. 6.C-2. As the efferent fibers travel from the postganglia to the effector organs, they branch repeatedly

so that many sites can be activated in cascade fashion by one initiating efferent neural impulse, Fig. 6.C-1a. Interestingly, the fibers from the sympathetic system synapsing to the skeletal muscles use acetylcholine as neurotransmitter, while the direct somatic synapses to the same muscles use the catecholamines. The various effector organs and sites also send afferent nerves back to the spinal cord and thence to the hypothalamus for input in the decision-making process leading eventually to their excitation.

The nerves of the sympathetic system are disynaptic, inasmuch as they synapse once at the paravertebral chain ganglia and a second time at ganglia far from the effector or-

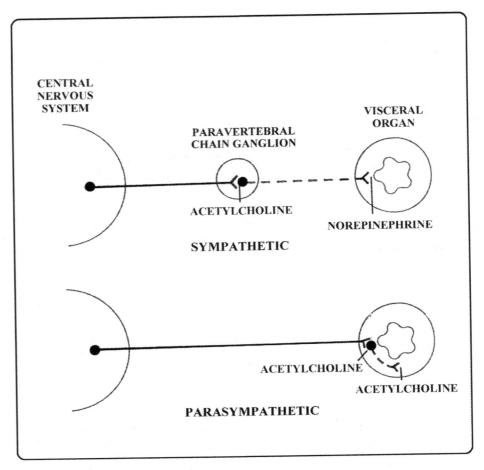

Fig. 6.C-2. Comparison of the innervation existing between the central nervous system and the visceral organs in the sympathetic and parasympathetic nervous systems. Note the different neurotransmitters used in the two systems and the relative positions of the synapses [195].

gans. By contrast, nerves in the neuromuscular system are monosynaptic, with nerves from the central nervous system traveling long distances to finally synapse at the relevant muscles. In the autonomic nervous system, the intermediate synapse allows for a modulating influence due to the dendrites from other neurons which contribute to the eventual neural signal. Thus the additional synapse allows for subtle fine tuning of the transmitted signal strength [155]. It follows that the motor control attained through the autonomic system may be of a finer sort than that possible through direct somatic control from the cortex. If so, then one possibly has an explanation for the quality of the performance when an athlete is in "the

zone", an unusual mental state in which the consciousness has shifted from the norm and is working in a rather independent way, as appropriate for the autonomic nervous system.

On the other hand, the axonic terminal at the neuromuscular junction is very precise in applying its neurotransmitters to just the intended receptor. In contrast, in the sympathetic and parasympathetic systems there is branching of the axonal terminal and a rather indiscriminate spraying of the neurotransmitters over a broad area of the innervated organ. The difference then is that muscles are capable of fine local control over just which muscle fibers are to be contracted, whereas the organs connected to the autonomic system tend to be activated in a global sense, *i.e.*, the bladder, for example, on command from the autonomic nervous system is emptied by the contraction of all of the muscles encircling it, rather than by a select few [155].

The Effects of Sympathetic Excitation

As can be seen from Table 6.A-2, excitations in the sympathetic nervous system favor blood flow to skeletal muscles, to the heart, and to the brain, all in expectation of an attack of some sort. At the same time, the epinephrine released by the sympathetic excitation directs blood out of the digestive system and into the muscles by inhibiting peristalsis in the gut, Chapter 18, THE GASTROINTESTINAL ORGANS AND DIGESTION, page 441.

As can be seen from the Table, the sympathetic nervous system readily initiates the flow of epinephrine and norepinephrine from the adrenal medulla into the blood stream, and these hormones by their actions can strongly affect blood flow. Rossi [389] states that the practice of focused attention, imagery, biofeedback, and therapeutic hypnosis (and presumably yoga under the category of focused attention) all involve redirection of blood flow. Arguing that this type of practice is a common factor in the resolution of most if not all body-mind problems, he lists 16 healing processes which are dramatically aided by redirection of the blood flow, all via the effects of the mind on the autonomic nervous system (see Section 6.F, The Effects of Emotions and Attitudes on Stress, page 160).

The autonomic nervous system affects blood flow by dilating some vascular components and constricting others using neurotransmitters in the sympathetic nervous branch. The only parasympathetic input to this is via the vagus nerve (cranial nerve X) to the heart which works to decrease the heart rate and contractility, Table 6.A-2. Once the hypothalamus is signaled by the cortex to do so, its release of hormones is rapid (on the scale of seconds), and affects target organs throughout the entire body. Because the postganglionic synapses of the autonomic nervous system respond strongly to nicotine, cigarette smoke is very effective in lighting up the sympathetic nervous system.

One can abstract Table 6.A-2 to list nine principal and immediate effects on the body/mind once the fight-or-flight response has been triggered [343]. Others, no less important, work on a longer time scale.

1) Sugar and fat enter the bloodstream as fuel for muscles and brain

2) Respiration rate increases to raise the level of oxygen in the blood

3) Heart rate and blood pressure increase to speed the delivery of oxygen to cells

4) Blood-clotting mechanisms are activated in anticipation of injury

5) Muscle tone increases in anticipation of muscular effort; sweating increases

6) Pituitary increases hormonal output; epinephrine and glucagon production also increase

7) Digestive processes (peristalsis, *etc.*) put on hold as blood is diverted from gut to muscles and brain

8) Pupils of the eyes dilate

9) Attention and alertness increase as beta waves become prominent in the EEG.

Release of the Catecholamines

The hypothalamus-mediated release of the important hormones epinephrine and norepinephrine upon stimulation of the sympathetic nervous system warrants a more detailed discussion. Once the hypothalamus is aroused by the appropriate signal coming either from below (via the reticular formation) or above (via the limbic and cortical systems), among other things, there is a direct neural signal to the adrenal medulla, a gland which sits on top of each of the kidneys. Actually, within each adrenal cap there are two glands, the adrenal medulla and the adrenal cortex, having different structures, embryonic origins and hormonal secretions. On command from the hypothalamus, the adrenal medulla releases a mixture of epinephrine (80%) and norepinephrine (20%) into the blood stream. This mixture of adrenalcorticoids is often called the catecholamines. A measurable amount of the analgesic pain-killer endorphin is also released from the adrenal medulla. As epinephrine preferentially binds to the beta receptors in cell walls and norepinephrine preferentially binds to alpha receptors in cell walls, and the materials are circulating freely throughout the body, these materials have several immediate effects as listed in Table 6.C-1.

As summarized in the Table, the catecholamines constrict the blood vessels in the skin and the viscera (mostly due to norepinephrine binding to alpha-cell receptors), thus leaving more blood for the muscles, the blood vessels of which are covered with beta receptors and so are dilated by the epinephrine*. The epinephrine (common in bronchial inhalers) acts to open the bronchioles, thereby making it easier for oxygen to come into the lungs and carbon dioxide to leave. At the same time, the heart rate and contractility are increased, the arterioles in the heart expand with more blood, and the blood pressure rises. The blood will now clot more readily (in case there is any spilled), and the pupils dilate so as to offer the widest field of view. The glycogenolysis turns glycogen in the liver into glucose for the brain, while lipolysis turns fatty acids into glucose, again for use by the brain in its time of emergency. At the same time, the brain is aroused and is unusually alert.

Activation of the sympathetic nervous system tends to turn all functions on (or off) together in one concerted action because the circulating catecholamines released into the bloodstream by the adrenals energize the synapses of all components of the sympathetic nervous system. Once triggered, it may take 20 minutes or so for the epinephrine and norepinephrine to be cleared from

TABLE 6.C-1. EFFECTS OF RELEASING EPINEPHRINE AND NOREPINEPHRINE INTO THE BLOOD

Effects of Epinephrine	Effects of Norepinephrine
Vasoconstriction in the skin, kidney, GI tract and spleen	Vasoconstriction in the skin, kidney, GI tract and spleen
Vasodilation in muscles	Decreased digestive action
Bronchiole dilation	Hair erection
Glycogenolysis	Glycogenolysis
Lipolysis	Lipolysis
Increased heart activity	Increased heart activity
Blood pressure rises	Blood pressure rises
Increased blood clotting	
Pupils dilate	

* By having two types of cell-wall receptors (alpha and beta), the body manages to constrict some blood vessels while simultaneously dilating others using the same epinephrine-norepinephrine mixture. The shift among those vessels that are vasodilated and those that are vasoconstricted acts to shift blood flow throughout the body as well as to change temperatures locally.

the blood stream and the synapses. Clearly, in this one stroke, the sympathetic nervous system has prepared the body for a physical/mental challenge of the sort we may face in our daily *yogasana* practice! But there is much more going on.

Cortisol

Even when the body is resting and there is no mental or physical stress on it, the hypothalamus slowly releases a hormone called corticotropin releasing factor (CRF) into a duct leading to the pituitary. The action of CRF in the pituitary is to release a second hormone, ACTH (adrenocortico-tropic hormone) into the blood stream and once ACTH reaches the adrenal cortex, three other corticosteroids are let go. The most important of these is cortisol (dihydro-cortisone) which is a potent stress reliever on a short time scale when working along with the catecholamines, as when doing *yog-asanas*.

ACTH acting on the adrenal cortex also produces aldosterone, which works within the kidney to maintain the proper concentrations of K^+ and Na^+ in the body fluids, and also regulates the sex hormones which in women are important sources of estrogen, but are much less important in men for whom the sex hormones come instead from the testes.

In the short term, cortisol in the blood relieves stress and its level is very sensitive to one's psychological state. In addition to being necessary for repeated muscle contraction, cortisol redirects glucose to the brain, breaks down protein into constituent amino acids for bodily repair, and raises blood pressure if stress happens to lower it (falling blood pressure is the instantaneous response to stress).

Were the hypothalamus to overproduce CRF, then high cortisol levels could result. However, at too high concentrations, cortisol acts to turn off the release of CRF from the hypothalamus and of ACTH from the pituitary, so that the body systems can be brought back into balance through negative feedback.* As the unstressed release of CRF from the hypothalamus is regulated by the circadian clock (Chapter 21, TIME AND BODY RHYTHMS, page 473), there is a diurnal variation in the body's cortisol level, being maximal in the early morning and minimal 12 hours later [309]. The traditional time for *yogasana* practice (4:00 to 7:00 AM) corresponds with the peak levels of cortisol in the body, *i.e.*, these are times of high energy and alertness.

In times of momentary high stress, the hypothalamus will flood the body with CRF, leading to very high cortisol levels. Such high levels of cortisol in the body are appropriate for real health emergencies such as freezing cold, hemorrhage, broken bones, wounds, *etc.* If the yoga practice is so intense as to reach this level of cortisol in the body, you have gone from the response-to-challenge mode to the response-to-threat mode, Subsection 6.F, *Emotion and Stress*, page 160, and should moderate your practice.

If the body is subject to chronic stress, then the cortisol levels will tend to remain high in spite of the negative-feedback effect of cortisol on CRF and ACTH production. In this case, the cortisol setpoint is reset to a higher level, and one can expect ulcers, lymphatic atrophy, protein imbalance, hypertension and vascular disorders along with the consequences of a depressed immune system [153].

In an interesting preliminary study [49], a one-hour *yogasana* practice with both experienced and inexperienced students showed

---

* However, the situation is a little more complicated, as leukocytes as well as the hypothalamus also are now known to release CRF.

significant lowering of plasma cortisol at the end of the hour (11:00 AM to 12:00 noon) in both groups, suggesting that the practice worked to reduce stress in these students. However, the study seems to have neglected the fact that cortisol is released in spurts and so is subject to rapid fluctuations (Fig. 21.B-9).

The hippocampus, an organ responsible for transferring short-term memory to long-term storage is studded with cortisol receptors, suggesting in some way, a role for cortisol in memory [153].

Renin

In addition to the catecholamines, the adrenal glands are able to excrete renin through the stimulation of the glands by the sympathetic nervous system, as when performing *yogasanas* or otherwise being under stress. Renin is an enzyme that acts on the angiotensins, eventually leading to the production of aldosterone, a hormone having an effect on the water retention abilities of the kidneys, and effecting the salt and water balance in the body. This is discussed further in Chapter 15, THE HORMONES, page 399.

SECTION 6.D. THE PARASYMPATHETIC NERVOUS SYSTEM

The parasympathetic branch of the autonomic nervous system is shown in Fig. 6.C-1b. If the sympathetic nervous system can be thought of in terms of "fight-or-flight", then the appropriate phrase for the parasympathetic nervous system is "relaxation response". Benson describes the "relaxation response" in prayer, meditation and yoga as due to "an integrated hypothalamic response resulting in generalized decreased sympathetic nervous system activity" [36]. The parasympathetic nervous system plays a more passive role in the body than does

the sympathetic, for its main job is to moderate sympathetic responses and to bring the body back to homeostasis once the sympathetic stimulation of an emergency is past. Actually, the two competing nervous systems are always "on" to some extent, with the relative proportions of each ready to change at a moment's notice, to accommodate whatever the situation. One sees in Fig. 6.C-1 that several organs are innervated by both the sympathetic and parasympathetic autonomic branches.

When the parasympathetic relaxation response is dominant, then the general physiologic and behavioral short-term changes are as follows [343]:

1) Decreases in heart rate, blood pressure and sweat production

2) Pupils of the eyes contract; many tears and much saliva

3) Increased peristalsis and digestive enzyme production; relative lack of control over defecation

4) EEG brainwaves shift toward the alpha state

5) Skeletal muscle tone decreases

6) Insulin production increases

7) Sense of inactivity, relaxation, drowsiness; lowered level of arousal

It is not unusual to find that as a *yogasana* class draws to an end and the students lie down for *savasana*, that a student will break into muffled sobs and copious tears. These tears and saliva are promoted by the parasympathetic response accompanying relaxation; the generally positive effect of parasympathetic relaxation on secretions (Chapter 14, page 393) is obvious as well in *sarvangasana* and *savasana* as a tendency to salivate excessively. It also appears that when the muscle tension is relaxed through the *yogasanas*, the previously-buried emotional upset that leads to muscle tension can be brought to the surface, again with sobs.

In the parasympathetic system, the proportion of afferent nerve fibers is unusually large, being as much as 85–90% in the vagus nerve, the main nerve of the parasympathetic system stretching from the neck almost to the genitals. These afferent nerves may be either myelinated or not, and can carry information on pain, distress or discomfort in the visceral organs. As discussed in Section 10.E, Dermatomes and Referred Pain, page 303, the visceral pain may be referred to the skin overlying another area of the body. As parasympathetic innervation does not extend to the sweat glands or the muscles which make hairs stand on end (piloerection), Table 6.A-2, there is only more or less sympathetic excitation in these cases.

Innervation

The nerve fibers forming the parasympathetic nervous system originate in the brainstem and then exit both from the brainstem (bypassing the upper vertebrae) so as to form part or all of the 12 cranial nerves, and exit as well from the lower region of the spinal column, between S2 and S4, Fig. 6.C-1b. Unlike the case with the ganglia in the sympathetic system, all of those in the parasympathetic system have synapses based on acetylcholine, Fig. 6.C-2, rather than epinephrine, and so they are not activated when the blood is rich in this latter neurotransmitter. The nerve structure of the parasympathetic system is different too from that of the sympathetic in that there is only one ganglion between the brainstem and the effector organ, and that one ganglion is quite close to the target organ. The various neuronal components of the parasympathetic nervous system and their effector organs and sites are listed in Table 6.D-1.

In contrast to the all-on/all-off aspect of the sympathetic nervous system, the parasympathetic nervous system is wired so that those parts of the system can be activated that are needed at the moment, while the other parts remain dormant.

TABLE 6.D-1. PARASYMPATHETIC NERVES AND THEIR EFFECTOR SITES AND ORGANS

Nerve-Fiber Bundle	Organ or Site
Cranial Nerve III	Ciliary muscle of the eye
	Sphincter pupillae of the eye
	Extraocular recti muscles of the eye
Cranial Nerve VII	Lachrimal gland
	Nasal and oral secretions
Cranial Nerve IX	Nasal and oral secretions
Cranial Nerve X (Vagus)	Heart
	Bronchioles of the lungs
	Stomach
	Liver, gall bladder and pancreas
	Intestine and colon
S2, S3, S4	Descending and sigmoid colon
	Rectum and bladder
	Genitals

The Vagus Nerves

Eighty percent of all of the parasympathetic nerve fibers in the body are found in the cranial nerve X, called the vagus nerve. Actually, there are two vagus nerves, the left and the right. Both go to the throat area, the lungs, heart and upper stomach, however the left stops at the upper stomach, whereas the right vagus nerve continues into the abdominal cavity and connects with digestive organs all the way down to the colon [343]. The word "vagus" is related to "vagabond", as the nerve seems to wander a great distance in the body [57].

The vagus nerves pass through the chest cavity and the motions of the chest while breathing seem to stimulate this nerve, with a subsequent effect on the heart rate. Thus it is known that on inhalation, there is a sympathetic excitation of the heart and the heart rate increases, whereas on exhalation, the effect is dominated by the parasympathetic response via the vagus nerves and the heart rate decreases [343]. This alternating effect of breathing on the heart rate is known as the "respiratory sinus arhythmia", and is discussed further in Subsection 12.A, *Innervation and Control of the Breathing Centers*, page 366.

The above illustrates the principle of reciprocal innervation of an organ. Both sympathetic and parasympathetic nerves innervate the heart, the first to raise the heart rate and the second to depress it. At rest, both are active and the resting heart rate is a reflection of this balance. In times of stress, the parasympathetic signal decreases in favor of the sympathetic, and the heart rate increases; the relative dominance of these two nervous systems shifts as the need arises.

The vagus nerve also passes through the center of the neck, and so it is possible that it is influenced as well by the pressure in the neck in *sarvangasana* [241], especially if the pose is done without blankets under the shoulders. Inasmuch as *sarvangasana* is considered to be a relaxing pose, we may take it to mean that the pressure on the vagus nerve in the region of the neck serves to stimulate a parasympathetic response. However, the vagus nerve plays an indirect role in the changes in respiration and blood circulation that occur whenever one is inverted in any *yogasana*. In brief, when certain receptors in the neck and chest (Section 11.E, Monitoring Blood Pressure with the Baroreceptors, page 339) sense the blood pressure is rising, they signal the hypothalamus as to the situation, and the response via the vagus nerve is to slow the heart rate and dilate the blood vessels accordingly. This is explained in more detail in Section 11.F, Blood Pressure in Inverted *Yogasanas*, page 343. The vagus nerve similarly is prominent in the stimulation of peristalsis and gastric secretion in the gut, however it should be noted that peristalsis takes place even after the vagus nerve is severed (Subsection 18.A, *Peristalsis*, page 447).

As discussed more fully in Subsection 7.D, *Other Reflex Actions*, page 220, the vagus nerve also plays a second but no less important role in regulating heart action in certain *yogasanas*. Thanks to the vagal heart-slowing reflex, pressure applied to various points around the orbits of the eyes (as when one performs *adho mukha svanasana* with the forehead resting upon a block) leads to a rapid shift toward parasympathetic dominance. This shift toward the relaxation inherent in parasympathetic dominance is most evident when infants (and adults) rub their eyes with the fists in preparation for sleep.

The Effects of Parasympathetic Excitation

Interestingly, all of the sympathetic reactions are bound together, so that if one of them is excited, all of them are excited, whereas the parasympathetic reactions are not necessarily bound to one another in this way. Consequently, if one particular body function can be turned from sympathetic dominance to parasympathetic dominance, it then can have the effect of turning off all sympathetic functions! That is to say, if we are sympathetically energized, and then consciously work with the breath so that the respiration rate becomes parasympathetically dominant, the other sympathetic functions will assume their subservient roles as well, and one has relaxed globally.

Our emotions are tied strongly to the momentary dominance of one or the other of the two autonomic branches. For example, recent experiments on the sites of brain function [385] show that the right prefrontal cortex is the site for negative, fearful thoughts, whereas the left prefrontal cortex is the site for positive thoughts. In depression, the EEG of the left prefrontal cortex is overly intense in the relaxing alpha-wave rhythm characteristic of parasympathetic dominance, whereas the right prefrontal cortex is deficient in this brainwave. In a sense, in depression, the left prefrontal hemisphere has gone to sleep, and the therapy for depression then is a *yogasana* routine which stimulates the sympathetic nervous system, leading to an alert state of mind (see Subsection 20.A, *Yogasana Versus Depression*, page 467).

It was mentioned above (Section 6.A, page 133) that the emotions of the hypothalamus are held in check by the prefrontal cortex. However, in those for whom the prefrontal cortex is under-developed, there is a strong parasympathetic dominance across the entire body/mind, and the emotional control takes an odd turn. In such people, sympathetic arousal is difficult, and the people are remorseless, lack any feelings of guilt, and lacking inhibitions, thrive on violence [327].

SECTION 6.E. AUTONOMIC BALANCE: STRESS AND *YOGASANA*

Stress

Stress is the reaction to any action or situation (called the stressor) which tends to unbalance a person either physiologically or psychologically, the effect being beneficial or harmful, or both in varying amounts. The thought that a particular stressor is either "good" or "bad" is not a useful one, because a stressor may be good for one person and bad for another, and in fact may have both good and bad aspects at the same time.

Though the fight-or-flight response may have been a very appropriate one for the circumstances in which it evolved tens of thousands of years ago, it is archaic today, for we live in a very different kind of world. In our world today, the most important aspect of stress is the time factor: is the stressor a momentary pressure or is it something that is chronic and longlasting? If it is the latter situation, then the sympathetic response that long ago was designed to protect us and keep us safe has become a stress today that is often harmful and even may be fatal.

The most common stressors today involve excitation of the sympathetic nervous system. Though originally developed in the course of human evolution as a life-saving response to the mortal dangers of living among wild animals in a violent environment, our stressors today are more psychological, and centered around our job, our family, traffic delays, *etc.* Nonetheless, the body's sympathetic response to a stressor, whether it be a genuine threat to our safety or just an annoyance, is fixed; our autonomic response is the same whether it is due to a python dropping out of the trees onto our head, or is due to a driver who insists on driving at 10 miles/hour below the speed limit and has traffic backed up for miles.

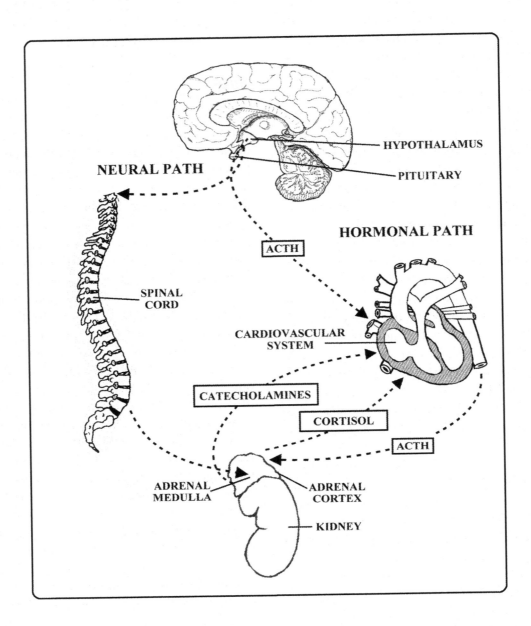

Fig. 6.E-1. The body's response to a stressor is both hormonal (using the endocrine pathway) and neural (using the autonomic nervous system). In the former case, the end result is the release of cortisol from the adrenal cortex, and in the latter case it is the release of the catecholamines from the adrenal medulla.

When reacting to a stressor, the body follows a hard-wired program, the fight-or-flight response, which follows two courses simultaneously, one of them hormonal and one of them neural, Fig. 6.E-1. In either case, the action begins in the hypothalamus [337], Sections 6.A, page 133, and 6.B, page 140.

In the case of the hormonal response to the stressor, the hypothalamus releases the hormone CRF directly into the pituitary gland, which in turn releases the hormone ACTH into the blood stream. On reaching the adrenal glands, the ACTH promotes the release of epinephrine and norepinephrine into the blood stream. Circulating then to all parts of the body, the epinephrine and norepinephrine act to increase heart rate, blood pressure, muscle tone, core body temperature, and the consumption of oxygen. Additionally, these hormones stimulate the liver to increase glucose and fatty acid levels in the blood, to divert blood from the digestive tract to the muscles, and to increase perspiration. The spleen is also activated to release more red blood cells, while blood-clotting ability increases and more white blood cells are produced. Psychologically, one has an increased level of anxiety and a sense of foreboding when in the stressed state. All of these automatic changes (and more; see Table 6.A-2 for a complete list) are in aid of protecting the body in the face of an emergency, either real or imagined.

The second route to sympathetic arousal, the neural route, is energized simultaneously with the hormonal route. Here, the hypothalamus energizes the spinal cord, which leads immediately to increased muscle tone, heart and respiration rates, blood pressure, and perspiration, while digestive processes and saliva secretion stop. Most importantly, activation of the sympathetic nervous system by intense stress can have an adverse effect on the immune system, leading to increased susceptibility to colds and minor infections.

If there is a perception within a person that the events of his/her life are so upsetting that the sympathetic nervous system is activated even though the events are not really life threatening, and the stimulation is ongoing and not resolved, then the physiological consequences of such constant stress may include hypertension, cardiac arrhythmias, indigestion, headache, backache, poor sleep, anxiety, depression, autoimmune dis-

ease, low resistance to cancer, and memory and cognitive deficits in old age [76].

It must be understood that stress is not necessarily a bad thing, for as Selye has said, "Stress...gives an excellent chance to develop potential talents, no matter where they may be slumbering in the mind or body. In fact, it is only in the heat of stress that individuality can be perfectly molded" [419]. Continuing in this vein, Councilman says, "We are what we are because of the stresses placed upon us and the adaptations we have made to these stresses, both physically and otherwise. The state of our bodies, our minds and our personalities is the result of this adaptation" [98]. All stresses leave us somewhat changed, sometimes for the better and sometimes for the worse.

Activation of the fight-or-flight response is useful in some situations, no doubt. However, Selye [419] has shown that the fight-or-flight response can be a first step in a four-stage process, the end result of which is catastrophic! Selye defines the four stages of response to stress in what he calls the general adaptation syndrome (GAS): Stage 1) The alarm reaction in which all aspects of sympathetic activation are turned on (Table 6.A-2) in response to a stressor. These are the short-term adaptations which our bodies make in doing the challenging work of the *yogasanas*. Stage 2) A resistance stage in which the body appears to resist the changes wrought by stage 1 by attempting to reverse its symptoms and so regain homeostasis. For students of *yogasana*, this takes place during our relaxation (*savasana, etc.*). Stage 3) If the stress of the stage-1 fight-or-flight situation is continual and on-going, then efforts to achieve homeostasis act to deplete the body's reserves and so lead to a state of exhaustion. As one has a depleted ability to adapt to the initial stressor, the body systems begin to break down in the long term. It is the chronic stress reached in stage 3 that can eventually prove to be a serious health threat. Stage 4) If sympathetic arousal continues beyond stage 3, the organism will die from the stressor.

All of the above assumes that there is no conscious control of the stress or of the reaction to the stress. However, as stated above, a person's response to a particular stressor and recovery from that stressor are each unique to that person, and so one cannot assign a particular quality to a stressor or a strategy of recovery and expect it to apply to everyone [188]. The response to stress can vary from individual to individual; in some, the response of the immune system is negative, reducing the resistance to both viral and bacterial attack. Those who respond to stress with extreme increases in heart rate and blood pressure are significantly more likely to have frequent minor illnesses, as compared with those whose response is more moderate.

The effects of stress are cumulative, and if we spend a certain amount of our adaptability on dealing with external stressors such as accompany bad living, anger, worry, *etc.*, the less will be available for handling the demands of *yogasana* practice. Should our levels of stress be sufficiently high and sufficiently long so as to enter Selye's stage 3, there will follow three general, nonspecific physiological long-term responses to the stress: a) Enlargement of the adrenal cortex with increased output of the catecholamines, leading to anxiety and hypertension. b) Shrinking of the lymphatic tissue, with a decrease of lymphocytes in the blood and a consequent decrease in the strength of our immune systems, and c) ulceration of the stomach lining, especially in the upper part of the duodenum, due to minor ruptures of small blood vessels.

Schatz [406a] has earlier pointed out how the global stress response can develop as a wide variety of body-function changes interact among themselves and with brain functions to place all of the body's systems on attack alert. It is excitation of the sympathetic nervous system due to stress that sets these changes in motion.

Not everyone reacts to stress in the same way. In fact, some respond to stress by withdrawal, *i.e.*, rather than fight-or-flight, these people roll over and play dead. When stressed, such people display decreased physiological function, loss of muscle tone, mental lassitude, inactivity and eventually depression. The totality of these responses implicates a parasympathetic response to stress rather than sympathetic [343].

Yogasana

In the 1950's, Wenger and Bagchi travelled to India to study in a most scientific way the claims that Indian mystics and yogis were able to voluntarily control aspects of the autonomic nervous system [481]. Their confirmation of these claims has somewhat opened the door of respectability to yoga in the West.

It is at this point, where discussion of the autonomic system intersects the discussions of stress, relaxation and *yogasana*, that the heart of this Handbook is revealed. In virtually all of the *yogasana* work that a beginning student may be taught by her teacher, performing the postures has a direct and understandable impact on the autonomic system. If one has an understanding of the physiology of the body at the level of the autonomic nervous system, and an understanding of the *yogasana* postures in terms of their alignment and their effects on the energy of the body, then one can work the postures so as to deliberately produce changes in the autonomic balance.

Referring to Fig. 1.B-1, we realize now that the psychological space labeled "unconscious" in the beginning student contains all of the autonomic adjustments of the body/mind, and that through the practice of

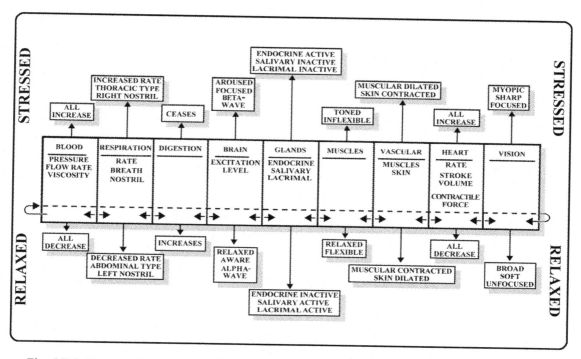

Fig. 6.E-2. Because the subsystems of the body/brain are strongly interconnected (center panel), a change in one of them toward either a more stressed state (upper panels) or a more relaxed state (lower panels) will drive the others in the same direction. Thus, through *yogasana* practice, the shift toward the relaxed state (or the stressed state) of one subsystem will act to pull all of the others more or less in the same direction.

the *yogasanas*, these factors, physical, mental and emotional, can be lifted into the conscious sphere. At the same time, certain of the deliberate, conscious actions of the *yogasanas*, after much practice will become intuitive and automatic.

As can be seen in Fig. 6.E-2, the concerted actions of many interacting body-mind functions can either conspire to make one stressed or the conspiracy can be reversed, leaving one calm and relaxed. The parasympathetic dominance that is necessary for this reversal can be attained through *yogasana* practice, most especially through the control of the breath and the tension in the muscles.

It is interesting to consider what the autonomic balance might be like for a beginning student performing *sarvangasana*, for example. To make the example even more concrete, consider the student's blood pressure in *sarvangasana* as representing the level of autonomic balance, with high pressure signaling sympathetic dominance and low pressure signaling parasympathetic dominance. The plot in Fig. 6.E-3 shows how one might expect the pressure to change year after year, as the student becomes more experienced. At first, the newness of the inverted position adds an element of panic to the posture and the pressure is higher than when standing. However, with several years practice, the essential relaxing quality of the position exerts itself, and the pressure drops. With more practice following this, one enters a period in which the conscious control over the autonomic nervous system is so complete that one can make the pressure either go up or go down, depending on one's will to have it rise or fall!

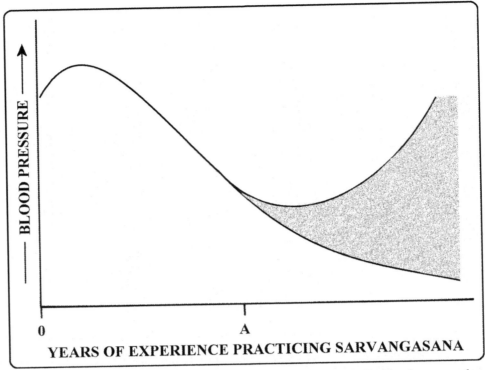

Fig. 6.E-3. With only a few years of practice, *sarvangasana* may raise the blood pressure, but with further practice, it becomes relaxing and the blood pressure falls. As one continues to practice and gains control over the autonomic system (point A), one can then consciously control the change of blood pressure in *sarvangasana*, making it either rise or fall (shaded area).

When the autonomic nervous system is working properly in a healthy body, it has a responsiveness that allows one to move easily between sympathetic and parasympathetic dominance in either direction. In contrast, in the unhealthy body, the dominant neural mode is set either too high (sympathetic) or too low (parasympathetic), and is unable to easily switch from one dominance to the other. Thus we see in Fig. 6.E-4, the healthy responsiveness of a balanced person as measured by fingertip temperature and muscle tension as he/she goes through cycles of stress and relaxation. The response is significantly different for the balanced person as compared with responses for subjects who are chronically excited either sympathetically or parasympathetically. Other health-related aspects of the responsiveness of the autonomic nervous system to changing dominance involve the respira-

tory sinus arrhythmia (Subsection 12.A, *Innervation and Control of the Breathing Centers*, page 366) and the alternation of nasal laterality in breathing (Section 12.C, Nasal Laterality, page 374).

In general, the beginner's practice of the *yogasanas* results in a stimulation of the sympathetic nervous system, with the challenge/threat of the asanas leading to all of the classic "fight-or-flight" responses on a rather short time scale. However, once we go from the active *yogasanas* to *savasana*, the parasympathetic nervous system then exerts its effect and brings the body back to a balanced physiological and psychological state, though not as rapidly as did the sympathetic system to create that imbalanced state. Obviously, the body's need is for a quick response to danger, but there is no rush to restore calm in the aroused body.

Often, the body seems constantly stressed, implying a certain rigidity in the autonomic balance in favor of sympathetic excitation. Through practice of *yogasana* with awareness, we can learn to relax through excitation of the parasympathetic system. In this, we build an autonomic/neural flexibility, in addition to physiologic/muscle and mental flexibilities. As described in Box 6.E-1, for example, occa-

sions may arise when the autonomic flexibility can be of great value.

The sympathetic and parasympathetic nervous systems affect every tissue and practically every cell in the body irrespective of function. By controlling the balance between sympathetic and parasympathetic actions through *yogasana* practice, we can control physiology at the cellular level [406a].

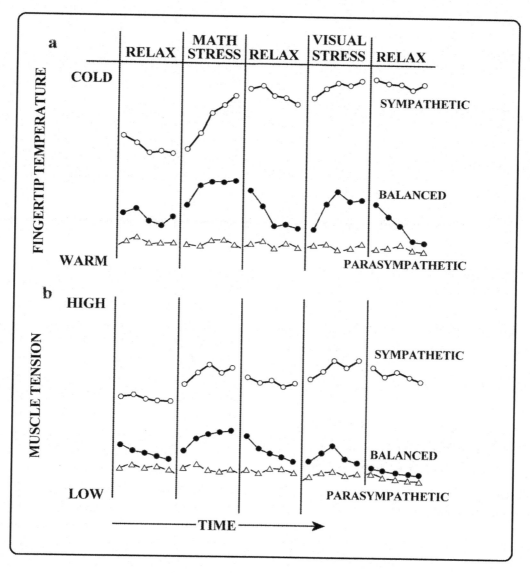

Fig. 6.E-4. Responsiveness of subjects having different autonomic types (sympathetic dominant, parasympathetic dominant, and balanced) to repeated stress/relaxation cycles as measured by (**a**) finger temperature, and by (**b**) muscle tension [343].

BOX 6.E-1: YOGIS CAN BEAT THE LIE DETECTOR

The lie detector works on the assumption that when one answers a question truthfully, there is little or no change in the level of sympathetic excitation in the body, but that when one lies in answer to a question, there is an unavoidable rise in the level of anxiety and a corresponding shift toward sympathetic excitation that can easily be measured as changes in palmar conductance, blood pressure, respiration rate, muscle tension, *etc*. The technique is generally practical for those suspects who cannot consciously control the balance in the autonomic nervous system [30].

On the other hand, it seems quite reasonable that a yoga student adept at sympathetic-parasympathetic shifting could easily manipulate his/her nervous system so as to foil the machine; see Section 3.E, Brainwaves and the Electroencephalogram, page 57. Such a student could raise the baseline readings during innocuous questions by right-nostril breathing, tightening the quadruceps, biting the tongue, compressing the chest, contracting the anal sphincter, *etc*. On releasing these autonomic tensions while lying, or going into a parasympathetic mode by left-nostril breathing, repeating a mantra, *etc*., the usual effects of the lie would be covered and the lie would go undetected.

Read Box 11.A-2, *Stopping the Heart by Conscious Control of the Vagus Nerve*, page 317, in regard Swami Rama and his exquisite control of the autonomic nervous system and then imagine the results of his lie-detector test! See also Box 14.A-1, *Using the Salivary Glands as Lie Detectors*, page 394, for further information on the use of the autonomic response as a lie detector in ancient times.

It is tempting to equate the three *gunas* (*rajasic*, *tamasic* and *sattvic*) as used broadly in describing the *yogasanas* [209] with the dominance of the sympathetic nervous system, the dominance of the parasympathetic nervous system, and a balanced state between the two extremes, respectively.

SECTION 6.F. THE EFFECTS OF EMOTIONS AND ATTITUDES ON STRESS

Emotions and Stress

In regard the question of the impact of one's attitude on stress, experiments show a great biochemical difference in the response when the stress is seen as a challenge *versus* the response when the stress is seen as a threat [389]. When the source of the stress is seen as a threat, both catecholamines and cortisol are released from the adrenal glands, whereas when the stress is viewed as a challenge, catecholamines are again released, but there is no increase in cortisol! As one works in yoga, it is clear that one always wants to regard the work as a challenge and not as a threat; one now sees that this distinction has a biochemical basis. That is to say, one wants the sympathetic nervous system excitation to travel from the hypothalamus to the adrenal medulla in order to release the catecholamines, but does not want the hypothalamic release of CRF, which leads to ACTH and cortisol. Note that this is accomplished by a shift in attitude; we must convert the negative stress of threat into the positive coping-experience of challenge. This is the basic principle of psychobiological therapy: "reframe threat into challenge."

Looked at in another way, one wants to avoid the sympathetic autonomic reflex that is the concomitant to dealing with a "threat", and instead use the responses dictated by the higher mental centers which are implicit in considering how to deal in a conscious, rational way with a "challenge".

Note that an external stressor does not necessarily create the autonomic response; it is the individual that does that, and so depending upon the individual's psychological makeup, the response can vary from person to person [337], being autonomic in some and involving higher centers only in others. In this regard, it is interesting then to note that the catecholamine level in men rises most sharply when triggered by competition and intellectual challenges, whereas for women, the most rapid rise is found to be during stressful personal situations. Men's catecholamine and blood-pressure levels also fall drastically when they leave the workplace, whereas women's levels for these two markers for stress stay elevated when returning home to face family responsibilities. For men, the rise in blood pressure is most rapid when angry, whereas it is most rapid for women when anxious. Still, women appear to be less vulnerable to stress because they are more likely to contemplate, discuss and then act on stressful problems than are men.

Though Gazzaniga [153] says, "...from a host of other studies we know that it is virtually impossible to teach the autonomic nervous system anything," Rossi points out that in fact the limbic-hypothalamus system is the connection between the mind and the body, and so can be a very active teacher in using the mind to modulate the functions of the autonomic nervous system [389]. The strong influence that the psyche can play on the operation and direction of action of the autonomic nervous system is clear in several phenomena. Two other striking examples besides that of Iyengar yoga will suffice to illustrate this point.

In voodoo death, a person of unchallenged authority decrees another person will die at a prescribed time, and the prediction comes true to the minute. The cause of death is psychological stress in which there are rapid shifts between sympathetic and parasympathetic dominance [389]. Collapse of the immune and endocrine systems also are involved in this.

On a longer time scale, there is the related phenomenon of the "defeat reaction" [195]. This is a pathophysiological syndrome brought on by repeated or prolonged psychic stress, which induces a complicated pattern of sympathetic and parasympathetic responses which eventually harm the blood vessels and decrease the level of sex hormones; while levels of ACTH and glucocorticoids rise, the immune system is depressed and infection or tumors follow.* The opposite effect also is well known. Further examples of the effects of mental attitude on the strength of the immune system, the ability to fend off disease, or to recover from an illness, are presented in Chapter 13, THE IMMUNE SYSTEM, page 383, while examples of the same approach in regard hypertension is given in Subsection 11.D, *Vasoconstriction, Vasodilation, and Hypertension*, page 334.

Though stress can be useful as a tool for learning or performance at a certain level, it can be overdone. When we overwork, the physiological effect is illness, whereas the psychological effects are boredom and a sense of anticlimax. In competitive sports and the performing arts, the boredom of

---

* Something reminiscent of this occurs with snakes, where males wrestle one another for the favor of a female, and the loser slinks off, turns brown and dies.

training is relieved by the excitement and release to be found in competition and performance, however in *yogasana* training we have no such avenues. It is then the responsibility of the teacher to be aware of incipient boredom, and to make every effort to keep *yogasana* practice fresh and interesting, both for herself and her students.

Considering the ease with which the breathing pattern can be changed by a simple emotional event, it is obvious that the autonomic nervous system controls the respiration process, influencing the respiration rate and the opening and closing of the airways. However, through *pranayama*, one can consciously control the breath, and in so doing, one thus gains conscious access to one of the functions of the autonomic nervous system. Control of the breath through *pranayama*, thus, is a doorway to conscious control over many if not all of the other processes of the autonomic nervous system [377].

Of course, consciously choosing to perform the proper *yogasana* will lead to predictable excitation of one or the other of the two autonomic branches. If one chooses, for example, to perform *yoganidrasana*, one can expect a general parasympathetic response from the body, for this pose takes one from wakefulness toward a state of sleep, and is used by yogis in high altitudes to generate superficial body heat (Table 6.A-2) to stay warm [209]. On going from a normal resting state to *yoganidrasana*, the blood flow in the brain shifts from the frontal lobes and the brainstem to cortical areas in the posterior brain [321a]. If on the other hand, one chooses to do *urdhva dhanurasana*, the body will shift toward sympathetic excitation, with all of its attendant characteristics, Box 7.D-1, *Why Are Backbends Energizing?*, page 216.

Another way to control the autonomic nervous system is through willpower [374]. By being single-minded and focused, one can direct the autonomic nervous system; however, the lungs and diaphragm are easier to control for most of us than is the will.

Rossi [389] lists the well-documented healing effects of increased blood circulation which are facilitated by modulation of the physiology by the mind:

- Warming and cooling of different body parts to lessen the pain of headache
- Controlling blushing and blanching of the skin
- Stimulating the enlargement and apparent growth of women's breasts
- Stimulation of sexual excitation and penile erection
- The amelioration of bruises
- Controlling the loss of blood during surgery
- Minimizing and healing burns
- Producing localized skin inflammations
- Curing warts
- Producing and curing forms of dermatitis
- Ameliorating congenital ichthyosis
- Aiding blood coagulation in hemophiliacs
- Ameliorating the fight-or-flight alarm response
- Ameliorating hypertension and cardiac problems
- Ameliorating Raynaud's disease (a vascular spasm of the superficial vessels)
- Enhancing the immune response

References to the original literature are given in Rossi's work [389].

Inasmuch as the blood's circulation can be stimulated and directed through the proper use of *yogasana*, one presumably can influence some or possibly all of the items in Rossi's list above through such practice.

Physiology Influences Psychology

There is abundant evidence (as stated above) that our psychology or frame of mind can have a direct and immediate effect on our body states or physiology. Similarly, one can influence the state of the mind by changing the state of the body in some way. The truth of this is clear to anyone who has practiced *yogasana* and been alert to the psychological changes that attend such practice. Thus within the *yogasana* practice, one has both energizing, arousing postures and those that are sedating and relaxing. With a proper choice and sequence of *yogasana*, one can play the body like a violin, exploring all of the notes possible in the course of several hours. As therapy for mental conditions, *yogasana* routines have been put forth for the treatment of depression and anxiety, Chapter 20, THE EMOTIONS, page 463.

Yogasana practice rivets our attention on the present moment as it energizes the body, and then leads to overall body relaxation; it is preferable to working out on a stationary exercise machine, for example, which is mentally defocusing, and so allows one to become tense as one thinks obsessively about one's problems.

Psychologists have shown that there is a connection between personality type and breathing type. But according to yoga experience, the breath and the mind have a mutual interaction, so that each can be influenced by the other. Thus one concludes that by changing the breathing pattern, one can change not only the mind but the personality [374].

Psychoanatomy

Given the close connections between the body and the mind, it is no surprise that there exist close connections between specific body areas and specific emotions, attitudes, and psychology. This is the field of psychoanatomy, with close relations to the ancient study of the *chakras* and their attributes (Section 4.F, *Nadis, Chakras* and *Prana*, page 100). A brief listing of these psychoanatomical body/mind connections is given below [152].

Feet: connect us to the ground and give us a sense of security.

Legs: mobilizers that stabilize us and keep us in touch with reality. The thighs are synonymous with independence, and strong legs imply one has a strong determination and may be excessively controlling.

Pelvis: the center of power, energy and sexuality. Relates to our sexual image and our relations to others.

Abdomen: the emotional center, expressing vulnerability and helplessness. The emotional responses are blunted by the overdevelopment of the abdomen.

Lower back: is the control center. When tight, behavior is compulsive, and when loose, behavior is impulsive.

Chest: is an amplifier and a form of muscular armoring, shielding one from emotional experiences of self such as a sense of inferiority or behavior that is assertive or aggressive.

Shoulders: are protective, with rounding indicating fear.

Arms and Hands: are clutching, reflecting our inability to hold on or to control.

Upper Back: an area of conflicted emotions (anger, rage, hatred, *etc.*) being held in check.

Neck: the mediator between the thought center and the feeling center. When the neck is very strong, there is a repression of the emotions.

Head: the locale for obsessive worry and self analysis, leading to bodily tension.

Given the above connections between body and mind, it is easy to see how the practice of the *yogasanas*, through stretching/releasing and through strengthening of specific areas of the body, can influence the emotions and attitudes.

The Placebo Effect

Because positive attitudes are known to effect cures in very ill patients, the "placebo effect", in which medically inert pills cure real illnesses, is not unexpected. The US Food and Drug Administration (FDA) reports, "People are often helped, not by the food or drug being tested, but by a profound belief it will help" [337]. This is in essence, the placebo effect. In fact, many in the medical field hold that our belief in our own health is the most important predictor of health outcomes [289], though strong religious beliefs also are a factor.

It is claimed that an average of 35% of the members of any large group will respond favorably to the administration of a "drug", when the "drug" in fact is nothing but water or sugar [153, 337]. Though the percentage of placebo effectiveness rises to 50% when the problem being treated is headache, it is seen to be exceptional even at 35%, considering that strong morphine is successful in only 75% of the cases for which it is prescribed [308]. As applied to somatic (muscle) pain, the taking of a placebo does reduce muscle pain to an extent beyond the statistical expectation [153]. The greater the implicit or explicit suggestion that pain will be relieved, the more effective is the placebo, however, it is less effective each time it is used thereafter [308].

It is thought that a specific mental state is promoted by being sold on a placebo "pain killer", and that this state releases endorphins, the body's own opiates. The endorphins in turn activate cells in the midbrain to block pain sensations, while suppressing the immune system [153] (Subsection 10.D, *The Endorphins*, page 303). Placebo effectiveness also has been related to the stress that many patients feel is released once they are in the hands of a warm, caring, and authoritative figure [456]; this is most true for patients suffering from asthma, hypertension, depression and anxiety. Placebos

---

BOX 6.F-1: EXAMPLES OF THE PLACEBO EFFECT

• Patients who were on blood-pressure medication were not told for three weeks that they would be given a placebo instead. In spite of this, their blood pressure returned to normal even though they were receiving placebo medication.

• Thousands of elderly Chinese Americans in California who were born in years with poor astrological qualities died sooner from cancer than did a similar group born under good astrological signs. Caucasians born in the same years showed no such tendency to die sooner when born in "poor" years as compared with "good" years.

• Patients who received pretend knee surgery but were not really operated on uniformly reported pain relief and said they would recommend the operation to their friends.

• Placebos do 75% as well as Prozac in relieving symptoms of depression.

• Saline injection was an effective anaesthetic for 30–40 % of the people it was given to who were undergoing wisdom-tooth extraction.

• Doctors today are relying on the placebo effect when they prescribe antibiotics for viral infections, and recommend drinking milk for gastric ulcers.

These examples show that people's expectation that they will get well, that cultural beliefs, and that the doctor's enthusiasm for the treatment are all contributing factors to the placebo effect.

are most effective not only in the treatment of pain and depression, but also for some heart ailments, gastric ulcers and other stomach complaints, achieving success rates of more than 60%. In some cases, the placebo success rate is even higher than that of the best drugs for the condition. See Box 6.F-1 for a wide variety of examples of the placebo effect.

It has been shown that the placebo effect can be effective in combating hypertension, stress, cardiac pain, blood cell counts, headaches, and pupillary dilation, all with the help of the placebo-induced activation of the autonomic nervous system. The placebo effect has been especially successful in treating depression and anxiety [308], with success rates that rival those of the best and most modern drug therapies [456], Chapter 20, THE EMOTIONS, page 463.

The efficacy of the placebo effect on the physical plane is shown by a study in which warts were eliminated by painting them with an innocuous but brightly colored dye, and telling the patients that the warts would disappear when the color of the dye wore off. Similarly, dilation of the bronchial airways results in many people when they are told that the inhaled substance is a powerful bronchodilator, though in fact it is a placebo [456].

The role of placebo in medicine revolves about the distinction between illness and disease: illness is what the patient feels, whereas disease is what the doctor finds. Placebos are effective in first softening the effects of illness by reducing the patient's distress; with this reduced level of distress, the body then has a better chance to heal

itself of the disease, Chapter 13, THE IMMUNE SYSTEM, page 383.

It has been determined that, with regard to the placebo effect, injections are more effective than pills, with capsules in between, and that among pills, small yellow ones are best for depression whereas large blue ones work best for sedation (see Subsection 16.D, *Color Therapy*, page 426); as might have been expected, the more bitter is the pill being swallowed, the stronger the placebo effect [346]. In the same vein, large placebo pills usually are more effective than small pills, placebo injections are yet more effective, and placebo surgery is the most effective course of treatment [456].

Rossi [389] proposes that about half of all the cures effected by Western medicine are due to the placebo effect, and involve the limbic-hypothalamic bridge between mind and body. Indeed, Western medicine in its earlier days operated totally on the placebo effect, and with strongly positive results, as both the physician and the patient were convinced of the efficacy of the treatments! Though a certain amount of credit must be given as well to the natural course of illness, which causes it to wax and wane, the placebo effect, nonetheless, is a real and useful tool, with results that go well beyond the natural cure rate.

The placebo effect is more effective with those who have right-cerebral hemisphere dominance, as is hypnotizability.* To the extent that our *yogasana* student-teacher relationship also involves a strong element of suggestibility, this will probably be true for yoga students as well. In this regard, it is known medically that a treatment can have

---

* In fact, the autonomic nervous system is regarded as a major factor in the physiological effects of hypnosis [389]. This must have some meaning for yoga. Notice that a therapeutic hypnotist uses phrases such as "getting more and more comfortable and your eyes close" which would be perfectly appropriate for a yoga teacher to tell the class when in *savasana*. This suggestion initiates a shift from sympathetic to parasympathetic dominance because the arousal of the reticular formation is lower, proprioceptive and kinaesthetic signals are sparse, while closing the eyes stimulates

an active healing effect just by the nature of the personal interaction between the doctor and the patient. It appears that the doctor-patient relationship may stimulate the innate self-healing powers within all of us [41], independent of the efficacy of the technological treatment. Inasmuch as the laying on of hands is one of the most basic actions offering human comfort, and the annual physical checkup is one of the tried and true bonding rituals between doctor and patient, it is no surprise that the bond between *yogasana* teacher and student also can be a curative one. As *yogasana* teachers, we in the United States are not allowed to function as doctors, however, it is within the law to state that certain poses are known to stimulate certain organs, for example, and to expect that though we do not prescribe them for our students, they nonetheless will take to heart what we say, and possibly heal themselves on the basis of the teacher-student (authority-patient) relationship.

Many other examples of the intimate connection between the mental centers and the autonomic nervous system quickly come to mind: thinking of delicious food promotes salivation via the parasympathetic system, embarrassment leads to blushing due to activation of the vascular system, sudden psychic stress leads to a change in the heart rate due to sympathetic excitation, *etc.* The repeated activation of some of the innocuous sympathetic reflex actions can lead to pathological changes in the visceral organs [195], *i.e.*, peptic ulcers, asthma, hypertension, coronary problems. The real importance of the placebo effect is in its demonstration that each of us has within ourselves a self-healing mechanism already in place, if only we can find a way to trigger it into action.

alpha and finally theta brain waves, Section 3.E, Brainwaves and the Electroencephalogram, page 57. The signals from awareness of feeling and imagistic experience shift one from external to internal awareness and the activity of the cerebral hemispheres (Section 3.D, Cerebral Hemispheric Laterality, page 49) shifts from the left to the right, all of this through the agency of the vascular system. Presumably, the hemispheric shift is accompanied by a corresponding shift in nasal dominance (Section 12.C, Nasal Laterality, page 374).

In hypnosis, as in *savasana*, once the eyes are closed there is generally considerable motion of the eyeballs and eyelids, suggesting a search of the inner landscape. Rossi [389] lists many such signs of "inner work" as they appear in a hypnotized subject; the list is not too different from what is observed in yoga students when in *savasana*. Hypnotized subjects are known to have a very high tolerance for pain [308].

Chapter 7

THE SKELETAL MUSCLES

SECTION 7.A. SKELETAL MUSCLE; STRUCTURE AND FUNCTION

Physical Structure

Skeletal muscle is the most abundant tissue type and the most adaptable tissue in the human body, undergoing large changes through either specific use or general disuse. The primary function of muscles is to move specific parts of the body with respect to one another. In the particular case of skeletal muscles, the movement involves the bones to which the muscles are attached, whereas with cardiac muscle, it is blood that moves, and for the smooth muscles of the viscera, for example, it is the contents of the intestines that move.

Because the two ends of a skeletal muscle in general are attached to different but adjacent bones, the contraction of the muscle which spans the joint acts to close the angle at the joint and so sets a part of the body in motion. However, there often is a second muscle spanning the joint in question, and activation of the second muscle can act to open the joint. Thus one has, for example, the opposing actions of the quadruceps and the hamstrings at the knee, the first opening the joint and the second closing it. Yet other muscles are joined to bones that are not in contact, as for example, the upper trapezius muscle, which is joined to the cervical vertebrae and to the top rim of the shoulder blade. Contraction of this muscle acts to pull the shoulder blade

toward the neck without changing any meaningful joint angle in the process. In the heart, there are strongly contracting muscles but no bones to anchor them, whereas in the skull, the bony plates are capable of movement with respect to the suture, but there are no muscles in place to move them. The respiratory diaphragm is a muscle anchored to bone at only one end. Thus there are a multiplicity of joint/muscle combinations active in the body.

Of the three general types of muscle tissue, this Section deals only with striated skeletal muscle; discussions of visceral (smooth) muscle and the cardiac muscle of the heart can be found in Chapter 18, THE GASTROINTESTINAL ORGANS AND DIGESTION, page 441, and in Section 11.A, Structure and Function of the Heart, page 310, respectively.

Our focus in this Chapter will be on the detailed mechanism which causes a skeletal muscle to contract, the neural circuits that activate the muscles on both the conscious and subconscious levels, how the contraction of certain muscles can be used to stretch other muscles, how muscles know when to stop stretching, and how the practice of the *yogasanas* leads to refinement of the poses while increasing our awareness of who we are and how our bodies function (*svadhyaya*).

With respect to *yogasana*, the skeletal muscles are used for (1) moving the bones in order to attain a new posture, (2) moving the bones in the new posture in order to open certain joints, and (3) holding the bones in place so that the bones support the body against the pull of gravity. In general, "a muscle action" in *yogasana* practice involves many muscles acting simultaneously. Though muscles have anatomic individuality (Figs. 7.A-l and 7.A-2), they usually do not function as individuals in beginners [222]. However, with the body control gained through the practice of the *yogasanas*, one can not only coordinate muscle actions, but also separate and individualize muscle actions on a very fine scale. With *yogasana* practice, these muscles can also be lengthened in ways that are either passive or active depending upon the circumstances.

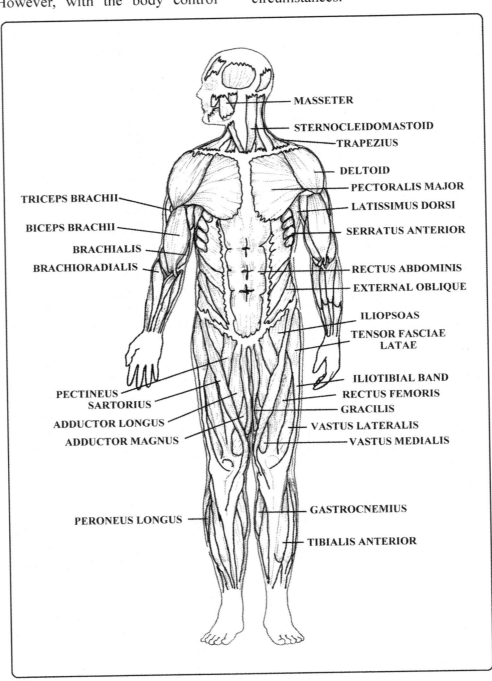

Fig. 7.A-1. The major muscles of the front body.

At the cellular level, muscle consists of elongated muscle-fiber cells containing cell nuclei and mitochondria, bounded by a fibrous-tissue membrane. In response to either electrical or hormonal stimulation, skeletal muscle tissue can contract actively by up to 30% of its resting length and because of the high demand for oxygen and glucose by its mitochondria, it is highly vascularized.

As an average adult, each of us has between 600 and 700 distinct muscles, which in the aggregate account for approximately 40% of our body weight (actually, 42% in

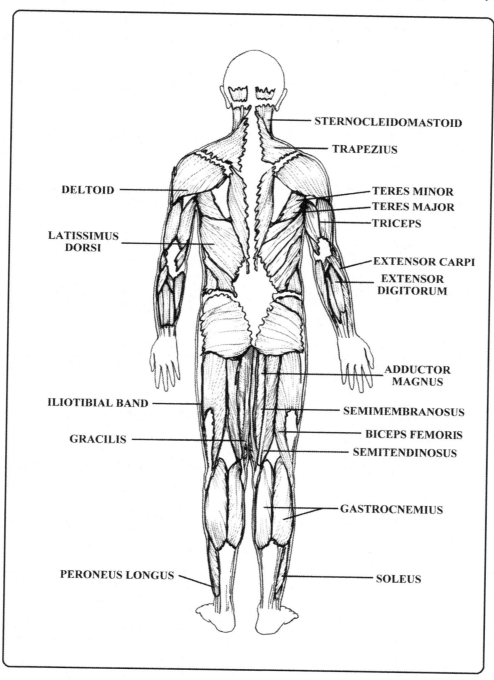

Fig. 7.A-2. The major muscles of the back body.

the case of males and 38% in the case of females). Discussion of muscle action in the context of the *yogasanas* would be most difficult without a map of the body's muscles and their identification according to their Latin names. The names and locations of the major muscles of the front body of interest to teachers of *yogasana* are given in Fig. 7.A-1 and those for the back body in Fig. 7.A-2. These muscles are shown again in Fig. 7.A-3, but labeled in regard to their modes of action. One clearly sees from the labels shown there, the opposing relationships between the placement of the flexors (muscles that fold up the body and close the joints, *e.g.*, the hamstrings) and their opposites, the extensors (muscles that open joints and work to keep us upright against the pull of gravity, *e.g.*, the quadruceps) and between the placement of the abductors (mus-

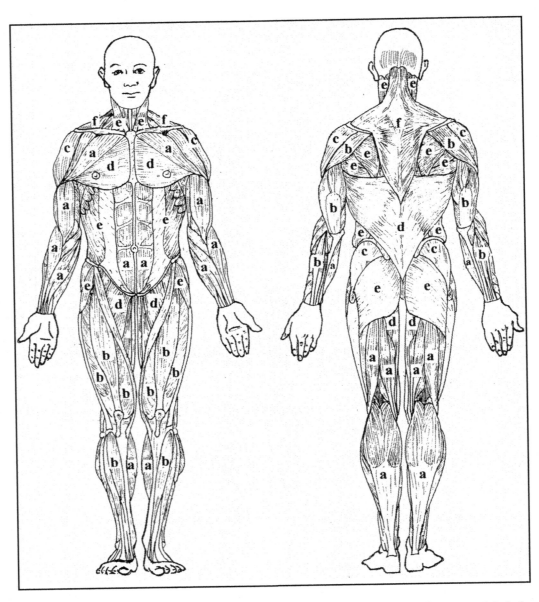

Fig. 7.A-3. The muscles of the body as related to their modes of action: the flexors are labeled **a**, the extensors are labeled **b**, the abductors are labeled **c**, the adductors are labeled **d**, rotators are labeled **e**, and the scapula stabilizers are labeled **f** [229].

cles that lift the limbs away from the center line) and the adductors (muscles that pull the limbs toward the center line). Pairs of muscles such as these that work in opposition to one another are discussed further below (Subsection 7.A, *Reciprocal Inhibition and Agonist/Antagonist Pairs*, page 193).

Though the contractile parts of the muscle fibers congregate toward the belly of the muscle proper, the connective tissue that envelops the muscle extends beyond the ends of the contractile muscle bundles to become woven into the fabric of the periosteum covering on the adjacent bones (Fig. 7.A-4a and Section 8.A, Bone Structure,

Development, and Mechanics, page 235). The bundle of connective tissue that connects the contractile part of the muscle to the bone is the muscle's tendon. The properties of tendons and ligaments, a related tissue, and the joints at the points of muscle attachment are discussed further in Section 8.E, The Joints, page 260. The two ends of a skeletal muscle most often are connected to adjacent bone. As they cross a joint, contraction of the muscle spanning the joint changes the angle at the joint, Fig. 7.A-4a, either opening it or closing it.

Certain skeletal muscles are constructed so as to be fit for rapid, short-term contractions (the biceps muscles of the upper arms,

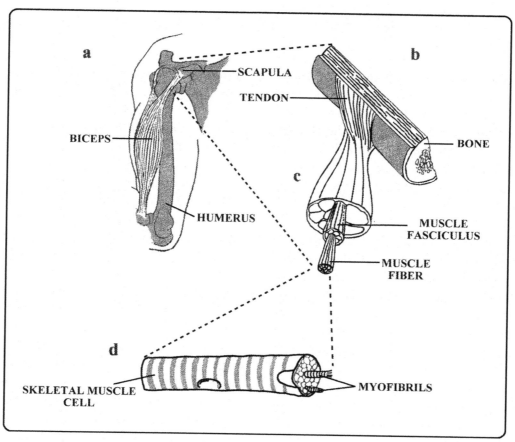

Fig. 7.A-4. (a) The biceps muscle is anchored at one end to the radius bone of the forearm and at the other end to the scapula, thereby spanning the elbow joint. (b) Looking more closely, the connective tissue within and around the muscle forms a thick band of tendon, which in turn becomes an integral part of the periosteum covering the bone. (c) A cross section of the belly of the muscle shows an array of smaller bundles within larger bundles, (d) with the skeletal muscle cell itself being packed with myofibril filaments of actin and myosin.

for example), whereas others are constructed so as to work best during slowly-developing, long-term contractions (the spinae erector muscles of the back body, for example). Though skeletal muscle is largely under voluntary control, even when at rest, there is an involuntary excitation of the muscles which maintains a certain nonzero level of contraction, called "muscle tone". This is discussed further in Subsection 7.B, *Resting Muscle Tone*, page 204.

The mechanism of muscle action becomes clear if we look at it at levels of increasing magnification. A cross section of a muscle taken through its belly shows it to consist of parallel bundles of fibers called muscle fasciculi, each within its own sheath of connective tissue called fascia (Fig. 7.A-4c). A closer look at the structure of a fasciculus bundle shows it to be composed in turn of up to 200 long, cylindrical muscle-fiber cells 5–100 microns in diameter (28,000 microns equal one inch), with each cell surrounded by a fascial sheath. The muscle fibers run the full length of the muscle, and thus the muscle-cell axes run parallel to the direction of movement that they initiate. Within each of the muscle fibers are bundles of yet finer fibers, called myofibrils, Fig. 7.A-4d, and within each of these there are two distinct types of filaments running parallel to one another over the entire length of the cell. It is these microscopic filaments, called myosin and actin, that contain the molecular machinery that is able to drive large-scale muscle contraction (Subsection 7.A, *Microscopic Muscle Contraction*, page 178). As with many other cells in the body, the number of muscle cells in the body is fixed at birth and does not grow as the body grows. Instead, muscles grow by packing more and more filaments of actin and myosin into the existing number of muscle cells [222].

The neural impulses that drive muscle action originate in the central nervous system (Chapter 3, THE BRAIN, page 21), a hierarchical structure built of lower centers which control involuntary body functions (including muscle contraction), and the higher centers of the brain, which direct the conscious actions of our bodies. These centers of the central nervous system, both higher and lower, activate muscles in response to signals sent to them from the sensors at the body's periphery. The nerves connecting the sensors to the central nervous system, called afferents, converge upon the spinal cord in order to send their information along the ascending pathway sequentially to the cerebellum, to the thalamus, and finally to the ultimate center, the cerebral sensory cortex, Fig. 2.A-1.

Once the afferent signal is processed, the consequent efferent (out-going) signal then descends from the cerebral motor cortex, through the brain stem and the spinal cord to eventually activate the appropriate muscles, but with many feedback loops for close control at many points in the descent. Many axons in the descending pathway (Fig. 7.A-5b) intercept the ascending fibers and inhibit or modulate their transmission to higher centers. These multiple interactions along and between the ascending and descending pathways of the central nervous system are important for us in yoga as they allow the subconscious actions to be sensed and altered by the conscious mind, *i.e.*, the interaction of higher and lower centers is the mechanism whereby we can increase our awareness and conscious control of the body at the most subtle levels. Note too that there is also a direct path from the cortex to the spinal cord, the pyramidal tract, Fig. 7.A-5b. Neural signals traveling this route activate muscles without interference from any of the lower brain centers. Efferent neurons that energize skeletal muscles are called "alpha-motor neurons".

As shown in Fig. 7.A-6, the axon of an efferent alpha-motor neuron terminates in

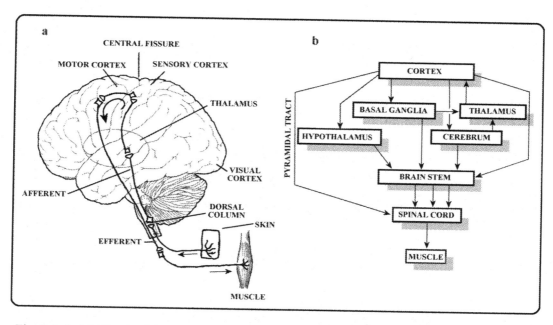

Fig. 7.A-5. (**a**) Sketch of the neural pathway connecting an initial sensation in the skin to the sensory cortex; the sensory signal then moves across the central fissure to the motor cortex, and then down the alpha-motor neuron to the relevant muscle. (**b**) Interconnections between several centers in the brain, other than the cortex, which can contribute to the final signal exiting the spinal cord via the alpha-motor neuron [195].

an end plate which contacts the skeletal-muscle fiber at the neuromuscular junction. Though the Figure shows a motor neuron innervating just a single muscle fiber, in fact, the branching of the neural axon is such that each alpha-motor neuron serves to energize between 3 and 300 muscle fibers simultaneously within a motor unit.

The contraction of skeletal muscle begins with an action potential moving down the axon of the associated alpha-motor nerve fiber toward the junction between the neuron and its muscle. In response to this action potential, Ca^{2+} ions are released in the myofibril of the muscle and contraction of that myofibril begins. This contraction lasts for between 5 and 50 milliseconds, after which time it relaxes to its original condition. In this relatively short time, the myofibril realizes only a small fraction of its total possible contraction.

The action potential (Section 5.B, Nerve Conduction, page 114) which stimulates muscle contraction is a voltage stimulus at the neuromuscular plate that consists of a series of spikes of equal voltage having a frequency (spikes per second) which expresses the intensity of the neural signal. The larger the number of voltage spikes in the signal per second, the more times per second the muscle fiber will be jolted into contraction. When sustained muscle action is required, the frequency of the signal in the motor neuron will be sufficiently high that the associated muscle fiber will be repeatedly jolted into action before it can relax again. These repeated contractions accumulate so as to produce a much larger contractile force than that achievable with only a single neural firing.

The strength of muscle contraction is governed by three factors: (1) the cross sectional size of the muscle and the sizes of the

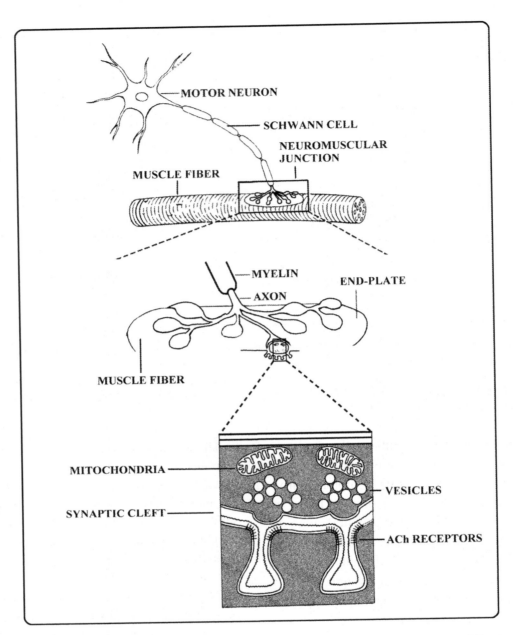

Fig. 7.A-6. Progressive enlargements of the junction between the alpha-motor neuron and the muscle fiber to be energized by it, showing the attachment of the motor neuron's axon to the receptor sites on the muscle fiber via the neuromuscular junction, at three levels of magnification [195].

muscle fibers of which it is composed, (2) the difference between its resting and fully contracted lengths, and (3) the amplitude of the action potential driving its contraction. The action potential necessary to excite contraction in a muscle fiber is smaller for the smaller (weaker) fibers. Thus at low action potential, only the small fibers of a muscle are excited. If the impulses are of such a low frequency that the time between impulses (longer than 50 milliseconds if the frequency is below 20 Hz) is longer than the muscle-fiber twitch time (5–50 milliseconds), then the muscle contraction will appear as a tremor because the number of excited fibers is minimal and its number oscillates in time. This mechanism may be responsible for the muscle tremor experienced by *yogasana* beginners in demanding poses. If the neural signal strength is raised, then so too is the action potential; in that case, both small and large fibers are excited, and contraction is then strong and continuous in time, *i.e.*, the tremor disappears as the nervous system is strengthened through practice of the *yogasanas*.

The activating neural axon will branch so as to serve more than one muscle fiber. Thus, in the case of small muscles with fine movement such as the ciliary muscles of the eyes, one nerve serves to activate fewer than 10 muscle fibers, whereas in the large but coarse muscles of the back, the ratio is more like 1:200 [131]. The motor neuron taken together with all of the muscle fibers that it innervates is called a "motor unit". In an amazing series of experiments, Basmadjian and coworkers [53] have shown that one can easily gain conscious on-off control over the excitation of a single motor unit! This is discussed more fully in Subsection 5.A, *The Motor Unit and Nerve Sensitivity*, page 113, and *Mental Control of an Individual Motor Unit*, page 113.

In the postural muscles such as the muscles paralleling the spine, the iliopsoas, and muscles of that sort, Fig. 7.A-l, where an extended action of low intensity is required but there is no need for fine-tuning of muscle action, each of the motor units can at some time relax and restore itself while other motor units become active, thus retaining the posture for long periods of time without undue overall muscle fatigue. When the task at hand requires the maximum strength of a muscle, then more motor units are recruited for the job.

In addition to the efferent alpha-motor neurons that energize skeletal muscle, these muscles contain sensors within them which relay many types of muscle-related information back to the central nervous system via afferent nerve systems, and the sensors themselves contain yet smaller muscles which are innervated by the gamma-motor neurons. Especially interesting to us are those sensors called mechanoreceptors which measure the state of tension in the muscle bundle (see Section 7.B, Muscle Sensors; The Mechanoreceptors, page 198), for the afferent signals from the mechanoreceptors form the basis by which the body controls the degree of muscle stretching/contraction and evaluates the positions of all of the body parts. Clearly, in our quest for both alignment and opening in the *yogasanas*, the mechanoreceptors will play a major role.

In the higher primates, there is a direct connection between the cortex and the motor neurons driving the muscles, so that individual muscles can be activated (Fig. 7.A-5b) at will without interference from the other lower centers. Specific areas of the right cerebral motor cortex, Fig. 3.A-5a, have been found experimentally by Penfield and Rasmussen [355] to correlate uniquely with the excitation of specific skeletal muscles. Thanks to this unique one-to-one correspondence, a "homunculus"-type gargoyle then can be drawn, with each body part of the homunculus given in proportion to the fractional amount of the cortex dedicated to control of the muscles in that part. It is no surprise that in humans, the parts of the cortex dedicated to moving the hand and the muscles of speech are disproportionately large in the motor homunculus. A related type of homunculus can be drawn as well for the sensory cortex (an adjacent area in the cortex, Subsection 3.A, *The Cortex: Seat of Conscious Action*, page 24), showing the relative numbers of neural sensors in each of the body parts, Fig. 3.A-5b.

Interesting sensory homunculi also have been determined for various other animals, as for example, the rabbit, in which the homunculus has a huge face and snout but very small feet, and the cat, which has a large face and snout, but compared to the rabbit, much larger paws. The monkey's homunculus seems most in proportion to its physical form while that for man shows huge tongue, lips, hand, and thumb, but very small feet [225]. One sees that the disproportions of the sensory homunculi reflect the neural adaptations made by each of these mammalian species in order to secure its niche and guarantee its survival.

As the afferent fibers in a nerve bundle ascend the spinal cord, its component fibers have a very specific spatial relationship to one another such that at every level of the spinal cord, the relationship is maintained. As this bundle terminates at some specific area on the sensory cortex, the result on the cortex is a map of the body parts, though not necessarily in the "real" proportions. Both the sensory and motor nerves are so bundled throughout, that many such maps are laid down in the body, *i.e.*, not only in different areas of the brain, but in the sole of the foot, the eye, and the hand as well.

Innervation Activates Muscles

Skeletal-muscle contraction is initiated only by electrical (nerve) impulses which flow to the muscle via the alpha-motor neurons and the gamma-motor neurons. The skeletal muscles are innervated by the swiftest afferent fibers (Ia and Ib) and the swiftest efferent fibers (A_{alpha}, A_{beta}, and A_{gamma}) in the body, Section 5.B, Nerve Conduction, page 114. The alpha-motor system is largely for the voluntary control of the muscles by higher centers in the brain, whereas the gamma system is largely for the involuntary control of the muscles by lower centers in the brain (Section 3.A, page 21). Chronic activation of the gamma system by the sympathetic nervous system is responsible for the resting-state muscle tone.

As regards motor units, only a few fibers per motor unit are involved in fine motor actions such as blinking the eye, whereas for coarse motor actions such as lifting the leg, the number of fibers in the motor unit will be much larger. The stronger a muscle is, the fewer the number of motor units recruited to support a given load, or to perform a given task. It is one of our eventual goals in *yogasana* practice to minimize the number of motor units engaged in performing the postures while making sure that those muscle units that are engaged are the appropriate ones. As a consequence of this, *yogasana* beginners may be defined as those who work with maximum effort and achieve minimum results, whereas advanced students work with minimum effort to achieve maximum results [350]!

Muscle tissue is not only activated by nerve impulses, but is metabolically dependent upon nerve action for its health; if the nerve to a muscle is cut, then the muscle atrophies in a few months, dies in one to two years, and the muscle tissue is eventually replaced by scar tissue [229]. Similarly, nerves have a short lifetime when they are removed from the vicinity of their target organs [225]. It follows from this that a muscle and its activating and sensing nerves which are only occasionally energized cannot remain healthy indefinitely. Because nerves do not in general regenerate, but instead tend to die off with increasing age (in the cortex, the number of cells decreases by 40% on going from age 20 to age 75, Section 3.B, page 35), muscle fibers must slowly but inexorably lose their innervation. As mentioned above, a muscle without its nerve will slowly die as well. Thus as we go into old age, muscles begin to thin as their fibers die off, especially in the legs [340].

In the corticospinal tract, a single neuron descends from the cortex to the base of the brainstem. At this point, 90% of the fibers decussate (cross over) and travel down the white matter of the lateral funiculus as part of the lateral corticospinal tract. At the appropriate spinal level, the nerve goes from the region of white matter into the gray region and there synapses with a motor neuron. These motor neurons have their cell bodies in the spinal cord, but extend their axons up to a meter to reach the appropriate muscles.

In a typical voluntary muscle action such as a *yogasana* that has been previously practiced, the train of neural pulses would be schematically as follows. The cortex consciously decides on the *yogasana* to be performed (*bakasana*, for example), and sends this information to the cerebellum and the basal ganglia, subconscious centers which orchestrate the various muscles, their timing, and degrees of contraction, as is necessary for the posture. Having been practiced repeatedly before, the neural circuitry for the performance of *bakasana* is well defined and in place. This master plan is then sent upward to the thalamus, and from there to the motor cortex in the frontal lobe, which in turn synapses with the alpha-motor neurons. Taking the direct route, the motor neurons relay the plan of action via the corticospinal tract, to the appropriate muscles, at the appropriate intensities, and at the appropriate times. With this, the pose appears! After a short time, the student voluntarily comes out of the pose, sensing that the strength of the muscles can no longer support it, however, this is not necessarily the case, for it might just as well be that the muscles are not fatigued, but that the nerves and the synapses that are involved in the muscle contraction instead have lost their strength. Indeed, practice of the *yogasanas* builds strength in both the muscular and the nervous systems.

Vascularization

Continuous muscular work requires a steady flow of oxygen (O_2) and glucose into the muscle tissue and a steady outward flow of carbon dioxide (CO_2) and other metabolic products. The vascular system of the body, consisting of the heart, arteries, veins and intermediate vessels (Chapter 11, THE HEART AND THE VASCULAR SYSTEM, page 309) and the blood that courses through them, provides the muscles with all they need metabolically in order to function. Because the activity of an organ depends upon its blood supply, those muscle fibers that are active are supplied by a substantial network of capillaries, whereas this is not so for inactive muscle fibers.

Muscle tissue appears red in part because of the extensive vascularization present in order to serve such a hard-working structure. The heavy vascularization leads in turn to excellent circulation and so accounts for the fact that muscle injuries heal much faster than those to less vascularized tissue such as ligaments, *etc.* [34]. One of the many health benefits of *yogasana* practice then is that the stretching done in the practice promotes the formation of new capillaries which in turn increase circulation in the stretched region. This in turn can speed healing and otherwise strengthens the region against injury or disease.

As discussed in Section 10.A, Structure of the Skin, page 283, the pipe-like elements of the vascular system serving the muscles have their own muscles within the pipe walls, and these muscles control the vascular diameters and therefore their flow rates. Autonomic control (Chapter 6, THE AUTONOMIC NERVOUS SYSTEM, page 133) of the vascular diameters locally can effectively readjust the relative amounts of blood flowing to the muscles, visceral organs, and the skin.

Thus, when a muscle is being used in a vigorous way, stimulation of the sympathetic nervous system will reroute blood from the digestive organs to the muscles. However, when a muscle is strongly contracted, the action tends more or less to clamp down on the vascular system locally and more or less to repress the flow of blood out of the muscle. Even when contracted strongly, the muscle cells continue their metabolism, and CO_2 and acids accumulate. Once the muscle tension is released, the accumulated metabolic products produce a dilation of the vascular system (termed vasodilation) so that, in a feedback loop, an accelerated blood flow then restores homeostasis as rapidly as possible [291] (see Section 11.D, Blood Pressure, page 334).

Vascularization does so much to support muscles, and muscles return the favor. Venous blood from the lower extremities is slow to travel upward against gravity, however, the contraction and relaxation of the muscles in the extremities acts to pump this sluggish blood and lymph back to the heart (Subsection 11.C, *Venous Flow Against Gravity*, page 332).

Microscopic Muscle Contraction

As shown in Fig. 7.A-7a, the inner part of the muscle fiber consists largely of parallel lengths of myofibril. Electron microscopy of the internal structure of such a myofibril shows that it consists of two types of filament, one thin and one thick, each running parallel again to the main fiber axis. The thicker filament, termed "myosin" is a polymer of the protein myosin, and the thinner one, called "actin", is a polymer of the protein actin. These myofibrils are constructed internally such that the actin filaments are interdigitated with the myosin filaments, with a packing pattern in which each myosin filament is surrounded by six actin filaments and carries appendages (cross bridges) which project toward all six actin neighbors. Each actin filament is surrounded in turn by three myosin-filament nearest neighbors (Fig. 7.A-7b). Over the length of the myofibril, the pattern of myosin/actin interdigitation is repeated over and over, with each unit (the sarcomere, a subunit

within the sheath of the sarcolemma, Fig. 7.A-7c) terminated at both ends by rigid endplates called Z lines or Z discs.

In the act of muscle contraction, neither the myosin nor the actin actually contracts, but the relative motion of the actin filaments with respect to the myosin filaments leads to the overall shortening of the distance between Z lines in the sarcomeres of the muscle. A similar statement holds for the case of the muscle being stretched, *i.e.*, when stretching, it is the relative motions of the actin and myosin filaments disengaging that leads to the change in muscle length.

In a muscle in the resting state, there is a third protein (troponin) which lies between the actin and myosin filaments of the muscle fibers, serving to keep them out of contact, Fig. 7.A-8. When the synapse at the neuromuscular junction is activated by the action potential brought to it by the motor neuron, there is an influx of acetylcholine into the synapse, followed by the movement of Ca^{2+} ion into the depolarized muscle fiber. This influx of Ca^{2+} temporarily removes the troponin which otherwise inhibits the myosin/actin interaction.

As shown in Figs. 7.A-7e and 7.A-8, the thick myosin filaments have numerous cross bridges, each of which consists of two joints and a head. When the muscle is relaxed, the angles at the joints of the cross bridges are such that there is no contact between the myosin heads and the corresponding attraction sites on the nearby actin chain, which are otherwise covered by the protective protein, troponin. When the neural signal for muscle contraction is received at the neuromuscular junction via the release of the neurotransmitter acetylcholine (Section 5.D, The Neurotransmitters, page 128), the troponin is removed, and a depolarized signal propagates down the length of the muscle fiber much as with the action potential in the nerve fiber (Section 5.B, Nerve Conduction,

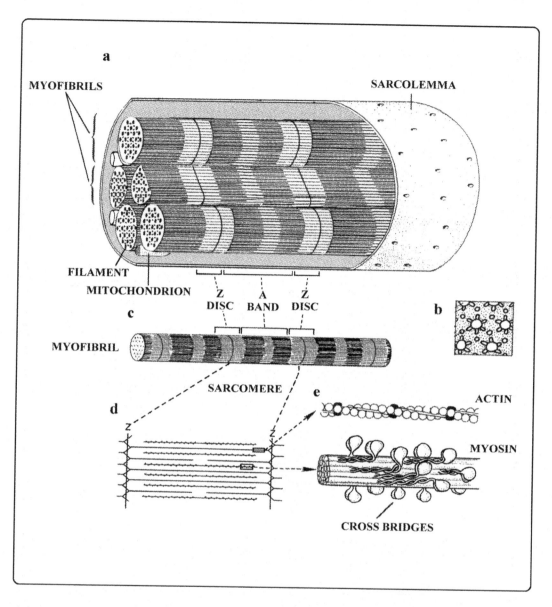

Fig. 7.A-7. Internal structure of a typical skeletal muscle fiber. (**a**) The myofibrils fill the sarcolemma sheath surrounding the fiber; each myofibril in turn is filled with filaments of the proteins actin and myosin. (**b**) End-on view of the myofibril, showing the relative placement and regularity of the actin (thin) and myosin (thick, star-shaped) filaments within it. (**c**) The banded structure of the myofibril bundle as seen from the side. (**d**) A schematic picture showing the interdigitation of the actin and myosin filaments. (**e**) Simplified molecular structures of the filaments. Note the cross bridges on the myosin filament.

page 114), but with much higher voltage so that no amplification is needed.

As the electrically depolarized signal propagates within the muscle, the joint angles at the cross bridge heads increase and the myosin heads are brought into contact with the corresponding actin molecules in the thin filaments. After the myosin-actin contact is established, the angle at the neck of the cross bridge decreases (the power

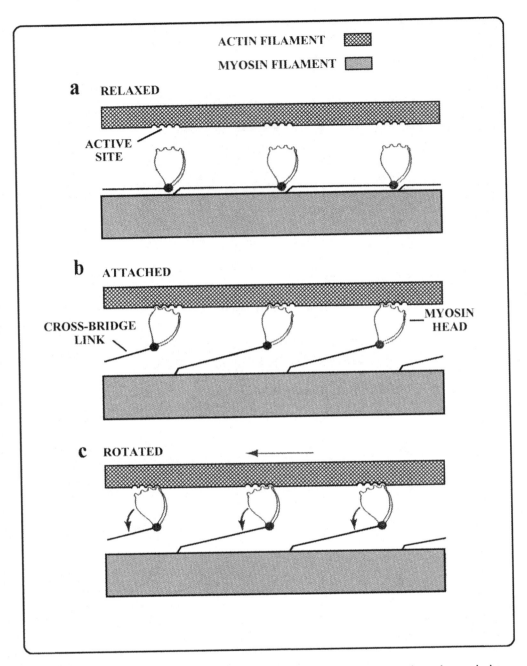

Fig. 7.A-8. Details of the three stages of the cross-bridge action between actin and myosin in muscle. (**a**) In the relaxed state, the cross bridges of the myosin do not engage the active sites of the actin filament because the latter are covered with the protein troponin. (**b**) When the muscle is energized, the troponin covering is shed at the actin sites, and the cross bridges become engaged. (**c**) The heads of the cross bridges then rotate counterclockwise, thus moving the actin filament from right to left.

stroke), thus pulling the Z discs of the actin chain toward one another, Fig. 7.A-9. The various cross bridges work independently of one another so that at any one moment, some are detached, some are in contact, and some are racheting their way down the actin chain. The net result of this is a smooth, continuous pulling of the actin filaments deeper into the spaces between the myosin filaments, *i.e.*, a shorter spacing between the Z lines of the sarcomere and overall shortening of the muscle. The chemistry driving the action of the cross bridges is described in the following Subsection, *Muscle Chemistry and Energy*, page 182.

The activation of a muscle fiber is an all-or-nothing affair, rather like a neural action potential (Section 5.B, Nerve Conduction, page 114), *i.e.*, it is either relaxed or contracted (for a period of about 50 milliseconds). However, a muscle fiber can be more or less contracted *on average* over a longer period of time, depending on the rate at which it is excited, relaxed, excited again,

etc. Though a particular muscle fiber is either activated or not, in an aggregate of such fibers which are not parts of a common motor unit, any and all degrees of activation of the aggregate are possible, depending upon just how many of the fibers are activated simultaneously, and how often per second they are activated. In this way, a large muscle can be energized to whatever level is appropriate to the task it is to perform. See the discussion *Macroscopic Muscle Contraction*, page 185, below for more on this.

It is clear from the above discussion just how the muscle contracts and shortens on a microscopic scale in order to do work. In contrast, on the macroscopic scale, we observe that as a muscle is shortened, it also

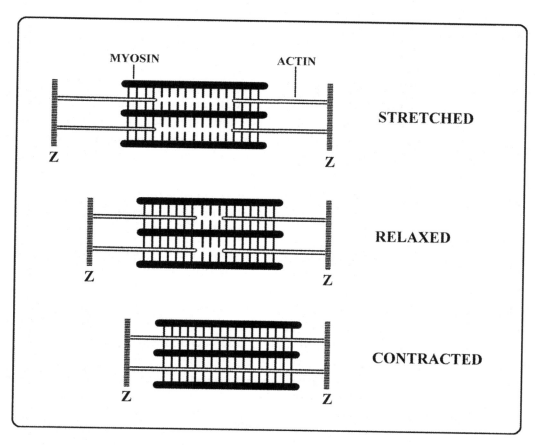

Fig. 7.A-9. The internal structure of a sarcomere showing the relative positions of the thin actin filaments, the thicker myosin filaments and the Z discs in the stretched, relaxed, and contracted states of a skeletal muscle fiber.

becomes larger in cross section, but this does not follow from what has been said up to this point. I postulate that in the relaxed state with the actin not filling the myosin channels, the channels are otherwise filled with a cellular fluid. On contraction, the actin moves into the channel and at the same time, the fluid flows laterally out of the channel into surrounding areas. It is this fluid pressed out of the myosin channels that expands the muscles in directions perpendicular to the shortening. Looked at this way, the muscle is seen to be an organ of constant volume, and if it gets shorter, then it must get thicker in order to maintain its volume.

Only those cells that are designed by Nature to circulate in the blood are able to avoid death without having to attach themselves to and spreading upon some sort of substrate. Experiments [62, 394] show that cells that have been forced to adhere to a solid surface and to spread out on the surface have higher survival and higher proliferation rates than do cells that stick to a surface but remain globular and compact. The conclusion that a mechanically-induced elongation of cells controls and promotes their survival and growth may have a direct connection at the cellular level with *yogasana* practice.

Muscle Chemistry and Energy

The overall chemistry of muscle action is complex, but it is sufficient for our purpose to say that the energy required for contraction involves the dephosphorylation of

adenosine triphosphate, ATP, and that the transport of small amounts of Ca^{2+} ions in and out of the muscle cells are essential elements of the contraction process (see Subsection 7.A, *Muscle Chemistry and Energy*, page 182). ATP, the fuel for muscle action, is a key product of the mitochondrial organelles* within every cell, muscle or nerve.

The molecular structures of the extremely important molecules ATP and its dephosphorylation product adenosine diphosphate, ADP, are shown below.

ATP   **ADP**

The energy for muscle action has its source in the cleavage and hydrolysis of the terminal $-PO_3$ group of ATP, thus forming ADP and the phosphate anion (PO_4^{3-}). There are then several other chemical processes that function to phosphorylate the ADP so that it can live again to help drive another actin fiber into the myosin channel. It is also known that the depolarization of the end-plate voltage and the propagation of the action potential down the length of the muscle fiber involve gates in the cell membranes for the transport of Na^+ and K^+ ions [225].

In the resting state, the ATP is bound to the head of the myosin cross bridges, but on approach to the newly uncovered actin sites,

*Mitochondria are organelles dispersed throughout the cytoplasm of all cells. Chemical reactions take place in the mitochondria (the oxidation of glucose by oxygen) that supply the energy to drive the cell's metabolic processes. They are the power sources for processes in the brain, muscles, all organs, the visual system, *etc.*, as they carry the DNA for producing the enzymes needed for energy production. Mitochondria multiply independently within the cell, not needing to wait for the cell itself to divide. When sperm unites with egg, the mitochondria of the sperm are absorbed and then destroyed by the egg, and so the mitochondria of all cells come only from the mother's side of the union [467].

the ATP is cleaved into ADP plus phosphate ion, both of which leave the cross-bridge head as it binds to the actin. It is the energy of this chemical reaction that is transformed into the mechanical energy of muscle contraction. Once this simple reaction is accomplished, there is a strong movement of the cross-bridge head (the power stroke) which is translated into actin filament motion. The presence of fresh ATP in the cellular fluid surrounding the filaments encourages the head of the cross bridge to disengage from the actin and bind again to the ATP once the power stroke is finished.

As long as there is Ca^{2+} and ATP in the cell, the heads of the cross bridges will continue to turn the ATP into ADP and to pull the actin filaments from the Z-disc endplates toward the centers of the sarcomeres. This process runs at about 10 to 50 cycles per second, but is limited by the amount of ATP which is available in the cell for re-attachment to the cross-bridge heads. In a dead body where the mitochondria no longer function so that there is no more ATP to recharge the cross-bridge heads, the contractile machinery is essentially frozen in place, *i.e., rigor mortis* has set in; see Box 7.A-1, *Muscular Life after Death,* page 184.

All muscle cells use ATP to fuel the work of the cell, but the cell at rest contains only enough ATP to fuel intense muscle activity for about 5–6 seconds. Obviously, this is not enough to sustain the more general needs of life and so other indirect sources of ATP may be called upon in times of need. As ATP is consumed by dephosphorylation and its decomposition product ADP is formed, the latter is readily rephosphorylated by the creatine phosphate in the cell to reform ATP.

Normally, there is enough creatine phosphate in the cell to extend the cell's working period to 20–25 seconds or so. For periods of time beyond 25 seconds, the cell relies instead on the anaerobic oxidation of glucose (or glycogen, a polymerized form of glucose) to help in reforming ATP. In this process, called glycolysis, for each new ATP molecule formed, there is also formed one molecule of lactic acid. As the muscle cell works using anaerobic glycolysis, it consumes glucose and generates lactic acid which accumulates in the cell and lowers its pH, eventually limiting its activity as the lactic acid buildup leads to muscle fatigue. Fast-twitch muscles (Subsection 7.A, *Types of Muscle Fiber,* page 189) when overused, take the glycolysis route in order to remain functioning.*

Anaerobic glycolysis can be active for only about 2 minutes, at which point, aerobic metabolism takes over. When one is exercising, the level of glucose in the blood falls, and in response to this, the glucostat in the hypothalamus activates the sympathetic nervous system so that both the catecholamines and cortisol are released from the adrenal glands (Section 6.C, The Sympathetic Nervous System, page 144). The epinephrine component of the catecholamines increases the mobilization of fatty acids by releasing them from their bound form as triglycerides in a chemical process called lipolysis. However, this lipolysis of the triglycerides by epinephrine is not possible in the absence of cortisol. Thus, through exercise, the sympathetic nervous system is activated and body fat is burned away through the intermediary action of the adrenal hormones [230].

*Realizing that lactic acid buildup was a negative factor in high-intensity exercise, athletes have turned to ingesting large amounts of sodium bicarbonate (as found in Alka Seltzer), and as hoped, the acid-buffering action of this compound has demonstrably improved performance [337]. In no way can one recommend "soda loading" to students of *yogasana,* but it might be possible to eat an alkaline diet [252] which will then tend to neutralize the lactic acid produced by prolonged work of the muscles in *yogasanas,* were that a problem.

BOX 7.A-1: MUSCULAR LIFE AFTER DEATH

Once the heart stops beating and the brain becomes quiescent, the body can then be said to have died physiologically. However, even in this state of death, there still remains a small quantity of ATP in the muscle fibers, and given an electrical stimulus from outside the body, the muscles can still be made to move until the ATP within them is exhausted. This muscle action in the dead can be stimulated for up to two hours after death. With the ATP in a dead body exhausted, the muscle action stops, leaving the actin-myosin machinery in a state of partial contraction (Fig. 7.A-9), with bridge heads in contact, but not able to either rachet forward or relax backward. This state of *rigor mortis* lasts for up to twelve hours, and then relaxes from that point [387].

This aerobic process also uses glucose and fatty acids as fuel for generating more ATP, "burning" them instead with the oxygen carried to the muscle fiber's mitochondria by the hemoglobin in the blood. In this case, ATP is produced, but without the lactic-acid penalty. Once into the aerobic regime, the muscle cell can work vigorously until the supplies of glucose, fatty acids and/or oxygen are exhausted. The shift into aerobic oxidation after 2–3 minutes of heavy exercise is evident as the athlete's "second wind". Yoga students benefit from this second wind when performing aerobic jumping routines such as *surya namaskar*, the Salute to the Sun, but are otherwise working in the anaerobic regime. When *yogasana* practice is working in the aerobic regime, it increases $\dot{V}O_{2max}$, and promotes the transformation of fast-twitch into slow-twitch fibers [23], Subsection 7.A, *Types of Muscle Fiber*, page 189. Because the amount of work that a muscle can do is strictly limited by the amount of oxygen that can be delivered to the mitochondria of its cells by the bloodstream, $\dot{V}O_{2max}$ is seen to be a measure of the body's ability to do work.

The effects of long-term exercise are even more interesting than those of short-term work. When the exercise is chronic rather than acute as with an intense daily *yogasana* practice, then $\dot{V}O_{2max}$ increases while the resting heart rate, the rise in blood lactate and the concentration of catecholamines in the blood (Subsection 5.D, page 129) are lower when exercising. Moreover, there is an almost 100% increase in the number of blood capillaries per muscle fiber [98, 337], and in the muscle cells themselves, the myoglobin and enzyme contents increase as do the size of the mitochondria. On prolonged, chronic exercise, the levels of stored glycogen and triglycerides increase and more fatty acids rather than carbohydrates are burned for energy, both of which lead to less glycogen being depleted, less lactic acid being formed, less soreness, less muscle fatigue and more endurance.

Cleavage of the high-energy-phosphate chemical bond in ATP results in only 25% of the energy being available for work, the other 75% appearing as heat (or entropy). Most of the sugar oxidized for energy in the mitochondria is stored first as glycogen in the liver, and is available for energy only when liver enzymes degrade the glycogen to glucose. Hormones from the brain activate these enzymes whenever we begin to exercise or even begin to think of exercising. Thus warming up not only loosens the muscles but gets the glucose flowing so as to keep the muscles well fueled.

It occasionally happens that when we practice certain *yogasanas*, a joint is severely closed in such a way that circulation is impaired and/or there is pressure applied to the nerve bundles. As regards circulation in such a compressed system, though the arterial side of the vascular system is strong walled and does not easily collapse under pressure, the same cannot be said for the venous side. Thus, under pressure, blood may be able to enter a compressed area, but it cannot leave through collapsed veins, leading to a condition called ischemia. In ischemia, the O_2 in the local blood is consumed but not replaced, leading in time to a hypoxic condition in which the oxygen level is severely diminished. Ischemia adversely affects muscles as they become starved for O_2 and yet cannot rid themselves of metabolic wastes.

It is difficult to detail the situation in regard to nerves (Subsection 5.C, *Mechanical Effects on Nerves*, page 125), but they also suffer O_2 depletion, moreover, they are soft mechanically and do depend upon material transport down their axons (by microtubules). When pressed, the axons become poor to nonexistent conductors of neural signals and so the muscles so innervated by these nerves may not be excitable; this too may involve ischemia and the concomitant hypoxia.

Macroscopic Muscle Contraction

Though the same muscle may be used to lift a one-ounce pencil or to lift a ten-pound sack of sugar, the amount of work performed by that muscle will be very different in the two cases. This can be understood if the number of muscle cells recruited to a task can be varied to suit the job. Lifting a pencil requires only a small percentage of the muscle fibers available in a large muscle, while lifting a heavier sack requires more. It is a specific benefit of *yogasana* practice that one can fine-tune just how many of the muscle fibers in a large muscle are called into action, as well as which ones they will be, and one can balance their effect by simultaneously activating their antagonist muscle groups (Subsection 7.A, *Reciprocal Inhibition and Agonist/Antagonist Pairs*, page 193). With such muscular discrimination available, the yoga student not only has precise control of body movement, but uses the body's resources in the most efficient way possible.

The strength of a muscle, or more properly the force (pressure per unit area) that a muscle can exert, depends upon its length. When a muscle is fully stretched, there is a minimal overlap of the actin and myosin filaments, Fig. 7.A-9, and so only a minimum force can be developed upon contraction. Similarly, when the muscle is tightly contracted, there is a jamming of the actin filaments in the channels of the myosin filaments, and only a weak contractile force is again possible. Muscle action is strongest when the muscle is at a length where all possible cross bridges can be realized but there is still room within the sarcomere for large-scale movement of the actin filaments.*

The "strength" of a muscle can be taken to be measured by the maximum force that it can exert or by its ability to do "work", a quantity defined as the product of the force exerted times the distance moved. As such, the ability of a muscle to do work is dependent not only on the microscopic details of the interaction between its filaments, as discussed above, but also on the more obvious

*As Lasater [275] has so eloquently pointed out, *yogasana* practice is involved not only with the strength of the muscles but also with the inner strength that one demonstrates in one's commitment to practicing what may be difficult. This is the motivational factor mentioned in Box 2.B-1, *Interactions of the Brain's Three Systems in the Teaching of Virabhadrasana I*, page 18.

factor: if the muscle at rest is already strongly contracted, *i.e.*, has a short rest length as is often seen in the weightlifting physique, then the muscle has a shorter range of motion through which it can work, and so is relatively impotent with respect to the same muscle having a longer rest length and a correspondingly longer range of motion. The ideal would seem to be the musculature of the *yogasana* student, for this type of work leads to muscles that are both forceful and supple so as to have large ranges of motion.

On the other hand, "power" is defined as the amount of work generated in a second of time. Because the practice of the *yogasanas* works to the advantage of the slower muscle fibers (see Subsection 7.A, *Types of Muscle Fiber*, page 189), the work done by these muscles may be high, but the power expended will be correspondingly low because *yogasana*-trained muscles are inherently slower moving.

Muscle strength is maximal at the resting length of the muscle, but drops to 50% of its optimal value when the muscle length is either shortened to 70% of the resting length or extended to 130% of that length [230]. From this, one sees that the very straight arm is relatively weak muscularly, for its biceps is totally extended and so has poor filament overlap, whereas the triceps is totally contracted and so has jamming of the filaments. For this reason, full-arm balance (*adho mukha vrksasana*) would be very exhausting were it not for the bones of the arms which support the weight of the body in the inverted position if they can be placed in the proper position, *i.e.*, vertically placed one above the other.

In this way, one also can understand the difficulty students might have in pressing up into *urdhva dhanurasana* from the lying position. With back on the floor and hands in position, the triceps are in an elongated condition, implying minimal contact of

cross bridges between myosin and actin in its muscle fibers. Thus not enough mechanical force can be generated by contraction of the triceps in order to start the shoulders moving away from the wrists. If the student is given a gentle lift at the shoulders at this point so as to help shorten the triceps, the contact between the sliding filaments of the triceps increases, the arms begin to straighten, and the chest and pelvis start to elevate. Triceps strength is maximal when the angle at the elbow is in the vicinity of 90°, as in *pincha mayurasana*, for example, or in *urdhva dhanurasana* when on the top of the head.

Complete contraction of the triceps in *urdhva dhanurasana* brings the body into the fully open position, however, once in this position, the triceps are fully contracted and so suffer a loss of force due to jamming of the filaments within the sarcomeres. However, at this point, the bones have been put into place to support the asana against the pull of gravity, and so the only triceps action required is that to keep the bones of the arms in their proper places. As one presses up into *urdhva dhanurasana*, a set of actions which are similar to those undergone by the triceps of the upper arms also takes place in the quadruceps muscles of the thighs.

Students of the art of *yogasana* make a distinction between a muscular movement and a muscular action. In the former, muscles are contracted, pull on the bones and move them in a particular direction. In contrast, when performing a muscular action, the muscles are contracted, but there is very little or no motion associated with the contraction. Thus, raising the arms overhead in *urdhva hastasana* is a muscular movement, whereas the lifting of the fingertips in this pose yet more upward while descending the shoulder blades is a muscle action. To the outside observer, it appears that "nothing is happening" during a muscular action, however, the *yogasana* performer knows that the pose is actually very dynamic, but balanced, with considerable muscle activity taking place in spite of the apparent lack of motion. As will be discussed more fully in the following Subsection, a muscular movement is an isotonic use of the muscles, whereas a muscular action is an isometric use of the muscles.

As muscles move with respect to one another, there is a need for lubrication just as there is when one bone moves with respect to another (Subsection 8.E, *Joint Lubrication and Arthritis*, page 265). To this end, where tissue moves over tissue, or tissue moves over bone, the body has placed about 150 pancake shaped, fluid-filled sacs called bursae, in order to lubricate and assist the motion. Thus when one sits in *virasana*, the ischium bones of the pelvis are protected from the hard floor by bursae, while there are other bursae between the ischium bones and the gluteus muscles. There are bursae as well within the tendons of the knees, Fig. 8.E-2, both above and below the patella, which bursae act to lubricate the mechanism. Over-use of the bursae leads to inflammation and bursitis.

The effects of exercise on muscle are manifold. As the strength of the muscle increases, so does its cross section (but not necessarily in young children). This increased size comes from the larger diameter of the fibers, as their number stays constant in adults. Practice of the *yogasanas* necessarily involves a certain amount of strength training, during which, both the strength and the diameter of the muscles increase. This increase in the size of a muscle with *yogasana* strength training again is due to an increase in the diameters of the muscle's fibers and not due to an increase in their number. However, as the fibers increase in girth, there is a corresponding increase in the amount of connective tissue binding them together [98]. Work that increases the bulk of a muscle but does nothing to stretch its connective tissue will result in a large muscle which can move through only a small range of motion. On the other hand, if a muscle is not used at all, it will shrink in size; this includes the heart (however, also see Subsections 11.A, *Effects of Western Exercise, Yogasana, and the Autonomic Nervous System on the Heart*, page 320, and 22.A, *Physical Aging*, page 495).

Types of Muscle Contraction

Viewed at an elementary level, there are three types of muscle contraction: isometric, isotonic, and isokinetic [337]. Isometric contraction involves working against a fixed, immovable object, as when one sits at a desk with the hands below it, and tries to lift it off the floor. The desk does not move and though the muscles involved (the biceps in this example) are working intensely, they do not shorten appreciably.

Because a real muscle is more than just a collection of muscle fibers, when speaking of muscle contraction, one must also consider all of the collateral structures such as tendons, connective tissue and cross bridges which have their own mechanical properties. In fact, when muscle fibers contract to shorten the muscle, the Z discs are pulled toward one another, but the attached collateral tissues are stretched! When the load on a muscle is very large, the lengthening of the collateral structures may just balance or slightly exceed the contraction of the sarcomeres, with the result that though the sarcomeres are contracted, there is no overall movement of the skeleton. This is the situation in an isometric contraction.

When isometric contraction is used to build strength, it should be done at several different joint angles, because the strengthening benefits earned at one angle do not transfer very effectively to other angles. That is, working isometrically with the elbow at 45° does little good for strengthening the arm when it is to be used at an angle of, say, 85°.

If the load on the muscle is light, the contractile force of the sarcomere is stronger than the forces that resist extending the tendons, *etc.*, and motion ensues. This is the case in an isotonic contraction. When a muscle contracts isotonically, its length changes appreciably when the load on the muscle is put into motion, as for example, the contraction of the triceps when pressing a bag of sugar overhead. If the length change in the isotonic contraction is a shortening, then the movement is said to be concentric (Fig. 7.A-10b), whereas if the change is lengthening, then the movement is said to be eccentric (Fig. 7.A-10c). As an example of the differences between concentric and eccentric isotonic actions, the lifting of straight legs from the floor into *sirsasana I* involves an isotonic concentric action of the muscles of the lower back (quadratus lumborum, *etc.*), whereas the slow lowering of the legs from *sirsasana I* to the floor involves an isotonic eccentric action of the same muscles. Throughout these motions, if the feet are kept broad and flexed at the ankles, then they are involved in isometric contraction.

In general, in practicing the *yogasanas*, various muscles pass through concentric and eccentric phases of isotonic action in arriving at the final positions and on returning from them to the initial posture, but while working in the *yogasana*, the contractions are all isometric, with little or no movement. In eccentric contraction, the muscle involved is stretched as it performs

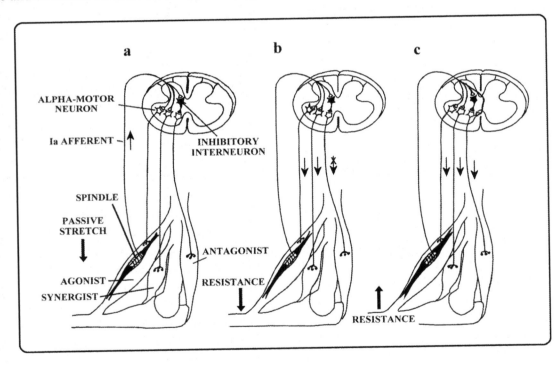

Fig. 7.A-10. Neural connections of the muscle spindle of the agonist biceps muscle to the spinal cord and thence to its agonist, synergist and antagonist muscles. (**a**) Under a slow, passive stretch such as traction, the muscle spindle sends its signal to the spine, but without a reflex reaction. (**b**) When working to lift a load, the alpha-motor neuron from the spinal cord to the biceps is energized, but not the muscle spindle; the synergist is also activated, but the antagonist muscle is inhibited by the spinal interneuron. This is an isotonic concentric action. (**c**) When working to lower a load as in an isotonic eccentric action, the agonist and the antagonist are co-contracted, but with the antagonist more strongly so than the agonist muscle.

its work, however, fewer muscle fibers are involved in the work of eccentric contraction as compared to concentric contraction. Though eccentric contraction requires 40% more force than the corresponding concentric contraction, it not only strengthens the muscle more quickly, but also places a much larger stress on the fibers involved while restricting bloodflow to the muscle, and so opens the door to excessive muscle soreness [5]. When working the *yogasanas* with beginners, the static, isometric nature of the poses will encourage them to hold their breath and so raise their blood pressures [90a], consequently they must be encouraged to keep the breath moving in the asanas even though the skeletal muscles appear not to move.

The final length of an elongated muscle, *i.e.*, the degree of the stretch, will depend upon the flexibility of the relatively inflexible connective tissue. As one's flexibility increases in the *yogasanas*, one is increasing the extendability of the connective tissue working in the isometric mode (see Box 7.A-2 for an interesting scenario in regard to what really stretches when a muscle is stretched). When the arm is bent and one tries to straighten it with the triceps, the load against which the triceps works in part is the inflexibility of the biceps. The antagonist of a pair supplies part of the load against which the agonist (Subsection 7.A, *Reciprocal Inhibition and Agonist/Antagonist Pairs*, page 193) can work in isometric extension.

Isokinetic contraction is done at constant velocity of the load being moved, regardless of the differences in the strength of the muscle at different angles, which can be appreciable: for example, the biceps are strongest at an angle of 120° at the elbow, and least strong at 30°. Isokinetic contraction is of no consequence for *yogasana* students as we make no particular effort to keep isotonic movements going at a constant velocity.

As mentioned on page 187, a muscle can be considered to be an organ of constant volume, whether contracted or elongated [473]. This means that as a muscle contracts lengthwise, it must broaden transversely, and *vice versa*. For example, the tip of the tongue can be shot forward by contracting the muscles that lie transverse to its axis, *i.e.*, if the volume of the tongue is to be kept constant and its width decreases, then the length must increase. Conversely, a relaxed tongue in *savasana* is broad.

Types of Muscle Fiber

There are three distinct types of skeletal muscle fiber, with every muscle in the body being a particular combination of the three types. Each of the three fiber types (here called Types 1, 2 and 3) is characterized by the unique form of its myosin myofibril at the molecular level. Because each of the fiber types has its strong and weak points, and because the proportions of the three fiber types within a muscle can be changed depending upon the type and intensity of one's exercise, over time, one can optimize the muscular action appropriate to one's performance or practice. All of the muscle fibers within a particular motor unit have the same fiber type, and all three types use acetylcholine as neurotransmitters. Each of the fiber Types 1, 2, and 3 is described in Table 7.A-l and Box 7.A-3, *Muscle Fiber Types in the Poultry World*, page 192. As can be seen in the Table, the fiber types can be distinguished by their color, speed of contraction, diameter, resistance to fatigue, and many other qualities as well.

Type-1 muscle fiber has a red-brown coloration due to its high content of myoglobin (a molecule much like hemoglobin) which strongly binds O_2 for eventual oxidation of the fuel in the muscle. These red fibers contract relatively slowly (maximum velocity of contraction only one tenth as fast as that for Type-3 fibers), and so are more numerous in those muscles which do not require a fast response, as with the postural muscles in the back body. The capillary networks serving the slow-twitch, red fibers are dense in order to supply abundant O_2 to the muscle in its extended period of work, and though the muscle is slow working, it can work at that pace for a long time. The slow-twitch Type-1 fibers are enhanced in the sort of isometric contractions met with in the *yogasanas*, and otherwise are most prominent in the postural muscles of the upper body. Actually, when doing *yogasanas*, all of the muscles become postural in a sense!

At the other end of the muscle-fiber spectrum, there are the Type-3 white fibers,

BOX 7.A-2: WHAT REALLY STRETCHES WHEN A MUSCLE IS STRETCHED, AND WHY DOES IT STOP STRETCHING?

In the contraction of a muscle fiber, the action potential that drives the contraction is triggered by a change in the permeability of the sarcomere membrane to specific ions, and the subsequent movement of the actin within the myosin channels. If the contraction is taken to the limit, the actin is fully driven into the myosin channels and no further muscle shortening is possible. In contrast, if the same fiber is being stretched, the fiber is relaxed and the cross-bridge heads are disengaged. In this scenario, it is easily imaginable then that continued stretching could pull the actin chain fully out of the myosin channel, and were this to happen, the sarcomere could not be reconstituted because the actin ends would no longer be in register with the channels of the myosin. In this situation, the stretch would have succeeded in essentially severing the muscle fiber, having separated the actin from the myosin.

It is clear from the above that there must be a brake on the stretching of muscle fibers if they are to survive *yogasana* work. Fortunately, there are two mechanisms that serve this purpose. First, as described above, the connective tissue bonded to the sarcomere offers significant resistance to lengthening of the muscle fiber, and so acts to hold the actin and myosin together. Remember that 30% of a muscle's bulk is connective tissue. Though an individual muscle fiber can be stretched to 150% of its resting length before tearing, the tendon attaching that muscle fiber to the bone can only stretch 4% before it fails, and so will offer considerable resistance to stretching. The lack of elasticity in the tendon is compensated by its very high tensile strength. Ligaments can be stretched only slightly more than can tendons [391].

Second, as is discussed in Section 7.B, Muscle Sensors; The Mechanoreceptors, page 198, there are mechanoreceptors called muscle spindles within muscles that trigger a muscle contraction if the extent or rate of muscle stretching exceeds certain limits.

Viewed in this way, we see that "how flexible a person is" depends upon the flexibility of their connective tissue and the sensitivity of their muscle spindles to stretch. As discussed in Subsection 9.A, *Collagen*, page 273, there is a strong hereditary factor dictating the flexibility of our connective tissue, making some of us contortionists and some of us inherently as stiff as flagpoles. The important question of how to overcome the resistance that muscle spindles have toward muscle stretching is discussed in Section 7.B, Muscle Sensors; The Mechanoreceptors, page 198.

TABLE 7.A-l. CHARACTERISTICS OF THE THREE SKELETAL-MUSCLE TYPES [6, 131, 230, 476]

Property	Type 1	Type 2	Type 3
Color	Red	Red	White
Twitch speed	Slow	Medium	Fast
Activation threshold	Low	Moderate	High
Contraction time, ms	100–120	40–45	40–45
Myoglobin content	High	Very high	Low
Innervation ratio	Low	Moderate	High
Type of efferent	B	A_{alpha}	A_{alpha}
Capillary density	High	High	Low
Muscle tension	Low	Medium	High
Duration of force	Prolonged	Prolonged	Intermittent
Size of force	Low	Relatively high	High
Resistance to fatigue	Very high	High	Low
Order of recruitment	First	Second	Last
Fiber diameter	Small	Medium	Large
Muscles high in this type	Postural muscles in back	Quadruceps	Biceps
Type of ATP production	Oxidative phosphorylation	Oxidative phosphorylation	Anaerobic glycolysis

which are most abundant in muscles which react quickly but for only a short time, such as the biceps. In these fast-twitch fibers, there is no myoglobin, for ATP production is via an anerobic mechanism (Subsection 7.A, *Muscle Chemistry and Energy*, page 182), which is to say, the oxygen for combustion is stripped from glucose rather than absorbed from the blood (see Box 7.A-3), for absorption would be too slow a process for the needs of these fast-acting fibers. Type-3 fibers are most often involved in muscle injury. The intermediate fiber, Type-2, is red and fairly-fast twitch, and is found in those muscles where both speed and endurance are factors, *i.e.*, in the muscles of the legs used for running.

As might have been expected, the fast-twitch Type-3 fibers are energized by those efferent nerves with the fastest conduction velocity, the A_{alpha} motor neurons, while the Type-l slow fibers are innervated by the slower Type-C neurons, Table 5.B-2. The A_{alpha} neurons are capable of delivering action potentials at a rate of up to 60 per second to the neuromuscular junction, whereas the figure for the C-type neurons is only about 10–20 per second [225]. Thus Type-l fibers are more powerful since their muscle fibers can be excited many more times in a second, but this can be maintained for only a few seconds. Such a muscular response occasionally may be advantageous, as when dropping straight body from *adho mukha vrksasana* into *chaturanga dandasana*, but is not often called upon when performing most *yogasanas*.

As shown in Fig. 7.A-11, the average couch potato has approximately equal amounts of the three types of fiber in the quadruceps muscles of the legs. By comparison, sprinters have four times as much fast fibers (Types 2 plus 3) as slow fibers (Type 1) in their quadruceps, and marathon run-

BOX 7.A-3: MUSCLE-FIBER TYPES IN THE POULTRY WORLD

Myoglobin is a red pigment which is found among (but not within) the capillaries of Type-1 and -2 muscles. Like hemoglobin, it too binds oxygen but more tightly, so that it is available to working muscle only slowly, but over a longer time period. As such, it is better suited for muscles that expend their energy slowly over a long time, *i.e.*, the Types 1 and 2.

The muscle types described in Table 7.A-1 may be more familiar to the reader when referred to poultry. In this case, the white breast meat of, say chicken, is largely the myoglobin-free, Type-3, fast-twitch fiber. As might be expected for a flightless bird, this muscle fatigues rapidly. The chicken does do a lot of walking, however, and so the muscle of chicken legs is dark, being loaded with myoglobin and not easily fatigued, as appropriate for Type-1 or Type-2 muscle. On the other hand, in the duck, this being a bird that both walks and flies, the muscles of both the breast and the leg are rich in the slow-twitch, high-myoglobin red fiber.

ners have twenty times as much slow fiber as the faster types [6]. In the case of extreme disuse, as for a person with paralysis of the legs, the muscles shrink, ironically leaving behind a preponderance of Type-3 fast-twitch fibers. Chronic exercise of the ordinary variety leads to an increase in the diameters of the slow-twitch fibers. See Section 22.A for the effects of aging on the proportions of muscle-fiber types in the body.

There is a preference in which the various muscle-fiber types are recruited in a muscular action. The slow-twitch fibers are the first to be recruited, and the fast-twitch are the last to be recruited, except in an emergency situation, where all types are recruited at once [131].

Interestingly, if the connectivity of the motor neurons is reversed so that a red slow-twitch fiber is energized by a fast neuron or *vice versa*, then the slow-twitch fiber slowly becomes fast or the white fast-twitch fiber slowly becomes slow [225]. These changes of muscle characteristics are paralleled by changes in the muscle's biochemistry and morphology. This implies that if

the higher levels of consciousness which control muscle action dictate a new role for a muscle, its responsiveness, chemistry, and morphology all will change in sympathy with the new demands made upon it by the altered neural signal activating it [88]. In this way, *yogasana* practice can change the muscular form and responses of the body.

Indeed, several recent experiments have shown that muscle-fiber Types 2 and 3 can be readily interconverted within a period of a month or so by the appropriate type of exercise [6]. Evidence for the conversions of the fast Types into slow-Type-1 fiber or the reverse are on less solid footing, but seem likely on a longer time scale. It is postulated for example, that if fast fibers suffer nerve death, the muscles could be re-innervated by the slow fibers nearby, thereby converting the fiber from fast type to slow type.

As the *yogasanas* are largely isometric positions, and isometric contraction encourages red slow-twitch fibers (Type 1), one can only conclude that *yogasana* practice in essence slows our internal clocks, re-tuning the muscles to a slower, more energy-effi-

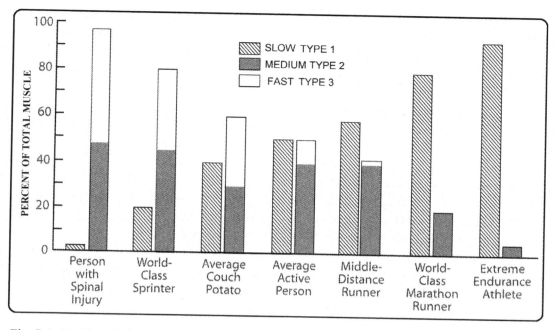

Fig. 7.A-11. The relative proportions of the three muscle-fiber types in the quadruceps of people with various athletic skills, or none at all. *Yogasana* students are closer to the right-hand side in this diagram.

cient mode, as appropriate for reaching higher meditative states. The fatigue felt by the student in a *yogasana* held for a long time is less of a factor when the muscle fibers in question are slow twitch, for they are both more economical energetically and so require less fresh blood to function than do fast-twitch fibers [473], and also are more highly vascularized. Note too that as the percentage of slow-twitch fibers increases in a muscle, its demand for O_2 decreases so that the relaxed state is promoted (slower heart rate, lower blood pressure, mind's external awareness relaxed, *etc.*), whereas the energized state is discouraged, *i.e.*, we become more laid back. Said differently, the nervous system moves from sympathetic to parasympathetic dominance as the *yogasana* practice retunes muscle fibers away from Type 3, and toward Type 1.

An experimental study supports these suppositions regarding *yogasana* and muscle-fiber type [23]. With *yogasana* practice, it was found that the aerobic power $\dot{V}O_{2max}$

increased significantly, whereas anaerobic power decreased significantly. These shifts are interpreted as showing the transformation of fast, glycolic fibers into slow, oxidative fibers, Table 7.A-1, as one practices the *yogasanas*.

Reciprocal Inhibition and Agonist/ Antagonist Pairs

Almost all muscles in the body are paired such that for every muscle action at a joint, there is an opposing muscle action possible which allows the motion at the joint to be reversed and thus controlled. See Fig. 7.A-3 for a display of muscle pairs with such opposing actions. Judicious excitation of these opposing muscle pairs, called agonist/antagonist pairs, then allows for fine-tuning of skeletal motions and reversal of motions. For example, the biceps muscle which flexes the arm at the elbow has the triceps muscle as its antagonist, which acts to straighten it. Working together, they allow a careful and graceful movement of the arm at the elbow, as when bowing a violin. In general, the agonist/antagonist muscle pairs control the motion of the joined bones in a single plane, while for a complex joint such as the shoulder (Subsection 8.D, *The Arms, Shoulders, and Shoulder Blades*, page 254), there are several pairs acting to make the allowed motion more spherical than planar.

There is a general state of mild contraction (the so-called resting muscle tone, Subsection 7.B, page 204) at all times in all of the muscles of the body. Even when the body seems to be doing nothing, as when standing, many muscles still play an active role in keeping the body upright rather than letting it collapse. If, in this state, the intention of the brain is to change the angle at a joint quickly, as by flexion of the arm to swat a fly on the nose, for example, then the instantaneous contraction of the flexor agonist musculature will be resisted by the ever-present muscle tone in the extensor antagonist musculature. In this case of sudden movement, the nervous system provides a mechanism whereby the antagonist muscle is relaxed by inhibiting its neural signal entirely, while the agonist is flexed quickly and maximally. Called reciprocal inhibition, this neuromuscular mechanism also is evident in the patellar knee-jerk reflex, Fig. 7.D-1. In the case of reflex actions, the reflexive contraction of one of the muscles in response to a stimulus elicits a simultaneous relaxation of its antagonist muscle. In a modified form, reciprocal inhibition also is a factor in the performance of many *yog-asanas*.

Nature manages to selectively activate one element of an agonist/antagonist pair by bifurcating the afferent nerve signal and sending each branch simultaneously to the efferent motor neurons of the two muscles in the pair, Fig. 7.A-12. The route to one of the muscles is direct and excitatory, whereas the other synapses instead with an inter-

neuron, the function of which is inhibitory (Subsection 5.C, *Excitation Versus Inhibition*, page 123). Thus, by interposing an interneuron in the synaptic gap of one of the muscles but not in the other, only the first is contracted while contraction in the second is inhibited. Of course, agonist/antagonist inhibition works the other way as well: if it is the second muscle which is excited, then excitation of the first will be inhibited.

Other muscles respond as well in this reflexive action. Thus, when the right leg lifts as in Fig. 7.A-12, the gluteus medius (origin at the iliac crest; insertion onto the greater trochanter of the femur) on the left also contracts so as to support the pelvis and keep it from dropping when the support of the right leg is no longer present. This interplay of excitation and inhibition within an agonist/antagonist muscle pair characterizes the situation in regard reflex actions, as described in Section 7.D, page 211.

The mechanism described above also works much in the same way when the muscle action is voluntary and slow rather than reflexive and fast, *i.e.*, when a muscle is activated voluntarily, its antagonist often is inhibited synaptically in support of the desired movement. For example, in *uttanasana*, one seeks to stretch and lengthen the hamstrings. The hamstring stretching can be facilitated by contracting the hamstring's antagonist, the quadruceps, for the reaction to quadruceps contraction is inhibition of the hamstring contraction, *i.e.*, lengthening. That is to say, when the agonist contracts, the antagonist relaxes and stretches. In the stretched state, the antagonist's forcefulness is very much reduced due to poor overlap of its sliding filaments (Subsection 7.A, *Microscopic Muscle Contraction*, page 178) and so it cannot generate much force to oppose the desired action, *i.e.*, full contraction of the agonist.

This mutual inhibition within the agonist/antagonist pair is of great value for

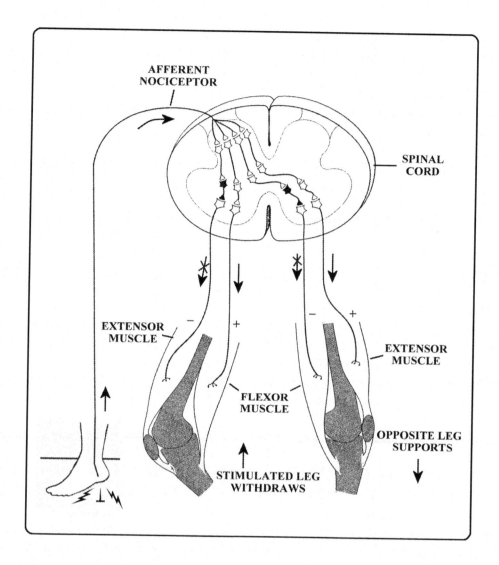

Fig. 7.A-12. When the right foot steps on a sharp object, the pain signal travels up the Type-II nerve fiber from the nociceptor into the spinal cord. Simultaneously, the flexor muscle (the hamstring) of the right leg is contracted so as to draw the foot upward, whereas the contraction of the extensor (quadruceps) on that leg is inhibited by the interposed interneuron. Meanwhile, to keep from falling with one leg lifted, the opposite scenario is being played out on the left leg, where the extensor is contracted to support the body, while the flexor is inhibited, again by the appropriately placed interneuron.

beginners, but when working at a higher level, both muscle groups of a pair are often worked simultaneously, for the inhibition can be overridden by influences from higher centers (see also Box 7.A-4, *The Hands Help Wag the Shoulder Blades in Adho Mukha Svanasana,* page 196). The simulta-

neous activation of both partners of an agonist/antagonist pair is called co-contraction. Though less energy efficient than reciprocal inhibition, co-contraction does allow for finer control of small movements by balancing the opposition of two active muscles rather than having one active muscle balanced against little or no resistance as in reciprocal inhibition. The practice of *yog-asana* allows for a sophisticated interaction of the agonist and antagonist muscles in a pair. Co-contraction of the muscles in an agonist/antagonist pair also can be used to immobilize a bone or joint for reasons of stability. For example, both the biceps and the triceps are active in *chaturanga dand-asana* in order to stabilize the elbows.

Joint Movements in Yogasana

Our goal in *yogasana* practice from the point of view of the muscles is to use them in a way that leads to an expansion of a joint or joints, even though the muscles them-selves cannot actively extend, but in fact can only contract. How can contracting muscles lead to expanding joints? As with everything in yoga, the answer is indirect (and paradoxical). Consider first the process of inhalation. On an inhalation, the dia-phragm contracts, and with its outer edge connected firmly to the lowermost ribs (T 12), one would reasonably expect the lowest ribs to move inward. Now take a deep breath with your attention on the lowest ribs, and you will see that, in fact, the low-est ribs move outward on inhalation! In order for the diaphragm to function proper-ly on inhalation, the points of attachment cannot move inward, for if they did, then the low pressure external to the lungs would not develop and the lungs would not inflate.

In fact, the inward movement of the low-est ribs during inhalation is resisted by the actions of the serratus magnus (intercostal) muscles (Fig. 7.A-l) that bind the outer sur-faces of the lower ribs to ones above; acti-vation of the serratus magnus acts to flare the lowest ribs outward. Thus it is seen that the action of the diaphragm is to pull the lowest ribs on the two sides of the chest

---

BOX 7.A-4: THE HANDS HELP WAG THE SHOULDER BLADES IN *ADHO MUKHA SVANASANA*

There are two muscles in the upper arm that work to flex the arm at the elbow: the brachialis and the biceps brachii. The former has its origin on the lower half of the humer-al shaft, with insertion on the ulna of the forearm, whereas in the latter, the origin is on the scapula with insertion on the radius of the forearm, Fig. 7.A-13. In *adho mukha svan-asana*, one wants the triceps of the beginning student contracted so as to straighten the arms at the elbows, and correspondingly, the biceps and brachialis should be released to allow the triceps to pull the bones of the arms into alignment. That is to say, one is look-ing for the reciprocal inhibition of the biceps and brachialis by the triceps. Now relaxa-tion/lengthening of the biceps comes from pronation of the forearm, *i.e.*, pressing down-ward through the base of the thumb and the base of the index finger. When the hand is worked in this way in *adho mukha svanasana* (and other poses such as *adho mukha vrk-sasana*), then a) the biceps are relaxed, b) the triceps can then contract with the greatest effect, and c) the tug of the biceps on the scapula pulling them toward the head is released so that the scapula can more easily be pulled down the back by the lower trapezius and latissimus dorsi muscles. In this way, the simple action of the thumbs and index fingers on the floor in *adho mukha svanasana* results in tangible consequences for the action of the shoulder blades on the rib cage!

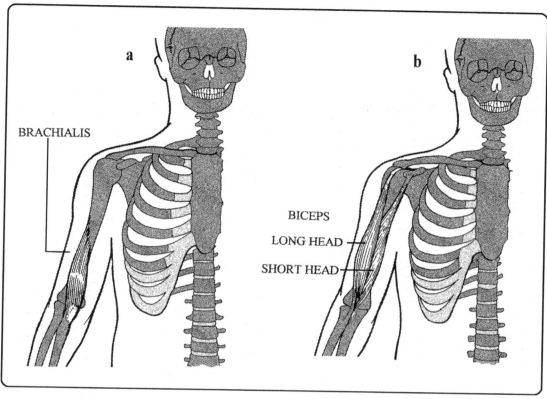

Fig. 7.A-13. The origins and insertions of (**a**) the brachialis muscles and (**b**) the biceps muscles of the upper arm and back.

toward one another, but that breathing also involves the top-to-bottom closing of the outer edges of the T12 and higher adjacent ribs in order to expand the lower ribs laterally. In this way we see how the contraction of muscles secondary to those spanning the bones in question can act to increase the distance between those bones.

Consider next how, with the arms held parallel to the floor and out to the sides, one can contract the muscles so that the fingertips on the left hand move away from the fingertips on the right, or to simplify it further, how one can open the shoulder joint. Let us assume that only the humerus and the scapula meet at the shoulder and form the shoulder joint. As the deltoid spans the space connecting the two bones, it clearly should be relaxed if the two bones are to move apart. But now, if the latissimus muscles pull the scapula closer to the spine,

while at the same time, the muscles of the forearm (brachioradialis and the triceps) pull the humerus toward the wrist, then the bones that meet at the shoulder will move *away* from one another, *i.e.*, the shoulder joint opens because the more-distant joints are pulled closed. This method of opening the shoulder joint is shown schematically in Fig. 7.A-14.

It would appear that all of the active joint openings in the body involve selective joint closing at nearby joints so that the selected joint is pulled open. Looked at in this way, it would appear that there is something of a zero-sum game here, with joints opening in one place only if joints in another place close. As extension in the *yogasanas* involves the interplay of muscles at a joint which is to open, and the closing of those at and around the joints adjacent to the joint in question, it does not seem possible to ac-

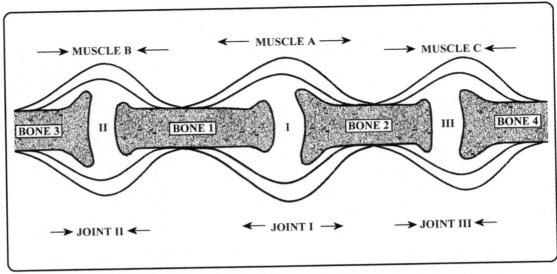

Fig. 7.A-14. In order to open joint I between bones 1 and 2, muscle A must first be relaxed, thereby lessening the resting muscle tone and opening the joint somewhat. However, it is the *closing* of adjacent joint II (between bones 1 and 3) and joint III (between bones 2 and 4) by contraction of muscles B and C, respectively, that substantially *increases* the distance between bones 1 and 2, *i.e.*, opens joint I.

tively open all joints simultaneously. That is not to say that all joints cannot be opened somewhat by relaxation in *savasana* or by anaesthesia, but these are passive openings, and we are here discussing the *active* opening of joints.

Mechanism aside, one should realize it is the muscles that support the skeleton in an erect position and not the other way around. As Juhan has stated [222], "Stability of the joints is maintained above all by the activity of the surrounding muscles. Ligaments also play a part, but they will stretch under the constant strain when muscles are weak or paralyzed."

SECTION 7.B. MUSCLE SENSORS; THE MECHANORECEPTORS

The Mechanoreceptors in Skeletal Muscle

There are a huge number of sensors both within and upon the body called mechan-oreceptors that are activated by mechanical stimuli, *i.e.*, by mechanical distortion due to pressure. The term "mechanoreceptors" refers to structures as varied as the muscle spindles within muscles that respond to stretch and rate of stretch of muscle fibers, and the baroreceptors within the heart that respond to changes of arterial blood pressure, again through mechanical deformation. In all of these receptors, the mechanical distortion is first transformed into a DC voltage which is transformed a second time into the frequency realm (Section 5.E, Transduction of the Stimulus into the Sensory Signal, page 131) and sent along an afferent neuron to the central nervous system. The end result of this process is that the degree of mechanical stress sensed by a mechanoreceptor is translated into an electrical wave in the nervous system having a frequency proportional to the stress: the large pressures felt by mechanoreceptors generate high-frequency electrical signals and low pressures generate low-frequency signals.

Among the most numerous and most important of these mechanoreceptors to *yogasana* students are the muscle spindles, the Golgi tendon organs, and the Ruffini corpuscles, the subjects of this Section. All of these mechanoreceptors are factors in sensing both consciously and subconsciously where the body is in space, what the degree of tension is in each of the striate muscles, and how these are changing with time as we stretch.

Notice that the sensory signals from the various mechanoreceptors are fundamentally identical. In every case, the sensory signal that is sent upward consists of a series of action potentials of constant voltage, but with frequencies that reflect the intensity of the stimulus. It is significant then that each sensory signal travels on a neural track dedicated to it alone (an afferent nerve) and heading to a specific point in the nervous system. The look-alike signals from different receptors are kept separate until they reach their appropriate destinations at higher centers, where they then can contribute to the competition for attention among all of the sensory-information inputs (however, see also Section 10.E, Dermatomes and Referred Pain, page 303).

Structure of Muscle Spindles

Our muscles are able to propel various body parts in various directions, while other muscles can work to reverse these motions (see Subsection 7.A, *Reciprocal Inhibition and Agonist/Antagonist Pairs*, page 193). These two actions can be thought of as being the accelerator and brake of an automobile. The two opposing actions must work in concert in the automobile if the ride is to be a smooth one, and so it is in the graceful movements of the yoga student as well. As a more pedestrian example, certain muscles propel the fork into one's mouth, while other muscles on the opposite sides of the relevant joints limit the motion so that

the fork does not jab the back of the throat. By what means are these muscle actions coordinated so that not only is the movement graceful, but its extent does not risk injury either to the muscles involved or to nearby muscles? And while we are in a questioning mood, let us also ask, "Does a muscle itself have anything to say in regard how far it is to be stretched, or is all of this under the jurisdiction of higher centers in the central nervous system?"

The answers to the questions above lie in part in the actions of receptors in the muscles and tendons that are interspersed throughout the contractile and noncontractile parts of all skeletal muscles, and that monitor muscle length, muscle tension, and the velocities with which these can change. Such receptors are found not only in the largest muscles of the leg, but also in the smallest muscles of the eyelid and all others in between.

There are so many receptors in so many muscle fibers constantly sending their messages upward that, were they to make their way to the conscious level of the nervous system, the system would be totally swamped. In fact, almost all of this data stream is handled by lower centers in the subconscious domain, with very little penetrating into our conscious awareness. Through *yogasana* practice, we can elect to bring a small fraction of this mass of real-time data into our consciousness and also to lower its intensity by relaxing the muscle tone (Subsection 7.B, *Resting Muscle Tone*, page 204).

Among the most important of such stretch receptors are the muscle spindles found within the body's skeletal muscles, and serving both to keep the muscles from over-stretching and to report on the state of muscle tension. The muscle spindles are elongate, fluid-filled capsules within which there are three types of sensor fibers: the static and dynamic nuclear-bag fibers and

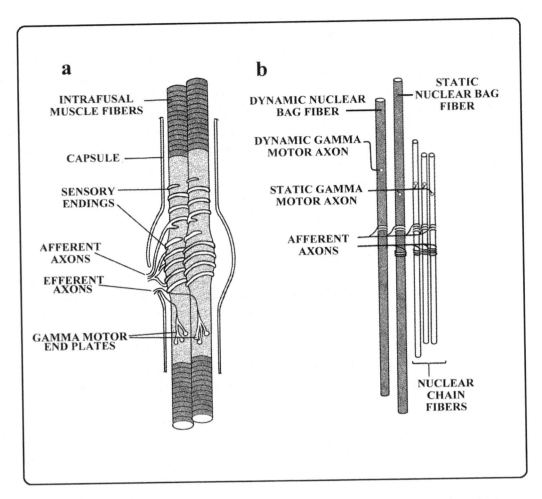

Fig. 7.B-1. A muscle spindle is shown as it would appear under the microscope (**a**), and schematically (**b**). There are three types of stretch sensors within the muscle spindle: the dynamic nuclear-bag sensors, the static nuclear-bag sensors, and the nuclear-chain sensors. All of the above are connected to afferent neurons. Additionally, each of the afferent-fiber types is innervated by a gamma-motor axon which can adjust tension in the spindle fiber by relaxing or contracting.

the nuclear-chain fibers, Fig. 7.B-1. The muscle fibers within a spindle are known as "intrafusal", to distinguish them from the fibers outside the spindle, which are called "extrafusal". The central portions of the intrafusal fibers contain stretch-sensitive structures wrapped helically around each of the fibers, whereas the ends of the fibers consist of more ordinary, striated contractile muscle operating through the actin-myosin interaction. A muscle spindle will contain between 3 and 10 stretch-sensitive fibers,

with each spindle much shorter than the muscle cells that surround it.

The contractile ends of the intrafusal fibers within the capsule are innervated by the gamma-motor neurons from the ventral horn of the spinal cord, whereas the extrafusal muscle fibers outside the spindle's capsule are activated by the alpha-motor neurons from the ventral horn. The alpha and gamma systems are efferent motor systems, with the alpha system generally controlling the skeletal muscles while itself being under the control of the motor cortex, whereas the gamma system is energized by the subconscious centers in the brainstem and controls the interfusal fiber tension within the skeletal-muscle spindles, which in turn dictates the level of resting muscle tone. Of all the motor neurons in the body connected to the vast number of muscle fibers, fully one third of them are hidden from our awareness as gamma-motor neurons [222]. It must be mentioned, however, that there are many neural interconnections between the alpha- and gamma-motor systems, so that they are not as independent as the discussion to this point might imply.

Of the three types of fibers within the spindle, the nuclear-chain fibers are innervated largely by Ib afferent neurons, whereas the nuclear-bag fibers are innervated largely by the Ia afferent neurons (see Section 5, THE NERVES, page 107). The Ia fibers are large in diameter and fast, while those of Ib are of a smaller diameter and slower, Table 5.B-2. Note though, that there are cross connections, with a few Ia fibers terminating at the nuclear-chain fibers, and a few Ib fibers also terminating at nuclear-bag fibers.

Function of Muscle Spindles

As the nuclear-chain and nuclear-bag intrafusal fibers are connected to the ends of the muscle spindle's capsule, which itself is nested firmly within the extrafusal fibers of the muscle tissue, any change in the length of the extrafusal muscle fibers is followed by a parallel change in the length of the intrafusal fibers. That is to say, the length of the intrafusal fibers increases as the muscle in question stretches, and decreases again when it relaxes. Referring to Fig. 7.B-1, the sensory endings spiraling around each of the three types of fiber function much like the spring in a sensitive spring balance. When a muscle is stretched, the intrafusal fibers within the spindles are stretched as well, thereby lengthening the spiral springs

attached to them. The lengthening of the springlike sensors is then transduced into an electrical signal that propagates along the afferent axons to the central nervous system; the muscle spindles function as stretch sensors.

Though the three types of intrafusal fibers share certain afferent pathways, Fig. 7.B-l, it appears that the function of the nuclear-chain fibers is to measure the static length changes attendant to muscle stretching, whereas the faster nuclear-bag fibers monitor the more dynamic rates-of-change of muscle lengthening.

Like other sensors (Section 11.E, Monitoring Blood Pressure with the Baroreceptors, page 339, for example), the muscle spindle encodes its information as a series of nerve impulses, the frequency of which increases as the intensity of the stimulus increases. In the simplest case, the afferent alpha-motor neurons from the intrafusal fibers have a single synapse within the spinal cord, the efferent end of which is the alpha-motor neuron activating the muscle unit in question, Fig. 7.A-10. If the muscle is being stretched too far or too fast so that the mechanical integrity of the muscle fibers is at risk, the high frequency of the muscle-spindle afferent signal then acts to stimulate the appropriate efferent alpha-motor neuron so that the muscle unit contracts, thereby releasing the tensile stress on the tissues. Operating in this way, the muscle spindles are able to regulate the amount a muscle is stretched and its rate of stretch, always keeping it in the "safe" range.

It seems reasonable that the nuclear-bag fibers are the first line of defense for a muscle being stretched. If the initial rate of stretch is too large for a cold muscle, then this fast-fiber alarm will sound, and the muscle will be thrown into contraction to slow the extension. On the other hand, if the rate of stretch is reasonable slow, then the nuclear-bag fibers are not excited, and the nuclear-chain fibers then monitor the slow stretch to see that even when done slowly, it does not proceed too far.

But even this is far too simple. Joints in general are crossed by more than one muscle, such that if a muscle acts to open the angle at the joint, another on the opposite side of the joint will act to close it. Such oppositely-acting pairs of muscles, called agonists and antagonists (Section 7.A, page 193), play an important role in muscle stretching; when the spindles of a muscle motor-unit signal that the stretching has gone too far, its mono-synapse to the alpha-motor neuron of the motor unit is energized, causing the muscle to contract, however, part of the afferent signal is also diverted through an inhibitory interneuron which then synapses with the alpha-motor neuron of the antagonist muscle, Fig 7.A-10. Through this dual action, the overly stretched (or too-rapidly stretched) muscle will begin to contract and the contraction in the antagonist muscle which was originally driving the stretch will then release in sympathy with the need to return the stretched muscle to its resting length. This mechanism, called reciprocal inhibition, is discussed further in the Section dealing with Reflex Actions, 7.D, page 211.

Reciprocal inhibition is met with both in the case of excessive tension on the muscle spindles and in the case of a noxious stimulus to the body from outside the body. Thus the neural diagrams in Figs. 7.A-10 and 7.A-12 look very much alike, as both involve reciprocal inhibition, but it should be noticed that in the latter case the stimulus for the reflex arc is a pain receptor lying outside the neural arcs of the relevant muscles, whereas in the former, the initiating receptor is not a pain receptor, but is a muscle spindle within the muscle it eventually will cause to contract.

The problem for the student of *yogasana* is how to achieve a deep stretch if the muscle spindles always react to contract the muscle each time the stretch tries to lengthen it. The solution to this puzzle is not at all clear on this key point of *yogasana* physiology, but it is likely to involve the following. Over a period of many seconds of constant extension, the afferent spindle frequency drops to a lower constant level as the gamma system resets the spindle tension by lowering the frequency of the gamma-motor efferent signal. Behaving in this way, the spindles are said to be slowly-adapting receptors (see Subsection 10.B, *Receptor Adaptation*, page 285) as are the mechano-receptors for joint position [230]. The adaptation of the spindles may be due to a viscous flow of the intrafusal spindle materials, or there may be a lessening of the gamma-motor action-potential frequency prompted from above. This gamma-motor frequency is known to be under the control of centers superior to the brainstem and is readily changed by various emotions, psychological attitudes, and body perceptions [222] (see Subsection 7.B, *Resting Muscle Tone*, page 204). It seems likely that a significant factor in the relaxation of the gamma-motor tension on the muscle spindles is the conscious relaxation of global body tension through conscious release and through relaxation of the breath.

As movements and limb positions become more familiar and are held for a longer time, the stretch receptors' sensitivities decrease through adaptation, and the movements and positions cease to impress us as much as they did on first meeting them [345]. At the same time, this allows for more and more extension of the extrafusal muscle fibers without triggering the intrafusal fibers of the muscle spindles.

The gamma-motor neurons within muscle spindles are stimulated by the cold center within the preoptic area of the anterior hypothalamus which acts to lower the body's temperature, and conversely, these neurons are inhibited by the posterior hypothalamus which acts to generate and conserve heat [225, 251], Table 6.B-1. As tension in the gamma-motor sensors is higher when the body is cold, it is more difficult to stretch at this time, whereas when the body is warm, tension in the spindles is inhibited and stretching is easier. As the anterior hypothalamus is also the center for pain, anxiety, and fear, these emotions also can stimulate the gamma-motor neurons and so make stretching more difficult, especially in backbends, Box 7.D-1, page 216.

There are really two muscle tones in a working muscle, that of the contractile muscle fibers and that within the muscle spindles. According to Kurz [251], there exists a compensatory mechanism in which the spindle tone tends to increase when the muscle tone decreases, which means that the muscle is least able to experience stretch without initiating a contraction when it is most passive and at rest. It is for this reason that we wake up stiff in the morning, for the contractile machinery has relaxed but the spindles have tightened in response to this. Based upon this idea, there is a simple (but non-yogic) technique that can work to overcome the spindle blockage of overstressed muscles. Called PNF, it is described in Box 7.B-1, page 204.

The signals from muscle spindles [225] in combination with other mechanoreceptor organs also are used by the body to determine static and dynamic limb position. These spindle receptor signals together with those from the joints and skin form the sensory net of the proprioceptive system, Section 7.C, page 208.

Sensory signals from the muscle mechanoreceptors do not easily work their way high enough to register in the conscious sphere, as they are more in the realm of sub-

conscious reflex action. Thus, they are not the carriers of pain signals sent by our muscles when we overstretch. These instead involve pain receptors (nociceptors) lying deep within the tissue, Section 10.D, Pain, page 294.

It is interesting to contemplate for a moment what the muscle-spindle situation might be in the hyperflexible body. Presumably, this type of body has very extendable collagen, which is to say, a small stress yields a large displacement (strain). As the hyperflexible student stretches, there is a relatively large lengthening of the relevant muscle, yet there is no inhibiting signal from the muscle spindles. It must be that the hyperflexible can stretch so far without triggering the spindle warning signals because the highly flexible collagen of their muscle fibers is incorporated as well into the spindle apparatus, so that it too is able to stretch abnormally without too large an increase in tension. This could result from the muscle components having a larger than normal amount of viscous matter in their viscoelastic makeup (see Subsection 7.E, *When Stretching, Time Matters, and Time Is on Your Side*, page 224), because strain on the spindle can be released by viscous flow. In any event, the intrafusal fibers of the muscle spindles must be at least as flexible as the extrafusal fibers, or the muscles would be in a constant spasm driven by the over-extended spindle fibers. Alternatively, the alarm points in the spindles may be set very, very high. In any event, the general feeling [268] is that the hyperflexible student is also the hypermobile student, and often is injured by over-stretching.

Stretch receptors are also found in the viscera, bronchi, bronchioles and the alveoli of the lungs. During the breathing cycle, these receptors are alternately activated and relaxed, and report their levels of stress to the brain using the afferents of the right

BOX 7.B-1: PNF, CONTRACTING IN ORDER TO LENGTHEN

In some situations, as one works to extend a stretch, the muscle spindles may become overstressed and signal instead for contraction of the muscle in question as a means of self-protection. In this situation, stretching can continue if the spindles can be momentarily convinced that the stretch has ended and so relax their grip on the muscle. This is the basic philosophy behind the proprioceptive neuromuscular facilitation (PNF) method of stretching [5, 337, 391]. Of course, PNF will be of no value if the stiffness is due to inelasticity in the muscle components, rather than to highly excited muscle spindles.

By way of example, stand with your back to the wall and let your partner raise your straight right leg to the horizontal position, stretching the hamstring on that leg as in *hasta padangusthasana*. With your partner firmly holding the leg by the heel in this position, press the leg *down* isometrically by contracting the hamstrings and thereby releasing the tensile stress in the hamstring spindles (but increasing the tension in the Golgi tendon organs, Subsection 7.B, page 206). Wait 30 seconds in this position with the leg elevated but the hamstrings contracted. With the spindle signals turned off by the apparent relaxation, next have your partner quickly raise the relaxed leg to a new height and engage the antagonist quadruceps muscles. It is known that after strong voluntary contraction, the resistance to stretching drops significantly; the resistance is minimal 1 second after the release and is still 30% less than normal 5 seconds after release [251]. Repeat the hamstring release again at the new height, followed by renewed elevation, slowly racheting your way toward placing your shin on your forehead. Blood pressure does not rise appreciably during PNF stretching as long as the stressful positions are not held for more than 10 seconds at a time [90a].

When practicing PNF without a partner, take the stretch to a submaximal position and then holding that position, deliberately contract the muscle for 30 seconds rather than stretching it. With the spindles relaxed due to the contraction, then shift into stretching mode and go deeper into the stretch. It must be pointed out that though the PNF technique is interesting and often effective, it is just stretching for stretching's sake, and is not yoga. Furthermore, as explained in Subsection 7.E, *Stress and Strain*, page 228, simultaneous stretching and contraction of a muscle does relieve stress on the belly of the muscle, but transfers it to the tendons, which may tear or pull away from the bone in the process.

vagus nerve. This in turn leads to shifts of heart action and blood pressure.

Resting Muscle Tone

As with all physical measuring systems, the nervous system is subject to certain levels of noise, *i.e.*, sporadic bursts of brief but random electrical activity not associated with any specific sensation, and also steady levels of useless neural activity associated with stress in the body/mind. Given this unavoidable level of noise (like the static in a radio), meaningful neural signals such as those from the proprioceptive sensors (Section 7.C, page 208) can be detected only if their amplitudes are larger than the noise level. This is important to *yogasana* practice because the more we are able to reduce the level of the background noise in the nervous system, the more easily we can become attuned to the weak signals characteristic of inner awareness. In the same way, it would be difficult to sense the effect of a lit candle in a room ablaze with bright lights, whereas in a dark room, the same candle becomes a beacon of light for the eyes.

One of the sources of the background noise in the nervous system arises from the ever-present tension in the muscles and the neural current that maintains this resting tension (tone) by energizing the muscle spindles (Subsection 7.B, *Structure of Muscle Spindles*, page 199). In this process, it is the gamma-motor system that energizes the muscle spindles, and the larger the noise in the gamma system that one must contend with, the higher is the tension in the muscle served by the gamma-motor system.

When there is a source of mental or physical stress in the body, the sympathetic branch of the autonomic nervous system is activated, and one consequence (among many) is that there is a neural stimulation of the gamma-motor systems within the body's skeletal muscles. Activation of the gamma-motor neurons contracts the intrafusal fibers of the muscle spindles, stretching them just as they would be if it were the extrafusal fibers that were being stretched in a *yogasana* posture. This stretch of the muscle spindles by the gamma system then stimulates the myotactic stretch reflex (Subsection 7.D, page 212) which works to contract the extrafusal muscles that appear to be stretching too far or too fast. The end result is that the stress and/or anxiety, via the sympathetic nervous system, has promoted a tonic, low-level contraction of the skeletal muscles, otherwise known as the "resting muscle tone".

Partial contraction as found in the resting muscle tone is called contracture. Chronic contracture shortens muscles, making them less supple, less strong, and less resilient to the shock and stress of various muscle movements. This leads to excessively short

muscles. Indeed, if a muscle were cut off from the bone and all surrounding structures, then its resting length would be 10% longer than its *in situ* resting length [5]. It has been found that exercise is more effective than meditation in reducing muscular tension, leading to longer resting-muscle lengths [5].

Even the more modest muscle contraction that characterizes the normal, resting-state muscle tone works in a significant way to reduce circulation. This can be especially significant because resting-state muscle tone is a 24-hour, 7-day-a-week stress on the system, wasting considerable amounts of both oxygen and energy in an activity that produces no useful work. Remember that "The more a skill is practiced correctly, the better the athlete learns to use only the muscles involved in performing this particular skill. The athlete thereby reduces the amount of energy necessary to perform a given amount of work" [98]. This applies as well to the *yogasana* student and his or her associated resting muscle tone.

Muscles that do not receive their proper circulation, as when the resting-state muscle tone is too high, suffer from ischemia. The cold feet that one often observes in extended inversions is a temporary form of ischemia, as is the situation when one muscle is pressed against another, as in *maricyasana III*.

Inasmuch as a positive muscle tone is a consequence of sympathetic activation of the autonomic nervous system (Section 6.C, page 144), which in turn is subject to intervention by higher brain centers, through *yogasana* practice and stimulation of the parasympathetic nervous system, one can consciously influence the intrafusal spindle tension even in the resting state, thereby lessening the muscle tone and achieving ever-deeper levels of relaxation. That is to say, through *yogasana* one can reduce stress in the body even when it is part of a tonic reflex such as the resting muscle tone; relaxing *yogasanas* that release mental anxiety also can make one looser in a muscular sense [88]. Working in this way can lead one from *yogasana* into higher-level meditative states. This is discussed more fully in Sections 6.E, Autonomic Balance: Stress and Yogasana, page 153, and 6.F, Effects of Emotion and Attitudes on Stress, page 160).

On the other hand, extreme stress can produce so much resting-muscle tension that the subtle signals from the kinaesthetic and proprioceptive sensors so necessary for *yogasana* practice are swamped by the tension signals, and one has no hope of going to a level of deeper awareness [98].

Sarno [402] takes a somewhat different approach to excessive muscle tone. He feels that emotions that are repressed result in muscle tension, and that pain may result from ischemia in the regions of tension. Most often the muscles so involved are the slow-twitch postural muscles of the back of the neck and the shoulders, the entire back, but especially the lumbar and the buttocks. The muscles that are responsible for posture 18 hours a day become painfully tense when the body is tied in emotional knots and is starved for oxygen due to poor local circulation. Accordingly, Sarno claims the cure for this painful muscular condition is psychological rather than physiological. Of course, *yogasana* is both psychological and physiological (Sections 6.E, Autonomic Balance: Stress and Yogasana, page 153, and 6.F, The Effects of Emotions and Attitudes on Stress, page 160), and so is consistent with Sarno's ideas.

The Golgi Tendon Organs

A second type of mechanoreceptor, the Golgi tendon organ, is found as a capsule embedded in the collagenous tissue of the muscle tendon, Fig. 7.B-2. Just as the job of the muscle spindle is to protect the muscle tissue from harm, that of the Golgi tendon organ is to protect the bones onto which such muscles are attached. That is to say, it is known that a muscle can contract with such force that its tendon is pulled from the bone, taking part of the bone with it. Remember now that when a muscle contracts, the tendons binding this muscle to the adjacent bone are being stretched. The Golgi organ's function is to monitor the tensile stress in the tendons of contracting muscle, and if the tension becomes too high, to initiate a reflex arc that terminates with the muscle unit being relaxed and the antagonist muscle contracting instead. Activation of the Golgi organ then leads to a lessening of the pull of the muscle's tendon on the bone to which it is anchored.

As shown in the Figure, the Golgi tendon organs are situated in the muscle rather differently than are the muscle spindles, for the afferent neurons of these receptors are intimately intertwined with the braids of the surrounding tendon fiber bundles. When the muscle contracts, the tendon-organ sensors are compressed by the stressed tendon and so transmit a signal having a frequency proportional to the tension in the muscle. The tendon organ's information is processed in the brainstem in tandem with that from the stretch receptors within the muscle spindles in order to coordinate complex reflex movements [195, 225], however, rather than being excitatory as it is with the spindles, the Golgi signal will be inhibitory, *i.e.*, it will act to relax the contraction. The Golgi tendon organs are far more common in extensor muscles than in the flexors.

The Golgi organs and the muscle spindles are alike in several ways and very different in others. Both have alarm levels that are set by unspecified factors; in both, the alarm levels are set by supraspinal feedback loops, and both are readily reset by emotional factors. Both function as well as sensors in the proprioceptive system of the body. On the other hand, one receptor promotes muscle

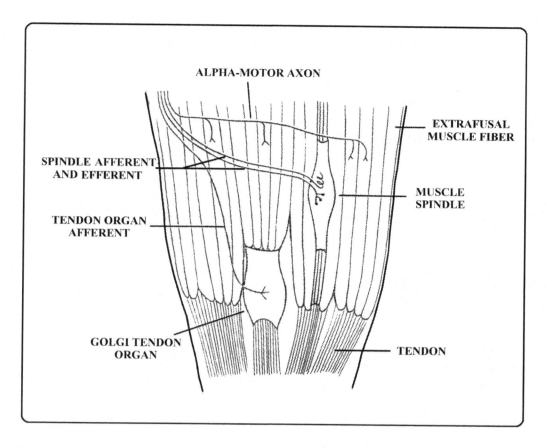

Fig. 7.B-2. Situation of the Golgi tendon organ within the tendon of a muscle. Note the relative size and position of the Golgi tendon organ with respect to a muscle spindle, and that the tendon organ has no neural efferent for readjustment of the tension on the organ.

contraction and the other, muscle extension. Furthermore one is adjustable in regard its alarm level and the other is not.

The tension on the tendon of an active muscle in general will increase as the muscle attempts to move against a certain resistance, usually a weight being lifted against gravity: the heavier the weight, the more the resistance and the more the tension. Thus, for the heavier body moving into *urdhva dhanurasana*, for example, the more tensile stress there will be on the tendons of the triceps as the student lifts into the final position. If the lifting is too rapid (I admit this is unlikely) in a heavy student, the triceps may avoid pulling the humerus apart by relaxing on signal from the Golgi organs within. In other *yogasanas*, the situation is more like

one muscle working to overcome the resistance of another to stretching (for example, the action of the forward arm against the forward leg to turn the upper body in *parivrtta trikonasana*). In all of these situations, we must be aware of the fact that, while certain muscles are being stretched and tend to react to this by contracting, other muscles in the body are being contracted and tend to react to this by relaxing.

Considering the protective actions of the muscle spindles in regard stretching and the protective action of the Golgi organs in regard contraction, it is a wonder that we can move at all! As Juhan points out [222], it is one of the fundamental jobs of the muscles' sensory system to resist any *sudden* changes, using the muscles' automatic reflexes. Fortunately for *yogasana* students, there are ways around these roadblocks, Subsection 7.E, *When Stretching, Time Matters, and Time Is on Your Side*, page 224.

In addition to the position and motion sensors in the tendons, there are complementary mechanoreceptor sensors in the ligaments and joint capsules which not only serve to monitor and limit the mechanical stresses at those places, but also contribute to the proprioceptive sense (Section 8.F, Mechanoreceptors in the Joint Capsules and Ligaments, page 268).

Ruffini Corpuscles

There are also stretch receptors called Ruffini corpuscles that respond to slow, steady stretching of the skin, Section 10.B, Sensory Receptors in the Skin, page 285. The Ruffini sensors are subcutaneous, residing in the dermis, below the epidermal layers. Though the Ruffini corpuscles are skin sensors, they are considered in the Section on muscular mechanoreceptors because they are quite responsive to the contractions of the muscles lying below the skin. As muscle is extended or contracted, the overlying dermis is extended or contracted along with the muscle, and the length of the muscle is indirectly sensed by the degree of dermal stretching of the Ruffini corpuscles. Ruffini corpuscles are slowly adapting (Chapter 5, THE NERVES, page 107) and have a large sensing field. Most interestingly, they can detect not only the degree of skin tension, but the direction of stretch as well. Related sensors are incorporated into the joint capsules (Section 8.F, Mechanoreceptors in the Joint Capsules and Ligaments, page 268).

The Ruffini corpuscles most likely are involved in Iyengar's sense of the "stretching of the skin" in the *yogasanas* [211]. It appears once again that Iyengar, through *yogasana*, has mastered the process of making conscious what is otherwise buried in the subconscious mind.

SECTION 7.C. PROPRIOCEPTION

Proprioceptors

All sensations come into our consciousness through our sense receptors. Thus a painting sensed by the retina can be a visual delight, to use the ear to hear a song sung can be an auditory delight, to receive a massage can be a tactile delight, to eat a great meal can be a gustatory delight, and to feel a cool breeze on the skin on a hot day can be a thermo-sensory delight. Moreover, the more discriminating these senses become, the deeper is the delight that we can feel through them.

Question: What sense is delighted when we do *yogasana*? Answer: The pleasure of doing *yogasana* must come from the appreciation of the kinaesthetic and proprioceptive sensors in the body which monitor the limb positions, motions and tensions within the muscles, joints, *etc.* As with the other senses, the delight of doing *yogasana* increases with increasing discrimination and sophistication in our practice.

The fact that we can perform *yogasana* in total darkness strongly suggests that we do have some "sixth sense" which reports on the motions and positions of our body parts even though we cannot see them. This sixth sense, in fact, is the positional sense called proprioception, in which the muscle spindles and other mechanoreceptors combine with the central nervous system to form a subsystem capable of knowing not only where all of the body parts are at any time, but also knowing the velocities and directions of their movements. This is the proprioceptive system; the majority of the body's proprioceptors are in the head and neck

[345], but extend to the soles of the feet as well.

Such sensory information as deduced by proprioception is absolutely essential to the student performing *yogasana*, especially as regards balance, degree of muscle tension, and correctness of position. Unfortunately, there is not much agreement as to how proprioception works, for the proprioceptive sense has a very short history by comparison with the other senses, being discussed first only in the early 1900's. Moreover, there is no unanimity as to just which mechanoreceptors are active in proprioceptive sensing.

It is agreed that there are two general types of proprioceptive sense, that of static limb position, and that of limb movement about joints, called kinesthesia [225, 230]. The proprioceptors for kinesthesia appear to be the slowly-adapting muscle spindles and Golgi tendon organs, Section 7.B, Muscle Sensors; The Mechanoreceptors, page 198, whereas limb position is assessed from joint angles as deduced in turn from the levels of muscle-spindle excitation. Experiments show that the accuracy of the proprioceptive signal is higher for limbs on the left side of the body, as appropriate for the superiority of the right cerebral hemisphere in handling proprioceptive and kinaesthetic information [250] (see Section 3.D, Cerebral Hemispheric Laterality, page 49). As the construction of a body map which is accurate in both space and time requires the simultaneous integration of information from several different sensors, the proprioceptive map is generated first in the right hemisphere of the brain which specializes in the parallel processing of information [250, 346].

Because *yogasanas* are more static than dynamic, the kinaesthetic mechanism of proprioception has less relevance for *yogasana* students, though it would be a factor in coming into and releasing from the *yogasanas*. Surprisingly, the joint-capsule sensors seem not to play a major role in sensing static limb position. However, they may be more important in signaling when at the extremes of limb position (as is often appropriate to *yogasana*) and may signal pressure changes within the joint capsules. A contrary view is put forth in [230], where it is felt that proprioceptors are special organs and do not involve either muscle spindles or pressure sensors in the skin.

Afferent fibers from the proprioceptors (type Ia, large, myelinated, and fast) are bundled with those for vibration sensing, fine touch and pressure in the human nervous system [230]. As these proprioceptive fibers ascend the dorsal column of the spinal cord, they leave the bundle at different levels [230, 345], as described below.

A) Those afferent fibers of the proprioceptive system that synapse with efferent fibers at the same level in the spinal cord may serve as elements of reflex arcs (Section 7.D, Reflex Actions, page 211), such as the patellar knee jerk.

B) Other fibers travel via the anterior and posterior cerebrospinal tracts to synapse on the cortex of the cerebellum. This leads to more complex subconscious reflex acts such as the shifting of posture to relieve muscular tension while sitting, but not falling off the chair in the process. A proprioceptive body map is on file in the cerebellum.

C) Yet other mechanoreceptor afferents move upward via the medial lemniscus and synapse instead in the thalamus; their activation registers consciously as pain or tension in specific areas of the body.

D) The highest level of proprioceptive awareness arises from those fibers that synapse at the thalamus at one end and then ascend to the postcentral gyrus of the cerebral cortex. Stimulation at this level results in a clear, conscious sense of body position and movement, with strong reference to earlier experiences. In this state, the mind is acutely aware of the physical orientations of the distant parts of the body and how they interact. In the sensory cortex, the information supplied by the proprioceptors in the skin, bones, muscles, ligaments and joints (Section 8.F, page 268) is synthesized into a body map of position and movement [157].

In addition to the proprioceptors mentioned above, two others are very important for sensing body position and rates of movement in space. Closely associated with the hearing apparatus and located within the inner ear are the balancing organs of the vestibular system (Section 17.B, The Vestibular Organs of Balance, page 437). The special sensitivities of the vestibular organs serve to sense the static and dynamic positions of the head, and so contribute valuable information for the formation of the proprioceptive body map. The first of these organs works on the basis of gravitational attraction, and the second on the basis of inertia, in each case using pressure-sensitive hairs within the organs. As discussed further in Appendix IV, BALANCING, page 525, the vestibular organs are critical to balancing.

Repetition of the *yogasanas* through dedicated practice results in a more facile transfer of the mechanoreceptor signals to the higher centers of the brain (Section 3.C, Memory, Learning, and Teaching, page 42), yielding in turn, more conscious awareness of where the body parts have been placed in the asana, where the muscle tension is, where the skin is being stretched, whether or not we are in balance or falling, *etc.*

Proprioception and Yogasana

Note how similar are the above physiological concepts and the statements of B.K.S. Iyengar [211] whose impressions are derived not by Western scientific study, but by closely watching the response of his own body while perfecting the *yogasanas*:

"As you work, you may experience discomfort because of the inaccuracy of your posture. Then you have to learn and digest it. You have to make an effort of understanding and observation: 'Why am I getting pain at this moment? Why do I not get the pain at another moment or with another movement? What have I to do with this part of my body? What have I to do with that part? How can I get rid of the pain? Why am I feeling this pressure? Why is this side painful? How are the muscles behaving on this side and how are they behaving on the other side?'

"You should go on analyzing, and by analysis you will come to understand. Analysis in action is required in yoga. Consider again the example of pain after performing paschimottanasana. *After finishing the pose you experience pain, but the muscles were sending messages while you were in the pose. How is it that you did not feel them? You have to see what messages come from the fibers, the muscles, the nerves and the skin of the body while you are doing the pose. Then you can learn. It is not good enough to experience today and analyze tomorrow. That way you have no chance.*

"Analysis and experimentation have to go together, and at tomorrow's practice you have to think again, am I doing the old pose, or is there a new feeling? Can I extend this new feeling a little more? If I cannot extend it, what is missing?"

A similar point of view can be found in [345], *"The more developed and thorough our capacities for receiving and responding to sensory information, the more choices we have about movement coordinations and body functioning."*

We see that the proprioceptive sense is the bridge between the "doing" of the asanas and the "awareness that comes from doing the asanas". Without the proprioceptive sense, it is impossible to refine the *yog-*

asanas, and it is difficult if not impossible to take pleasure in getting deeper into the pose.

As we stretch in the *yogasanas*, the resting length of the muscle gets longer. Thus after practice, the muscle tension in the spindles and other receptors must be less than before practice, meaning that the relationship between muscle tension and limb position must change as the muscle's resting length changes. This recalibration of the muscle-tension *versus* geometric-position relationship is important in constructing the proprioceptive map, and must happen unconsciously in order to accommodate yogic transformations.

SECTION 7.D. REFLEX ACTIONS

Reflex actions involving the muscles are important as they are always with us, sometimes working in our favor, and sometimes not. Such reflexes usually operate in the realm of the subconscious and can have profound effects on our body, in and out of yoga. However, through attentive *yogasana* practice, these reflexes eventually become amenable to conscious control from higher brain centers.

There are in general, two types of muscular reflex. The first is a phasic reflex, in which a fast-twitch fiber is involved in a rapid, momentary action, *i.e.*, step on a tack and withdraw the foot. The second is a tonic reflex, in which certain slow-twitch postural muscles are activated by ill-defined stimuli, to produce a long-lasting postural imbalance. In both cases, the muscular responses to the aggravating stimuli are largely subconscious ones, and in both cases, a simple neurological scheme can be put forth to "explain" the reflex. However, it is also clear that all of the simple neurological reflexes actually take place within a web of complexity, as all such neurons involved in reflexes are directly or indirectly connected to all others.

General Definition of Phasic Reflex

A phasic reflex is a pre-programmed, hard-wired reaction in response to noxious or painful stimuli in the muscles, joints, or skin. Being preprogrammed and hard-wired, phasic reflexes are with us at all times, and as will be shown, can have a profound effect on how we perform the *yogasanas*. There are five basic steps involved in a phasic reflex action:

1) A receptor receives a stimulus which may be pain, pressure, chemical, thermal, rate of stretch, *etc*. If the stimulus is strong enough,

2) An afferent fiber carries the stimulus signal directly to the spinal cord and indirectly to higher cerebral centers

3) The reflex center in the central nervous system acts swiftly and appropriately on the stimulus signal

4) Via one or more synapses, an efferent neuron is activated

5) An effector organ (skeletal muscle, *etc*.) is then energized.

In general, a phasic reflex is rapid, brief, and involves an intense muscular contraction; in contrast to this, a tonic reflex is long-lived and of low intensity.

By the criteria given above, the responses of the muscle spindles and the Golgi tendon organs to rapid muscle extension and muscle contraction, respectively, (described in Section 7.B, Muscle Sensors; The Mechanoreceptors, page 198), qualify as phasic reflexes. Note too, that by these criteria, reflex reactions bypass the higher brain centers, having a trajectory from the sensor to the spinal column and back to the region of sensation. Only after the entire reflex arc has been traversed might the awareness of it appear in the consciousness.

The above description of the reflex arc is most relevant in the new-born, but on maturation, control of the reflexes by higher cerebral centers becomes more and more possible. Thus, for example, when the stretch receptors in the bladder signal fullness, the infant urinates reflexively, whereas the adult can control and/or delay the release for a more convenient time and place. With practice of the *yogasanas*, more and more of the purely reflexive actions of the body, phasic and tonic, come under the control of the more conscious centers of the brain.

The mechanism for bringing a reflex under control is straight forward. In general, an alpha-motor neuron may synapse simultaneously with several afferents, so that the overall signal at the neuron is an algebraic sum of the action potentials coming from the reflex stimulus, the inhibitory interneurons, and the descending fibers originating at the supraspinal centers. Other combinations also are possible, in which the descending fibers synapse with the interneuron and modulate its effect on the alpha-motor neuron, for example. Given connections of this sort, it is possible then to interrupt and redirect the reflex arc using conscious signals (will power) from the higher centers, providing their action potentials are large enough to compete with those originating at the lower centers, and provided they can be activated quickly enough to compete with the more subconscious tendencies.

Note that the ideas of "reflexive action" and "voluntary movement" are not mutually exclusive in practice, for there is a strong element of reflexive action even in a voluntary movement. Thus, deliberately moving into *trikonasana* with great awareness still involves considerable reflexive action as many agonist/antagonist pairs adjust their muscle tones accordingly, but with little or no conscious control. As a corollary to the above, the line between "conscious" and "subconscious" also becomes blurred as we practice our *yogasanas* (Subsection 1.A, *Reconciling the Rationality of Medicine with the Sublimity of Yoga*, page 4).

The Myotactic Stretch Reflex

As its name implies, the "myotactic" stretch reflex involves a muscular stretch induced by a tactile stimulus, and the phasic response to this stimulus. In the most famous example of the myotactic stretch reflex, the classical knee-jerk phenomenon [434], the reflex is excited by striking the patellar tendon of the knee with a rubber-tipped hammer just below the quadruceps in the relaxed bent leg, Fig. 7.D-1. The impulsive blow acts to rapidly stretch the quadruceps muscle, and in response to this, the muscle spindle at the top of the knee senses a muscle stretch that is developing too rapidly, and so sends distress signals along afferent neurons terminating in the region of L3 and L4 in the lumbar spine. The neural alarm is sounded because the stretching is occurring at such a rapid rate that were it to continue at that rate, the muscle would be over-stretched and possibly injured. To prevent this from happening, the afferent signal takes the quickest route and synapses in the region of the gray matter of the lumbar vertebrae; an efferent signal in response is then sent via an alpha-motor neuron to contract the quadruceps and straighten the leg.

Simultaneous with the contraction of the quadruceps, a branch of the quadruceps afferent bundle also goes to the region of L5 where it synapses with an inhibitory interneuron, the purpose of which is to inhibit the contraction of the hamstrings (biceps femoris, Fig. 7.A-2), which would otherwise tend to bend the leg and stretch the quadruceps even more. The net result of such a simultaneous excitation/inhibition is that the leg is immediately straightened without any resistance from the hamstrings

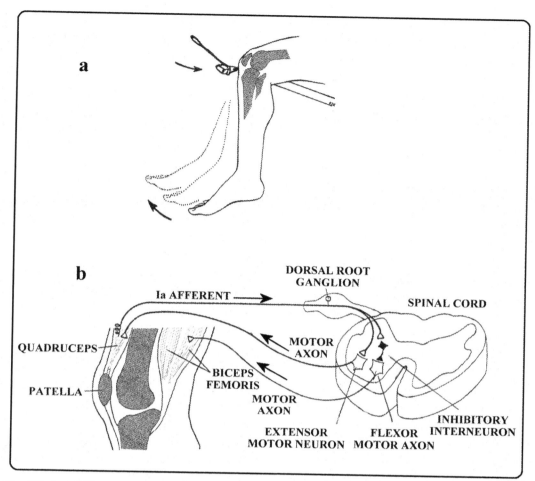

Fig. 7.D-1. (**a**) The patellar tap that initiates the patellar (knee-jerk) reflex. (**b**) The Ia afferent axon from the dynamic nuclear-bag fiber of the muscle spindle within the quadruceps (rectus femoris) muscle is too rapidly stretched by the tendon tap. This signal enters the spinal cord via the dorsal root ganglion in the lumbar region and bifurcates into two branches, one synapsing with the efferent quadruceps motor neuron, and the other synapsing with an inhibitory interneuron which synapses in turn with the efferent motor neuron leading to the biceps femoris (the hamstrings), the antagonist to the rectus femoris (Figs. 7.A-1, -2, -3). The reflex does not occur if either the Ia afferent or the quadruceps motor neuron is severed [313], and is minimal in those who are in a depressed mental state [343].

and apparently without any input from the supraspinal centers. Similar stretch reflex arcs are observed at the biceps tendon, the styloid process of the radius, the triceps tendon, and the Achilles tendon. The stretch reflex is stronger in the extensor muscles than in the flexors because the extensors are on almost constant duty in regard to gravity.

In the case of the knee-jerk reflex, it is observed that if the brain is injured so that inhibition does not take place from higher centers, then the reflex is clearly exaggerated. This is interpreted as showing that higher centers actually do contribute in an inhibitory way to reflex arcs normally supposed to be localized in the spinal cord [340].

The myotactic stretch reflex in the above example is stimulated by an external factor (the hammer) that causes an unacceptable stretch to a particular muscle. There is no essential difference between this reflex arc and that precipitated in *supta virasana* for example, where rapid stretching of the quadruceps muscle by virtue of the body position induces it to contract and the antagonist to relax. Thus we see that the discussion of muscle spindle action given in Subsection 7.B, *Function of Muscle Spindles*, page 201, in many ways is equivalent to the myotactic stretch reflex.

Because the myotactic stretch reflex is a primary means by which all muscles resist stretching, all efforts at elongation in the asanas must deal with this reflex. Being strongest in the extensor muscles and weakest in the flexors, the stretch reflex is of special importance in *yogasana* work. Activation of the stretch reflex, thereby impeding the stretch, may incorrectly be attributed to a lack of strength, but a lack of control over the muscle spindles may be closer to the truth. The yoga method for overcoming the myotactic reflex is discussed in Subsection 7.E, *When Stretching, Time Matters, and Time Is on Your Side*, page 224.

Returning to the knee-jerk reflex for a moment, note that the reflexive jump of the lower leg does not occur when the hammer is pressed slowly but firmly into the patellar tendon. In this case, the muscle attached to the tendon is stretched so slowly that the relevant muscle spindles are able to re-set the muscle-spindle tension via the gamma neurons so that the alarm signal is never sounded (Section 7.B, Muscle Sensors; The Mechanoreceptors, page 198). This then is the secret to stretching in the *yogasanas* without resistance from either the muscle in question or its antagonist muscle: *move slowly so that muscle spindles have time enough to re-set their tension to a level where the reflex arc is not triggered.* See Subsection 7.D, *Yoga and the Conscious Control of Reflex Action*, page 222, as well.

Yet another variety of myotactic reflex is driven by mental/emotional factors, rather than external or internal muscle stretching.

For example, in the normal course of life, we experience a certain amount of unavoidable anxiety. Because activation of the gamma-motor nerves by the sympathetic nervous system can be induced by emotions, anxiety can drive the sympathetic nervous system to stimulate increased gamma-system discharge that leads to a general tightening of the muscles, *i.e.*, a shortening of their resting lengths, Subsection 7.B, *Resting Muscle Tone*, page 204. In this way, anxiety acting reflexively through the sympathetic nervous system really can make one feel "up-tight". The nonzero tension of the skeletal muscles in the body when at rest is a tonic reflex reaction rather than phasic, in that it is long lived and not very intense.

The Flexional Tonic Reflex

The flexional tonic reflex is an especially interesting one, with many ramifications [95, 195]. In general in this reflex, the limbs draw rapidly away from the noxious stimulus and in toward the body. As expressed in the full-body muscle tone, the flexional reflex tends to fold the knees into the chest, heels to buttocks, forehead onto the knees, and arms around the shins, in this way protecting all the vulnerable places in the body from attack from the outside. This reflex, like all others, is spinal, not cerebral, so that even a brain-dead animal will show the flexional/withdrawal reflex.

When the flexional reflex is more local (lifting the bare foot off of a sharp stone, for example), there is an associated extensor reflex on the opposite side of the body in aid of keeping postural balance, Fig. 7.A-12. As seen in the Figure, the reflex arc goes no higher than the relevant vertebrae in the spine, and involves the interplay of the excitation of certain muscles and the inhibition of others. Note that in the myotactic reflex example given in the Subsection above, the initial stimulus came from the muscle spindle and resulted in the leg being reflexively bent, whereas in this case of the flexional reflex described here, the stimulus is from a subcutaneous pain receptor in one leg, and the reflexive response is to bend that leg and straighten the other.

The flexional reflex begins *in utero*, as the fetus assumes this shape in order to conform to the shape of its container. Babies born prematurely can more or less miss this phase of neurological development, and as adults may show a tendency toward lumbar hyperextension in backbending and chronic lower-back pain as a consequence. The psychology and physiology of the fetal state can be regained in *karnapidasana* [137].

A person with a strong flexional reflex will have generally stronger muscle tone in the front body than in the back. In this case, it is then easier to fold forward in a ball, but more difficult to extend the front body as in backbends. Consider too that a backbend implies action in the back body, a mysterious and little-known region for the beginner.

Those who display the flexional reflex will have one or more of the following physiological symptoms [349]: incontinence and impotence, increased heart rate and cardiac output, internal organ dysfunction, lower-back pain, abdominal tension, anal contraction, rounded shoulders, hyperkyphosis (dowager's hump) and a pelvis with the lower aspect rotated forward, Fig. 4.E-4a. The assumption of the flexional reflex posture may be the result of trauma, disease, repetitive motions, or the result of emotional states such as depression or fear [349]. Understandably, a student who has such a reflexive posture would work on those postures that open and stretch the muscles of the front body and strengthen the muscles of the back body.

In keeping with the union of body, mind, and spirit, the self-protective flexional reflex is also present more or less in response to grief, fear, emotional pain and sadness [95]; when we experience these psychological states, the tendency is for the body to fold inward in an act of self-preservation and self-protection.

Since the bridge between spirit and body can be crossed in both directions, it is possible as well that not only does fear inhibit backbending, but that backbending can elicit the negative feelings associated with the flexional reflex. To open up in backbends can be fearful because one is then instinctively vulnerable in all of those soft places otherwise protected in the reflex: the face, the throat, the breasts for women, the abdomen, and the genitals. Moreover, to lean backward into a backbending position is to fall into a dark and scary place, going in a direction in which the eyes are of no use, and into a place about which one knows little or nothing. No wonder that backbending can be so frightening and counter to the instinctive reflex. No wonder that forward bends cool the body-mind (soft parts protected and parasympathetic nervous system activated), whereas backbends are arousing and warming (soft parts unprotected and vulnerable, with the sympathetic nervous system activated as a defense; see Box 7.D-1). From this, the meanings of the phrases "You've got me over a barrel" to express a vulnerable position, or "I am bending over backward to help you" to express maximum effort, difficulty and stress [265], are obvious! In yoga, the trick is to try and stay as cool in backbends as one is in forward bends (or even *savasana*).

For some students, the flexion reflex is so intense that even *savasana* can feel like a backbend! In this case, a relative level of relaxation can be experienced in *savasana* only by bending the knees, resting the hands on the abdomen and slightly raising the back of the head [95], *i.e.*, by assuming the flexional posture.

In opposition to the tonic reflex of the flexional case discussed above, one has the situation shown in Fig. 4.E-4b, where the tightness is in the back body rather than in the front. In this case, the posture is associated with neck and back pain, sciatica, and headaches [349]. The tension here is such as to make the top of the pelvis roll forward, creating a lordosis in the lumbar spine. Given muscle tension in the back body, the *yogasana* therapy will involve considerable forward bending to stretch the back body and to strengthen the front so as to bring the front and back bodies into postural balance.

What then of those yoga students who love to do backbends from the very beginning? It could be that they also feel the same vulnerability, but being thrill seekers, they enjoy the threat rather than run from it. These are the same people who ride motor-cycles, hang glide, do headstands on elevated surfaces, *etc.*, claiming that the action makes them feel "more alive". It is also true that backbending can be sexually stimulating; perhaps some students enjoy the sexual self-stimulation that backbends can provide (body open, genitals pressed forward), or use it instead as a substitute for sex [234]. The arguments for why backbends might elicit the reactions that they do are discussed in Box 7.D-l.

Because the sleep centers in the brain may be aroused by backbending and so lead to a poor night's sleep, it is wise to follow backbends with spinal twists in order to release any tension in the back.

It is interesting that in spastic paralysis of the lower extremities, the flexional reflex is hyperactive. In this case, passive flexion of the big toe drives the full-body flexion

---

BOX 7.D-1: WHY ARE BACKBENDS ENERGIZING?

From the Ayurvedic perspective, the center of our fear complexes rests at the core of the body, at the level of the solar plexus in front and at the level of the kidneys in back [242], Table 1.A-1. According to Kilmurray [242], fear and anxiety manifest themselves not only as muscular tension in the region of the solar plexus/kidneys, but as tight breathing as well. As we attempt to open the region between the collar bones and the kidneys in *yogasanas* such as *urdhva dhanurasana* and its variants, we are forced to come face-to-face with our inner fears. When in a fearful state such as this, the breath and the organs and muscles of the mind/body contract. That is to say, the reflex reaction to such a situation is the postural reflex described above. By what physiological or psychological mechanism does this come about? Let us hypothesize that many beginners show what appears to be an innate fear of backbends ([233, 242] among many others), that the rise in energy level is related to the release of the catecholamines into the bloodstream from the adrenal glands (Section 5.D, The Neurotransmitters, page 128), and that the immediate effects of backbends can be reversed by appropriate *yogasanas*. Let us then discuss three possible mechanisms by which these "facts" might come about.

1) Perhaps the backbending action simply squeezes the adrenal glands on top of the kidneys to release the catecholamines. Without doubt, backbend action is certain to increase fluid circulation in the area of the kidneys, which will have a long-term benefit, but this is not the way endocrine glands work in the short term. Endocrine glands are not wet sponges waiting to be wrung out by a squeezing action, but instead they are activated by either neural or hormonal signals (Chapter 15, THE HORMONES, page 399). On

receiving such a signal, the gland releases vesicles filled with hormones to the surface of the gland and the hormones within the vesicles then are released into the extracellular fluid in much the same way as is the case for neurotransmitters [57], Fig. 5.C-1. In contrast, the eccrine tear glands can be made to release their contents by squeezing.

2) Perhaps the nerves that stimulate the adrenal glands on the kidneys are somehow activated by the compression in the kidney area. But the nerves in question are efferent nerves, and the general effect of compression on an efferent nerve is to weaken its signal or shut it off all together (Section 5.C, Nerve Connections; Synapses, page 121 and Subsection II.B, *Neurological Damage*, page 513). Moreover, if mechanical pressure in the lower back were the determining factor as in argument 1), then spinal twisting also would be expected to have the same energizing effect, whereas spinal twists are antidotal for backbending.

Furthermore, if backbending pressure on the adrenal glands can activate them, then in *sarvangasana*, the pressure on the thyroid gland should activate it as well. Because thyroid secretions promote increased metabolism, *sarvangasana* should increase body heat, whereas it is known to be cooling and relaxing. The benefit of *sarvangasana* in regard to the thyroid is that it increases circulation to the area, but it does not necessarily force an immediate glandular secretion.

3) If one accepts the catecholamines as being responsible for the energizing effects of backbends, then one is talking about stimulation of the sympathetic nervous system, Section 6.C, The Sympathetic Nervous System, page 144. Now, as noted in the discussion above, the sympathetic nervous system can be activated by the flexional reflex, which is essentially a fear reflex in which the more vulnerable parts of the body are shielded from attack from the outside by a full-body anterior flexion, whereas backbending places one in full-body anterior extension.

It seems more likely that the primary reason backbends are so stimulating is that there is a *psychological* fear of opening the front body, and in response to this, the sympathetic nervous system is activated and epinephrine and norepinephrine flood the blood stream. As with all sympathetic excitations, there then follows all of the standard consequences, *i.e.*, increased heart rate and respiration, redirection of the blood supply to the muscles, sweating, *etc.* (Section 6.C, The Sympathetic Nervous System, page 144). That the characteristic physiological consequences of backbending are related to fear is supported by the fact that in many cases, the consequences appear even before the backbending is begun.

Yet another possible factor in backbending is that the position most often involves tipping the head and eyes up and back. However, the eyes-up position is a well-known one among hypnotherapists for promoting a dissociation in which the subject feels that he or she is leaving the body [279]. This may be a contributing factor to the element of fear among some students when in this type of *yogasana*.

However, with practice of the backbends, it is also true that the panic felt by many of us in *urdhva dhanurasana*, for example, can be considerably reduced by relaxing the muscles of the face and front body, and by *consciously* relaxing the breath. This strongly implies a conscious control and reining in of the sympathetic nervous response and a corresponding heightening of the parasympathetic influence. With practice, the fear aspect decreases and so the level of sympathetic response decreases as well. These ideas do not resonate well with scenarios 1) and 2), but do agree with scenario 3). Moreover, with practice, the fear and pain of backbending can be moderated, as learning and control by the more conscious centers of the brain gain dominance over the purely reflexive. Finally, with relaxation following the backbending practice, the parasympathetic system then has a chance to become fully dominant, and so brings one back into hormonal and emotional balance in a matter of 10–20 minutes, just the time it takes for the catecholamines to clear the body.

reflex even harder. In the *yogasanas*, we would seem to be working the other side of this coin, often stressing extension of the big toe in aid of opening the body and so avoiding the flexional reflex. Perhaps these two phenomena are related.

In view of the discussion above, it is interesting then to consider that in Lasater's book, *Relax and Renew: Restful Yoga for Stressful Times* [269], many of the relaxing, renewing and restful poses are backbend variations! Though seemingly at odds with what has been said in this Subsection, note two things about her suggestions. First, the backbending is very gentle, being only a lift of the thoracic chest. Second, the backbending is always *supported*. Thus, it must be that in this case, the phasic aspects of flexional reflex are minimized when the backbending is minimal and the vertebrae are supported comfortably from below. If it were otherwise, relaxation would not follow. It would appear reasonable to assume here that the stimulation of the deep-pressure sensors in the skin and muscles of the back when supported in a backbending position (Subsection 10.B, *Deep Pressure*, page 290) in some way inhibits the triggering of the fearful flexional reflex. It is also relevant that in almost all of the upward-facing poses in Lasater's book, the head is supported such that the eyes are tipped downward toward the heart. As explained in the following Subsection, this position of the head and eyes is another posture promoting reflexive parasympathetic relaxation.

A Reflection on the Cervical Flexion Reflex

As explained above, when the front body is put into the open, vulnerable position as in backbends, the reflexive response is excitation of the sympathetic nervous system in anticipation of any threat that may appear while vulnerable and exposed. In all of the *yogasanas* that elicit the flexional response, the head is thrown back and the eyes turn inward and toward the eyebrows. The head posture that is counter to that associated with backbending is that in which the chest and head are pulled toward one another so as to protect the vulnerable area of the throat [349]. In this position, Fig. 7.D-2, the head is dropped forward and the eyes look down to the heart. Once in the safe and protected position, what then is the reflex response, if any?

Experience shows that poses done passively with the chin pulled into the sternal notch as in *jalandhara bandha*, Fig. 7.D-2, and with the eyes looking toward the heart are calming and so probably excite the parasympathetic nervous system. Indeed, contraction of the inferior recti muscles of the eyes (Fig. 16.A-2), which act to turn the eyes downward and outward, is driven by excitation of cranial-nerve III, a branch of the parasympathetic nervous system. As might have been expected, the eye's upward-and-inward action as when backbending strongly involves the superior recti muscles of the eyes, actions not coordinated by the parasympathetic system. We might call the relaxation that comes with tipping

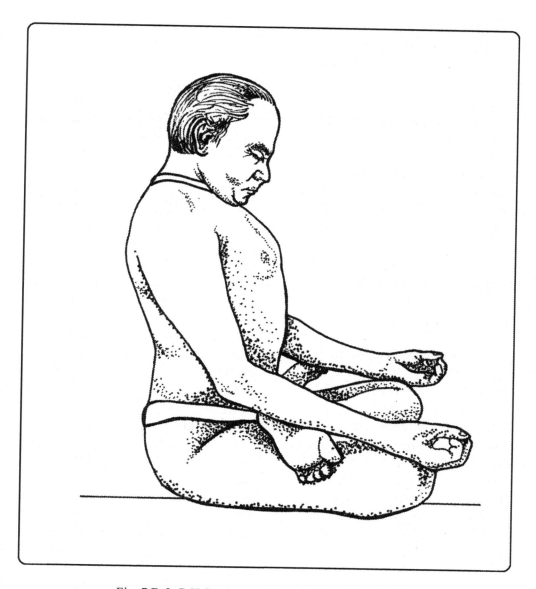

Fig. 7.D-2. B.K.S. Iyengar sitting in *jalandhara bandha*.

the head forward and turning the eyes outward and downward, "the cervical flexional
reflex". Consider the following examples:

1) In *savasana*, if the head is tipped
backward so that the chin is further from the
floor than the brow, then there is a strong
excitation of extraneous mental processes
which interfere with the relaxation. It is best
to place a folded blanket under the head so
as to adjust the head toward *jalandhara
bandha* [215], thereby allowing the brain to
relax.

2) Lifting the chest and hips somewhat
with respect to the head while the legs are
up the wall as in *viparita karani* leads to
both the relaxing effect of having the
chin/chest in the *jalandhara bandha* position and the calming effects of the semi-
inversion (Subsection 11.F, *Blood Pressure
in Semi-Inversion*, page 348).

3) The *jalandhara bandha* action appears
with increasing prominence in the passive,
supported versions of *setu bandhasana, halasana*, and *sarvangasana*.

4) When the seated forward bends are done passively with head support, then the *jalandhara bandha* reflex stimulation of the parasympathetic system is reinforced by the ocular-vagal heart-slowing reflex action that follows when the weight of the head rests on the forehead (see Subsection 7.D, *Other Reflex Actions*, page 220).

5) To the list given above must be added the meditative seated poses in which full *jalandhara bandha* plays a large part [215].

In all of the examples quoted above, the parasympathetic system will dominate only if the conscious will does not enter the picture. Though the head and neck are in the *jalandhara bandha* position in *ardha navasana*, for example, the pose is quite strenuous and so will activate the sympathetic system much more than the parasympathetic.

According to Iyengar [215], the *jalandhara bandha* position is stimulating to several centers below the chin, but the chin-lock aspect of the posture keeps the energy and pressure from rising into the head where they might otherwise cause dizziness and tension. From the western medical perspective, it is likely that when the chin is dropped into the sternal notch, there is a local pressurization of the baroreceptors in the carotid sinuses (Subsection 11.E, *The Baroreceptor Reflex Arc*, page 341) and the body's response to this is to try to regain homeostasis by lowering the heart rate and blood pressure. This chain of events in *sarvangasana* would act to make it a much more relaxing *yogasana* than *sirsasana I*, even though both are fully inverted, and would make cervical flexion a welcome accessory to any pose otherwise intended to be relaxing.

The physiological effects of *jalandhara bandha* have been studied [168], but when done with breath retention (*khumbaka*), and so is not relevant to a pose such as *sarvangasana*. Still, with *khumbaka*, no change in carotid pulse was observed, but there was reported to be easy venous drainage through the neck.

Other Reflex Actions

Cole [80] mentions a rather interesting and pertinent reflex; when pressure is applied to the forehead or the orbits of the eyes, there is a parasympathetic vagal heart-slowing reflex that becomes operative. Thus, when infants and small children rub their eyes with the backs of their hands, the pressure applied to the rectus muscles of the eyes (Subsection 16.A, *External Structure of the Eye*, page 411) stimulates the vagus nerve to slow the heart beat and thus prepare for sleep. The reflex slowing of the heart rate is useful in many *yogasanas*, as for example, in *sirasana I*: if one rests with the forehead on the floor for a few minutes before inverting in this asana, the lower heart rate so induced will keep pressure from building up too rapidly behind the eyes. Many other *yogasanas* that are downward-facing when performed in a passive way, are done with the weight of the head supported on the brow of the forehead [269]; presumably, the vagal heart-slowing reflex is at work here. The reduced tension felt in child's pose (*garbhasana*) also may be attributed to this reflex.

Approximately 90% of headaches are of the "tension" variety, and involve a super-pressurization of the arteries of the brain due to vasodilation of the arterial walls (Subsection 3.B, *Headaches*, page 37). In many cases, the vasodilation can be released by placing weight on the forehead and/or orbits of the eyes, either by letting them rest on a hard surface in a downward-facing pose (*adho mukha svanasana* with the head on a wooden block, for example), or resting a weight on these features, as with a wooden block balanced on the forehead/eyes in *savasana*. In either case, one is taking advantage of the vagal heart-slowing reflex in order to reduce the arterial pressure, Subsection 3.B, *Blood Flow through the Brain*, page 35.

Yet another reflex of interest to the *yogasana* practitioner is illustrated in Fig. 7.D-3. When the head is tipped to one side, the reflex reaction to this is to straighten the leg and arm on that side, but to bend the arm and leg on the opposite side [225]. As such reflex actions would be most apparent in beginner students, their tendency in *trikonasana*, for example, would be to drop the head toward the floor and in doing so, the upward-pointing arm and the back leg would be encouraged to bend! Moreover, as the head drops toward the floor in *parsvakonasana* to the left, the tendency of this reflex would be to encourage straightening of the left leg and the bending of the right arm, whereas just the opposite is the

goal. This reflex is rather primitive, and so may be more active in children and beginner students. Otherwise, higher centers will inhibit such reflexes in the more practiced student.

In many situations, the application of sharp pressure in a direction perpendicular to the fibers of a muscle in contraction will act to release its tension [350]. This is most apparent in a pose such as *ardha baddha padma paschimottanasana*, where the shin of the bent leg presses crosswise on the belly of the quadruceps of the straight leg. In this case, it takes a great effort of the will to keep the quadruceps activated, as the reflexive response to this pressure is to release the contraction of the muscle being pressed. Using the pressure of a judiciously placed pole, this reflex action can be used to great advantage in releasing stubborn con-

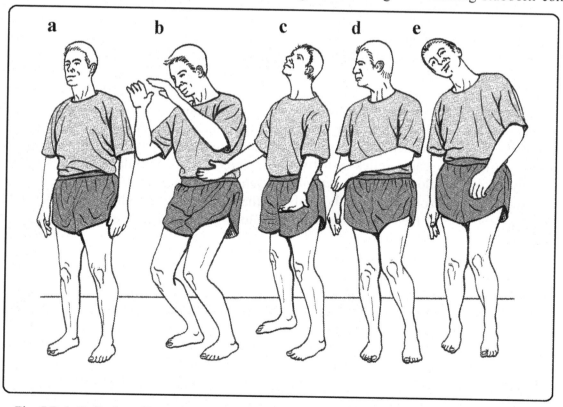

Fig. 7.D-3. Reflexive effects of neck bending on the muscles of the limbs. (**a**) Normal standing. (**b**) Tipping the head forward elicits the flexional reflex, whereas tipping it backward (**c**) opens the front body. (**d**) Turning the head to one side or tipping it in that direction (**e**) tends to bend the arm and leg on the opposite side, but straighten the arm and leg on the same side.

tractions in large muscles [350]. However, in working this way, one should be aware that in pressing the pole perpendicularly across the belly of the muscle, there is a throttling of the alpha-motor neuron by the pole so that the efferent signal driving the muscle contraction is strongly diminished, and that there would seem to be a risk in regard to damaging either nerves or the walls of the blood vessels when doing this type of work too vigorously (Subsection II.B, *Vascular Damage*, page 515).

The effects of emotions on muscle tone and reflexes are well known. Thus, for example, when the tibial nerve is stimulated, there is a monosynaptic reflex lifting of the heel as the soleus muscle contracts. This reflex action disappears almost completely when the subject is told a joke and is laughing [348]. This is related perhaps to the state of cataplexy, a sudden state of bilateral muscle weakness brought on by strong emotional feelings, as when laughing. See also Box 11.F-3, *Inversion (and Laughing) Can Lead to Urination*, page 351.

When we get out of bed in the morning and first place the feet on the floor, pressure on the soles of the feet triggers a reflex action that acts to strengthen the legs so that we do not fall. The same reflex is active when lying on the floor in *supta padangusthasana*, and helps to straighten both of the legs if the sole of the foot of the horizontal leg is pressed into the wall while the sole of the foot of the vertical leg is belted.

A muscular reflex occurs in a rather unexpected place. When the intestine is pressurized from within as when filled with food, the smooth muscles of the gastrointestinal tract reflexively begin to contract so as to push the food mass from the oral to the anal end of the intestine (see Subsection 18.A, *Peristalsis*, page 447). This action occurs in sections of gut that are totally severed from any connection to the central nervous system, showing that the gastrointestinal system has a self-contained nervous system of its own, and can function without control from the central nervous system [155].

Yoga and the Conscious Control of Reflex Action

The ends of both types of fibers within the muscles are contractile (Subsection 7.B, *Structure of Muscle Spindles*, page 199), with subconscious activation by the gamma-motor system adjusting the intrafusal spindle sensitivity, while conscious activation of the alpha system contracts the extrafusal muscle fibers. Focusing on the gamma-motor system, which activates the ends of the intrafusal fibers within the muscle spindles, the presence of this contractile tissue within the spindle implies that gamma-neuron activation can cause spindle length and tension to be set independently of the extrafusal length and tension in the muscle fibers. However, because there are several neural connections between the alpha and gamma systems, interactions of the alpha (the conscious) and gamma (the subconscious) systems is possible, *i.e.*, the higher centers of consciousness can influence the sensitivity and response of the spindles. Since the alpha and gamma systems do co-activate, the linkage between them is flexible and allows for independent alpha and gamma excitation as well. As with the autonomic situation, higher centers can be brought into play, thus bringing the automatic reflex under more conscious control. As shown in Fig. 7.A-5, if the muscle-spindle afferent gets as high as the thalamus, there are then many opportunities for conscious cortical influence on the efferent that finally reaches the spinal cord (see Box 7.D-2, *Conscious Action Pays Off in Yogasana*, page 223).

In the case of reflexive actions, the afferent signals go as far as the spinal cord and then return via efferent motor fibers to the

BOX 7.D-2: CONSCIOUS ACTION PAYS OFF IN *YOGASANA*

Try this experiment put forth by Coulter [96]. After warming up, sit in *baddha konasana* and then press down sharply and heavily on the knees and release as quickly. Done in this way, the knees spring up reflexively as the rate of stretch was just too great to let the stretching continue. If instead, the knees are depressed slowly and then released, they stay down. In this case, the rate of stretch was acceptably slow and the reflexive contraction did not materialize.

The point here is that if the stretch is not done too fast, there is a constant re-setting of the spindle trigger point which allows an on-going stretching without triggering a reflexive contraction. Thus it is possible through conscious action to redirect or modulate reflex actions through the spindle response to stress.

Beginners often confuse the warmth generated by bouncing in a stretch with the muscle relaxation and lengthening that only comes with slow, steady action. Though stretching while bouncing is inhibited by the muscle spindles, the work still can be of some use as it warms the muscles and lubricates the joints in preparation for serious stretching.

As another example of the impact of consciousness on stretching, the knee-jerk reflex appears only if the leg is relaxed and there is the conscious will to let the reflex happen. In a similar way, the reciprocal contraction/relaxation action between agonist/antagonist muscles that occurs reflexively can be augmented in the *yogasanas* by a willful action which will contract both muscles simultaneously (Subsection 7.A, *Reciprocal Inhibition and Agonist/Antagonist Pairs*, page 193).

appropriate muscles, Fig. 7.D-1. Note however, the several inputs to the spinal cord from higher centers such as the cerebellum, basal ganglia, brainstem, *etc.*, extending all the way from the cerebral cortex. These centers encourage, moderate, modulate, and inhibit the efferent signal, and so add an element of conscious choice to the muscle action.

At this point it must be mentioned that some reflexes do go directly into the brain where decisions are made as to what motor neurons are to be activated reflexively [230]. Thus, when falling, for example, the accelerations of the fall stimulate the vestibular organs (Section 17.B, The Vestibular Organs of Balance, page 437) and their afferent signals are sent directly to the cerebellum where a plan of action is computed and the proper motor neurons excited to pre-serve balance. All of this is done with a speed close to that of the knee-jerk reflex.

Coulter [95] states that we "can read the record of past traumas in the rawness of our flexion reflexes. This is best done in the course of a regular hatha yoga practice carried out with an attitude of self-study and non-attachment. In this attitude, we can separate past from present, and can re-program our nervous systems to meet our current needs rather than continue to live as though we were still in danger of being visited by ancient traumas."

SECTION 7.E. RESISTANCE TO MUSCLE STRETCHING

If there is no signal transmitted from the alpha-motor neurons to the muscle fibers of a motor unit, then the actin-myosin cross bridges are disengaged and the motor unit is relaxed. In this case, the actin-myosin filaments will readily slide past one another as the sarcomere is stretched. If, on the other hand, there is a significant muscle tone to the motor unit, this implies that the cross bridges are more or less engaged, and that the toned muscle will show significant resistance to sliding the actin-myosin filaments past one another. Thus it is seen in this simple way, that a relaxed muscle will show less resistance to stretching than will a toned muscle.

At a somewhat more realistic level, actual muscle consists of both the sarcomeres discussed above and the endomysium connective tissue that binds each muscle fiber to its neighbors. Even in a relaxed muscle in which the cross bridges are disengaged, stretching sooner or later comes up against the resistance of the connective tissue (Section 9.A, Connective Tissues, page 273). It is the nature of this intramuscular connective tissue that it is only barely extendable, *i.e.*, it can be strained only a few percent and then breaks. Given the make-up of relaxed muscle tissue as a composite of an easily stretched material inhibited by its wrapping of a largely inextensible material, how then can one practice the *yogasanas* and effect a permanent change in the structures of the relevant muscles? The answer to this important question is provided below.

When Stretching, Time Matters, and Time Is on Your Side

How have we come to regard time as our enemy? Why do we need to "kill time" or "hold back the tide of time" or "beat the best time" in everything we do? Whether we can answer this or not, it is still good to know that in the *yogasanas*, time is our friend, and that time spent soaking in the *yogasanas* is time well spent.

The stretching of a "muscle" is readily seen to be a complex affair, for muscle is far more than the sarcomere on which we have been fixated for the past 57 pages. It is the connective tissue between the muscle fibers that both limits the extent of stretch of a relaxed muscle and allows the resting state of the muscle to lengthen. Because mild stretching of the muscle and its associated connective tissues is essentially elastic, it can not lead to a permanently lengthened muscle unless there is an element of viscous compliance to it. In fact, real muscle is viscoelastic, meaning that for short-term stretches it behaves as an elastic band and does not show any permanent lengthening once the stretch is released, whereas when the stretch is extended in time, the muscle flows in a viscous manner, and will have a permanent change of length when the stretch is released. Thus it is seen that spending a prolonged time in the *yogasanas* works both to disarm the muscle spindles and also allows viscous flow of the connective tissue to occur, again leading to an extended muscle in the long term.

Though muscle is a complex mixture of different entities, each with its own mechanical properties, for ease of discussion, let us assume that each of the relevant elements of a muscle is either elastic or viscous, that elements of like property can be grouped together, and that the two types of element are in series in a muscle, as in Fig. 7.E-1. We can model a real muscle containing both elastic and viscous elements as shown in Fig. 7.E-1a, wherein the viscous element is represented by a piston within a cylinder, with the piston filled with a viscous liquid (say, honey) and connected to the cylinder by a small hole. A spring is connected to the cylinder and represents the elastic element in our viscoelastic composite. When a load is applied to the end of the spring, Fig. 7.E-1b, the spring responds immediately and lengthens while the viscous element shows no response. Were the load disconnected at this point, the spring, being elastic and hav-

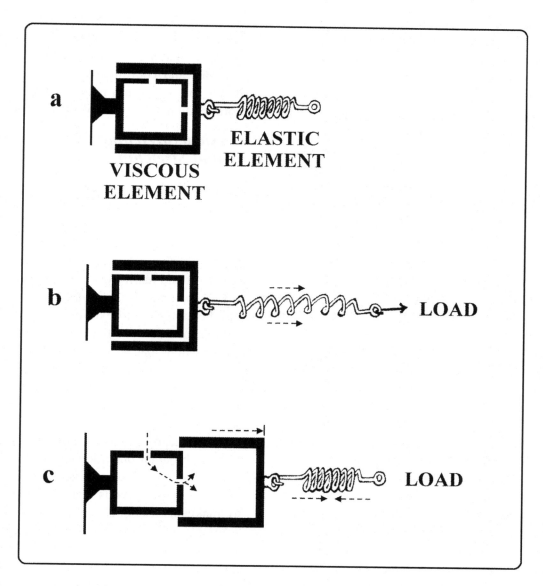

Fig. 7.E-1. (**a**) A mechanical model of a viscoelastic muscle, consisting of a piston fixed to the wall at the left and filled with a viscous fluid, a cylinder surrounding the piston and an elastic spring with no load. (**b**) A load is rapidly applied to the spring and only the spring responds by lengthening. (**c**) After a longer time, the cylinder also moves away from the piston as the viscous fluid flows toward the load through the hole in the piston. At the same time, the spring slowly releases to its original state of zero tension.

ing perfect memory, would quickly return to its original length. However, after a long time in the loaded state, the viscous element will have leaked honey from the inner to the outer cylinder, thereby releasing the tension in the elastic element and lengthening the muscle, Fig. 7.E-1c. When the load is released as in this case, there is no return to the original condition as the viscous element has no memory whatsoever.

Thus, when a muscle is stretched ballistically, it has an elastic resistance to stretching, whereas when the muscle is stretched slowly, the resistance to stretching changes to viscous compliance. In the latter case, the tissue fibers lengthen without returning to their original length, *i.e.*, without biomechanical memory. That is to say, if the stress on the muscle is held for a sufficiently long time so as to allow viscous flow, then the change in length will be permanent; moreover, a relaxed muscle can change its length more easily than a tense muscle [469].

In the case of muscles being stretched, our goal is to affect an overall lengthening of the muscle, with little or no return to the initial length, *i.e.*, we want to stretch the muscle in a way that accentuates its viscous properties and minimizes its elastic properties. To this end, yogic stretching should be done in a slow way and the final position maintained for a reasonably long time so that the viscous elements within the muscle have every opportunity to reach their maximal length. On releasing from this stretch, the muscle will have a longer resting length. The effects of stretching on muscle and tendons is discussed quantitatively below (Subsection 7.E, *Stress and Strain*, page 228).

In contrast to the situation where one stretches slowly, rapidly moving in and out of position as when bouncing in the stretch will generate warmth as the muscles work, but the only thing being stretched will be the elastic elements of the muscle, and these, by definition, return to their original lengths once the exercise is finished. When bouncing, the stress does not last long enough for the viscous component to contribute to a permanent deformation, and the impact of rapid motion will trigger the muscle spindles which then throw the muscle into contraction rather than extension. However, see Kurz [251] for an opposite opinion in regard to the flexibility advantages of ballistic stretching.

When we take our time in stretching the muscles, moving slowly and staying longer, the fast-twitch fibers are transformed into slow-twitch fibers (Subsection 7.A, *Types of Muscle Fiber*, page 189), with the result that

our internal clock is slowed, and while in the asana, we feel no impetuous rush or a feeling of having to move. When done in this way, and coordinated with the breath, the *yogasanas* form a natural bridge to the more meditative aspects of yoga practice.

Physical Stretching Can Lead to Mental Stretching

Our willingness at the mental level to go into uncomfortable places on the physical plane eases the discomfort, allowing us to go more willingly into other uncomfortable places, whether physical or otherwise. If we can profit and learn from the initial discomfort of beginner's *yogasana* practice, we may be able then to extrapolate to uncomfortable positions in the social, emotional, and spiritual spaces of our lives, believing that there too, there is something interesting to be learned about ourselves if we will bear the discomfort and seek its source within ourselves.

As we learn to broaden our bodies, we learn to broaden our minds as well. At the same time, stretching physically calms and strengthens the nervous system and in doing so, makes us less likely to react impetuously to unexpected events. Thus, for example, *halasana* not only defuses anger in the present, but doing *halasana* now will make anger a less likely response to unexpected events in the future.

Complementing these effects of the body on the emotions, there are similar effects of the emotions on the body. Thus, for example, when the mind is occupied with thoughts that are sad and depressing, the muscle strength at that time is lessened, whereas if the thoughts are switched from sadness to joyous and positive, the muscles are strengthened again [354]. See Box 16.D-1, *The Effects of Color and the Emotions on Muscle Strength*, page 429, for a demonstration on this point. One can assume from this, that if *yogasana* students are met at the door with a few happy words from their teacher, they may be put into a mood more conducive to working their asanas with more energy, purpose, and strength.

If stretching a muscle resets the spindle tension to a lower level and reduces the resting muscle tone, then not using a muscle resets the spindle tension to a higher level and so increases the resting muscle tone. As a result of this, after a rest, our muscles can feel stiff and tense. When such a muscle is finally stretched, one experiences a satisfying feeling because the stiffness and tension are released as fresh, oxygen-laden blood pours through the muscle, displacing the stagnant, depleted blood of the resting state.

The emotional component of stretching is implied in B.K.S. Iyengar's comment "selfishness means rigidity; selflessness means pliability" [213].

Warming Up

Certain aspects of yoga exercise more or less conform to the normal understanding of exercise physiology, and this is especially true in regard to warming up in order to avoid injury. Peterson [358] lists ten good reasons for warming up before more vigorous exercise, and these will apply to the *yogasana* student as well.

1) To increase the decomposition of oxyhemoglobin, the oxygen-carrying molecule in the blood. When oxyhemoglobin decomposes, the O_2 set free is more available to the exercising muscle.

2) To increase the body's temperature, thus reducing the risks for injuries to the otherwise cold skeletal muscles and connective tissue. If we stress joints and muscles that are cold because there is no flow of warm blood through them, then small muscle tears and muscle spasms will be the result.

3) To increase blood flow to the muscles to be exercised, thereby bringing glucose and fatty acids where they are needed for exercise. The elasticity of muscle, tendon and ligament depend upon the level of blood saturation; cold muscles have a low blood saturation level.

4) To increase the flow of blood to the heart, thus reducing the risks of exercise-induced cardiac abnormalities.

5) To decrease the viscosity of the muscles, thereby making their actions more efficient and powerful. Without the warmth of flowing blood, the elasticity of the connective tissue will be inhibited. Warming up shifts the tension from the muscle attachments to the belly of the muscle.

6) To promote early sweating so as to cool the body before heavier exercise.

7) To increase the speed of nerve impulses so that neuromuscular coordination improves.

8) To increase the blood saturation of the muscles, thus making them warmer and more elastic for stretching.

9) To bring the cardiovascular system up to speed for the tasks that are to come.

10) To ease into more strenuous work so that muscle soreness is minimized.

All of the ten points above are reasonable factors for the *yogasana* student to consider when ready to begin the daily yoga practice, however to the ten points listed above, one should add

11) to increase lubrication of the joints prior to moving them to the limits of their range of motion.

12) to enhance the activity of muscle enzymes.

These twelve points are most effectively taken advantage of by the yoga student when he/she moves quickly from side to side (for example, *trikonasana* right, *trikonasana* left, *trikonasana* right, *etc.*, [350]) or moves quickly between poses as in *surya namaskar*.

Douillard [125] has presented a list of long-term and short-term benefits to be derived from the practice of *surya namaskar* as either a warm up or a regular part of *yogasana* work: it deeply massages internal organs, takes the spine through its full range of motion, breaks adhesions in the rib cage that inhibit deep breathing, coordinates movement and breath to send *prana* to every cell, increases strength, flexibility and endurance of every major muscle group, reproduces PNF naturally (Box 7.B-1, page 204), and improves one's circulation, energy, and vitality.

Stress and Strain

The concepts of physical stress and physical strain are relevant to a discussion of muscles, but in general these concepts often

either are confused with one another, or are thought to be synonymous. Let us look at the situation first from a purely didactic point of view, and then consider the case of stress and strain in a real muscle.

In Fig. 7.F-1a, a block of material of length X_1 inches and cross-sectional area A square inches (in^2), is left to hang under its own weight. When a 10-pound (lb) weight is then hung from the block, it is stretched to length X_2. In this situation, the material is under a stress defined as $10/A$ (lb/in^2). For the sake of concreteness, let the area of the block be 2.5 in^2, so that the stress then is $10/2.5 = 4$ $lb/in^2 = 4$ psi. Because (X_2-X_1) is positive in this example, *i.e.*, the two ends move away from one another, the stress is a tensile stress. Were the ends to move toward

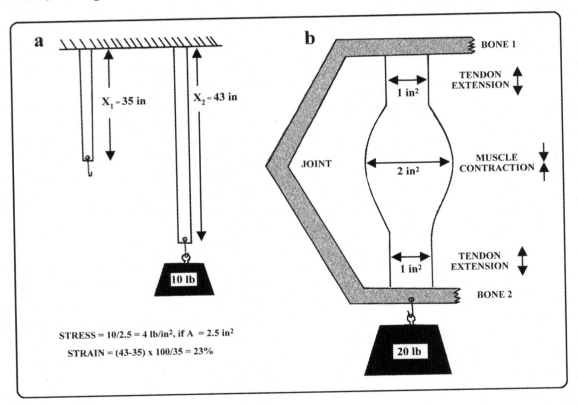

Fig. 7.F-1. (**a**) A block of cross sectional area 2.5 in^2 increases its length from 35 in to 43 in when a ten-pound weight is hung from it. The stress on the sample is 4 lb/in^2, and the strain is 23%. (**b**) An idealized muscle with a cross sectional area of 2 in^2 at the belly and 1 in^2 at the tendons is stretched by a 20 pound weight. The muscle lies between two bones joined at the point labeled "JOINT". Though the muscle is stretched by the 20-pound weight, it is also contracting isometrically.

one another, then the stress would be a compressive stress. In response to the 4-psi tensile stress, assume the length changes from 35 to 43 inches. The strain is then defined as the percentage increase in length due to the stress, *i.e.*, (43 - 35) X 100 / 35 = 23%. Thus it is seen that though stress causes strain, they are not the same thing.

Let us now replace the unspecified material in Fig. 7.F-1a with an idealized muscle, Fig. 7.F-1b. Let the weight be increased to 20 lb, but assume the cross-sectional area of the belly of the muscle is 2 in^2, and that of the tendons is only 1 in^2. In this scenario, the tensile stress on the belly of the muscle is 10 psi, but that on the tendons is 20 psi. The stress is much higher in the tendons than in the belly of the muscle because of the smaller cross-sectional area of tendon *versus* muscle (see Fig. 7.A-11, for example).

The tensile strength of a material is defined as the smallest tensile strain that is sufficient to break the material. For most tendons, the material in question is essentially collagen, which breaks when the strain typically reaches 8% [4]. However, this figure is variable, for tendons may contain more or less of the material known as elastin (Subsection 9.A, page 274), which has a strong effect on the tendon's strain. For example, the ligamentum nuchea that spans the cervical vertebrae in the neck can be strained by up to 200 % as when in *sarvangasana*, presumably due to its high elastin content.

It is often said that in an ideal stretch of a muscle, the strain is totally in the belly of the muscle, and little or none appears in the tendons. This would appear to be a situation over which we have no control, for both the muscle and the tendons experience the 20-lb tug of the external weight, and they respond as their molecular structures allow.

Consider now a more realistic model of muscle, Fig. 7.F-1b. In this case, the two ends of the muscle (area 2 in^2) are attached by their tendons (area 1 in^2) to two bones forming a joint. Additionally there is an antagonist muscle that spans the same joint. As a source of stress, we pull on one of the bones with a force of 20 lb as we try to stretch the muscle isometrically. At this point, the stress on the muscle is 10 psi, and that on the tendons is 20 psi. If now the muscle is contracted isometrically, the tensile stress on the belly of the muscle drops below 10 psi as the two ends of the muscle move closer together, however, simultaneous with this, the muscular contraction acts to pull the tendons away from the bone and so the tensile stress on the tendons goes up above 20 psi. In this way we see the danger of contracting a muscle while it is in the act of being stretched: the two forces of contraction and stretching work together to put the tendons under tremendous tension, perhaps exceeding the tensile strength of either the tendons or the bones to which they are attached. Should a tendon be torn by such an action, it can be very slow to heal due to the poor vascularization of such tissue, and may require surgical repair. Though we often think of "a muscle" as contracting when active, only the belly of the muscle contracts, whereas the tendons of the muscle are being pulled longer as the belly shortens! It is this pull of the tendons on the bones that helps build bone density (Subsection 8.G, *Yogasana, Western Exercise, and Osteoporosis*, page 271).

Even if a muscle and its tendons are only slightly toned, if they are stretched too rapidly as in a reflex motion, then the tendon may tear before the spindle's reflex arc is active, just because the tendon has a relatively small cross-sectional area with which to bear the stress. However, if the stretching is carried out slowly so that the muscle spindles can reset their alarms, thereby allowing time for viscous flow, then the muscle can be lengthened without putting undue stress on the tendons. Said differently, we stretch slowly and without bouncing, so as to keep the stress of the stretch on the belly of the muscle and off the tendons.

Though there is no quantitative meaning to stress and strain in the emotional or mental spheres, the terms stress and strain still can be used. There are stressors in our lives that place us under stress (job, relationships, money, time, *etc.*), and if these stresses change our mental or physical states, then the change is the strain under which we work and live.

SECTION 7.F. ASPECTS OF MUSCLE DISTRESS AND INJURY

Muscle Fatigue and Soreness

Muscles tend to stiffen with time if there is no movement, leading to a state of stationary rigidity wherein blood flow and O_2 concentration in the blood decrease while the concentrations of CO_2 and metabolic products increase. The squeeze/flood cycle of stretching in the *yogasanas* brings fresh blood to the muscles and with that, a strong "feel good" sensation. However, in our quest for that sensation, we can overindulge in our work, and the result is often muscle soreness.

There are two types of muscle soreness, prompt and delayed. Prompt muscle soreness occurs during or immediately after the exercise, whereas delayed onset of muscle soreness (DOMS) only appears on the following day or two, and can then last for four or five days beyond the initial event [337]. In prompt soreness (or acute soreness), the physical work expands the relevant muscle so that blood flow is impeded and lactic acid and potassium accumulate in the muscle tissue. The excess of these materials in the tissue then stimulates pain receptors (Subsec-

tion 10.D, *The Physiology of Pain*, page 296).

For *yogasana* students, most practice sessions will not drive the physiology into the region in which excess lactic acid is produced in the muscles, and so this is not likely to be a source of soreness. More likely for *yogasana* students is delayed onset soreness due to torn muscle, torn connective tissue or spasm [5]. Predisposing factors for DOMS include the performance of eccentric contractions, poor physical condition and insufficient warm up.

Soreness that persists for days after the exercise is due to muscle-fiber damage, in particular to damage of the sarcolemma membrane surrounding the muscle, Fig. 7.A-7, allowing cell contents to leak out and extracellular fluid to leak in. This type of damage occurs most often during isotonic eccentric movements, *i.e.*, when muscles produce force while lengthening during which blood flow is restricted (Subsection 7.A, *Types of Muscle Contraction*, page 187), as for example, when slowly lowering from *adho mukha svanasana* into *chaturanga dandasana*.

DOMS is often the result of overly vigorous exercise for someone unaccustomed to its intensity, and can be avoided by making only gradual changes in the types and intensities of the normal practice patterns. A study shows that for a given eccentric hamstring stretch, the least flexible athletes have the strongest DOMS reaction, and lose isometric strength in the process [38]. It is suggested that because muscle-fiber damage is caused by the strain of lengthening stiff muscles during eccentric contraction, the more flexible you are, the longer and harder you can work without suffering DOMS.

Easing the pain of musculoskeletal injury involves binding the area so as to control edema and swelling while periodically cooling the affected area with ice. Heat is to be avoided, as it promotes hemorrhaging and the inflammatory response [337]. When faced with a case of DOMS, consider a very light practice to reduce stiffness and pain, but do not directly challenge the sore spot. If you rub or gently massage a DOMS injury that is not swollen or inflamed, the action can act to stimulate a flood of touch-sensor signals that act to drown out the pain signal and so offers some immediate pain relief.

A sudden or violent stretch may lead to ligament or tendon damage about a joint. Called a strain, it is more often observed in those involved in percussive actions, as with the inflammation of the lateral epicondyle of the elbow of the racquet arm of tennis players or the medial epicondyle of the elbow in golfers. Tissue injuries of this sort are discussed further in Subsection 7.F, *Paying the Price for Stretching Too Far and/or Too Fast*, page 232, in Section 10.D, Pain, page 294, and in Subsection II.B, *Muscular Damage*, page 518.

Muscle Cramping and Spasms

In the contraction of a muscle doing work, the biceps for example, the various motor units are energized in a random way, so that as one relaxes another begins to contract, with the result that the overall contraction is smooth and sustainable. If however, the neural connection stimulates the contraction of all of the motor units simultaneously, then the result is a painful muscle cramp if it lasts for a minute or less, or spasm if it lasts for a day or more.

There are undoubtedly several mechanisms responsible for muscle cramps and spasms. In the case of heavy exercise, the prime cause of cramping would seem to be the buildup of metabolic waste products in the overworked tissue. This could in turn result from insufficient blood flow into and out of the muscle due to the intense contraction it undergoes in doing its work. If, for example, the arterial blood supply to the heart is inadequate, painful signals are sent to the brain as the cardiac muscle spasms until either the work load on the heart is lowered, or the blood supply is returned [308]. Dehydration and electrolyte imbalance also can raise the risk of cramping [304].

In *yogasana* practice with beginners, the most frequent cramp seems to be that of the foot while going into or sitting in either *virasana* or *vajrasana*. In this case, it is likely that the cramp is a reflexive response to the contraction of the muscles in the soles of the feet, however, the cramping certainly is not helped by the small angle at the knees which can act as a tourniquet to keep circulation from passing beyond the knees.

Given a muscle cramp in the body, one can often release its grip by breathing so that the exhalation is sent mentally to the point of cramping, so that the relaxation of the exhalation can work on the contraction of the muscle. This allows one to stay in the pose while working on the cramp. If this is not possible, then coming out of the pose to allow more blood circulation and massaging the cramped area so as to overload the neural circuitry in that area with skin sensations can be of some short-term help [304]. Cramps also can be relieved by the passive stretching of the affected muscle or by active contraction of the antagonist muscle.

It is conjectured that a systematic program of stretching will prevent cramps from occuring [5], and I have found this to be true in my *yogasana* practice. It is said, for example, that regular stretching of the pelvic area by *baddha konasana, upavistha konasana, supta virasana, etc.,* will reduce or eliminate the pain of menstrual cramping associated with dysmenorrhea in women [216].

Spasms may occur in muscles as an automatic and protective response to an injury in a related part of the body [34]. The spasm is triggered when a movement in the body threatens to impinge upon an already injured structure. Most often the injuries that can trigger a spasm involve torn muscles, ligaments and tendons, a disc pressing upon a nerve, irritation within a joint, or an infected organ [34]. Thus, for example, if one sleeps in an awkward position which strains the ligaments of the neck, one might awaken with spasms in the neck muscles which act to immobilize the neck and so protect the ligaments from further stretch.

Paying the Price for Stretching Too Far and/or Too Fast

As a muscle is stretched, signals are sent by the various mechanoreceptors in the muscle as to its length, muscle tension, and rate of lengthening. As long as these quantities are within reasonable bounds, the conscious sensation is only that of stretching, *i.e.*, muscle tension. However, done too far or too fast, reflex signals normally are sent to the spinal cord which in turn activates the stretched muscle, leading to a contraction, Section 7.D, Reflex Actions, page 211. Nonetheless, through willpower or sheer speed of action, one can continue to stretch in spite of the reflex attempting to inhibit further muscle lengthening, and this can lead to torn muscle fibers. Once torn, a second type of muscle sensor will be activated, the nociceptor, sensitive to injury and signaling pain. Details of how injury leads to a pain signal, and the neural pathways open to this signal are discussed in Section 10.D, Pain, page 294. At the same time that the injury initiates a pain signal, it also initiates a local chemistry that leads to inflammation of the injury site.

In a muscle which has never been injured, all of the fibers run parallel to the line between the insertion and the origin. However, once some of the fibers have become separated from the others by overstretching or by some other mechanism, the healing process often joins loose fiber ends

to neighboring fibers in a haphazard way. The result is scar tissue in which the fiber axes within the scar are not parallel to those of the uninjured fibers. The scar is then a point of weakness in that it often is the site of further tearing and scarring. Most often, there is more scarring in the tendons and ligaments than in the bellies of the muscles [34]. This is understandable in terms of the stresses displayed in Fig. 7.F-1.

Needless to say, the inelastic scar tissue so formed will inhibit muscles from stretching to their full potential. Immediately after an injury is signaled by a sharp, piercing pain, one should turn to rest, ice and compression [34], however, mild stretching is also advised once healing is well underway, as it acts to break up adhesions in the muscle tissue that can lead to inflexible scar tissue.

In treating the pain of a *yogasana* injury, it is best to allow for a rest period so that tissue can recover and rebuild [164]. As shown in Table 7.F-1, there are specific time intervals recommended for the rest period, depending upon the injury. The rest phase of recovery can be as short as one day for a minor muscle strain and as long as eight weeks for a lower-back strain with complications of a herniated disc. Most importantly, once the times stated in the Table have elapsed, one should then begin an activity phase in which the affected muscle is brought back into use. To begin exercising in the active phase also can be painful, but this pain is in part emotional (Section 10.D, Pain, page 294), is secondary to the original injury, and is a healthy part of the recovery process. If one allows the resting phase of the healing to go much beyond the times quoted in the Table, then the affected area starts to atrophy, the muscles shorten and stiffen, and even more pain is in store once the area is activated.

TABLE 7.F-1. RECOMMENDED RESTING INTERVALS FOR VARIOUS MUSCLE INJURIES [164]

Injury	Rest Period Prior to Active Phase
Minor muscle strain	1 to 10 days
Upper back, shoulder or neck muscle strain	Up to 7 days
Lower-back strain	1 to 14 days
Lower-back strain with complications	2 to 8 weeks
Torn muscle	3 to 4 weeks

Muscle Memory, Yogasana Detraining, and Over-Training

The most meaningful benefits of *yogasana* practice are hard won, and once they are in hand, we begin to worry about losing them if we skip a few practice sessions. It is of interest then as to what the effects are of going from intense, regular practice to less intense irregular practice or to no practice at all. Moreover, if we stop practicing (detraining) and then start again, will we continue to learn as quickly as when we were practicing? Answers to questions such as these are not known with any certainty in regard to *yogasana* practice, however, they should not be too different than those referring to resistance exercise in general, and answers abound in this case [51].

In an activity such as *yogasana* practice, muscle strength increases not only from structural changes in the muscles, but also from a learning process in which more motor units become involved in the work and various muscles learn how best to work with one another in the postures. It is the case with beginners, that the strength increase is largely due to the "muscle education" process. Because a significant amount of the strength gain from *yogasana* practice comes from the education of the muscles and from muscle memory, strength is maintained for a significant period after quitting practice. Thus young people can retain full strength for up to five weeks after quitting, however, noticeable weakening occurs for those over 60 years old after only two weeks of detraining. For young people, 30–60% of the strength gain will have vanished by 12–30 weeks, but even after 30 weeks of detraining, they will still be stronger than they were before training was started. 100% of top strength can be maintained for 20 weeks with a once-a-week practice that is as intense as those leading up to detraining. Breaks from practice of 5 weeks or less will leave a student largely where they were before the break.

It is known as well that in spite of regular and intense exercise when young, it is of no value whatsoever in regard sickness and long life if not continued into old age (however, see Section 8.G, Osteoporosis, page 269, for a counter example). On the other hand, even if there was no exercise when young, beginning in old age still can add years of good health. It is never too late to start a *yogasana* practice!

For young children, it has been observed that their strength will increase with physical training, but without any noticeable increase in the size of their muscles, and it is thought that the effect is one involving a more complete and efficient use of the nerves driving the muscles, *i.e.*, muscle memory. There is a general inhibition of the alpha-motor nerve pulses from the brain, but with exercise, more motor units can be activated on demand and there is a better integration of the work patterns of the motor units. One can think of all of this as a long-term warm-up benefit, comparable to those listed by Peterson [358] for short-term exercise, however, the gains of chronic exercise are lost through lack of activity about as fast as they were gained.

In some sports, it is possible to train so intensely, that the effects on the body are overall negative rather than positive. Such overtraining will result in the generation of chronically high levels of cortisol and growth hormone, leading to muscle wasting, loss of bone, stress fractures, and a suppressed immune system unable to fight even minor infections. Compare this situation with the statement of Samantha Dunn in regard the gift of *yogasana* training, "If I did any kind of exercise too much, my immune system would crash, and I would get sick. Yoga was the only thing I could do that would not make me sick" [127].

Chapter 8

THE BONES

SECTION 8.A. BONE STRUCTURE, DEVELOPMENT, AND MECHANICS

Most people equate "bones" with "skeleton" and so come to think of bones as hard, inert, dead objects, Mother Nature's steel reinforcing rods. However, though Rolf [386] states, "The function of bone, any bone, is to serve as a sophisticated, curved thrusting bar, holding softer myofacial tissue apart," its importance goes far beyond being an inert structural element [319].

True, bone is the mechanically rigid scaffolding holding the body upright against the forces of gravity and other accelerations, and it acts as well as the lever arm for muscle action, however, the bones of living animals are themselves very much alive. Compared to flesh, it is easy to think of bone as rigid, but in fact, it too is elastic and can be bent and stretched. In response to internal and external stimuli, bone can be removed and replaced in the processes of growth and repair (Section 8.C, Bone Repair and Remodeling, page 244). In addition to holding the body erect, bones such as the ribs and those of the skull also offer protection to more vulnerable internal organs such as the viscera and the brain.

Bones also play major roles in many other important biochemical processes in the body. As we shall see, several important components of the blood are manufactured within the long bones of the body, components which are critical for both respiration and immunity. Finally, the bones are the body's storehouse of calcium and of phosphorus, elements essential to skeletal stability, to nerve conduction and hence to muscle action. Bone is found only in vertebrate animals; teeth are a form of bone [4]. Most relevant to a discussion of the functioning of bones are the joints formed by two bones which come into end-to-end contact, the ligaments which act to join one bone to its neighbor, and the tendons and aponeuroses which connect the muscles to the bones.

Bone Structure and Development

In the mesoderm phase of fetal development (approximately the first two weeks after fertilization), the tissue is a soft, jelly-like mass of collagen protein containing areas of more rigid cartilage (Section 9.A, Connective Tissues, page 273). Where this cartilage is penetrated by blood vessels, inorganic hydroxyapatite crystals begin to form and ossification (bone formation) takes place, with different long bones forming at different times. Thus the cartilaginous tissues are models for the long bones which are to be formed from them [222, 386, 473]. In contrast to the growth pattern of the long bones, the flat bones of the skull, the jaw bone and the collar bones form directly from a tissue called periosteum without going through the intermediate process of cartilage modeling.

The bones of the adult human body can be divided into two groups: those 80 bones of the skull, vertebral column and ribs that form the axial skeleton, and those 126 bones of the upper and lower limbs that form the appendicular skeleton. The 206 bones of the adult skeleton are derived from the 270–300 bones of the infant skeleton by fusion of many bone pairs. This implies a corresponding decrease in the number of joints in the body on reaching maturity. The major bones of the body are named in Fig. 8.A-1.

Mechanically, the collagen component of bone offers a material which is strong in tensile stress, which is to say, it can be stretched reasonably without breaking, however on compression, it buckles easily. On the other hand, because the hydroxyapatite component of bone is a ceramic material which is strong in compression but weak in tension, the composite matrix of hydroxyapatite crystals suspended within the collagen matrix, *i.e.*, bone, has the beneficial mechanical properties of each of the component substances. Furthermore, the tensile strength of collagen is doubled by the addition of the mineralization [4]. Compared to cast iron, mature bone is almost as strong, is far more flexible and is considerably lighter. Bone is also able to resist shearing stresses such as those encountered in twisting, in addition to compressive and tensile stresses.

The major components of the immature long bone are shown in Fig. 8.A-2. The long bones of the body (those in the arms and legs) consist of a long hollow shaft (the diaphysis) constructed of high-density cortical or compact bone, and end caps (epiphyses) which are constructed of a rather open network of spongy bone called cancellous or trabecular bone. The diaphysis structure is ideal for resisting bending forces as the outermost layers of cortical bone have mutually perpendicular fibril orientations for maximum strength. On the other hand, the struts of cancellous bone of the epiphyses are arranged so as to optimally support the compressive loads placed on them, while being light in weight. Furthermore, the

flared ends of the long bones offer large surface areas over which to distribute the forces of loading.

Up to age 20, the diaphysis and the epiphyses are separated by a cartilaginous region (the growth plate or epiphyseal line, Fig. 8.A-2) into which they both grow when driven to do so by the growth hormone secreted by the pituitary [473], see Subsection 8.B, *Hormonal Control of Ca^{2+} in the Body Fluids*, page 242. Once sexual maturity is reached, the two growing faces on each end of the bones fuse under the action of sex hormones, and bone growth is terminated [461]. However, this is not to say that mature bone is otherwise inactive, for bone repair and remodeling of extant bone continue into old age. Moreover, even after the cessation of bone growth, a relatively small amount of virgin cartilage is left in the joints of the arms and legs, the front ribs, at the nose and ears, and in the intervertebral discs. The cartilage remaining in the joints serves as a lubricant insuring frictionless motion about the joints.

In the cancellous bone at the ends of long bones (and in the vertebrae of the spine), the internal structure of the spongy bone mass at first seems to be randomly aligned, but in fact, the lattice is oriented so as to support external stresses, with struts crossing at right angles for maximum strength, Fig. 8.A-2. Moreover, cancellous bone in fact slowly can change the orientation of its struts in order to accommodate new stresses over time (Subsection 8.C, *The Remodeling Response to Mechanical Stress*, page 245). The bone surface just beneath the periosteum is a thin shell of cortical bone in all bones.

Long bones contact one another end-to-end at their articular surfaces, Fig. 8.A-2. These surfaces are covered with cartilage and though pressing on one another, their relative motion is lubricated by the cartilage and by the synovial fluid secreted by the lin-

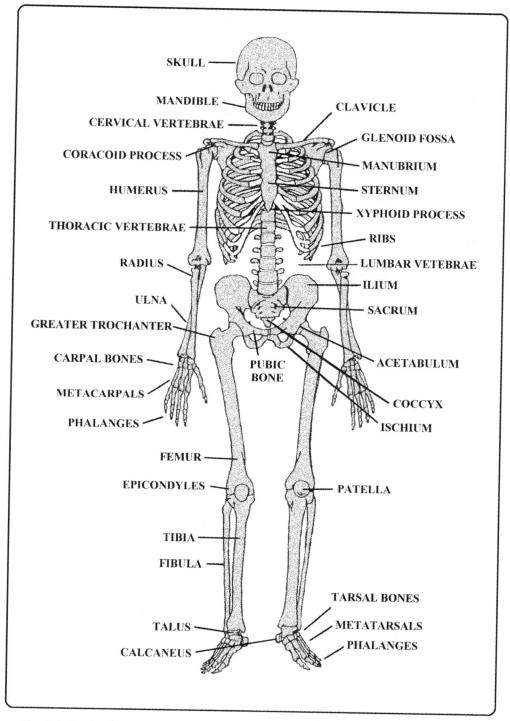

Fig. 8.A-1. The major bones of the human body (shaded) and the cartilage of the ribcage (unshaded); the scapulae are not visible in this frontal view.

ing of the joint's capsule (Subsection 8.E, *Joint Lubrication and Arthritis*, page 265). In contrast, the skull and shoulder blades are plate-like bones and derive their strength from a structure in which two layers of stiff bone are sandwiched around a third layer of spongy bone, much like corrugated cardboard [4]. This offers a high degree of compressive strength against blows from outside the body.

The sculpting of a bone into the shape ideal to fit its intended function is accomplished using two complementary cell types, the osteoblasts which deposit cortical bone, and the osteoclasts, which reabsorb it. During the growth phase of a long bone, it is covered on the outside by the periosteum, the outer layer of which is intimately interwoven with the tendons and ligaments bound to the bone, and the inner layer of which is responsible for radial bone growth; the corresponding covering on the inside of the bone is known as the endosteum [473]. In immature bone, solid cortical bone is first deposited in the region of the epiphyseal line (Fig. 8.A-2) by the osteoblast cells in the endosteum and on the outer bone surface by osteoblasts in the inner layer of the periosteum. However, osteoclasts in the endosteum then work from the inside out to thin the bone shaft (diaphysis) and to convert cortical to cancellous bone in the epiphyses. As we shall see, these two bone-cell types, the osteoblasts and the osteoclasts, are active throughout our life, the first depositing bone substance and the second reabsorbing it.

The central channel of long bone is filled with marrow; in adults, the marrow is yellow and fatty, and has no recognized function in the body. However, red marrow persists in adults in the spine, ribs, and skull. The marrow of the bones of the skull, ribs, and spine produce blood platelets at the rate of ten million per minute, all in aid of fighting invading organisms and repairing any breaks in the vascular plumbing (Subsection 11.B, *Platelets*, page 324). Thus, the red marrow within the bones is a chemical factory of great importance to our health and well being.

The outer covering of bone (periosteum) and the inner covering of bone (endosteum) form a continuous sheath of connective tissue. These inner and outer coverings of the bone are much like the bark of the tree; if the periosteum is breeched, the internal bone mass slowly leaks to the outside. Interwoven with this covering is the connective tissue of the ligaments and tendons, the latter of which is contiguous with the connective tissue surrounding the muscles, blood vessels and organs.

Because all muscles are tethered at their ends to different bones, the continuity of the connective tissue extends from one joint to the next *ad infinitum*. In this way, there is formed a continuous head-to-toe web of connective tissue to which bones contribute significantly [345]. The muscle attached to the bone comprising half of a joint has its connective-tissue fibers so tightly interwoven with those of both the periosteum and the endosteum, that a contraction of the muscle sufficient to fracture the bone will not pull the muscle's tendon free of the bone. The importance of bones and their connections to other body parts cannot be overestimated. See Rolf [386] and Juhan [222] for further comments on this.

Innervation and Vascularization

As the cartilage of the fetal bones is calcified, narrow passageways are formed so that blood vessels and nerves have access to both the outer and the inner regions of the bone. On the microscopic level, the bony material of the cortical bone is laid down as concentric layers in a cylindrical pattern, each cylindrical unit of which is called a Haversian system, Fig. 8.A-3. These systems have open central channels which provide space for vessels and nerves, and which run not only along the length of the bone, but transversely as well so as to connect the periosteum and endosteum. Haversian systems are not found in the more open structures of cancellous bone [229].

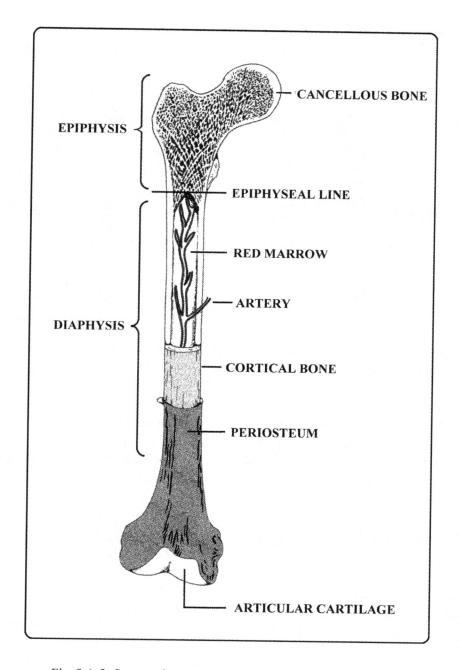

Fig. 8.A-2. Structural components of a long but immature bone.

The blood vessels carry raw materials and products to and from the chemical factories active within the bones, while the nerves sense the nature of the mechanical stresses on the bone and carry neural signals directing the actions of the cells which build bone (osteoblasts) and those which destroy bone (osteoclasts). The relevance of *yog-asana* practice to maintaining a balance between the opposing actions of the osteoclasts and the osteoblasts is discussed in later Subsections of this Chapter.

Though the epiphyses are covered with thin layers of hyaline cartilage which help the bones at the joint to move easily, and with a minimum of friction, those parts of

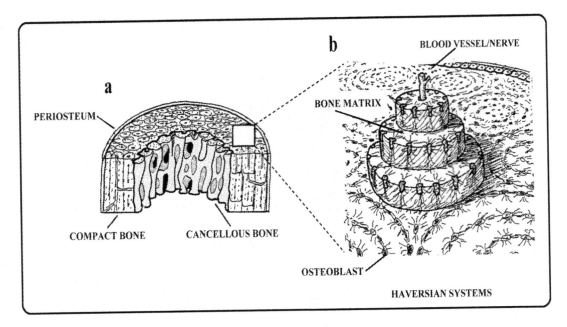

Fig. 8.A-3. Microscopic bone structure, showing the Haversian channels carrying the blood vessels and nerves [230].

the bones not in contact with one another are covered by periosteum. This outer layer carries both blood vessels and nerves (afferent and efferent) which penetrate to the inner layers of the bone, Fig. 8.A-3.

Bone Mechanics

Tubular construction is generally favored for long bones, with the thickness of the bone wall often being 6–20% of the bone-shaft radius. A bone with a strong, compact shaft offers some resistance to overloading as it bends and twists. However, the apparent strength of long bones is very much dependent upon the tone of the muscles attached to and surrounding the bone in question. Thus when an inebriated person falls, they are much more likely to break bones than others would, because in the inebriated state the muscles do not react quickly enough to support the stresses on the bones generated by the fall [200].

To function in a broad range of situations, bone has to be strong in both compression and tension, and it must combine strength

with lightness for reasons of speed and energy. Mother Nature has met these criteria using a composite structure consisting of collagen, a flexible organic meshwork (Subsection 9.A, *Collagen*, page 273), in which hard microcrystals of the mineral hydroxyapatite are embedded.

As discussed more fully in Section 8.B, Bone Chemistry, page 242, the collagen in the body takes the form of helical cylinders, called fibrils. The relative orientation of the fibrils in the layers of bone can change in response to local stress. Usually, a layer is composed of, say, right-handed collagen helices, while adjacent layers are built of left-handed helices [4]. Additionally, some bone layers may be rich in collagen in response to the need to support tensile loading, whereas others may be richer in hydroxyapatite in order to supply more compressive resistance locally.

In order for a bone to be strong in all directions, all the fibrils in a layer must lie parallel to one another, whereas in adjacent layers the fiber directions are skewed with respect to that of the first. In this way, the bone structure gains strength in the same way that plywood does, *i.e.*, by using a layered structure in which the direction of highest strength varies from one layer to the next due to the orientation of rod-like fibers.

As applied to the *yogasanas*, consider first the practice of *adho mukha vrksasana*, the full-arm balance. When performing this asana, though there is a compressive load on the humeral bones of the arms (Fig. 8.A-1) as they support the weight of the trunk and legs, these bones do not bow outward under their load, for the hydroxyapatite within strengthens them so that they can resist compressive forces. Moreover, the practice of this compressive type of posture promotes the formation of a higher proportion of hydroxyapatite within the humeral bones. In contrast, when doing *paschimottanasana* with the arms vigorously extended so as to bring the hands beyond the feet, the tension in the arms is more tensile than compressive, and the effect of the posture on the bones of the arms will be to increase the proportion of collagen in them. Similarly, the bones are under tensile stress when hanging from the ropes, and under compressive stress when in *adho mukha svanasana*.

Stress is the force per unit area that is applied to an object, causing it to deform, *i.e.*, to lengthen if the stress is positive or to shrink if the stress is negative (Subsection 7.E, *Stress and Strain*, page 228). A positive stress, as in $\leftarrow X \rightarrow$ is a tensile stress, whereas a negative stress as in $\rightarrow X \leftarrow$ is a compressive stress. In response to the stress, the object's fractional change of dimension, *i.e.*, its percentage-wise increase or decrease in length, is called the strain. Due to its collagen component, bone is mechanically strong under tensile stress and due to its mineral component, bone is also strong under compressive stress.

When muscular action is constantly drawn upon to hold the bones in place in a

yogasana, the muscles are pulled onto the bones, and become more bone-like in their hardness, compaction and density. Moreover, with the bones and the muscles acting this way, there is no opportunity for openness or fluidity within the body, no flow of the pranic energy, no release of the tension, no relaxation, no meditation. Working as we do in the gravitational field (see Appendix V, GRAVITY, page 553), we must work with the bones in such an intelligent way that the gravitational force is resisted by the skeleton, while the muscles not only do minimum work in holding the bones in their proper positions [237], but also work to keep the joints from collapsing.

Bone Density

Bone density is defined as the mass of a bone of a given volume; the density of cancellous bone is understandably low due to its open, low-mass structure, whereas that of cortical bone is high, for there are no open spaces in it to lower the density. The question of bone density is especially relevant to the condition of osteoporosis faced by the elderly, Section 8.G, Osteoporosis, page 269, and should not be confused with bone mass, which considers the total weight of bone, but not the weight per unit volume. Thus the bone mass of a large person may be large, all the while the bone density may be only normal or even small.

When a bone is compressively stressed at a level below that of its breaking point, the general reaction is a thickening and strengthening of the bone to raise its density in the region of maximum stress. This higher bone density is the general benefit of *yogasana* practice to the skeleton from the health point of view (Subsection 8.G, *Yogasana, Western Exercise, and Osteoporosis*, page 271).

Humans lose bone mass rapidly when gravitational or muscular stress is removed from legs, as in weightlessness, bedrest, or spinal-cord injury. The loss of bone mass amounts to 1% per week of bedrest, but when stress is applied to bone, the piezo-electric effect promotes bone growth (Sub-section 8.C, *The Remodeling Response to Mechanical Stress*, page 245). The mineral mass of the femur bone is largest in weight-lifters, and decreases then in shot and discus throwers, in runners and soccer players (who do run considerable distances but who only support their bodyweight while doing so), in cyclists, and is least in swimmers, whose skeletons experience very little grav-itational stress due to their neutral buoyancy in water [288]. The truth of the "use-it-or-lose-it" aphorism with respect to bone den-sity is shown clearly by studies of the two arms of tennis players; in these athletes, the bones of the racquet arms have significantly higher bone densities (by about 20%) than those of the other arm [44, 337]. The ques-tion of the impact of exercise on bone den-sity is addressed further in Section 8.G, Osteoporosis, page 269.

SECTION 8.B. BONE CHEMISTRY

Collagen

Chemically, the bony substance when fully developed is a mixture of 35% organic matter (collagen and cell components) and 65% hydroxyapatite $\{Ca_{10}(PO_4)_6(OH)_2$ or $3Ca_3(PO_4)_2 \cdot Ca(OH)_2\}$. If the inorganic component of bone (hydroxyapatite) is removed by soaking in acid (try a chicken bone in vinegar, for example), the remain-ing cartilaginous "bone" is so flexible that it can be tied into a knot! Correspondingly, a bone deprived of its organic content by incineration is easily broken by twisting or bending. Within the spectrum of connec-tive-tissue elements based on collagen (Subsection 9.A, *Collagen*, page 273), bone is the hardest of them all.

Focus for a moment on the structure of collagen. Collagen is a protein composed largely of units of the amino acids glycine and proline, strung together in long chains. In the body, the collagen chains intertwine three-at-a-time to form rod-like fibers known as triple helices. In the formation of bone, the hydroxyapatite microcrystals are laid down in the 400-Angstrom gaps that exist between the ends of one triple helix and its neighbor.

The bones and several of the internal organs of the body function in part as store-houses for chemicals intentionally and unin-tentionally present in the body. On occasion, these stores may be emptied on a relatively short time scale, with the release of high lev-els of toxins. See Box 8.B-1, *Detoxification*, page 243, for a discussion of this process.

Hormonal Control of Ca^{2+} in the Body Fluids

In contrast to the bone-building action of the osteoblasts, the osteoclasts within bone function to demineralize bone by locally excreting concentrated hydrochloric acid [473], which acts both to loosen the colla-gen matrix and to dissolve the hydroxyap-atite. This destructive action can be good or bad depending upon many factors, but gen-erally serves an important and useful pur-pose: the bones are the body's storehouse of Ca^{2+}, and on receiving a hormonal signal, the osteoclasts can be activated to deminer-alize the bones, and so supply Ca^{2+} to the body fluids. Similarly, the action of the osteoblasts removes Ca^{2+} from the body fluids and ties it up in the hydroxyapatite of the bones. As seen from the chemical for-mula for hydroxyapatite given above, the removal or deposition of hydroxyapatite is accompanied by the corresponding removal or deposition of phosphorus as $(PO_4)^{3-}$ ion.

Ninety-nine percent of the body's Ca^{2+} is stored within the bones. In order to maintain

BOX 8.B-1: DETOXIFICATION

Because the chemistries of calcium (Ca^{2+}) and lead (Pb^{2+}) are very similar, a portion of the Ca^{2+} in hydroxyapatite can be replaced by Pb^{2+} if and when Pb^{2+} should be ingested. This sequestering of the lead in the bones is fortunate, for Pb^{2+} otherwise interferes with brain function, most especially in young children. However, as the bones demineralize in the osteoporotic process (Section 8.G, page 269), there is a rapid release of stored Pb^{2+} into the body fluids, which can lead to lead intoxication and neuropathy if the lead is not otherwise chelated [473]. On the other hand, as *yogasana* practice promotes bone mineralization and so works against osteoporosis, it is prophylactic for lead poisoning from bone demineralization.

In a way similar to the situation in the bones, ingested pesticides and other organic toxins are stored in part in body fat, and may be released during extreme dieting. The effects of *yogasana* work can be similar to dieting, in that *yogasana* work may promote a short period of detoxification as both the liver and the body fat release their toxic burdens into the circulatory system. The detoxification is evident in beginning students as a momentary nausea following a demanding *yogasana* practice centered on backbending and spinal twists, both of which tend to have a wringing action on the liver. Concomitant with this detoxification in beginners, there is a foul odor released into the air through the skin and breath, such that the studio must be aired out before others can come in to work. This detoxification reaction may be present for a month or two, until the body finally clears itself of its toxic burden.

Ca^{2+} homeostasis in the body fluids, there is an on-going absorption of Ca^{2+} from the body fluids into the bones and a release of the Ca^{2+} from the bones, each driven by hormonal regulation of the osteoblasts and osteoclasts [229, 461]. The parathyroid glands release a simple polypeptide (parathyroid hormone, PTH) when the concentration of Ca^{2+} is too low in the blood; PHT simultaneously represses the bone-building of the osteoblasts while activating the Ca^{2+}-releasing actions of the osteoclasts. If the Ca^{2+} concentration were to remain too low in the blood due to an inactive parathyroid, then muscle twitching, stiffness, spasm and convulsions can follow. On the other hand, if the parathyroid is overactive, too much Ca^{2+} is leached from the bones and they become weak and brittle, while the muscles

also weaken. A second hormone, calcitonin, originates in the thyroid gland, and acts to counter the effects of excess PTH, *i.e.*, it inhibits osteoclast activity and leads to a stabilization of the concentration of Ca^{2+} in the blood.

The importance of maintaining the proper levels of Ca^{2+} throughout the body cannot be exaggerated, for not only is Ca^{2+} a major constituent of bone, but is an important player in muscle and nerve function, is involved in the release and actions of many hormones, neurotransmitters and enzymes, affects membrane permeability and is essential for blood clotting [461]. As the fetus develops within a pregnant woman, it too will draw Ca^{2+} from the mother's skeleton in order to form its own bones.

SECTION 8.C. BONE REPAIR AND REMODELING

Injury and Repair

When, in the normal course of an active life, a bone suffers a microfracture, the local osteoclasts first clear damaged material from the site by re-absorption, Fig. 8.C-1. The bone-building osteoblasts then fill the cavity formed by the osteoclastic action with an organic matrix (hyaline cartilage) which is then mineralized to form new bone [288]. This process of absorption and redeposition of bone works not only to repair fractured bone, but also to remove bone from areas of little use and then to redeposit it in distant areas needing more mechanical support.

The wear-and-tear of an active lifestyle leads unavoidably to small cracks and tears in our bones and these microfaults are under constant repair. However, if there is unrea-sonably high stress for a long time on a bone without a rest period for repair, a stress fracture may occur in which the bone crack finally becomes a bone fracture.

Once a bone is fractured, primitive bone cells and macrophages gather at the point of fracture in order to span the gap with colla-gen bridges. At the same time, the osteo-clasts and osteoblasts work in the area of the break in order to remodel nearby bone dam-age. Growth hormones then work to strengthen the new bone growth. The direc-tions of the Haversian channels (Fig. 8.A-3) in the new bone growth do not necessarily follow those of the surrounding older bone, and so will resist fracture along the old fault line. Though formal bone growth (lengthen-ing) ceases at about age 25, the osteoblasts and osteoclasts remain active as the agents for repair and remodeling, albeit at a slower rate as we age.

Bones generally respond to submaximal stress by becoming thicker and stronger,

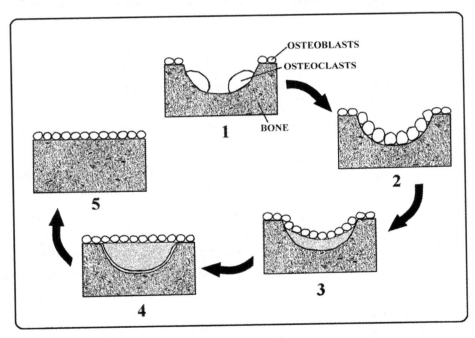

Fig. 8.C-1. The bone-remodeling process begins with the site of a microfracture being cleared by osteoclasts (**1**), followed by osteoblastic activity at the site to backfill the cavity with organic mate-rial, (**2**) and (**3**), which is then mineralized (**4**) to form new bone (**5**).

with osteoblasts more active than osteo-clasts. However, the balance between these two cell functions is reversed when there is no stress on or use of the bone in question. Disuse of the bone as a structural element promotes demineralization and consequent weakening. Thus in both space flight and in horizontal bedrest, osteoblast activity declines and bones weaken, often along the lines of previous fractures.

With respect to the repair of broken bones, perhaps the largest benefit of *yogasana* practice would be in the extra circulation of body fluids that occurs during the practice. Thus, for example, one would not want to do *vrksasana* on a leg having a badly injured ankle bone, but *viparita karani* (as well as other inversions) would be non-threatening to the injury yet would encourage healing by promoting the flow of blood through the injured area.

The Remodeling Response to Mechanical Stress

As was pointed out above, there are several ways in which bone is alive. To this list must be added the remarkable property of "remodeling", a process most active before reaching sexual maturity. At any one time, it is estimated that 5% of the bone mass of the body is undergoing regular reabsorption and redeposition through remodeling [473].

As an example of bone remodeling, suppose a foot injury causes one to walk on the left outer heel. Under direction of the autonomic system, bone remodeling then will commence with reinforcement of the bone strength in that area by dissolving bone from the left inner heel where it is no longer needed, and redepositing it on the left outer heel. Assuming that the bone deposition was "normal" before the injury, one sees that after bone remodeling, the bone has been encouraged to take an abnormal shape (strong on the outside, weak on the inside) which in special situations may prove to be a problem (say, balancing on that foot and ankle in *virhabhadrasana III*).

As with the bone remodeling described above, the conversion of cartilage to bone is directed by the mechanical forces on the tissue in question. Thus, for example, the shapes of the infant and adult vertebrae are significantly different, for those of the infant lack bony processes (Fig 4.A-3), however, as the infant sits and then stands, the use of the spinal muscles molds the vertebrae so as to form strong anchors for muscle action [386].

The remodeling of bone in response to an externally applied stress has its analog in the world of trees, where Japanese horticulturists hang weights on tree limbs in order to coax them into more aesthetic positions. In this process, the wood structure of cellulose and lignin slowly is altered to accommodate the stress, much as in the case of collagen and hydroxyapatite in bone.

If the stress on a bone changes slowly in magnitude or direction, the affected bone can change its internal architecture through remodeling so as to accommodate or resist the shifting stress. In this way, bones can be reshaped, lengthened and realigned (or misaligned, too), even though there has been no separation of bone substance as in a fracture. It is estimated that the shape of a bone can be changed by remodeling if the stress driving the remodeling is applied for between 7 and 10 years.

How would the osteoclasts know where to dissolve bone and the osteoblasts know where to lay down a cancellous web of bone so that it is mechanically most supportive? I hypothesize that this is accomplished using the known piezoelectric properties of bone [283]. A large number of biological materials are known to be piezoelectric, which is to say, when these materials are deformed mechanically, they develop a significant electrical voltage on their surfaces in proportion to the extent of the deformation, with the voltage having a sign dependent upon whether the deformation is compressive or tensile. Because bone shows the piezoelectric effect, previous to the remodeling the normally applied stress on the bone leads to a particular pattern of induced local voltages due to the particular local pattern of compression. When the stress pattern changes, signaling the need for remodeling, the afferent nerve endings within the bone detect these stress-induced voltage changes, and the signals are sent to the brain for processing. Following this, the proper nerves are energized via the autonomic nervous system to activate the osteoclasts to remove bone in areas of lowered stress and the osteoblasts to deposit bone in areas of higher stress, thus remodeling the bone so as to be more supportive of the stress. It is known that the osteoblasts and osteoclasts in the body communicate with and influence one another using two neuroproteins that bind to the receptor sites on the bone-cell surfaces [466].

It should be pointed out that the bone remodeling process involving both osteoblasts and osteoclasts is a distinctly different process from that involving these cells to change the Ca^{2+} levels in the blood. In the latter situation (Subsection 8.B, *Hormonal Control of Ca^{2+} in the Body Fluids*, page 242), there is hormonal activation/inhibition on a global scale in order to satisfy the body's need for Ca^{2+} homeostasis in the blood, while in the case of remodeling, the action is local, probably is driven by neural signals, and is aimed at reconfiguring bone structure in order to resist new stresses.

It is obvious from what has been said above, that if one were to always carry a heavy weight from the left shoulder while walking, that there would be a slow but definite asymmetric response of the bones in the skeleton in support of the load in question. What is not as obvious, but is just as true, is that the "load" on the skeleton can just as well be chronic tension in the muscles which results in a chronic pull on the bones to which they are attached, resulting in a slow but definite asymmetric response (remodeling) of the bones to the perceived loading. In this way, the shapes of bones and the orientations of their structural elements can be changed by excessive and chronic muscle tension [222].

As a corollary to the above, when the muscular stresses on the bones are released or realigned as through *yogasana* practice, the internal structures of the relevant bones will change to accommodate the shifting stress. In this way, the proper practice of *yogasana* with attention to elongation and alignment will slowly pull the elements of the body into a new and more functional shape.

The normal pull of the muscles on the bones is sufficient over time to remodel the bones to suit the particular pattern of stress that they apply to the bone. That level of stress can be multiplied and the remodeling speeded if the muscles so involved work in an active way to stress the bones. This occurs for the ankle, for example, when one stands on one foot in *vrksasana*, or on two feet on a vibrating platform [371], where in both cases one works the muscles about the ankle to maintain balance.

Yet another factor in bone health is mentioned by Lasater in [397]; when the body is under stress, the acidity of the blood increases (pH decreases) and this tends then to slowly destroy bone much as the osteoclasts use hydrochloric acid to thin bone, however, in this case, performing the relaxing asanas will bring the pH back to the basic side.

SECTION 8.D. THE SKELETAL APPENDAGES

In Chapter 4, the skeletal structures of the spine and the attachments thereto, the skull and the pelvis, were presented. In this Section, the bones forming the appendicular appendages (the arms and legs) are briefly outlined. The topic discussed below also is treated in part in Subsection 4.E, *The Pelvis*, page 96.

The Legs and Feet

The femur or thigh bone of the leg is the longest bone in the body, and is a most active bone, having both a two-dimensional ball joint at the hip allowing 360° angular motion and a one-dimensional curved surface at the knee for extension and flexion. The combined motion about these two joints allows a wide range of position for the leg. There is a rather unexpected geometry of the femur close to the point at which it enters the hip joint: when standing in proper alignment, there is a near-vertical plumb line between the centers of the hip joint, the knee joint and the ankle joint, however, the largest part of the femur lies well to the outside of this plumb line, Fig. 8.D-1a, and then turns sharply inward at the upper end to enter the hip joint. The short bone segment that forms an angle with the long shaft of the femur is known as the neck. This arrangement of femur and pelvis allows an approach of the neck of the femur at an angle of 125° with respect to the vertical [227], which in turn allows the pelvis to swing front-to-back between the femur necks, like a bucket between the ends of its handles [345] or like a seesaw, Subsection 4.E, *The Pelvis*, page 96. The most lateral point of the femur is called the greater trochanter, Fig. 8.D-1a, this being the bony point on which we lie when performing *anantasana*; the hemispherical knob of the femur rests within the socket of the hip

called the acetabulum, thus forming the ball-and-socket hip joint. Notice how far inward the hip joints are set with respect to the greater trochanters.

Considering the plumb line between the center of the ankle and the center of the hip joint when standing with the legs straight, the centers of the knee joints can fall either on this line, to the inside of the line, or to the outside of the line, leading to straight and aligned legs, bowed legs or knock-knee legs, respectively, Figs. 8.D-1b and 1c. The latter two conditions can arise when there is an insufficiency of vitamin D in the diet in the early years, and the long bones of the legs, being overly flexible, bend either outward or inward under the compressive stress of gravity [473]. As shown for the right leg in Fig. 8.D-1b, in bowed legs the knee joint bears unbalanced stress on the inner aspect of the joint, and *vice versa* for the case of knock knees, Fig. 8.D-1c. Unless the knee joints can be brought back into alignment, the asymmetrical stress shown in the Figure can be an open door to osteo-arthritis at the points of stress. The benefits of rotating the femur in certain *yogasanas* are discussed in Box 8.D-1.

Strangely, there is a muscle (known as the psoas major) that directly connects the lumbar spine to the femur! This muscle attaches to T5 and L1–L5 at the spine and then moves diagonally through the pelvis, over the rim of each pubic bone and inserts on the lesser trochanter of each femur. Being a key player in integrating the actions of the spine, pelvis and upper legs, the psoas flexes the lower back when the legs are stable, and flexes the hips when the lower back is stable. When the beginning student holds her legs up in *urdhva prasarita padasana*, for example, the superficial abdominal muscles are active, the ribs are pulled toward the pelvis and the belly is pushed upward to the ceiling. Through *yogasana* practice, she will learn instead to release the abdominal mus-

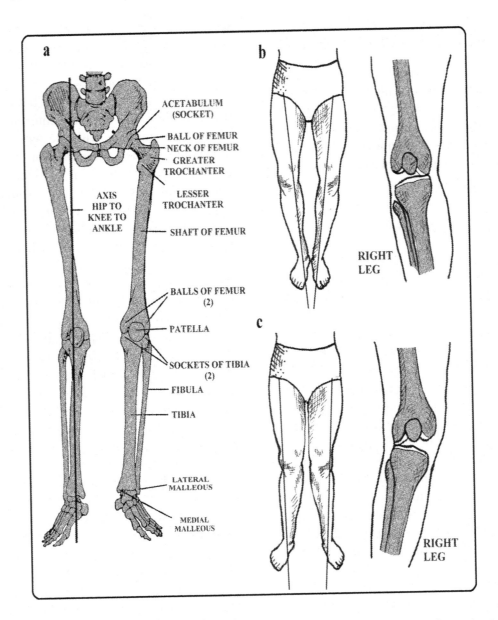

Fig. 8.D-1. (a) The bones of the lower extremities in proper alignment, showing the near-vertical line passing through the center of the acetabulum, the knee joint, and the ankle joint, on the right leg as seen from the front. (b) In the case of bowed legs, the centers of the knee joints lie outside the lines connecting the hip sockets to the ankles, resulting in an articulation of the femur and tibia at the knee joint which is heavy on the inner epicondyle, as shown for the right leg. (c) In the case of knock knees, the centers of the knee joints lie inside the lines connecting the hip sockets to the ankles, resulting in an articulation of the femur and tibia at the knee joint which is heavy on the outer epicondyle, as shown for the right leg.

cles, and to support the legs with the psoas instead, so that the ribs can be moved away from the pelvis and the abdomen dropped toward the floor as the lumbar is pulled somewhat upward.

Because the psoas is oriented diagonally left to right and diagonally front to back, contraction of the psoas on just the right side in *upavistha konasana*, for example, will both tip the torso to the right and rotate

BOX 8.D-1: THE BENEFITS OF ROTATING THE FEMURS IN *YOGASANA*

The unique shape of the femur allows for some exceptional yogic positions. As shown in Fig. 8.A-1, when standing in *tadasana*, the femur is angled outward from the knee, and at the point of the greater trochanter, it abruptly turns inward to settle into the acetabulum. The transverse section, known as the neck, is terminated by the hemispherical femoral head, which in turn fits into the hemispherical socket of the acetabulum. Taken together, the acetabulum and the head of the femur form the hip joint.

In general, the range of motion of side bending at the hip joint is limited by the pressure of the rim of the acetabulum on the upper surface of the femoral neck. You can test your range of motion in this regard in the following way: standing with your back to the wall, legs separated as for *trikonasana*, place the feet parallel to one another and perpendicular to the wall. Keeping the spine straight and back to the wall, bend to the right side at the hip joint (closing the bottom hinge, but keeping the top hinge open, Subsection 4.E, *The Pelvis*, page 96), slide the right hand down the right thigh, and note how far down it can go with respect to the knee. This displacement is limited by the contact of the rim of the acetabulum with the femoral neck, and will vary from person to person, depending upon the angle between the shaft and the neck of the femur. Next, rotate the right femur outward so that the right foot, knee, and thigh point fully to the right, as when doing *trikonasana*. Bend again to the right, and note how much farther one can descend, again keeping the back to the wall and the top hinge open.

How does this increased range of motion come about? Stand in *tadasana* and place the fingers of the right hand on the greater trochanter. Then rotate on the right heel so as to send the right foot fully to the right, and note how this outward rotation of the thigh takes the greater trochanter backward. In regard side bending, the femoral neck is also rotated backward by rotation of the femur shaft, and being rotated out of the path of the descending acetabulum as it rotates over the head of the femur, the rotation allows a deeper bend to the right side.

When the femur is rotated in *trikonasana*, three significant things happen in the pelvic area: 1) the femur neck and greater trochanter are rotated backward, 2) as the greater trochanter is rotated backward, it presses the right groin forward and so opens it up, and 3) with the femoral neck out of the way, the deep bend to the right is unencumbered by bone-to-bone contact. Similar consequences when rotating the forward leg backward in both *parsvakonasana* and *ardha chandrasana* are to be noted.

With one leg rotated outward, the groin on that side is pressed forward. With both legs rotated outward, the entire pelvis is pressed forward, and the lumbar spine tends to become lordotic as a consequence. In this way, it is seen that the "natural" action of the body when backbending to have the feet, knees and thighs rotate outward is an accommodation of the legs to the lumbar lordosis; this again is a consequence of the length of the femoral neck and its angle with the femoral shaft, as well as the peculiar way in which the psoas is connected to both the lumbar spine and the inner femurs (see below). Similarly, when in *baddha konasana* with strong outward rotation of the thighs, there is a simultaneous tendency toward pulling the lumbar spine forward. In an analogous but opposite way, inward rotation of both thighs presses the groins backward, as appropriate for all forward bends such as *uttanasana*, *adho mukha svanasana*, etc.

As the femurs are rotated inward or outward as seen from the front body, the weight on the heels can be felt to move either to the inner edges or the outer edges, respectively. In the standing poses, one should try to work with just enough inward or outward rotation of the femurs so that the heels are evenly balanced on the floor with respect to the inner and outer edges [482a].

As upright, bipedal animals, one might at first expect the human femurs to be long, straight bones with hemispherical ball-and-socket joints at the hips. Though there would be strong vertical support of the upright body with this arrangement, bending forward again would be hampered by the pressing of the rim of the acetabulum against the shaft of the femur, the more so the joint is deeper, and it is very deep in the hip. The femur head is set deepest into the acetabulum when one is on hands and knees, bent 90° at the waist [54]. That forward bending should be an important factor in our skeletal structure is clear from the fact that our quadrupedal ancestors must have spent considerable time in postures on all fours with their spines parallel to the ground, bent at the waist and with their noses to the ground. This forward bending action is best accommodated by femurs that enter the hip sockets from the side rather than from below, and so allow easy rotation about the left-right pelvic axis without the limiting contact of the two elements of the joint. In her wisdom, Mother Nature has given us an intermediate form: largely straight and vertical femurs for the support necessary for a vertical stance, and nearly horizontal femur necks for the unrestricted rotation of the forward bend.

A somewhat similar situation obtains for the head of the humerus when lifting the arm overhead. In this case, the greater tubercle of the humeral head can collide with the acromion, a portion of the scapula that contributes to the formation of the shoulder socket (Fig. 8.D-6). This bone-on-bone contact can be minimized by descending the shoulder blades in those poses requiring the arms overhead, i.e., urdhva hastasana and adho mukha svanasana, for example.

it to face upward, as appropriate for parivrtta janu sirsasana to the right. Because the psoas is bound to the inner, posterior aspect of the femur, stretching it as in backbending will tend to roll the front thighs outward, a common predicament among beginners.

The knee joint is protected from outside forces by the patella or kneecap, Fig. 8.D-1a. This bone is free floating, but is embedded in the tendon that binds the four quadruceps muscles to the lower leg. Unlike the other bones of the leg, the patella does not bear any weight in standing postures, but would do so in kneeling postures such as ustrasana, parighasana, etc. Because the patella is inserted in the tendon of the quadruceps, firming of the quadruceps noticeably lifts the patella toward the pelvis as the muscle contracts. Awareness of the "lifting of the kneecap" as the quadruceps straighten the leg can be of great help to the beginning student trying to find the leg-straightening action in the yogasanas. Inserted as it is in the tendon of the quadruceps, the patella increases the mechanical efficiency of that muscle and also keeps the tendon from rubbing against the femur [476].

Each of the lower ends of the femur bones forms two hemispheres (condyles), side by side, Fig. 8.D-2, and correspondingly, each of the upper ends of the tibia (the major bone of the lower leg) has two shallow sockets which can accept the hemispherical balls of the femur condyles in forming the knee joint. However, as the shapes of the condyles and the top of the tibia are rather incongruent, considerable stress would be applied to their point of contact were it not for the meniscal discs that separate and lubricate them, Fig. 8.D-2b. As the knee is flexed and extended, the femur heads roll and glide across the top of the tibia, and the intervening menisci deform to accommodate the stress. Just as with the intervertebral discs (Section 4.C, page 87) during rest, when the loading on the menisci of the knees is relaxed by lying down, the menisci flow back into their unstressed shapes.

Improper action at the knee joint also can act to destroy the menisci that otherwise keep the femur and tibia from rubbing directly against one another. Should a menis-cus become frayed, loose particles of tissue may then float freely within the joint, and then become painfully enmeshed between the bones of the joint, inhibiting motion at that place. This seems to be a rather common injury among those who insist on pulling the legs into *padmasana*-type poses while stiff in the hips (see Box 8.E-1, *A Safe Way to Teach Padmasana*, page 266).

When abnormal rotation of the lower leg as in *padmasana, etc.,* acts to tear the menisci in the knees, most often it is the medial meniscus, Fig. 8.D-2b, which is injured [476]. The risk for such knee injuries is much lower when the knee does not bear weight in such maneuvers.

The cartilaginous menisci between the tibia and femur serve as both shock absorbers and as lubricants between the bones. Internal to the knee joint, there also are

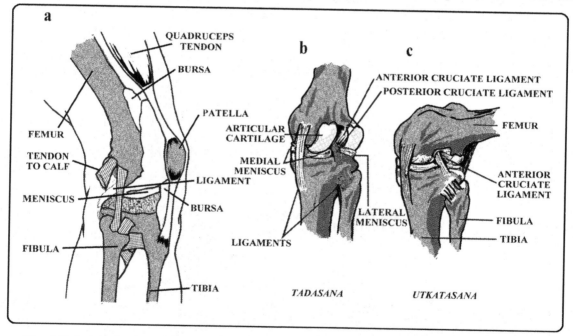

Fig. 8.D-2. (**a**) The internal structure of the knee as seen laterally. In this area, four bones come together with over a half dozen cartilaginous pads (menisci) and cushions (bursa) to protect the epiphyses from rubbing against one another, synovial fluid to keep the apparatus lubricated, and ligaments to hold the structure in place while allowing a certain mobility of the joint. Structures of the knee joint when standing erect in *tadasana* (**b**), and when the knee is bent, as in *utkatasana* (**c**). In *tadasana*, one stands on the bottoms of the condyles of the femurs, whereas in *utkatasana*, the condyles roll within the discs of the menisci and slide forward as well, so that one stands on the back of the condyles of the femur, with the meniscus pressed forward.

crossed ligaments connecting the balls to the sockets (the cruciate ligaments), and the whole is surrounded by a synovial joint capsule (Subsection 8.E, *Joint Lubrication and Arthritis*, page 265).

Thanks to the structure of the joint at the knee, only flexion and extension of the leg at the knee are allowed formally. Other actions at the knee, such as axial rotation of the lower leg with respect to the upper will act to over-stretch the ligamentous structure at the knee, and so should be practiced with great care. If the ligaments and tendons at the knee become over-stretched, then the knee can be easily hyperextended posteriorly or medially (pressed backward so that the center of the knee joint lies *behind* the plumb line of Fig. 8.D-1a, or to one side of it). In that case, the ligaments do not reach the level of tension necessary for supporting the joint, and the students end up "hanging on their joints", further stretching them, as

often happens for example, on the forward leg in *trikonasana*.

Just below the knee joint, one has the tibia, the straightest bone of the body, connecting the knee joint to the talus bone of the foot, Fig. 8.D-3. The second bone of the lower leg, the fibula (Fig. 8.A-1), does not articulate with the femur, but lies parallel to the tibia and is connected to it by a web of interosseous connective tissue.

As can be seen from Fig. 8.D-2, the tibia by far is the larger of the two bones in the lower leg, and carries most of the load between the foot and the femur. In fact, the fibula is relatively weak and of not much use, and there is little or no movement between tibia and fibula.

The gastrocnemius or calf muscle, Fig. 7.A-2, is most interesting in that it spans two joints, the knee and the ankle, and can act on either one separately but not on both simultaneously. When the toes are pointed,

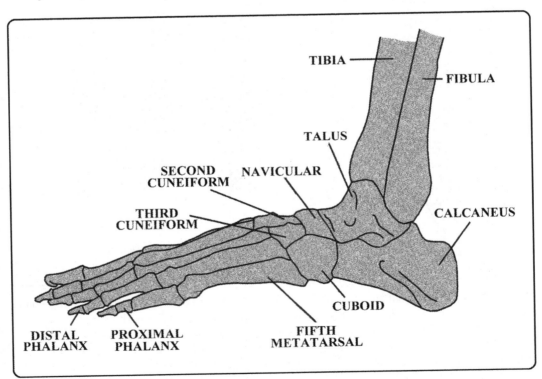

Fig. 8.D-3. The bones of the lower leg and the foot, showing how the tibia and fibula articulate with the talus of the left foot.

the ankle is extended but the knee joint at the same time tends to be flexed, whereas when the heel is pointed so as to dorsiflex the ankle, knee flexion is inhibited (Subsection 7.A, *Reciprocal Inhibition and Agonist/Antagonist Pairs*, page 193) [429]. In virtually all of the *yogasanas*, the extension of the inner heel and the base of the big toe are basic to straightening the leg and to spreading the toes laterally. The range of dorsiflexion of the ankle is larger when the knee is bent and the gastrocnemius is relaxed. This ankle flexion is of great value in straightening the leg, as Kapandji [227] states that the rectus femoris is not strong enough by itself to fully extend the leg. On the other hand, the quadruceps muscles are said to be twice as strong as the hamstrings [448].

Being bipedal animals, it is our feet that connect us to the earth, and it is here that so many pressure sensors are to be found (see Box IV.E-1, *You Have More Sensitivity in Your Big Toe Than You Ever Imagined*, page 539). These pressure sensors contribute significantly to the input data from which the body's proprioceptive map is constructed. This is especially so in regard to balancing on the feet.

The connection of the foot to the tibia and fibula of the lower leg is through the talus, using a joint that allows limited motion in almost all directions, Fig. 8.D-3. The talus is supported by the action of the bases of the toes on the floor, with the front of the talus most supported by the downward action of the innermost three toes, and the back of the talus supported by the downward action of the outermost two toes. Thus when standing in *tadasana* with the bases of all five toes of each foot actively engaged with the floor, both the front and the back edges of each talus are being lifted upward.

Kapandji [227] describes the foot as "the plantar vault", consisting of three arches connected by strong but elastic muscles and ligaments, Fig. 8.D-4, the combination serving as an efficient shock-absorbing system. The three arches span the distance between the heel and the base of the big toe (first metatarsal), between the heel and the base of the little toe (fifth metatarsal), and between the base of the big toe (first metatarsal) and the base of the little toe (fifth metatarsal). The last of these is the shortest, lowest and weakest of the arches, whereas the first of these is the longest, highest and strongest of the arches. When the weight of the body in *tadasana* presses into the talus, the pressure is distributed among these three arches so as to flatten them somewhat and to broaden them. The heights of the arches are sustained by ligaments and muscles in the sole of the foot, with the ligaments handling short-term compression of the arches, as when the foot strikes the ground while jumping into a straddle-leg position, and the muscles handling long-term compression, as when standing in *trikonasana*.

The short length of the first metatarsal of the foot (that of the big toe) is thought to increase the efficiency of the arches of the foot. It is this part of the foot that we activate in order to lift the arches from the floor.

Kapandji [227] gives an exhaustively complete discussion of the various actions of the muscles, bones, ligaments, and tendons in the legs; as only a brief synopsis of this information is given here, the student interested in a deeper discussion is referred to that encyclopedic work. Figure 8.D-5 from Kapandji shows the ranges of motion typical for the legs of those who do not practice *yogasana* or ballet, and so gives *yogasana* teachers a rough guide as to what their beginning students will be capable of doing. For example, outward rotation of the bent-leg thigh in beginners as seen from the front will be about twice as large as the inward rotation, *etc.*

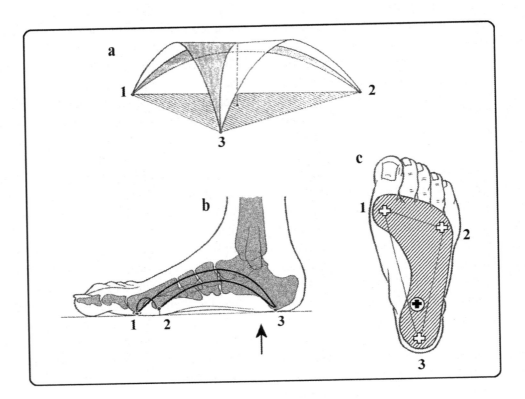

Fig. 8.D-4. (a) A systematic display of the three arches of the foot between points 1–2, 1–3, and 2–3, with the point of applied pressure (where the body weight comes into the foot), represented by the vertical dashed line. (b) The three arches of the foot as drawn appropriate to the anatomy of the foot. The arrow represents the position of the talus. (c) The floor plan of the foot, with the open crosses showing the lowest points of the three arches, and the filled cross marking the point of application of the body weight when standing in *tadasana* [227].

The Arms, Shoulders, and Shoulder Blades

The bones of the arm are rather like those of the leg up to a point. Corresponding to the femur bone of the upper leg, we have the humerus of the upper arm, Fig. 8.A-1, however, the shoulder joint is rather different from the hip joint in structure and function. As with the hip, several bones also join together to form the shoulder socket (the glenoid fossa) into which the hemispherical head of the humerus will fit, Fig. 8.D-6. The joint so formed is called the glenohumeral joint. Specifically, the shoulder girdle is formed from the three bony structures, the

scapula, the clavicle, and the humerus, and their associated muscles, ligaments, and tendons.

The most important of the connections in the shoulder is that between the humeral head and the upper, outer edge of the scapula, forming the glenohumeral joint [226, 429, 449]. The particular part of the scapula involved in this joint is called the acromion process. Also involved in forming the shoulder joint is the lateral end of the clavicle or collar bone, connected at the medial end to the manubrium of the ribcage (Subsection 12.A, *Using the Diaphragm and Ribs to Breathe*, page 362). This latter connection is the only one connecting the arms to the cen-

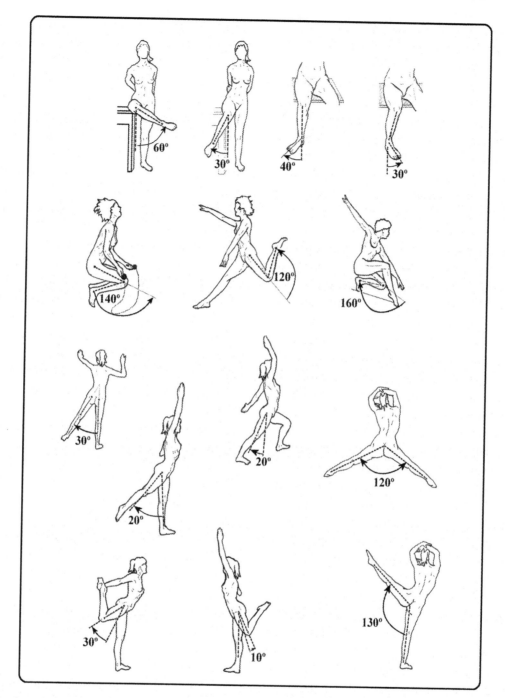

Fig. 8.D-5. Angles of the legs as found by Kapandji for normal, untrained subjects in various body positions [227].

tral axis of the body. The four muscles which hold the humeral head in the shoulder socket are known collectively as the rotator cuff.

The head of the humerus has a surface area approximately three times larger than that of the glenoid fossa into which it can be fit, and as a consequence of this, the shallow joint has a wide range of motion in several directions. As is the case with the other long bones, the epiphyses of the humerus are large and expanded in order to decrease the compressional stress at the ends of the bones, as when supported in *adho mukha vrksasana, purvottanasana,* etc.

The three bones of the glenoid fossa (the humerus, the scapula and the clavicle) are lashed together by an array of muscles and ligaments to give strength and a wide range of motion to the shoulder, the most mobile joint in the body. However, the shallow depth of the shoulder socket also makes it easy to dislocate. In contrast, the hip joint is the most stable joint in the body with respect to dislocation, however, in compensation, the arm and shoulder are capable of motions that are totally forbidden for the leg and hip. Due to the large number of components in the shoulder girdle, in which the spine, neck, shoulder and arm are interconnected, this is a very complex and easily injured part of the body. As is the case with the knee, the shoulder is further destabilized if stretching extends to the inelastic ligaments binding the shoulder joint.

Each of the scapulae lies close to the ribcage, but rather than articulate with it, each floats on the back ribs, suspended in a web of muscle, tendon and ligament. Using various muscles bound at one end to the scapula and at the other end to either the ribcage or the shoulder, the scapula can be elevated, depressed, pulled toward or away from the spine, and can be rotated either inward or outward [54]. Most often, the upper trapezius (Fig. 7.A-2), are chronically tense, resulting in the scapulae and shoulders being lifted upward, toward the ears. This tendency should be countered in all of the *yogasanas* by depressing the scapulae using the lower trapezius muscles.

Notice that the head of the humerus, Fig. 8.A-1, is very much to the medial side of the long axis of the bone, much like the head of the femur, Fig. 8.A-1, and much like the femur, when the humerus is rotated about its long axis, the off-center head pushes its appendicular joint either forward or backward, depending upon the sense of rotation. Imagine that the arm is hanging straight down with the biceps facing forward. If the rotation of the humerus is such that it will take the biceps to face laterally, then this rotation acts to press the scapula onto the back ribs from behind, and to lift the ribcage upward and forward while also spreading the collarbones. Because this open-chest position is that appropriate for almost all *yogasanas,* this lifting and opening of the chest induced by humeral rotation will be an important element of almost all *yogasanas.* Regardless of the arm position, if the biceps are rolled outward, the scapula will be depressed and will press into the ribcage to lift it.* This arm-shoulder action is quite similar to the rotational action of the femur of the right leg, for example, when in *trikonasana* to the right, in order to bring the right groin forward.

As with the foreleg, there are two bones in the forearm, the radius and the ulna, Figs. 8.D-1 and 8.D-7, and beyond these bones, the bones of the hands. When lying down with the arm horizontal and the palm turned up, the bones of the forearm are parallel, with the ulna on the inner (medial) surface and the radius on the outer (lateral) surface. The ulna and radius are bound together by the interosseus membrane. In the forearm, the ulna articulates with the humerus, whereas the radius articulates with the carpal bones of the wrist.

As the hands hang down at the pelvis, palms facing inward in the neutral position,

---

* Actually, in order to get the upper-arm rotation to press the scapulae into the ribcage, it is necessary to stabilize/immobilize the shoulder girdle by activating the pectorals and the muscles of the rotator cuff. If the arms are lifted to the sides, this is most easily accomplished by extending the ring fingers of each hand away from one another [161].

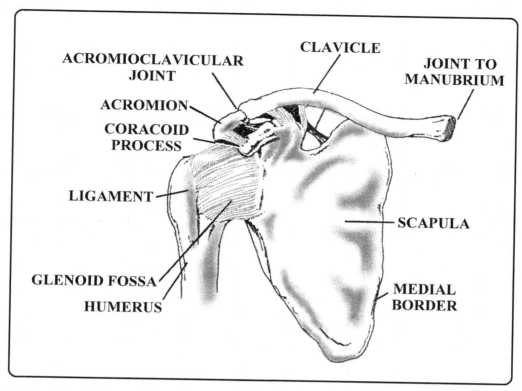

Fig. 8.D-6. The clavicle, acromion and the coracoid process of the scapula are bound together so as to form a shallow cavity into which the head of the humerus can fit in forming the shoulder joint (the glenoid fossa). The anterior view of the right shoulder is shown.

the ulna and radius are more or less crossed over one another. In fact, these two bones of the forearm can be rotated with respect to one another by more than 180º [226], and in large part, independently of any rotation of the humerus. With the arms pendant, the radius and ulna are parallel to one another when the palms are facing forward and are fully crossed when the palms face backward (Fig. 8.A-1); the radius is curved so that it can curl about the ulna without making strong bone-to-bone contact with it in the crossed position. When shoulder rotation is added to forearm rotation, more than 360º of rotation about the long axis of the arm can be achieved with the arms hanging down, but only 180º when the arms are extended overhead [226].

On rotation from the neutral position (with palms toward thighs and arms hanging at the sides) to the palms-forward (supinate) position with the arms still hanging down, the two bones of the forearm tend to unwind, and in the process, tend to rotate the humerus from a biceps-forward position to a biceps-outward (lateral) position. Remember that the insertions of the biceps are on the radius and ulna, Box 7.A-3, so that rotations of the hands can influence shoulder orientation. This action of the hand and forearm on the humerus, through the agency of the shoulder musculature, then takes the scapulae down, toward the spine, and forward onto the back ribs, yielding, in the end, a lift upward and outward of the chest and a lateral broadening of the collarbone. This palms-turned-forward, supinate action of the forearms when in *tadasana* is the appropriately arm/shoulder/chest action for virtually every *yogasana* that we practice, whereas the palms-backward position of the fore-

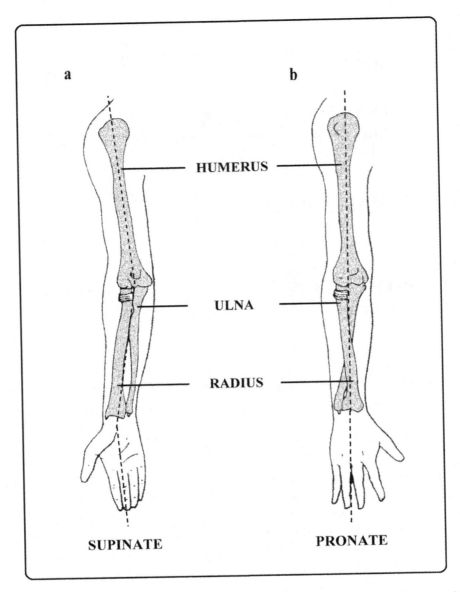

a   b

HUMERUS

ULNA

RADIUS

SUPINATE   PRONATE

Fig. 8.D-7. (a) Relative positions of the two bones of the right forearm as seen from the front when the right palm is turned to face forward (supinated), and (b) when it is turned to face backward (pronated). Note how the centers of the joints at the shoulder, elbow and wrist are colinear when the arm is pronated, but when supinated, the elbow is very strongly displaced to the medial side of the line between the shoulder and the wrist. See Fig. 8.D-1c for the corresponding situation in regard the legs.

arms and hands induces an opposite rotation in the upper body and so works to close the chest.

More correctly, it is the distal end of the radius at the thumb-side of the wrist that rotates about the distal end of the ulna (little-finger side of the wrist) on going from a palmar-supinated to a palmar-pronated posi-tion. The muscles that rotate the forearm into the supine position are stronger than those that rotate it into the pronate position. Because the forearm and humeral rotations can be consciously uncoupled from one another (in *adho mukha svanasana*, for ex-ample), the forearms can be rotated inward as seen from the back body to bring more weight onto the thumb and index finger sides of the hands, whereas the biceps and deltoids can be rolled outward to bring the scapulae into the ribcage and broaden the collarbones.

The outward-spiraling action of the biceps as seen from the front is appropriate regardless of whether the arms are down, forward, lateral, or lifted overhead, and regardless of the body position, be it erect, bent forward, bent back, inverted, twisted, *etc.* One can get the proper sense of arm rotation in any *yogasana* position by first doing the proper rotational action with the arm hanging at the side, and then slowly bringing the rotating arm into the position appropriate to the pose in question. Notice in Fig. 8.D-7 that when the arm is pronate, the centers of the shoulder, elbow and wrist joints are co-linear, whereas when the arm is supinate, the elbow is deviated inward (medially) from this line as the medial epicondyle of the humerus is pulled toward the center line of the body; the angle between the shoulder, elbow and wrist on the lateral side of the arm is termed the carrying angle. The carrying angle is often assessed by having the subject place the palms upward, outer edges of the little fingers touching and the arms then straightened. A large percentage of students (almost always women) will display such large deviations from 180° that their elbows will touch when the arms "straighten"! The carrying angle in women is said to be 165° on average, whereas the corresponding angle in men is 175°.

The significance of the difference of the carrying angle from 180° is not known, but it is a factor in many *yogasanas*. In those students with small carrying angles, the elbows will tend to drop out of alignment with the wrists and shoulders even though the arms are being held in the pronate position. For such students, the elbows will drop toward the floor in *adho mukha svansana*, and fall forward into the room in *adho*

mukha vrks-asana done against the wall. In these cases, the elbows must be pressed into place mechanically using blocks, *etc.*, in an effort to straighten the arms.

Do note, however, that the "inward-outward" description of an appendage's sense of rotation depends upon one's point of view. Thus, for example, rotating the upper arm outward as seen from the front body corresponds to rotating the upper arm inward as seen from the back body, just as clocks appear to run clockwise when viewed from the front, but counterclockwise when viewed from the back. This point must be kept in mind when instructing students to rotate their appendages in a certain way, for it is totally ambiguous to ask them to "rotate your thighs inward" when in *tadasana*, for example, without specifying whether it is the front thighs or the back thighs that are to be rotated "inward".

Interestingly, when in *adho mukha vrks-asana*, it is the ulna that forms the weight-bearing joint with the humerus at the elbow, whereas it is the radius that forms the joint with the lunate bone of the hand at the wrist. Thus there is a shearing action of the interosseous membranes between the two forearm bones when standing inverted on the hands which tends to collapse the forearms, and there also is the opportunity to extend the forearms by moving the ulna up and the radius down. Entrapment of the ulnar nerve at the elbow is discussed in Subsection 5.C, *Mechanical Effects on Nerves*, page 125.

Though the possibility of hyperextension of the knee is controlled by the tension in the joint capsule and by the ligaments and tendons surrounding the joint, in the case of the elbow, the hyperextension is limited by bone-on-bone contact, and so is much less frequently a problem [227].

In those *yogasana* postures in which the palm of the hand presses the floor, the relative amounts of thumb-side and little-finger-side pressures will dictate the extent of pronation versus supination of the ulna and radius of the forearms. As described above, these actions eventually find their way to the scapulae, and influence the actions of these bones with respect to the ribcage and shoulders. Thus, for example, in *dandasana* with the hands cupped and fingertips on the floor, fingernails forward, preferentially pressing the thumb and index fingertip to the floor leads to the action of pressing the inner edges of the scapulae forward and upward into the ribcage to lift it further. Instead, when the little finger is pressed to the floor, the outer edges of the scapulae are pressed forward. Thus in a sense, the actions of the hands are mapped onto the back of the ribcage by the scapulae.

As with the discussion of the legs and hip joints, Kapandji also has written an exhaustive volume on the arm and shoulder [226], and the interested reader is referred to this book for an in-depth discussion.

SECTION 8.E. THE JOINTS

The Bones Form the Joints

Adjacent bones are in contact at their articular surfaces, thereby forming a joint; the joints between bones are generally of two types [170, 229, 345]. In the first type, there is little or no motion intended (as between the plates of the skull, or between adjacent vertebrae, or between the tibia and fibula of the lower leg), and the joint is held together by strong bands of fibrous or cartilaginous tissue. In the second type of joint, movement of the bones is relatively large (as with the knee, hip and shoulder joints), and though the ends of the bones are covered with a smooth cartilaginous coat, the joint is further provided with an internal system of lubrication. Called synovial joints, such joints are encapsulated by a stout outer covering called the joint capsule, and an inner synovial membrane that lubri-

cates the joint by exuding synovial fluid into the joint capsule, Fig. 8.E-1a. This fluid not only reduces the friction between the bones in a joint when moving against one another by keeping the coverings of the ends of the bones soft and moist, but also is the medium by which nutrients move from surrounding tissue into the cartilage of the joint, which otherwise has no direct access to nutrients as it has no blood vessels. The synovial fluid (only 3.5 milliliters in the knee joint) also contains phagocytes of the immune system to remove cellular debris and to envelop any invading organisms [54].

By widening the bones at their ends (the epiphyses), bones are better able to resist oblique compressive stresses transferred across synovial joints [473, 476]. Because the forces are spread over a large area at the epiphyses, the ends of long bones can be built lighter, which is to say, they can be made of cancellous bone; in this way larger joints are more easily stabilized and cushioned. As described more fully in Section 7.B, Muscle Sensors; The Mechanoreceptors, page 198, the joints play a major role in the body's proprioceptive system, for they carry important sensors for determining body position and motion.

Most synovial joints place a concave surface of one bone onto the convex surface of the other, so as to more or less simulate the ball-and-socket arrangement, a configuration of high mechanical stability [473]. For example, this principle is evident in the knee joint, Fig. 8.E-1a, and to a much greater extent in the hip joint, where the ball (the femur head) is set deeply into the socket (the acetabulum), Fig. 8.A-1. In the former, motion is allowed only about one axis as in a hinge, whereas in the latter it is allowed in two directions, as with a true ball and socket.

Interestingly, even in the hip joint, the archetype of the synovial joint, there is a ligament between the center of the femur

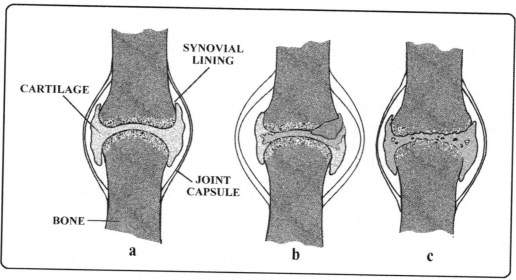

Fig. 8.E-1. (**a**) The internal structure of a synovial joint, showing the two bones separated by a cartilage coating and the synovial lining which fills the joint with lubricating synovial fluid. (**b**) In rheumatoid arthritis, the synovial lining is inflamed and the joint is over-pressured with excess synovial fluid. (**c**) In osteoarthritis, the cartilage is degenerated and painful spurs may form as the eroded bone in the damaged area attempts to repair itself.

head and the back of the acetabulum which helps bind the two together, much as with the fibrous type of joint. Integrity of the hip joint also is maintained by atmospheric pressure against the partial vacuum within the joint. Because there is no equilibration of the gas pressures on the outside and inside of the joint capsule, changes in atmospheric pressure may be felt in sensitive joints as the capsules swell or shrink. There are no pressure or pain sensors in the articular tissue at the ends of the bones, but there are many of these in the joint-capsule tissues.

There would appear to be a reciprocal relation between the stability and the mobility of a joint. Thus, for example, because the shoulder joint is much more shallow than the corresponding hip joint, the shoulder joint is much more mobile in allowing motion of the attached arm as compared with the motion allowed by the hip joint to the attached leg. On the other hand, the shoulder is much more unstable than is the hip, which is bound by large muscles for

stability but which muscles inhibit motion [261].

Flexibility is joint specific [5], which is to say, the range of motion achieved in one joint is no indicator of the range of motion achievable in the other joints. Flexibility in the right hip joint is no indicator of flexibility in the left hip joint, and the flexibility for one shoulder movement is no indicator for flexibility of another movement in the same shoulder. For the *yogasana* beginner, one can in no way assess whole-body flexibility by looking at just one joint in one particular movement; this will be less true as the beginner progresses in the *yogasanas*.

If there is pain in a synovial joint, then we tend to avoid moving it. However, when a synovial joint is not used, the joint capsule shrinks and stiffens, and the range of motion about that joint tends toward zero. The end result of shying away from a painful joint in the long term is a "frozen joint" in which little or no motion is possible [402]. If a joint has been injured and is in pain, it is best to accept that this is the body's way of insuring sufficient rest for the injury, but if it is allowed to rest so completely that it goes into retirement, then its action may be lost forever.

The proper alignment of the bones comprising a joint is important in that misalignment can lead to swelling and/or thickening of the surrounding tissue, which in the vicinity of the joints is rich in both nerves and blood vessels. Compression of these tissues can be deleterious, especially in the vertebral joints [222]. A particularly obvious misalignment of a joint often is seen in women who insist on wearing pointed shoes. In this case the result is a big toe (the hallux) which is strongly angled inward toward the second toe, while the joint between the big toe and the foot moves outward, forming a bunion; technically, the condition is known as hallux valgus. The corresponding condition resulting from the inward turning of the little toe is called a bunionette. The misalignment can be reversed by working the feet in the *yogasanas* so as to broaden across the base of the foot, by wearing non-tapered shoes, and by inserting and leaving spacers between the toes at night so as to encourage the toes toward alignment. Lacking this, the solution is surgical. Yet another shoe-related joint problem stems from the wearing of high heels by women (see Subsection 8.E, *Joint Lubrication and Arthritis*, page 265).

When practicing *yogasana*, it is useful to remember that the range of angular motion at a synovial joint is largest when the joint is most open, *i.e.*, when the ball and socket are most disengaged. Thus in *baddha konasana*, first extend each femur from the groin to the knee, and with the hip joints opened in this way, then rotate the thighs so as to bring the knees toward the floor. Similarly, in *ustrasana*, while upright, lengthen the spine by lifting the ribcage up and away from the pelvis, and with the vertebrae disengaged in

this way, then maintain this opening as the spine is bent backward.

It is especially important that students of *yogasana* realize that hypermobility at the joints (hyperextended knees, *etc.*) is very dangerous, as this can easily injure nearby soft tissue or allow catastrophic collapse of the joint when the student works at maximum intensity. Such collapse is resisted in part by the ligaments about a joint which act as collagenous straps to maintain its integrity. Improper practice of the *yogasanas* over a long period of time can overcome this safety factor, with disastrous results. In this regard, see, for example, Lasater's work [270] on spinal rotation, Subsection 4.A, page 75.

Ligaments and Tendons

Two adjacent or nearby bones are joined by one of three different types of collagenous strap. A joint may be spanned by a muscle, with the two ends of the muscle being tightly interwoven with collagenous material which in turn is interwoven with the periosteum of the bones. If the collagenous material of a muscle that is bonded to the bone is a relatively narrow strap (as with the biceps), it is called a tendon, but if it is a broad band (as with the latissimus dorsi), then the structure is called an aponeurosis. A third possibility is that the collagenous band contains no muscle yet spans the two bones in question; in this case, the structure is called a ligament. Ligaments cannot contract, but are supplied with many stress sensors, the outputs of which are used in the construction of the proprioceptive map in the brain.

Collagen is one of the main constituents not only of bone, but of many ligaments, tendons and cartilage as well. Indeed as described in Section 8.A, bone is formed by the incorporation of microcrystals of the mineral hydroxyapatite into a matrix of collagen fibers. Being collagenous materials, but totally lacking in mineralization, ligaments and tendons are somewhat elastic, but not overly so: untreated tendon can extend only 8% before rupturing, *i.e.*, it can be strained only 8% before rupturing, whereas the comparable figure for rubber is 300%.* However, see Section 9.A, Connective Tissues, page 273, for more on the chemistry and structure of connective tissue such as is found in ligaments and tendons. This semi-rigidity of the ligaments and tendons serves us well, as these elements are used as straps to hold one bone close to another (ligament) or to tie a muscle onto a nearby bone (tendon). As collagenous material can withstand strong tensile forces with minimum strain, it is ideal for this purpose, but of course, it buckles immediately under a compressive force.

It is worth repeating that, though a ligament is unable to contract on its own the way a muscle can, when stretched, a ligament can return to its unstretched length if the initial stretch was not too extreme, *i.e.*, did not exceed the elastic limit. If, on the other hand, the strain approaches 8% or so, the elastic limit is exceeded, and the ligament will be permanently lengthened or torn apart.

At several places in the body, the muscles and their attendant tendons are forcefully pressed onto nearby bone when the muscle is contracted. In order to soften the contact of bone on muscle and tendon, the body has incorporated about 150 small sacs, filled with synovial fluid, at these critical points which serve to lessen the friction of the motion of the soft tissues against the bones. So, for example, there is such a sac in the pelvic area where the gluteus maximus muscle crosses the greater trochanter of the femur bone. These sacs are called bursae, and when they become inflamed and sensi-

tive, one has the corresponding bursitis. The discomfort of trochanteric bursitis will be apparent in forward bends such as *prasarita padottanasana, parsvottanasana, etc.*

In general, the ligaments and tendons lack distinct vascularization and are nourished by diffusion. In fact, were they vascularized, they would have been converted into bone in the fetus! Because of this lack of vascularization, once broken or ruptured, ligaments and tendons heal only by a long, slow process. Note that since the ligaments are essentially collagenous, they do not have the ability to contract rapidly as might a muscle. As a consequence, if they are over-stretched as when poses are done by hanging on the joints (as when doing *trikonasana* with the quadruceps limp, for example), they can be fatigued and in pain long after the stretching has ended [260].

The mechanical integrity of a joint will depend upon the proper tensioning of the stabilizing ligaments and tendons, which in turn will depend upon proper alignment of the relevant bones. If one performs *yogasanas* with the bones of the joints out of alignment, over time there will occur a corresponding misalignment and relaxation of the relevant ligaments and a corresponding destabilization of the joint [238]. As often happens with students doing "hang-out" yoga, the ligaments about the joints can learn the wrong lesson, be stretched excessively, leading to serious joint problems down the line. In fact, an entire treatment protocol for joint pain has been developed based on the idea that joint pain is the result of weak, loose ligaments, and that tightening of these structures by injection of innocuous substances (sugar, *etc.*) reduces the pain [132].

Laxity of the ligaments is synonymous with hyperflexibility [268]. Joints that are

---

*Actually, the ligamentum nuchea in the neck stretches by almost 200% when the neck is flexed so as to place the chin on the chest as in *sarvangasana*, but this is quite atypical of ligaments.

hyperflexible do not hold chiropractic adjustments very well, and because high levels of estrogen promote such laxity, it can become more of a problem during the menstrual period and during pregnancy. Hyperextension is especially serious when it occurs in the sacroiliac joints, for these joints have no other muscles to hold them together, and if the ligaments are overstretched, the result is certain back pain.

The instability at the joint extends to the muscles as well. If the bones of a joint do not bear weight properly, then muscular action will be called upon. Over time, this incorrectly used muscle will become short and hard (like a bone), while its antagonist (Subsection 7.A, *Reciprocal Inhibition and Agonist/Antagonist Pairs*, page 193) at the same time will become weaker through lack of use. This muscular asymmetry will then work further to destabilize the joint, with the problem eventually spreading to other joints in the body [238]. On the other hand, proper alignment can release the tension at the joint and restore the proper weight-bearing relationship between bone and muscle.

The largest and strongest tendon in the body is the Achilles tendon behind the ankle, this being 6 inches (15 cm) in length. As with most tendons, there are few nerves in the Achilles tendon, so that total rupture may be painless! Rupture of this tendon is more likely in middle age, when tendons are stiffer and more easily over-stretched to the point of damage. Though damage to the Achilles tendon can occur if the stress on the tendon is applied rapidly and is intense, as when the high heel on a woman's shoe breaks off and the heel instantly drops several inches to the floor, this would not seem to be much of a problem when stretching the same ligament slowly, as when the heel of the back leg descends to the floor in *parsvottanasana*. Lacking vascularization, a torn Achilles tendon heals slowly if at all, and often has to be repaired surgically.

Keeping this tendon long and flexible along with its associated muscle (the gastrocnemius) through practice of *yogasanas* such as *parsvottanasana* will help in avoiding such a tear. Of course, if any pose is done to the extent of having gone from discomfort into pain, one then runs the risk of tearing a tendon rather than strengthening it.

It is generally held that the popping and cracking of the joints is due to the formation of a gas bubble within the fluid of the joint on pulling the two bones away from one another [5]. Bubble formation is then followed by an explosive collapse of the bubble and the generation of sound waves. Once popped, the joint is in the open position for about 20 minutes, as the remainder of the gas bubble re-dissolves. During this time, the joint is unstable and is subject to trauma. If this indeed is the mechanism, it would appear that cracking of a joint does not release any tension in the body, and otherwise leaves the joint susceptible to damage for a short time after the cracking.

Vertebral joints often crack the first time one goes into *urdhva dhanurasana*, but it is difficult to see how these joints are pulled apart to form bubbles. Perhaps it is better to view this cracking sound as due to the realignment of overlying muscles and tendons after a night of relaxation.

One can estimate the relative importance of ligaments and muscle tendons in holding a joint together from a comment made by Juhan [222]. He notes that when a hospital patient is given a general anaesthetic which relaxes the muscles, hospital personnel must be very careful in moving the patient, as without the ordinary muscle tone (Subsection 7.B, *Resting Muscle Tone*, page 204), the patient's joints can be easily dislocated. Assuming that the noncontractile ligaments are unaffected by the anaesthetic, this then can be taken to demonstrate that the muscle tendons play an important role in stabilizing joints with respect to dislocation.

The effects of pregnancy on joints and ancillary structures are discussed in Subsection 19.B, *Muscles, Joints, Ligaments, and Tendons During Pregnancy*, page 457.

The Knee Joint as an Example

The knee joint is one of the largest, most fragile, and most abused joints in the body, being stressed from above by our weight and from below by the impact of walking, jumping, *etc.* The fragility of the knee joint arises from the fact that the epiphyses of the three long bones (femur, tibia, and fibula) which meet at the knee, along with the patella, Fig. 8.D-2, are in relatively poor contact. The joint is held together instead by four ligaments, the cruciate ligaments at the back of the knee and at the patella, and two collateral ligaments at the sides of the knee joint. As the primary task of the ligaments is to bind the knee and keep it stable, there is no elastic tissue in these ligaments, and they do not stretch without consequences [448]. The ends of the bones not only are covered in smooth-sliding cartilage, but are separated in part by thick, cushioning cartilaginous pads (the menisci), and the entire structure is bathed in synovial fluid. Bursae also contribute to the cushioning within the knee joint. Of the two menisci in each knee, it is the inner (medial) one which is more easily damaged. In fact, the inner knee is devoid of any tissue which can either contract or stretch elastically [448], which is to say, if the tissues of the inner knee are stretched in *yogasana* practice, they will not return to their original lengths, and the joint will be correspondingly destabilized.

The fact that the femur shaft is angled with respect to the vertical line of the lower leg, Fig. 8.D-1a, implies that the knee joint will be subject to several types of mechanical stress due to motions at the hip joint. Indeed, of the eleven muscles that cross the knee, seven of them also cross the hip joint (three hamstring and four quadruceps), thus coupling hip and knee actions [448].

The momentary load on the knee joint when the foot strikes the ground while walking is four times the body weight, and this increases to eight times body weight when running. Done to excess, these activities can break down or irritate the cartilage of the knee and lessen the extent of lubrication, possibly leading to arthritis (see below) and/or bursitis in and around the joint.

Because the joints are not highly vascularized, they are cooler than surrounding muscular tissue. This is especially true of the knee joint [220]. Thus, a joint that feels as warm as the surrounding muscles is inflamed.

It is of prime importance to *yogasana* students and their teachers that they understand that the knee is constructed to bend like a hinge; rotation about any axis other than the hinge axis, which goes laterally from the outside of the knee to the inside, risks damage to the ligaments and/or menisci. Realization of this limitation on the motion permissible about the knee joint is of special importance when performing an asana such as *padmasana*, where tightness in the hip joint can force the knee into a risky position if force is used to cross the legs (see Box 8.E-1, page 266, for a discussion of a safe way to approach *padmasana*).

Joint Lubrication and Arthritis

The two general types of joint degeneration, called rheumatoid arthritis and osteoarthritis, are shown graphically in Figs. 8.E-1b and 8.E-1c. In the former, there is an inflammation of the synovial capsule due to an autoimmune reaction in which the immune system mistakenly recognizes the collagen within the joint as a foreign substance and attacks it. This reaction leads to over-production of synovial fluid, the swelling and stretching of the joint, and the

BOX 8.E-1: A SAFE WAY TO TEACH *PADMASANA*

The following prescription will take a student toward full *padmasana* without endangering the knees due to unnecessary torque. The scheme is based on the idea that putting the first leg into *ardha padmasana* is relatively safe, and that injuries arise from bending the second leg and then trying to lift its foot high enough to rest on the thigh of the first. It is this lift and rotation that should come totally from the hip joint, but often involves too much improper rotation at the knee joint and so puts it at risk [211]. Students should move through the steps in order, only moving on when they have mastered the previous steps.

1) Start in *dandasana* and bend the right knee toward the right shoulder, pulling the right heel to the right buttock. Keeping the deep bend at the knee, roll the knee to the right, and holding the ankle from below, lift the bent leg so that the right heel rests high on the left thigh, with the right heel in the left groin (*ardha padmasana*). If the student is unable to do this, sit the student on a block and practice going in and coming out of *ardha padmasana*.

2) Now bend the left leg and let the full length of the left shin, ankle to knee, rest on a bolster.

3) With the left knee held above the floor by the thickness of the bolster, can the student release the right groin and take up the slack in the right buttock so as to bring the right knee to a level below that of the left foot? If so, then

4) Slide the left foot horizontally into its place on the right thigh without lifting its ankle with respect to its knee. Adjust the feet so as to keep the knees as close as possible; tip back momentarily and push the bolster away so that both thighs can rest on the ground. *Padmasana* is achieved without risk to the knees by first depressing the thigh of the bent leg in *ardha padmasana*, so that the second shin does not have to be lifted to be put in place.

5) Once in *padmasana*, the top shin often presses strongly on the bottom shin so that when coming out of the pose, it is tempting to first lift the top shin. Resist this temptation, for it will torque the knee in the manner we are trying to avoid. Instead, slide each knee sideways so that there is no upward motion of the top shin. The pose ends in a cross-legged sitting position, much like *swastikasana*.

An intermediate position which helps to loosen the relevant muscles of the pelvis without threatening the knee is a useful preparation for full *padmasana*: from a seated position, bend the right leg so that the shin is parallel to the front edge of the mat. Place the left ankle at the right knee and then slowly depress the left knee toward the right ankle using the action appropriate to *baddha konasana*. Eventually, the shins will come to rest one over the other.

When the legs are placed in *padmasana*, each of the ankles presses inward on the upper-inner thigh of the opposite leg, *i.e.*, upon the femoral artery of that leg, Fig. 11.C-2. This pressure on a major artery is thought to restrict the flow of blood to the lower body, and thereby to alter the flow of blood throughout the body. The well-known meditative state of mind induced by this posture may well be related to the altered course of blood flow induced by the placement of the ankles on the femoral arteries. Note that *padmasana* would be counterindicated in someone with pre-existing circulation problems in the legs, such as varicosities (Subsection 11.C, *Venous Flow Against Gravity*, page 332).

Unfortunately, placing the feet as described above also puts pressure on the sciatic nerves running from the lower spine to the toes of each leg. The case of a meditator who fell asleep for more than three hours in *padmasana* (Appendix II, INJURIES INCURRED BY IMPROPER *YOGASANA* PRACTICE, page 511) is instructive: there was eventual loss of nervous sensation in the right lateral femoral cutaneous nerve (tingling became numbness) as witnessed by the loss of sensitivities to pinprick, temperature, and light touch on the skin on the inside of the right thigh [301]. A similar report of a meditating student in *sukhasana* for two hours, showed that the compression on the medial components of the sciatic nerve (right leg) caused demyelination and axonal degeneration of this nerve, leading to foot drop [472]. Unfortunately, in neither case was it reported which leg was placed over the other. In any event, one must be wary of remaining for a matter of hours in any of the *yogasanas*, or falling asleep in them, if there is any pressure on the nerves.

An approach closely related to that presented here for teaching *padmasana* in a safe way is presented by Farhi [136], along with appropriate warm-up asanas to loosen the hips in preparation for lifting the second leg into place.

weakening of the ligaments and tendons in its vicinity. Once the ligaments and tendons have loosened, the alignment at the joint is compromised, the bones fall out of alignment, and the characteristic joint distortions then become evident. The effects of rheumatoid arthritis are usually right-left symmetric in the body, and are three times more prevalent in women than in men [220]. The lubrication quality of the synovial fluid also declines in rheumatoid arthritis and with that, so too does its ability to supply nourishment to the joint's cartilage. Several experts in the field consider rheumatoid arthritis to be caused by an infectious organism, but this has not been proved [476].

When the barometer is reading low as it would be when a storm is approaching, the low pressure experienced by the hermetical-ly-sealed joint allows the tissue cells to expand and irritate any inflamed tissue in the joint. When coupled with high humidity and atmospheric electrical disturbances (phase 4, meteorologically), this combination can be very painful to those with rheumatoid arthritis.* There is evidence that *yogasana* practice can work to increase the strength about joints afflicted with rheumatoid arthritis [193], but the inflamed joints must not be worked directly.

In osteoarthritis, there is an erosion of the cartilage and the epiphyseal surfaces leading eventually to spurs or projections which are painful when the joint is moved. The erosion is initiated by overloading of the joint as often happens in obesity, or by poor alignment of the joint surfaces which causes the protective cartilage to wear away. This in turn can lead to a rubbing of bone on

---

* Other physical and mental responses to changing weather have been reported [254]. For example, alertness and wakefulness as measured by response times both noticeably decreased in a period of phase-4 weather, possibly involving parasympathetic excitation. Industrial accidents rise noticeably when the temperature goes outside the range 12–24° C (54–75° F), and the effect of cold weather on many people is to increase the blood pressure. It also is known that very small changes in atmospheric pressure of the order of 0.001 atm can have demonstrable effects on the abilities of test takers to solve puzzles, *etc.*

bone, with little or no intervening lubrication. Erosion of the epiphyses is promoted by chronic muscle tension which acts to close the joints [9].

It is the knee joint that is most commonly affected by osteoarthritis, this particular problem being experienced by twice as many women as men, whereas osteoarthritis of the hip joint is more common in men than in women. Experiments show that walking in high-heeled shoes reduces torque at the ankle as compared with walking barefoot, but increases it at the knee. It is conjectured that the significantly higher incidence of bilateral osteoarthritis in the knees of women can be traced to their frequent walking in high-heeled shoes [235].

The tendency in osteoarthritis to avoid movement in order to avoid pain quickly leads to immobility. For those with osteoarthritis, it is best to do range-of-motion exercises, which at the same time do not stress the joints. All of these movements should be low impact, smooth and rhythmic. Clearly, *yogasana* has a great potential use here in maintaining range of motion [138] and in reducing muscle tension at the joints so that bone-on-bone contact is minimized.

Practically everyone who is 20 or more pounds overweight will show signs of osteoarthritis due to the added pressure of the weight on the joints, which acts to wear away the protective coating on the ends of the bone, especially at the knee [220]. *Yogasanas* done with special attention to keeping the joints open can work to resist the collapse of the joints and so reduce wear on their protective cartilage.

As shown in Fig. 20.B-1, the symptoms of rheumatoid arthritis are most intense at 6:00–7:00 AM, whereas those of osteoarthritis are most intense at 6:00–7:00 PM. The time between 6:00 and 7:00 AM is the hour during which the sympathetic nervous system becomes active, whereas the time between 6:00 and 7:00 PM is the hour during which the nervous system converts from sympathetic to parasympathetic dominance.

SECTION 8.F. MECHANORECEPTORS IN THE JOINT CAPSULES AND LIGAMENTS

Alter [5] presents a concise description of the four types of mechanoreceptors that are found in and about the joint capsules (Fig. 8.E-1) surrounding all of the synovial joints within the body. The first three types of joint-capsule receptors (types I, II, and III) essentially monitor mechanical stress at the joint, whereas the fourth (type IV) registers pain. Signals from these receptors provide input to the proprioceptive centers in regards to joint position and movement, and so aid the construction of the proprioceptive map.

Type-I receptors are found in the tissue of the joint capsules, more so in the tissues of the hips and spine than in the more distal joints. As they are highly sensitive, are active for every joint position whether moving or not, and are slowly adapting, they will be easily activated in every *yogasana*, and the signal will be long lasting. Type-I receptors signal joint angle, velocity of joint movement, and changes in joint pressure.

Type-II receptors are found in the deeper tissue of the joint capsule, and because they respond only when the joint is in motion, and are rapidly adapting, they will be most active when moving into and out of the *yogasanas*. Presumably, type-II receptors will play a role as proprioceptive elements when balancing.

The type-III receptors function much like the Golgi tendon organs, except that they are located in the joint capsule and the ligaments of each joint. Being dynamic sensors, with a high threshold and slow adaptation, the type-III sensors work largely at the extremes of joint angle position, and may act as inhibitors of joint motion if such motion is extreme. In this sense, they function much like the muscle spindles and the Golgi tendon organs in protecting the musculoskeletal system from overwork.

When joint motion is extreme and the surrounding tissue is injured, then high-threshold, slowly-adapting pain receptors (type IV) are activated in the articular tissue, and joint pain is sensed. These sensors are present in synovial tissue, menisci, and the ligaments of the joints, however, by a pain-gate mechanism (Subsection 10.D, *Neural Aspects of Pain*, page 298), their pain signal can be inhibited by mixing with the signals from type-I sensors.

SECTION 8.G.
OSTEOPOROSIS

Definition, Statistics, and Causes

As women pass middle age (50–51 years) and go through menopause, the levels of estrogen and progesterone in their bodies fall precipitously. Because estrogen activates the osteoblasts, inhibits the osteoclasts and speeds the absorption of Ca^{2+} into the bones, its loss following the onset of menopause often leads to thinning of the bones, a condition called osteoporosis [450]. Osteoporotic bones have a density (Subsection 8.A, *Bone Density*, page 241) substantially lower than the norm for younger but adult bone.

Figure 8.C-1 illustrates the manner in which osteoclasts and osteoblasts normally work together to remodel a flaw in bone structure. However, with increasing age and hormonal shifts due to menopause, a state of osteoclastic overactivity and/or osteoblastic underactivity often leads to the formation of deep fissures in the bone and a dangerously low bone density, *i.e.*, osteoporosis. As the demineralization of osteoporosis proceeds more rapidly with cancellous bone than with compact (cortical) bone, a person with osteoporosis has heightened risk of stress fractures of the cancellous bony features such as the spinal vertebrae, pelvis, and wrist [288, 409, 473]. The differences between normal and osteoporotic bone structure are shown in Fig. 8.G-1.

If only Ca^{2+} is leached from bones, then the result is osteomalacia, a softening of the bones. However, in osteoporosis, there is a

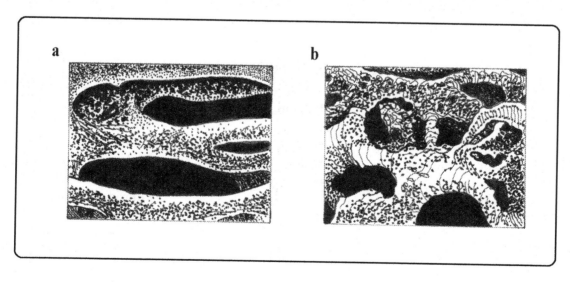

Fig. 8.G-1. Comparison of the structure of normal cancellous bone (**a**), and the same bone afflicted with osteoporosis (**b**).

loss of Ca^{2+} and a loss of the organic collagen matrix as well, resulting in brittleness. As the countries with the highest level of dairy consumption in the world also have the highest rates of hip fractures among its older citizens, it is clear that fighting osteoporosis may involve more than just ingesting dairy products.

If bone loss is not stopped, 90% of women and 50% of men will have osteoporosis by age 80 [288]. Elderly women subject to osteoporosis will eventually lose 50% of the Ca^{2+} in their cancellous bone and 30% in their cortical bone. For elderly men, the corresponding figures are only 30% and 20%, respectively. For women who are 5–10 years postmenopausal, the bone loss can amount to 2–3% per year. Elderly men also incur a bone thinning with age and increased risk of fracture, but at only half the rate experienced by women [409]. Osteoporosis becomes a heightened risk for men having low levels of testosterone [409].

It recently has been found that activation of the T cells of the immune system (Subsection 13.A, *The T Lymphocytes*, page 384) leads to the production of an immunotransmitter that is preferentially stimulating to the osteoclasts of the bone, leading to osteoporosis. Action of this immunotransmitter is blocked by estrogen [466].

Symptoms and End Results

There are no obvious symptoms in the early stages of osteoporosis, but with advancing age, osteoporosis becomes more and more of an important health factor. At age 40, bones inevitably begin to lose mass, though not as fast as after age 50. Nieman [337] presents a table of risk factors for osteoporosis, divided according to the strength of the evidence supporting each claim, as shown in Table 8.G-1. Schatz [409] also lists a more complete list of such risk factors, but does not comment on how conclusive these various factors might or might not be.

It is very interesting to note from the Table that it is well established that, though old age, alcohol and smoking work to increase the risk of osteoporosis, the risk is also increased by bedrest and decreased by obesity! This is understandable from the point of view that bedrest essentially negates the gravitational pull on the skeleton and so promotes bone weakness, whereas the extra weight carried by obese people stresses the skeleton and so leads to an increased growth of the weight-bearing

TABLE 8.G-1. RISK FACTORS FOR OSTEOPOROSIS[a] [337]

Well Established	Moderate Evidence	Inconclusive
Age (+)	Alcohol (+)	Moderate exercise
Removal of ovaries (+)	Cigarette smoking (+)	Asian ethnicity
Use of steroids (+)	Low dietary Ca^{2+} (+)	Diabetes
Bedrest (+)	Heavy exercise (−)	Progestin use
Obesity (−)		Fluoridated water
Black ethnicity (−)		Caffeine
Estrogen use (−)		Lean body
		Short stature and small bones

----

[a] The (+) sign signifies an increased risk, whereas the (−) sign signifies a decreased risk for osteoporosis.

bones. It is felt that an exactly parallel situation results from performance of the *yogasanas*, with the bones of the skeleton being stressed in a beneficial way so as to provide an antidote to osteoporosis.* It is known [450] that if the bone mass of a young woman is low due to a lack of exercise, she will have a much higher risk of severe osteoporosis in her later years. Thus, the years of *yogasana* work done by young women in their premenopausal days is bone density in the bank for a later day.

Yogasana, Western Exercise, and Osteoporosis

Though walking and running provide weight-bearing for the legs of the aging but active senior, only *yogasana* can do as much not only for the legs, pelvis and spine, but for the arms and upper body as well through the practice of inversions and hand balances. To the increased bone strength created by *yogasana* practice should be added the increases in neuromuscular control and balance which make a fall less likely, and the increased muscle strength which can make the impact of a fall less serious. The importance of avoiding if possible such an accident is clear in the statistics [288] which show that for the elderly, the morbidity following a hip fracture is 20%! Note too that it has been found recently that in middle-aged and older women, hip fractures are reduced by 30% in those women whose diets are rich in vitamin K (the blood-clotting factor), as found in leafy green vegetables. A similar beneficial effect of vitamin K is found in astronauts in space.

Of course, the strengthening of osteoporotic bone or the maintenance of high bone density will depend upon the diet supplying an amount of calcium adequate for serious bone building. Schatz [409] gives a detailed *yogasana* program for those having osteoporosis, or who are at risk for this condition.

Interestingly, fluoride ion at the 1-ppm level has a strongly positive strengthening effect on teeth, making them resistant to dental caries, through the formation of fluorohydroxyapatite. At much higher levels (4–50 mg), fluoride ion seems to stimulate osteoblast formation (especially in the spine!) and renewed bone formation, though it is still an open question as to whether the new bone is strong or not [44, 288].

It must be noted however, that whereas hip and wrist fractures often result from falls by the osteoporotic, fractures and collapse of the spinal vertebrae can occur without falls [44]. Thus, the osteoporotic woman can fracture vertebrae just bending over to pick up the newspaper, or even can awaken to find her vertebrae broken during sleep. A multiplicity of such fractures in the vulnerable senior can result in a deep spinal kyphosis (also called dowager's hump, Fig. 4.A-4) and the loss of several inches of height. The care with which such vulnerable *yogasana* students must be guided by their teachers is obvious.

When osteoporosis is active, there is a gradual collapse of the spinal column which is outwardly evident as a loss of height as one ages. However, even without osteoporosis, if the musculature is atrophied, weak and sagging, then it is not able to support the bones, and there will be a general collapse of the skeleton even though the bones themselves are healthy.

---

* Note however, that in the obesity situation, the extra weight that promotes stronger bones also acts to collapse the relevant joints, rubbing bone against bone thus promoting osteoarthritis as well (Section 8.E, Joint Lubrication and Arthritis, page 265) whereas in the practice of *yogasana*, one works to keep the joints open and well lubricated so that the conditions for the formation of arthritis are discouraged. Interestingly, the physical symptoms of weightlessness can be mimicked by resting with the head inclined downward by 6 degrees [482].

Osteoporosis is less of a problem for older men because as children they were on average more active physically, and so have a larger bone mass to start with, and also because the decrease in testosterone levels in men is not as precipitous as the decrease of estrogen levels in women [44]. With almost equal certainty, it can be said that the postmenopausal risk for osteoporosis among women can be avoided by taking an external source of estrogen [44], and it is now known that the hormone therapy so effective for older women also works for older men.

Though heavy exercise does increase bone density, young women who are extremely active physically and so have low fat-to-muscle ratios still may suffer from osteoporosis. Under heavy exercise, a young woman can become amenhorreic because the body acts to prevent an under-nourished woman (one with a low fat-to-muscle ratio) from becoming pregnant; in losing her menstrual period, this woman also loses the protective effect of having estrogen released into her system [450, 473].

Note that the bone-building effects of exercise are site specific, *i.e.*, running strengthens the bones of the legs but not of the arms, and that the exercise must be weight bearing, *i.e.*, swimmers' bones are not strengthened at all by their exercise, as only their cardiovascular fitness increases [44]. The phenomenon of a 20% higher bone density demonstrated in the racquet arms of active tennis players can be a positive factor against osteoporosis in all of the long bones in the bodies of *yogasana* students.

The power of *yogasana* to build a stronger/more-dense bone mass is evident in the variety of weight-bearing positions it takes. In what other activity is weight placed for a long period of time on the head so as to load the cervical vertebrae? In what other activity is the spine twisted for an extended time while in alignment? *Yogasana* practice is good as well because the weight-bearing positions often can be held for relatively long times, rather than just being experienced impulsively, as when one swings at a tennis ball. In contrast, a complete lack of loading, *i.e.*, no work done against the force of gravity as when confined to bedrest, acts to thin and weaken bone. Arguing in reverse, it seems likely that bone also will demineralize if one does only "hanging" poses while holding weights, which poses put bones under tensile stress rather than compressive stress. This will be a small effect unless one hangs often for hours at a time using heavy weights.

It is almost certainly true that larger, stronger muscles do lead to larger, stronger bones because the pull of such muscles on the bones when they do work, acts as loading on the bones and so strengthens them. In this regard, *yogasana* is again valuable for it will strengthen the bones as it strengthens the muscles. On the other hand, while a large frame does signify large bones, it does not necessarily signify a high bone density, which is the more relevant factor for osteoporosis [184].

Chapter 9

CONNECTIVE AND SUPPORTING TISSUES

SECTION 9.A. CONNECTIVE TISSUES

The Body's Glue

Unlike the situation in tissues such as muscle, nerve, *etc.*, where there are dense concentrations of the relevant cells, in connective tissue one finds relatively few cells otherwise present in a large excess of noncellular components, *i.e.*, large numbers of collagen and elastin fibers floating in a semifluid gel called ground substance or extracellular fluid. These three components (collagen, elastin, and ground substance) are produced by cells floating within the tissue, and the wide variety of mechanical properties found within this tissue type are the direct result of the various proportions of the components.

Though the connective tissues form a continuous web throughout the body, the proportions of ground substance, collagen and elastin may vary widely from point to point, depending upon the task they are to perform locally. Thus connective tissue, subject to strong tensile loading but which nonetheless should stretch only slightly, will be high in collagen, a molecule which is strong but rather inextensible. Other areas of the body may require much more flexibility in the connective tissue and so will be high in elastin instead. In yet other connective tissues, it will be the ground substance that predominates. In general, connective tissue functions as a mechanical support and/or binder for other tissues, as the medi-

um for the intercellular exchange of cell metabolites, nutrients, wastes, *etc.*, and as a lubricant [476].

Connective tissue is the body's glue; in its different forms, it works to keep various organs in place, to bind groups of cells together to form organs, plexi, *etc.*, to surround and cushion every cell in the body, and ultimately to define the overall shape of the body [386]. The supporting tissues are closely related to the connective tissues, but they are constructed such that they can help support the weight of the body.

Collagen

Collagen (the most abundant protein in the animal world) is a long-chain polypeptide, with the chains wrapped three at a time into triple helices (also see Subsection 8.B, page 242). There are at least five types of collagen; type I is the most common type in the skin, bones, ligaments and tendons. In all five types, the triple helices of the collagen molecule are bound together to form collagen fibrils, and the fibrils then are bundled to form fibers. When properly aligned, connective tissues formed with a high percentage of collagen fibers have very high tensile strengths, but relatively low extensibility, and so are able to resist strong pulling (tensile) forces. The collagen fibrils are manufactured by special cells called fibroblasts within the connective tissue.

The collagen strands within the triple helix are joined not only by the relatively weak hydrogen bonds between amino acids on adjacent strands, but by stronger crosslinks which are chemical in nature. The crosslinks between collagen strands resemble somewhat the cross bridges between the actin and myosin of muscle fibers (Fig. 7.A-7), however in the case of connective tissue, the crosslinks act to prevent the relative motions of the strands rather than promote it as with muscles.

Because the collagen strands even though crosslinked are still overall wavy and crimped, there is a certain limited elasticity to them as the crimps are ironed out in elongation. However, once this elongated state reaches 10% beyond the original length, further elongation will require work against the crosslinks that inhibit motion, and this is hard work indeed. In fact, attempts to increase the length of collagen by more than about 10% often will result in rupture of the fibers. The more the collagen chains are crosslinked, the more rigid they become, and the harder one must work to extend them. It appears that the crosslinking of the body's collagen with glucose is an important factor in the loss of flexibility with aging (Subsection 22.A, *Physical Aging*, page 495).

When animal flesh or bone is boiled with acidified water, the collagen helices unwind to give a solution of polymer chains which are then randomly intertwined. On cooling, this solution forms a semisolid gel called gelatin, or Jello commercially. When the collagen of our skin is present as triple helices, the skin itself is vibrant and resilient, however, on aging, the helices again tend to unwind and the skin sags under the pull of gravity.

Among the five different types of collagen, there is one that is "normal", one that is unusually stiff and one that is unusually elastic [5, 485]. These distinctions are largely hereditary. Those who inherit the very loose form of collagen can become contortionists and more or less show the Ehlers-Danlos syndrome, in which the flexibility of the collagen is so extreme that joints easily become dislocated, skin is very elastic but very fragile, wounds are slow to heal and the internal organs and blood vessels tend to collapse from lack of support. Both nutritional and hereditary flaws in collagen biosynthesis can lead to Ehlers-Danlos symptoms without involving any change in the elastin content of the tissue.

If, on the other hand, the fibroblasts run wild and generate excess collagen, then the result will be skin which is extremely tough and inflexible (a condition known as scleroderma), and ligaments which pull the joints out of alignment. This condition would clearly pose great problems for the *yogasana* student. By far the stiffest and strongest form of collagen-based connective tissue is bone, a composite material formed from collagen (30%) and bone minerals (70%). This tissue is discussed in detail in Chapter 8, THE BONES, page 235.

Elastin

Elastin is another fibrous material found in connective and supportive tissues, in this case, having the ability to deform to a large extent and then return to its former size and shape. Elastin is also highly resilient, which is to say, when it is stretched it stores energy, and when the stretch is released, a large fraction of the stored energy is returned as heat. Though the structure and composition of elastin fibers are not well understood, they are thought to be rather smoother proteins than are the forms of collagen, with fewer crosslinks and interchain binding. This "smoothness" allows elastin chains to readily slide past one another, and so allows the strain in elastin to reach 200% before the fibers separate, whereas the corresponding figure for collagen is only about 10%. Moreover, when the elongation of elastin is released, the fibers return to their original, prestressed length.

The connective tissues of the body are variable blends of the collagen and elastin fibers. Those structures such as the ligaments and tendons that are overwhelmingly collagenous are strong and rigid, whereas those that are overwhelmingly made of elastin are supple and extendable, like the ligamentum nuchea and ligamentum flavum of the cervical vertebrae. All connective-tissue structures are a blend of these two extremes. Because of its extreme elastic property, tissue high in elastin is found surrounding those sites in the body where expansion is of utmost importance, *i.e.*, in the walls of arteries and veins, the air cells of the lungs, in some ligaments and in erectile tissue.

Ground Substance

Ground substance is a viscous gel, forming the matrix within which the collagen, elastin, and cells function. Being fluid, ground substance serves largely as the agent for intercellular transfer of various cellular materials, for the connective tissues otherwise are without any of the blood vessels which normally serve this function. Being glue-like, ground substance does serve to bind cells together in muscles, *etc.*, which is to say, connective tissues high in ground substance are flexible and binding, but offer very little support against outside mechanical loads. Ground substance may also function as a lubricant within moving muscle, as when *yogasana* poses are held for several minutes [391].

Though ground substance is largely formed from carbohydrates in solution, in some situations the basic component of the ground substance is a proteoglycan, this being a huge molecular complex between a protein, a sugar and considerable water. When proteoglycan is combined with more or less collagen or elastin, the result is a range of substances called cartilage. Cartilage is a tough, rubbery material which is not only strong in tension, as are the regular connective tissues based on collagen, but also can be strong in compression, shear, bending and torsion, unlike regular connective tissues, Section 9.B, page 280.

Ligaments and Tendons

Collagen predominates in those connective tissues which require great mechanical strength. Tendons, ligaments and joint capsules consist almost totally of parallel bundles of collagen fibers interspersed with fibroblasts which produce the collagen. Such collagen-rich structures will be very strong in regard to tensile stress, but will be very rigid.

The collagen polymers that form the ligamentous and tendon tissues are in a pleated form in the resting state, but when stressed positively, the pleats are ironed out and the tissues extend. This elongation is accompanied by the generation of a significant amount of heat, which in turn acts to further soften the tissue [262]. However, because ligaments contain a higher percentage of elastin (see below) than do tendons [251], less heat is generated on stretching ligaments than tendons, and so ligaments have a higher resistance to prolonged stretch and resume their normal folded configuration more quickly than do tendons. Some ligaments can be stretched 25–30% of their resting length (that is, the strain equals 0.25–0.30, Subsection 7.E, *Stress and Strain*, page 228) and some in the cervical spine can be elongated to 200% to allow flexion of the neck! [262] In contrast, the ligaments that bind the knee, for example, have little or no elastic content, and stretching them leaves them permanently loose and ineffective in stabilizing the knee (Subsection 8.E, *The Knee Joint as an Example*, page 265). In general, there is no need to stretch the ligaments in the *yogasanas*, for stretching them can destabilize the associated joint.

Ligaments, tendons and joint capsules are among those connective tissues that are very high in collagen, that are naturally stiff, and that serve the body as inextendible substances. If in our *yogasana* work, we mistakenly take these materials beyond their mechanical limits, the results will be torn tissue that is extremely slow to heal and unstable joints that can readily cascade into all manner of bodily misalignments.

Myofascia

Fascia is the tough connective tissue that holds us together, enveloping all structures of the body, from the tiniest blood vessel to the largest bone. Meaning "band" or "bandage," the fascia most often occur as membranous sheets, dividing the body into compartments. The totality of the fascia in the entire body is a single system, for one can travel from any point in the body to any other point without ever having to leave the fascial highway. Because all body parts are interconnected by fascia, any tension or stretch in one part of the pattern will be rapidly transmitted from the point of application to further parts, as in Fig. 9.A-1.

In general, the fascia of the body have their fibers oriented longitudinally, however the orientation in some places is transverse, where it acts as a flexible support (as with the thoracic and pelvic diaphragms), and to control lateral spreading. Yet other fascia may be randomly oriented. The fascia have some mobility and elasticity as witnessed by any ballet performance, however, where the fascia is under constant stress, there is a hardening and thickening of the tissue. If the muscles are strongly exercised, they may outgrow their fascial sheaths, leading to very restricted ranges of motion.

Of the three facial layers of the body, our focus is on the myofascial layer which covers the muscles, muscle fibers, bones, and blood vessels [5]. Approximately 30% of the muscle mass is attributed to the connective tissue about and within the muscle. In such dense fibrous connective tissue, or myofascia, the relative amount of collagen is very high, with the fibers packed tightly around the fibroblasts, either in an orderly parallel array or more randomly. When packed in the parallel arrangement, this tissue has a very high tensile strength and so is found in most ligaments and tendons. In the tendons, the connective tissue blends smoothly and seamlessly into the various layers of the myofascial connective sheaths which surround the muscle fibers (see Section 7.A, Skeletal Muscle; Structure and

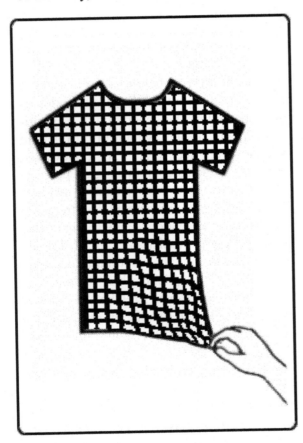

Fig. 9.A-1. An elastic medium when pulled at one point as with the hand and shirt shown above, transmits the strain to distant parts of the system. A similar distortion-at-a-distance is produced by stress in the myofascial system of the body.

Function, page 167). This layer of fascia lies just below the surperficial layer.

With respect to muscles, the myofascia perform three functions [5]:

1) They bind the muscle fibers together and orient them in a common direction, along with the blood vessels and nerves serving the muscle. At the same time, they serve to separate the muscles from surrounding structures.

2) Should the muscle be less than totally contracted, the myofascial connective tissue serves to spread whatever stress there is from the muscle action over a large area, and so offers a safety factor for the muscles.

3) They serve to lubricate the muscle internally, so that the component parts can move easily with respect to one another when the muscle changes shape.

As was discussed in the case of muscles, Subsection 7.E, *When Stretching, Time Matters, and Time Is on Your Side*, page 224, connective tissue is a viscoelastic material. That is to say, it has properties of both the ideal viscous and elastic materials. When the myofascia are weakly stretched and then relaxed, the original length of the tissue is fully recovered, as appropriate for an elastic material. In contrast, when the stretching is done slowly and held for a long time, on release of the tension, the material is permanently elongated, as appropriate for a viscous material. If muscle were only elastic, one could never change its length by stretching it, for an elastic material will always return to its original length after releasing the stress on it. On the other hand, the ability of a viscous material to flow under stress allows it to be permanently lengthened following a tensile stretch and release. It is this latter characteristic of the viscoelastic muscle leading to a permanent lengthening which we exploit in *yogasana* practice, provided the muscle and/or myofascia are not injured in the process.

As students of *yogasana*, it is most interesting to note that in a relaxed muscle being slightly stretched, the resistance to stretching can be apportioned as follows: 47% to the connective tissue (ligaments) in the joint capsule, 41% to resistance from the fascia, 10% to resistance by the tendon and 2% to resistance from the skin overlying the muscle. This shows that a very significant portion of the energy required to stretch a relaxed muscle is expended in stretching the myofascia surrounding the muscle as a whole and each of the muscle fibers as well. Furthermore, when a muscle is exercised and the muscle grows in girth, the amount of fascial tissue also increases, so that the muscle becomes yet more difficult to stretch, unless equal time is given to this end. As explained in Box 9.A-1, there is an economic aspect to myofascia as well as a yogic one.

When a material such as connective tissue is stressed in one dimension, a one-

BOX 9.A-1. WHAT PRICE MYOFASCIA?

In the meat market, the prices on the various cuts of muscle vary inversely as to the proportion of myofascia in the cut, *i.e.*, the most expensive cut of meat has the least amount of myofascia and so is the most tender. In the cow, this honor falls to the fillet mignon, which is the psoas muscle (Subsection 8.D, *The Legs and Feet*, page 247) of the animal. In bipeds, this muscle is depended upon for posture much more so than in quadrupeds, and so our psoas may not be as myofascia-free and tender as the cow's.

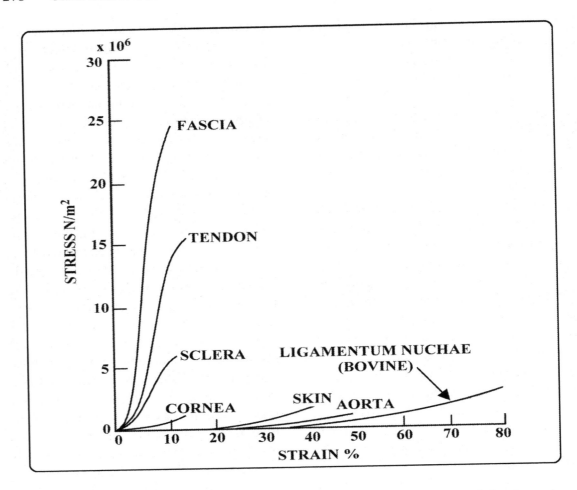

Fig. 9.A-2. Stress-strain curves for various connective tissues. The stiffness of the tissues is defined as the slope of the stress-strain curve; at between 0 and 10% strain, myofascia is seen to be stiffer than tendon, and both are far stiffer than skin or the aorta.

dimensional deformation (strain) is induced in its shape. These two quantities can be plotted against one another as in Fig. 9.A-2 for various body tissues; the slopes of these lines are equal to the stiffness of the body parts. Obviously they differ from one another and are different depending upon the extent of the stress, *i.e.*, a soft structure can become stiff when extended too far. The resistance of a tissue to tensile stress is a measure of safety, for truly stiff structures are not easily injured. Stiff students in *yogasana* practice may not feel that they are stretching very far, but on the other hand, they rarely sprain a ligament or strain a muscle, whereas the hypermobile students

have very soft tissue, can easily overextend, and so can be more easily injured by their stretching.

How far should one then stretch in the asanas? Speaking physiologically and psychologically, the answer as given by Alter [5] is to stretch to the point of pain, but not beyond it. However, as discussed in Section 10.D, Pain, page 294, pain is a very subjective sensation, and so Alter's answer to the question will have a different meaning for different students. Furthermore, if one is already injured, stretching to the point of pain may be going too far and so can cause further injury. Iyengar [210] also answers this question, stating, "When practicing asanas, go beyond thoughts of pleasure and pain.... When you feel that you have obtained the maximum stretch, go beyond it. Break the barrier to go further."

What is somewhat more certain with regard to stretching connective tissue is that the time factor can be very important, as can the temperature. If a stretch is held at a constant elongation, with time the tensile stress will relax by itself. Similarly, if the stretch is conducted at constant stress, then the elongation (called "creep" when done at constant stress) takes place naturally as one waits. It is also known that a strong stretch held for a short time yields largely an elastic deformation, while a more shallow stretch held for a longer time will result in a viscous lengthening of the muscle that is more or less permanent. High temperatures encourage myofascial elongation, especially if the muscle is heated while stretched and is then cooled while in the stretched condition [5]. Muscle strength is yet another factor to consider. When a muscle is stretched strongly at a low temperature but for a short time, the loss of strength on relaxing is larger than when the stretch is softer and longer, and done at a higher temperature. It is admittedly difficult to apply these facts gathered from isolated muscles in a science lab to living students in the yoga studio, but it strongly suggests that not too deep stretches held for long times would be the most effective, especially if the room is warm.

Following Kapit, *et al.* [229], a few of the other relevant connective-tissue types are described below.

Other Connective-Tissue Types

In loose connective tissue, a viscous fluid (the ground substance) forms the organic matrix, within which several different cell types float, along with a loose tangle of collagen fibrils and a few elastin strands as well. The loose connective tissue is found under the skin as superficial fascia, and allows the skin to roll back and forth over the deeper myofascial layers.

In adipose tissue, the cells of the tissue are largely fat cells, clumped together, and with only a scant amount of collagenous fibers present. Adipose tissue usually is found under the skin and covering the surfaces of some of the viscera.

Effects of Age on Connective Tissue

The effects of age on collagen and elastin appear to be the same. In both, the amount of crosslinking between chains increases with increasing age, resulting in a loss of flexibility. Simultaneous with this, the ground substance loses water with age (ground substance is 85% water in infants *versus* 70% in adults) and becomes more viscous. Immobilization of a joint also leads to connective-tissue crosslinking and rigidity. As one might hope, it appears that exercise and regular use of the joints can work to decrease crosslinking in the associated connective tissue and so increase flexibility. This is where *yogasana* practice can become a very important factor in one's quality of life as one ages.

Connective-Tissue Injury

According to Benjamin [34], the cruciate ligaments of the knee can be damaged by fatigue of the thigh muscles which then fails to keep the knee joint open and in alignment. This fatigue of the thigh muscles (as one might experience in the standing poses) places too much weight on the cruciate ligaments and as they fatigue, they slowly tear. *Padmasana* also can stretch and weaken these ligaments, which makes them then more vulnerable to this type of injury from fatigue of the thigh muscles. Benjamin describes this type of injury as "horrid", and I agree. Once damaged in this way, one must forego all forms of *padmasana* and any sort of deep knee bend for a long while. However, see Box 8.E-1, *A Safe Way to Teach Pamasana*, page 266, for a relatively safe way to learn, to approach learning, and/or to teach *padmasana*.

Though such injuries to the ligaments of the knee are very slow to heal, Benjamin does point out that such healing can be speeded greatly through the use of proliferants, largely innocuous substances like dextrose, which when injected into the joint space, strongly stimulate new cell growth in ligamentous tissue [132].

When the integrity of the skin is breeched due to a cut of any sort, the healing process involves the activation of fibroblasts and the generation of a tangled web of collagen fibers at the site as a skin patch. A hypertrophic scar is then formed at the site of tissue injury at great cost to the local flexibility of the skin at that point. If the injury is deep enough to have severed muscles as well, the collagenous binding of the muscle tissues and fascia as they heal will result in a significant tightening of the muscle as the internal scar will impede the relative motions of the muscle fibers with respect to one another. Most often, when a muscle is torn, it is the ligaments and/or tendons that have suffered the injury, and which must therefore bear the scars [34].

Myofascial coverings of the muscles serve to separate the muscles and to ease the movement of one muscle past another. Myofascia are not meant to bear weight, so, for example, if the feet tire in standing poses and the arches of the feet then collapse, then the plantar fascia across the bottoms of the feet needlessly bear the body's weight and plantar fasciitis results [34]. Stretching the calf muscle, as when extending the heel away from the knee in straight-leg poses will aggravate plantar fasciitis. Obesity too can be a factor here.

SECTION 9.B. CARTILAGE

Cartilage plays a dual role in the body: it is both a rather stiff material capable of helping to support the weight of the body (as with the intervertebral discs, Section 4.C, page 87), and also serves as lubricant at the points where bone meets bone (as in the knee joints, Section 8.D, page 247). In regard stiffness (technically, the ratio of the stress to the strain in a structure, Subsection 7.E, *Stress and Strain*, page 228), cartilage is more stiff than regular connective tissue, and less stiff than bone. A rather lax form of cartilage is found in the external ear, but is of no significance to yoga. Cartilage is a more primitive tissue than bone [319], as one might guess from reading Box 4.A-1, *Ontogeny Recapitulates Philogeny*, page 69.

The early fetus is composed largely of hyaline cartilage (see below), allowing a high fetal flexibility and a safe delivery for both mother and child. This cartilaginous skeleton of the neonate at first resembles the cartilaginous skeletons of sharks and rays [473] (Box 4.A-1, *Ontogeny Recapitulates Philogeny*, page 69), but is then slowly transformed into the bony skeleton of the infant as it is vascularized (Section 8.A, *Bone Structure, Development, and Mechanics*, page 235).

As described in Subsection 8.A, *Bone Structure and Development*, page 235, the cartilage of the infant is the model for the later formation of the bones. The fetal cells known as chondrocytes (or chondroblasts) generate cartilage so as to form the model skeleton. Once this is penetrated by the vascular system, bone-growth proteins become active and the chondrocytes are transformed into osteoblasts which excrete the inorganic salts that mineralize and further stiffen the cartilage, and so turn it into bone [222].

Like bone, cartilage is piezoelectric, and so is able to display the momentary pattern of mechanical stresses on it as a pattern of voltages. However, though bone has an extensive system of blood vessels and nerves, neither of these is found in cartilage.

Because not all of the fetal cartilage is vascularized, a certain fraction remains in the adult body to serve various functions. Nonetheless, not being vascularized means that if it is in some way injured, there will be very little support for healing and repair. Injuries to cartilage (as well as to avascular ligaments and tendons) are very slow to heal.

As with the regular forms of connective tissue, different forms of cartilage can have differing amounts of collagen, elastin and ground substance, and depending upon the relative amounts of these three substances the resulting composite can have widely varying properties.

Another form of cartilage, fibrocartilage, is much like dense regular connective tissue, but with the parallel collagen bundles interspersed with chondroitin sulfate and parallel bundles of matrix-producing cells, the chondrocytes. This tissue forms the outer casing of the intervertebral discs (Section 4.C, Intervertebral Discs, page 87), and also is found in the areas of the joint capsules and ligaments.

The weight-supporting tissues, *i.e.*, cartilage, are dense tissues of great strength and high water content. In hyaline cartilage, one again has collagen fibers, this time embedded in a gelatinous matrix, the whole being rather solid yet flexible. Such hyaline cartilage is found capping the epiphysial ends of bones (Fig. 8.A-3), and also is prominent in the ribcage. The sliding of one hyaline-covered bone with respect to another is eased by the lubricating synovial fluid exuded within the joint capsule. In joints of relatively low mobility, there also are cartilaginous connections between bones which function as ligaments. Thus, the intervertebral discs are largely cartilage and function as ligaments, and there is a cartilaginous connection within each hip joint binding the femur head to the acetabulum.

When the cartilage-covered surfaces of the bones in contact at a joint are sliding well, the forces are compressive only. However, if the surface becomes sticky, then there is a tendency for the forces to become more shearing in nature, and the result can be ripped cartilage [34, 473]. This can happen most easily to the meniscus cartilage of the knee in *padmasana*, or when twisting the knee while it is bearing weight, as in *mulhabandhasana*.* If injured, this avascular cartilage is nourished by diffusion of nutrients via the synovial fluid. However, this diffusion can be aided greatly by repeated cartilage compression and release of the joint [5, 473], for this pumps the surrounding fluids in and out of the pore spaces of the tissue, just as with the diurnal compression and extension of the intervertebral discs (see Section 4.C, Intervertebral Discs, page 87).

When cartilage is kept under a constant load, it creeps to a region of lower compressive stress, is permanently deformed, and suffers from poor nutrition. On the other hand, cartilage health is maintained by a dynamic compression which first squeezes and then releases the cartilage. Looking at the misaligned knee joints in Fig. 8.D-1c, one would expect the cartilage covering of the bones to be chronically thinner at the points of contact, and therefore to be less well-nourished at those points.

---

* This suggests that, for safety reasons, poses such as *mulhabandhasana* be learned from a sitting position so that there is little or no weight on the knee as it is being twisted and bent.

Chapter 10

THE SKIN

The paradox of the skin is that it is both a barrier between one's self and the outer world, and at the same time, it is one's window onto the world that lies beyond the self [222]. As the former, it is key to keeping all sorts of toxins and predatory species from entering the body, and key to keeping the life-sustaining chemicals within the body in their places. Not only is the skin largely waterproof in both directions and tough enough in most situations to be puncture-proof as well, but it is also an important element of the body's temperature-regulation apparatus, an organ of purification and an organ of metabolism. Moreover, it is a gland of sorts, for vitamin D is manufactured in the skin.

Though it is not widely realized, "the skin" does not stop at the entrances to the body's orifices. Skin continues over the lips and into the mouth, goes down the throat into the stomach, through the intestines and to the anus. All of our "insides" in fact are firmly and seamlessly attached to the outside skin, but with modifications to suit particular functions. This Chapter deals with what we can consider to be the outer skin, whereas the inner skin is considered in Chapter 18, THE GASTROINTESTINAL ORGANS AND DIGESTION, page 441.

The skin also serves as the interface to the experiences of the outer world beyond the skin, thanks to the large numbers and many types of sensors located within it. In this Chapter, the many aspects of the skin's function will be discussed, along with the special properties of its sensors, and how they relate to the practice of *yogasana*.

SECTION 10.A. STRUCTURE OF THE SKIN

The skin is one of the largest organs within the body, accounting for about 8 pounds of an adult's body weight and spanning an area of 18 square feet. At the lowest magnification, skin is seen to consist of three distinct layers, the epidermis, the dermis, and the subcutaneous layer, Fig. 10.A-1. The outer-most layer of the skin, the epidermis, is an avascular layer consisting of a lower layer of living cells (the basal cell layer) covered by an outer layer of dried, scaly cells (the horny layer). These two layers are separated by a third layer of maturing cells, the squamous layer. Cells of the horny layer contain a large amount of keratin, and are being constantly sloughed off as dead skin and replenished from below. Within and through the epidermis grow the nails, hair, and various superficial glands of the body. The thickness of the epidermis is largest in those places that bear the most weight (the soles of the feet and palms of the hands), and varies from about 4 mm in the sole of the foot to about 0.1 mm in the eyelids. Ridges in the epidermal layers of the skin on the palms of the hands and the soles of the feet aid in gripping the sticky mat in poses such as *adho mukha svanasana*.

A closer study of the epidermal layer shows it to consist of at least four layers, the deepest of which, the Malpighian layer,

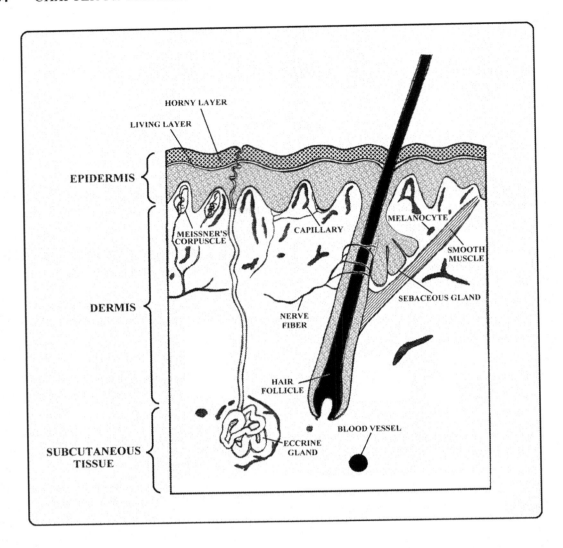

Fig. 10.A-1. A cross section of skin showing the three layers, the epidermis, the dermis and the subcutaneous layer, and several of the other structures found in those layers [222].

gives birth to epidermal cells which diffuse upward as they mature, to eventually become the dead scaly cells of the horny layer (Fig. 10.A-1). As the horny layer sloughs off (more than a million dead cells are cast off every hour), new cells are being produced at the same rate in the deepest layer. Formation of a new cell in the Malpighian layer requires only about 2 hours and such a newly-born cell has an average lifetime of about 27 days [222] before it is cast off. With a lifetime of only 27 days, a 70-year-old person will have made and discarded approximately 850 skins in a lifetime!

The layer just below the epidermis is known as the dermis. It is vascularized, and being made largely of connective tissue (collagen and elastin, Subsection 9.A, *Myofascia*, page 276), it functions largely as the skin's supportive layer. This basal layer of the skin is the thickest, and contains vessels for both blood and lymph, as well as nerve endings sensitive to touch, pressure, pain, heat, *etc*. The vascularization of the dermis plays a strong role in the regulation of the body's temperature, whereas the connective tissue works to hold the upper layers of the skin in strong contact with the deeper layers of fat and muscle. The dermis also contains the melanocytes, cells bearing pigment which can give skin the outward appearance of pink, yellow, brown or black, depending upon the quality and quantity of the pigment. Below the dermis lies the third layer, subcutaneous tissue, which is both muscular and the storehouse for the body's fat, which serves both as fuel and as cushioning.

The two chief structural components giving skin both its strength and resiliency are collagen and elastin, two proteinaceous substances, Chapter 9, CONNECTIVE AND SUPPORTING TISSUES, page 273. Exposure of skin to sunlight weakens these proteins. As we age, the skin loses water, connective tissue becomes more dense and less elastic, and the skin loses about 30% of its thickness as it becomes dried, wrinkled and flaccid. Because skin in this state is easily bruised, teachers of *yogasana* must use care in adjusting students having this condition.

One's ability to move deeply into a *yogasana* in some part depends upon the resistance to stretching of the skin overlying the muscles being stretched. This resistance of the skin to stretching is smallest in students with large, round bodies and largest in students who are thin. This stretching of the skin in *yogasana* offers an external signal to the *yogasana* teacher and an internal signal to the alert student as to what is happening in deeper layers of the student's body.

Scars in the skin are formed when the skin is cut, and the cut edges are then bridged by collagen fibers which contract to pull together the two sides of the wound. Scar tissue is the remnant of the bridging collagen, and will severely impede the stretching of the skin.

Two types of specialized cells that are found in the skin, the receptors for surface sensations and the glands, are described more fully in their respective Sections below.

SECTION 10.B. SENSORY RECEPTORS IN THE SKIN

There are a variety of sensory receptors populating the skin, with the abilities to record sensations not only of touch and pressure at the surface and at deeper layers, but superficial sharp pain, deep tissue pain, heat, cold, and tension as well. The largest number of receptors are for sensing pain while the least number are for sensing temperature. There are an estimated 50 receptors in a patch of skin 1 cm square, however, the number is closer to 200 per cm^2 at the tip of the tongue [356]. It is important to point out that the sensors for light and deep pressure (this Section) are totally different functionally from the receptors for pain (Section 10.D, page 294) in the same skin areas.

Skin also serves as a channel for communication between humans [320], and as such is closely linked to our emotions (Subsections 10.B, *The Skin, Emotions, and Touching*, page 291, and *Yogasana and Touching by the Teacher*, page 291). Because of this, the *yogasana* teacher must be aware of the possible emotional content that can accompany the touching that often is a part of *yogasana* teaching.

Receptor Adaptation

When considering the skin and its multitude of sensors, it is important to understand the concept of adaptation in regard to the receptor signals. Should any receptor be activated with a stimulus which is constant in time, it appears to fatigue more or less, such that its response falls with time, Fig. 10.B-1. This is called adaptation. As shown in the Figure, a receptor with a rapid adaptation has an output which falls rapidly to zero, in spite of the constant stimulus, *i.e.*,

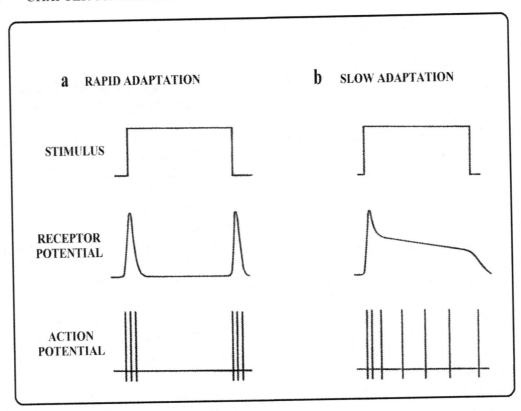

a RAPID ADAPTATION   **b** SLOW ADAPTATION

STIMULUS

RECEPTOR POTENTIAL

ACTION POTENTIAL

Fig. 10.B-1. Comparison of the receptor and action potential responses for (**a**) a rapidly-adapting receptor and for (**b**) a slowly-adapting receptor, both responding to the same square-wave stimulus. In the latter case, the receptor potential falls only slowly during the stimulus and the action potential remains above threshold over the full course of the stimulus, but with decreasing frequency. In the former case, the action potential is above threshold only at the rapidly rising and rapidly falling ends of the stimulus, and so the receptor potential is zero at all places except at the points of rise and fall.

its response is nonzero only when the stimulus is rapidly changing, as when it is first applied or removed. In contrast, a receptor with a slow adaptation has an output which only slowly decreasing; the frequency of its receptor potential falls with time, albeit slowly, even though the stimulus level is constant. For example, if you place your fingertip on the lip, there is a momentary sensation as they come into contact, but this fades rapidly to zero because of the rapid adaptation of the touch receptor. On the other hand, the sensation persists as the fingertip is drawn over the lip.

The significance of the differences in adaptation is that a rapidly-adapting receptor only gives a momentary signal whenever the stimulus switches on or off, but not in between. Thus it is useful in tracking a stimulus that moves rapidly across the skin, but is ineffective in staying in touch with a constant stimulus. In contrast, a slowly-adapting receptor will give a signal of almost constant amplitude for a long period, but has no use in tracking a signal that varies rapidly in time or space. These consequences are presented below in the context of the touch receptors of the skin [222, 225].

Anticipating receptors to be met in the following Subsections, the Meissner, hair receptors and the Pacinian corpuscles are all rapidly-adapting receptors, whereas the Ruffini and Merkel receptors are slowly adapting [222, 308]. Note that the rapidly-adapting sensors do not adapt due to a rapidly-developing fatigue, but that they are constructed to be inherently sensitive to the changing character of stimuli and to be insensitive to constancy [57]. Such rapidly adapting signals would be especially useful when trying to balance, as they would activate only when falling (Appendix IV, BALANCING, page 525).

As we come into a *yogasana* posture, the proprioceptors (Section 7.C, page 208) are actively sending their messages regarding body position and movement to the brain for synthesis into a complete body-posture picture. Because the neural signals adapt toward zero amplitude in time, one's sense of postural alignment fades. However, in the Iyengar approach, one first poses and then reposes [22] by continuously making slight adjustments. This constant readjustment keeps the pose dynamic and from the proprioceptive point of view, would seem to repeatedly refresh the proprioceptive pic-

ture in the subconscious. Rapidly-adapting sensors would be important in this situation.

Light Touch

Several types of receptors occupy the more superficial layers of the skin, receptors such as Meissner's corpuscle, Merkel's disc, the Pacinian corpuscle, and the nerve plexi at the hair roots, Fig. 10.B-2. The sensitivity of such surface sensors to light touch depends upon their depth beneath the skin's surface, but also upon the density of touch-sensing units, or equivalently, the reciprocal of the distance of separation D between neighboring sensor units, *i.e.*, 1/D. Simple experiments with pins, a ruler, and a willing subject show that the tongue, genitalia, tips of fingers and lips have only a 1–3 mm separation between sensing units, whereas on the back of the hands, on the back body itself and on the legs, the separation can be as large as 50–100 mm, Fig. 10.B-3. Because the density of touch sensors in the fin-

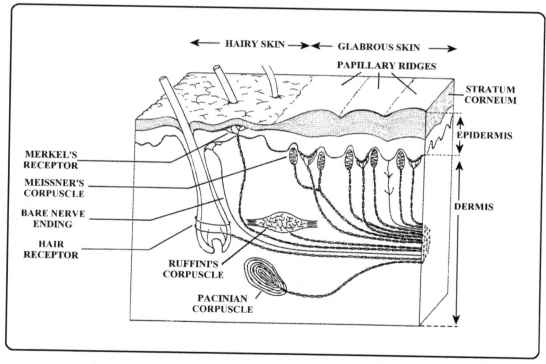

Fig. 10.B-2. The various mechanoreceptors found in hairy and glabrous skin at various depths, with afferent neurons myelinated with Schwann cells.

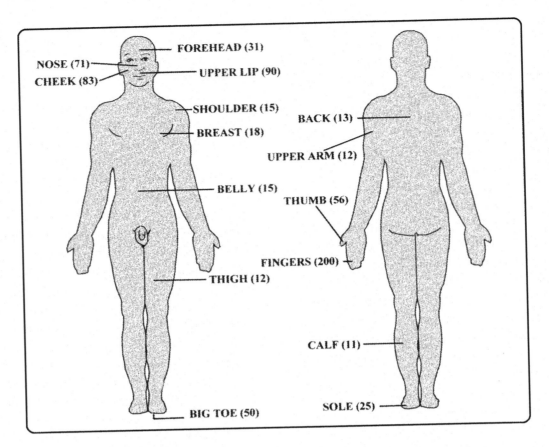

Fig. 10.B-3. Relative measurements of the densities (number per square centimeter) of receptor cells for surface pressure in the skin of the human body. The highest densities of such receptors are on the hands, face and big toes, in agreement with the relative proportions of the sensory cortex devoted to these areas, Fig. 3.A-5b.

ger tips is 15 times as large as that on the legs, the area in the cerebrum for finger sensations is larger than that for leg sensations. Similarly there are more than 15 times as many touch sensors on the tongue than on the back of the hand [192]. Consequently, the skin-sensation map in the cortex is highly distorted from the body form with which we are familiar. These differences in the degrees of spatial discrimination are reflected in the proportions of the sensory homunculus of Penfield [229, 355], Fig. 3.A-5b. There is no representation of the heart, liver, or kidneys in the sensory homunculus, as sensations from these are referred to other skin areas [313] (see Section 10.E, Dermatomes and Referred Pain, page 303).

In the case of Meissner's corpuscles (sensitive to very light touch, especially plentiful on the lips and fingers, but found on all surfaces of the body), the receptors are solidly in the rapidly-adapting category [222]. When in a *yogasana*, the parts of the body touching the floor will report pressure signals from the Meissner's corpuscles for proprioception, but only for an instant as these sensors are rapidly adapting. Such proprioceptive signals can be refreshed in time by slight shifting of the weight on the floor as when making small adjustments, but not when in *savasana*.

The afferent nerves carrying the signals of light touch and pressure utilize type-A fibers, *i.e.*, thick, myelinated and with rapid signal conduction (about 10 m/second), as is characteristic of the newest biotechnology available to primates and humans (Section 5.B, Nerve Conduction, page 114). One clearly sees the effect of age on skin sensitivity, for the average number of light-touch Meissner's corpuscles per mm^2 is 80 in the three-year old, 20 in the young adult, and falls to 4 in old age [320].

The signals from pressure and touch receptors that are rapidly adapting ascend the spinal cord to the thalamus and then radiate to the postcentral gyrus in the sensory cortex. However, just before entering the spinal cord, the sensory nerves branch so as to provide collaterals to the alpha-motor neurons participating in reflex-arc circuits (Section 7.D, page 211). The ascending fibers from the light-touch receptors also send branches to midbrain motor centers and to centers in the reticular formation to influence involuntary motor activity. The sensory nerves from different parts of the body are bundled more and more as they ascend, but they still keep their sense of order, with the nerves from the legs on the inside of the spinal cord and those from the arms, neck and face on the outer edge. These packing patterns are then resolved into a coherent picture of the body in the higher centers of the brain.

That signals from the light-touch receptors can be factors in conscious intelligence is shown by Braille reading, wherein one can learn to read patterns of raised bumps on paper using the fingertips, and these patterns are then understood by the conscious mind as letters. Other forms of "dermographia" are discussed by Montagu [320]. Perhaps this is a form of the skill developed by Iyengar [211], for whom reading the messages of the skin in *yogasana* plays such a large role. One can imagine in his case that the muscle tensions generated in the *yogasanas* pull on the skin so as to stimulate the light-pressure and deep-pressure sensors, and that he is consciously aware of the pressure patterns in the skin generated by both the muscles upon the overlying skin and by the pressure of the floor.

It is worth noting that Iyengar [211] places great stress on the skin as both an organ of perception and as the body's outermost boundary. In the work of the *yogasanas*, he strives to connect the intelligence of the mind to sensations in the skin and the underlying flesh. All the while, he remains relaxed so that the skin is not overstretched to the point of becoming painful. Once the link between skin sensations and the intelligence of the mind is established, then one can begin to move from the skin toward the soul, the innermost level of the body.

Tickling on the other hand is random stimulation of nerve endings, registering as confusion in the cerebellum [345], but it is strange (and meaningful) that you cannot tickle yourself, nor can someone tickle you if you dislike them; only someone you like can elicit the laughter of tickling [320]. This suggests that in the over-abundance of touch signals going upward to the spine, those involving self touching are discarded as unimportant, whereas those with a stronger emotional content (a lover's caress or an insect crawling up one's leg) register more insistently in the conscious sphere.

Sensors of the skin often are involved in reflex arcs, as when one steps barefooted on a sharp object and instantly lifts the foot, or tries to pick up a hot potato and immediately drops it. See Section 7.D, Reflex Actions, page 211, for details on the neural circuitry involved in such arcs.

Deep Pressure

The Pacinian corpuscles, Fig. 10.B-2, are located in the deeper layers of the skin and respond to heavy pressure at those deep layers [230]. These receptors consist of a sensory nerve ending surrounded by a collagenous capsule. When deformed by external pressure, the capsule walls change their permeability to Na^+ ions, thus leading to a DC voltage change within the capsule which is proportional to the pressure. As with many such mechanoreceptor signals, it is transduced into the frequency domain so that the pressure is proportional to the frequency of the signal rather than its DC magnitude, and the modulated signal then is sent to the central nervous system.

Because the deformation of the Pacinian capsule is quickly relieved by a readjustment of the layers of the capsule, the signals from the Pacinian corpuscles are rapidly adapting, and as such, they produce a signal only when the stimulus is rapidly changing.

Pacinian corpuscles use type-C neural fibers {slow (1 m/second), thin, unmyelinated} for afferent transmission, as found in the basic primitive sensory systems of all vertebrates [230]. These type-C fiber bundles synapse at the dorsal spine and then terminate at the thalamus. As discussed in Section 7.C, Proprioception, page 208, signals from the Pacinian corpuscles may help in constructing an instantaneous proprioceptive map of the body in motion because they do extend all the way to the thalamus, and the thalamus is known to share information with many parts of the brain involved with construction of such a map.

Pressure on the skin so intense as to produce a wheal involves the sympathetic nervous system in the case of white wheals and parasympathetic vagal hyperactivity in the case of red wheals [320]. White wheals immediately result from pressure on the skin, for at this time, blood is absent from the tissue as superficial blood vessels contract in expectation of a large letting of blood to the outside. However, after about 7 seconds, blood does flow to the injury site and it becomes red and swollen as fluids leak from the affected cells, forming a red wheal [387].

Up to this point, it is a question as to what sensor is slowly adapting such that it can continue to give a pressure signal from the skin on a long-term basis. It would appear to be the Merkel cells, which are slowly adapting and are sensitive to skin indentation. When the student lies down for *savasana*, there are immediate sensations from the Meissner, Pacinian and Merkel receptors, but the first two fade rapidly to zero and only the sensations from the Merkel cells persist. After five minutes or so, even the Merkel-cell sensations have adapted and one loses totally the sensation of the back body pressing on the floor, unless the muscles are periodically reactivated. When in poses held for long periods of time, such as *sirsasana, etc.*, sensations of pressure from the floor after 5 minutes or so will involve the Merkel cells, unless there are frequent readjustments of the posture. It is rather strange that we *yogasana* students spend so much time walking around in bare feet, for one generally hardens the soles of the feet in this way, thereby making them less sensitive to pressure.

As discussed in Section 7.B, page 208, the Ruffini corpuscles are subcutaneous sensors, sensitive to the magnitude and direction of skin deformation as the muscles below flex and relax. Such slowly-adapting and direction-sensitive sensors of skin deformation are assumed to play a large role in the construction of the proprioceptive map.

Other Receptors in the Skin

It is thought that the temperature receptors are just free nerve endings in the skin [230], but they must be more than that, since there are two distinct types, Krause corpuscles for sensing temperatures below 33º C (91.4º F) and Ruffini corpuscles* for sensing temperatures above 33º C (91.4º F) [195]. Both use slow (less than 2.5 m/second conduction velocity) types-C and A_{gamma} fibers. As with other skin receptors, the information from the temperature sensors is presented to the brain as a frequency representation. These sensors are intimately involved in the thermal regulation of the body, Section 10.C, page 292. Nociceptors for pain sensing (Section 10.D, page 294) seem to be just free nerve endings, as are the temperature receptors.

The Skin, Emotions, and Touching

It is no surprise that tactile stimulation of the skin can be of great importance to our emotional stability. Thus actions such as head scratch, rubbing of the chin, rubbing of the eyes, *etc.*, are self-comforting and help to reduce tension. Because clasping of the hands also releases tension, both facial self-massage and light hand clasping can be recommended when doing *savasana* with tense beginner students.

Montagu [320] discusses several examples of how the body may express psychosocial and cultural stress as skin disorders. Thus soldiers bombarded repeatedly in World War I developed a darkening of the skin called "fear melanosis". In other cases, pent up anger and frustration precipitated itching which was satisfied by scratching. The waxing and waning of many diseases of the body are expressed through eruptions through the skin.

Yogasana and Touching by the Teacher

One can do no better than to read Montagu's monograph on the skin [320] in order to learn how absolutely crucial touching is to the proper socialization and maturation of the infant. This is true in different cultures, at different times and in different species. Babies who are cuddled, pressed to their parents' breast, wrestled with, tossed and caught, swaddled, *etc.*, are much more outgoing, sociable and happy as children and adults than are their touch-deprived brothers and sisters.

Even as adults, the innocent touch can be a life-affirming gesture for those who are otherwise untouched for whatever reason. This can be especially true for the elderly. To be touched in a sympathetic way by another person is to connect with them not only on a yogic level but on a personal level if they need to feel that. *Yogasana* practice with a teacher offers the opportunity for such touching as a side benefit to proper *yogasana* instruction, but also for its own sake. Somewhat the same comforting effect can be got when the student holds himself or herself as in *pasasana* or *pavan muktasana*.

The object in touching the student in *yogasana* is either to try to reconnect the student's consciousness with the muscular action in a particular region of the body or to aid a particular motion from the outside. If the teacher wants to stress the rolling inward of the upper thigh for example, then it is sufficient to use the fingertips to brush the flesh of the thigh in the proper direction, giving a student a clear signal of what is to be done. In this situation, it is the rapidly-adapting Meissner's corpuscles that respond to the touch and transmit its sense of movement to the brain.

When placing the hand on a student with the intention of moving a limb, *etc.*, the full

---

*These temperature-sensitive Ruffini corpuscles in the skin are not to be confused with the Ruffini corpuscles also within the skin, which function as stretch receptors, Subsection 7.B, *Ruffini Corpuscles*, page 208.

length of the hand (fingertips to palm) should be placed on the limb, and the fingers should point in the direction in which you wish the student's flesh to move. The teacher's hands should never press on flesh that is not supported by bone, *i.e.*, never press on the eyes, throat, lower abdomen, *etc.*, and never hold or press at a joint, but rather at the belly of the muscle. Physiologically, when the skin over a muscle is stimulated, the large muscle fibers are activated more quickly and used more efficiently, leading to an increase of muscle strength [390].

When the student is adjusted manually by the teacher, and the student is receptive to that touch, then a bond of sorts begins to develop between the two. This bond can be strengthened if the teacher adjusts his/her breath so as to be in synchrony with that of the student. In this case, the signal for movement on the student's part is on the exhalation [266].

In working to move students appropriately, you will find some students who clearly like the touching aspect of the adjustment, or at least like where the adjustment is taking them, as witnessed by their sigh of pleasure. On the other hand, there also will be students who for whatever reason, do not like to be touched, especially women by a man. Teachers must remain alert to this possibility and respect the student's wish without seeking clarification or further comment. If you are rebuffed, rather than taking it personally, consider instead that the woman may have been abused by a man as a child or as an adult, and is not ready to be touched in any way by a person in authority. Many times, demonstration on the teacher's body rather than on that of the student, or use of a prop will suffice to get the yogic point across without violating a student's personal space.

In this regard, there is a general confusion among many people that equates tactile touching with sexual touching. The differences between these two kinds of touching are described very clearly by Juhan [222], and should be clear in the minds of *yogasana* teachers if not in the minds of their students.

SECTION 10.C. THERMAL REGULATION BY BLOOD VESSELS AND SWEAT GLANDS IN THE SKIN

Metabolism of fuel within the body continuously generates more or less heat, whereas homeostasis within the body demands that the core temperature of the body (98.6º F, 37.0º C) remain relatively constant. The general problem in regard to body heat is that of transferring more or less of this internal heat to the external environment, thus keeping the core temperature constant. The importance of temperature regulation is clear once it is realized that if the temperature of the body rises beyond 106º F (41.1º C), there is danger of kidney dysfunction, muscle breakdown, loss of brain function and death. The skin is an active participant in the mechanics of thermal regulation.

The skin, as the body's largest organ, plays a central role in the temperature regulation of the body's core, using two mechanisms [230]:

1) There are special blood vessels in the dermal layer of the skin that do not serve to nourish skin cells, but serve only for thermoregulation. Depending on whether these vessels are dilated or constricted, they bring more or less blood from the warmth of the core to the surface of the skin where the blood is cooled by contact with the surrounding air and by radiation into space. Blood flow at the skin can vary by as much as a factor of one hundred depending upon the diameter of these vessels, and under normal conditions with the body at rest, 70% of

the body's excess heat is lost by radiative and conductive cooling through the skin.

Our skin is a very responsive organ to the state of balance in the autonomic nervous system, Table 6.A-2. When the sympathetic nervous system is dominant, the blood vessels at the skin surface constrict so as to send the superficial blood to large muscles [195, 229, 319], and with this, the skin temperature drops [80]. At the same time, sweating is copious [195, 229, 230, 319] and the electrical resistance of the skin decreases [80]. This latter is the basis of the lie detector, predicated on the idea that the stress of lying generates a sympathetic response and sweaty palms (see Box 6.E-1, *Yogis Can Beat the Lie Detector*, page 160). When instead, the parasympathetic nervous system becomes more active, the blood vessels in the dermal layer are dilated, the skin temperature rises and the shivering response to cold is inhibited [343]. The skin temperature at the fingertip is often taken as reflecting the relative activities of the sympathetic and parasympathetic nervous systems [80, 343]; the greater the stress (physical or mental), the greater the sympathetic arousal, and the colder the fingertip.

2) At temperatures below 37° C (98.6° F), water passes from the pores of the skin directly to the vapor phase without really becoming the liquid we know as sweat. However, when one is physically active and the body temperature rises above 37° C (98.6° F), Fig. 10.C-1, sweat droplets form on those parts of the skin having an abundance of sweat glands; only the tip of the penis, the clitoris and the inner labial lips have no sweat glands, (Section 14.C, Sweat, page 395). Sweating is not only an essential part of the body's attempt to maintain thermal homeostasis, but the sweat glands are also a part of the body's purification system. This is discussed further in Section 14.C, Sweat, page 395.

Due to the high heat of evaporation of water (0.6 calories/gm) the evaporation of the aqueous component of sweat leads to a substantial evaporative cooling of the skin and of any blood-laden vessels close to the skin. Evaporative cooling normally is called upon to deal with only 15% of the body's heat loss, but in a hot, dry climate, this can increase to 90% [43]. This second mechanism ceases to be of much utility when the relative humidity is high, as high humidity retards evaporation.

The two mechanisms of controlled blood-flow to the skin and evaporative cooling are so efficient when working in tandem [109] that the thermal output of the body may be increased twenty-fold by vigorous physical exercise, yet the core temperature rises by less than 1° C (1.8° F)! Note too, that whereas the core temperature of the body is held to a constant value, the skin temperature will vary over the body and that this variation will depend upon the temperature of the outside air, as seen in Table 10.C-1. As might be expected from its location, the foot's temperature most closely follows that of the outside air, whereas the temperature of the head, chest, and body core are the most resistant to such changes of air temperature.

Physical exercise as a way to keep warm is excellent in the short term, but quickly leads to exhaustion and thence to dire straits. In very cold weather, the hairs of the body hug the skin and the skin shivers in order to generate heat at the surface.

As with all animals, just how effective the body is in ridding itself of excess internal heat depends upon the extent of its effective surface area with the surrounding air. As this effective area can change with body posture, it will be different in different *yogasanas*. That is to say, cooling of the core can be less efficient in folded but otherwise cooling poses such as *paschimottanasana* where the upper and lower parts of

TABLE 10.C-1. VARIATION OF SKIN TEMPERATURE OVER THE BODY AT TWO DIFFERENT AIR TEMPERATURES.

Skin of Body Part	Temperature when air is 21° C (70° F)	Temperature when air is 35° C (95° F)
Hand	28° C (82.4° F)	35° C (95.0° F)
Head	33° C (91.4° F)	35.5° C (95.5° F)
Upper Chest	32.5° C (90.8° F)	35.5° C (95.9° F)
Foot	21° C (69.8° F)	34.5° C (96.8° F)
Core	36.1° C (97.0° F)	36.5° C (96.8° F)

the body press on one another, as compared with *savasana*, where they do not. *Savasana* in hot, humid weather should be done with the arms well separated from the torso for this reason. Contrarywise, when performing the *yogasanas* in a cold room, it is more heat-conserving to work with the body in folded positions than in open positions, all other things being equal. In a parallel way, the sweat pores of the skin automatically close in cold weather and open when it is hot. Note too, that long, thin bodies will cool more quickly than short, stout bodies because their ratio of surface area to volume is larger.

Emotions also have a profound effect on the temperature of the skin. Fear and anxiety lead to a lowering of the skin temperature, to pallor and dryness (the first two of which signal excitation of the sympathetic nervous system), whereas embarrassment and pleasure raise the skin temperature with obvious blushing.

The effects of a regular *yogasana* practice on thermoregulation have been reported by Bhatnagar, *et al.*, [40] who find that the resting core temperature decreases by 1° C after several weeks of beginner's practice, and that the rise of the core temperature following strong exercise is less in those who practice *yogasanas*. These results support the idea that *yogasanas* slow the metabolic processes and so these processes produce less heat in the body per unit time. A com-

parison of two groups of trainees, one in "physical training" and one doing *yogasana* instead, showed that the *yogasana*-trained students were more resistant to cold, shivering less and shivering only at a lower temperature than those taking the physical training [418]. This is in accord with *yogasana* practice raising the level of parasympathetic excitation in the autonomic nervous system, for parasympathetic excitation raises skin temperature and inhibits shivering, Table 6.A-2.

The general factors involved in generating and dissipating heat in the body while exercising are summarized in Fig. 10.C-1. The magnitudes of the in-flowing and out-flowing heats will depend upon many factors, but will be adjusted automatically so as to keep the core temperature constant.

SECTION 10.D. PAIN

The yoga practitioner who is committed to teaching often will find herself enmeshed in other people's pain, and will quickly come to see how much pain there is in the world, and how great are our efforts to avoid pain if we can. Understandably, it may very well seem that the world would be a much better place if pain could be banished from our lives, however, that view ignores the fact that pain is a useful signal, alerting us to something going wrong in the body, and that those without any sensitivity to pain are

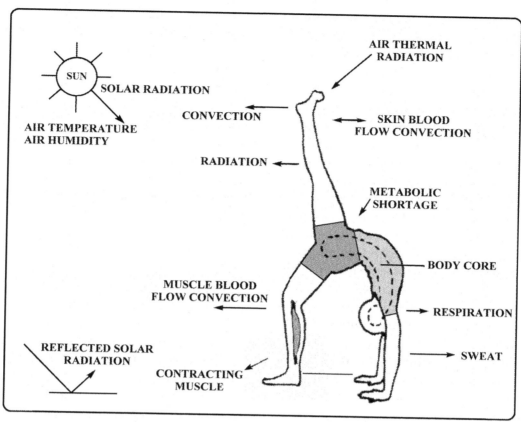

Fig. 10.C-1. Several factors that influence the heat balance within the body as modulated by the skin. In-flowing heat is represented by inward facing arrows and out-flowing heat is represented by outward facing arrows.

at great risk for harming themselves because they do not receive the alarm signals. Touch a hot object and the pain of the contact goes immediately to the somatosensory centers in the spine and leads to an immediate withdrawal of the hand before further damage can be done; without the pain signal, the damage to the hand might otherwise be catastrophic. Conversely, pain is not only uncomfortable, but often causes muscles to contract and so blocks the responsiveness of the tissues involved. Frequently, there is strong activation of the sympathetic nervous system when we are injured and feeling pain.

Because pain is both a sensation and a perception, perhaps more so than with any other sensation, pain brings the body and the mind together at the level of the central nervous system. Pain often has two major components: 1) the sensation of pain at the site of physiological damage, and 2) the emotional responses to the pain, such as worry, anxiety, and agitation which can act to keep the pain gates open, or exercise, relaxation, and understanding the sources of pain, all of which act to keep the pain gates closed. Component 1 of pain involves the somatosensory cortex and reflexive activation of the relevant muscles, whereas component 2 goes to the limbic system in the brain (Subsection 3.A, page 33) and there adds an emotional component to the sensation. *Yogasana* practice can be of great use in regard point 2), as with practice, one can learn to more or less control the pain (Subsection 10.D, *Yoga, Injury, and Pain*, page 301).

Still, one of the lessons of our *yogasana* practice is that some pain is an inescapable part of life, and that one can learn how best to handle such times of unavoidable pain by practicing pain control in the *yogasanas*, by learning how to minimize the pain, how to deal with that part of pain that cannot be ignored, and how to get on with one's life.

Though the topic of "Pain" is discussed under the heading of "The Skin", pain receptors are to be found not only on the skin, but deep within the body, and unlike the situation with pressure and touch, the pain signals are slowly adapting and therefore long lasting. When the pain signals are delivered to the brain, there is a diffusion of the signal to many different areas simultaneously, *i.e.*, pain involves a highly-distributed processing system within the central nervous system. It can be difficult to launch a pain signal unless one is supersensitive, and once launched, it can be difficult to turn it off.

The Physiology of Pain

The sensations of normal stimuli are reported to the central nervous system using the normal sensory routes of the peripheral nerves. However, if the stimulus is so intense as to injure the tissue at the site of stimulation, then a chemical reaction ensues which results in the stimulation of pain receptors, called nociceptors, which have their own sets of dedicated neural pathways into the central nervous system. The brain itself has no pain receptors [230], however, see Subsection 3.B, *Headaches*, page 37.

The nociceptors as found on the skin, in the joints and muscles, and in the viscera, can be triggered by thermal (both hot and cold), mechanical and chemical insults to the body tissue. Unlike all of the other mechanoreceptors (Section 7.B, Muscle Sensors; The Mechanoreceptors, page 198), those for pain are simply the free nerve endings of the pain-conducting nerve fibers,

Fig. 10.B-2. Some endings are specific for thermal or mechanical pain stimuli whereas others are polymodal, responding to all forms of pain-generating stimuli.

The nociceptor fibers in general are either the A_{gamma} myelinated fibers (Section 5.B, Nerve Conduction, page 114) having high conduction velocity and giving the sensation of sharp, stabbing pain, or the more slowly-conducting C fibers, which are polymodal. It appears that signals of intense pain travel more quickly than those for slight pain [190]. Once tissue is injured and the pain signal is sent upward, then inflammation is initiated.

The free nerve endings of the nociceptors have relatively high thresholds for activation, so that those noninjurious stimuli which can strongly excite touch receptors, for example, do not excite the pain receptors. If the stimulation is so strong that the tissue cells are injured, then the affected cells burst and immediately release chemicals into the surrounding tissue. Two of these released chemicals that are of the most interest to us are the prostaglandins and histamine.

The prostaglandins (a group of 14 different substances), when released from injured cells, act to sensitize and to activate the free nerve endings of the nociceptors in the vicinity of the injury. With this sensitization, exposure of the nerve endings to substances at the injury site such as serotonin, bradykinin, or histamine leads immediately to a pain signal launched along the nociceptor toward the spinal cord. From there, the nociceptor signal may become active in a reflex arc (withdrawal of the foot from a sharp object, say), and/or may branch upward toward the cortex, to be registered psychologically and consciously as pain. Aspirin and NSAIDS (nonsteroidal anti-inflammatory drugs) work to block prostaglandin production and so can lessen the pain sensation. Prostaglandins not only stimulate uterine contractions during childbirth, and during the active phase of the menstrual cycle, but are prominent in the brain during headaches at the times of menstruation [118].

Histamine acts not only to trigger the pain reaction, but also to promote inflammation, the first stage of healing following an injury. Histamine vasodilates the blood vessels locally so that the injured tissue is flooded with fresh blood, making the affected area redden and rise in temperature. It also promotes a super-permeability of the vessel walls, so that extra lymph (Section 11.G, page 352) is produced and swelling appears. The inflammatory response can be inhibited by cortisone. Once a tissue site is damaged, the threshold for generating a nociceptor action potential is lowered below that of the initial threshold, *i.e.*, the injured area becomes more sensitive to pain stimuli.

In general, repetitive sensory signals command the brain's immediate attention and then are dealt with in one of two ways. If the signal is only mildly bothersome (as with a loud radio in the next room when one is trying to practice), then the central nervous system becomes habituated to the signal and its sensation fades with time. In contrast, if the sensation is truly noxious (pain from a stone in the shoe or worse), then the central nervous system becomes sensitized to the signal, and it becomes even more painful over time. See Subsection 3.C, *Consolidation and Long-Term Memory*, page 45, for a further discussion of the effects of sensitization and habituation on neural morphology. In the case of the noxious stimulus, the neural circuitry associated with the action that is persistent over time changes so as to make the neural path easier to traverse. This is called learning (Section 3.C, *Memory, Learning, and Teaching*, page 42). Unfortunately, if pain signals are transmitted for a sufficiently long time, the neurons learn this lesson too, and then are able to

transmit pain spontaneously. Called chronic pain, this condition is often associated with psychological/emotional problems [186].

In the case of chronic pain, the neural circuits may be cut surgically, however, even severed nociceptors seem to find new paths to the brain and so can re-establish the pain signal. Over time, the nociceptors also can develop resistance to the most powerful opiates.

The above discussion focuses on nociceptive pain, *i.e.*, the pain arising from tissue injury which is sensed by the nociceptors in the vicinity of the injury and then transmitted as a pain signal to the central nervous system. On the other hand, it is also possible to have neuropathic pain, wherein the nerve itself is injured, and the pain signal is spontaneous and on-going. Even in this case, psychology is a large factor in one's response to the pain. It appears that men and women use different neural circuitry in sensing pain.

The flip side of pain is pleasure. The centers for registering both intense pain and intense pleasure are found in the hypothalamus. Though the locus ceruleus is known to be the center for pleasure, the concept is poorly understood, other than to say that pleasure is a driving force in humans, much like hunger, thirst, sex, *etc.* The centers for pain and pleasure are linked to the motivational system in the limbic area (Box 2.B-1), and encourage certain behaviors, rewarding some with pleasure, and discouraging others with pain. Being motivationally driven, we can never get enough pleasure. This drive differs from homeostasis (Subsection 6.A, *Homeostasic Control; Feedback and Feedforward*, page 133), where there is a driving force only when the system is out of balance [120, 225, 357].

The Psychology of Pain

The interaction between the body and the mind is perhaps nowhere more evident than in the area of pain perception, for examples abound of how one person's intense physical pain is unbearable, whereas another person with the same injury but with a different attitude toward it is able to bear the pain with grace and good humor, or perhaps not even be aware of it at all. Box 10.D-1 below lists several examples of the cultural and psychological factors that can influence our perception of pain.

Factors such as the above will be at work more or less in all of the students in *yog-asana* class, and the teacher must be open to the wide range of pain responses possible among the uninitiated. As a *yogasana* teacher, one must be aware of how suggestible our students might be and how open they are to suggestions about "good" pain and "bad" pain. This is discussed further below in Subsection 10.D, *Yoga, Injury, and Pain*, page 301. A second type of pain is discussed in Section 6.B, The Hypothalamus, page 140.

Sarno [403] takes a different approach to pain. He argues that unresolved emotional problems lead to a sympathetic excitation in the nervous system that raises the resting muscle tone, Subsection 7.B, page 204. As a result, there is an ischemic (low blood flow) condition in the soft tissues (muscles, nerves, tendons) and the affected tissue responds to the oxygen deficit with sensations of pain. In his view, the "herniated disc" problem is a nonstarter in regard lower-back pain, for the problem is emotional rather than mechanical, and the cure is mental rather than surgical.

Neural Aspects of Pain

The neural fibers for nociception enter the spinal cord and then travel upward, some passing through the thalamus, and some passing through the reticular formation (Subsection 3.A, page 31) on their way to the cortex. Attempts have been made to map the pain loci in the cortex, as has been done for tactile sensation (Fig. 2.A-6), however, no regularities could be found. It appears that at the conscious level, pain signals are processed in parallel and at widely distributed points in the cortex.

Sensations originating in the skin and muscles travel into our consciousness using the spinothalamic tracts of the central nervous system, these being nerve bundles in the white matter at each of the two sides of the spinal cord. The tract is bilateral because the skin and muscles that it serves are bilateral. By contrast, pain signals from the internal organs use the dorsal tract of the spinal cord [430], an area on the back side of the cord.

The conclusion that the level of pain perceived is very dependent upon other circumstances (emotional and psychological) is well documented. For example, fear raises the sensitivity to pain, while thinking deeply sexual thoughts erases pain. This is rationalized by noting that the nociceptor axons are synapsed with many non-nociceptor neurons (both ascending and descending) in the central nervous system, thus affording ample opportunities for modulation or even blocking of the ascending pain signal through the intervention of inhibitory interneurons (see the discussion below on the endorphins). The reticular formation also integrates ascending and descending neural information, and so would be able to lessen or block totally the nociceptor signal as it attempts to pass upward from that point, just as it suppresses or transmits neural signals from any of the other sensory receptors.

The gate-control hypothesis of pain-lessening is outlined schematically in Fig. 10.D-1. In this theory, both the C-fiber nociceptor and some non-nociceptor neuron (A_{alpha} for touch, for example) are energized simultaneously as with a pin prick. Being adjacent in the skin, these afferent

BOX 10.D-1: CULTURAL AND PSYCHOLOGICAL FACTORS IN PAIN

Abundant evidence exists that the psychological component of pain is huge, that our mental and cultural attitudes toward pain greatly influence the magnitude of the sensation we sense as pain, and that our response to pain is a learned behavior. Listed below are several examples of these aspects of pain gleaned from a large body of work in this area [153].

* Mediterraneans tolerate pain poorly.

* A level of heat that northern Europeans consider as merely warm is considered by Israelis and Italians as intolerable.

* Jewish women increased their tolerance to a pain stimulus after they were told that Jews have a low tolerance for pain. When told the same thing, the pain threshold for Protestant women did not change.

* Jews are big complainers about pain, wondering about its meaning and what the implications might be for their having been chosen to suffer. Italians are also big complainers about pain, and wonder how they can gain relief.

* Nepalese porters carry heavy loads to the tops of the world's highest and coldest peaks without complaint. Tests show that these people are just as sensitive to stimuli as Westerners, yet they can endure much higher levels of pain. The Nepalese have been taught by their culture to stoically endure pain levels that Westerners consider unbearable.

* If an infant sees its parent scream at the slightest pain, that infant will learn and execute similar responses in its own life.

* Chronic pain can generate psychological neuroses; when the pain is relieved, the neuroses vanish.

* People often experience horrific war wounds yet rarely complain about the pain while the same sorts of injury incurred in a peacetime situation often involve intense pain and anguish.

* When one is angry and the sympathetic nervous system is activated, one is less sensitive to pain, whereas on the other hand, when one is afraid and anxious, the sensitivity to pain increases [404]. A vicious cycle is set in motion, for pain promotes anxiety, which acts to intensify the pain.

* Pain is often more intense at night, when there are no other distracting influences and we can focus on the sensation. Rubbing a painful spot can diminish the pain signal by adding many other non-pain signals to the area.

* Men may react more strongly to serious pain than do women because they feel powerless in the face of something society expects them to endure silently, and because they resent having to depend upon others for relief.

* *Yogasana* students in India appear to have a mental point of view that allows them to bear significantly higher levels of discomfort than do the corresponding students in America, however, the Indian students are less energetic and less committed to their practice.

nerves are in the same nerve bundle and enter the spine through a common dorsal horn, where they synapse onto an interneuron in the spine. The effect of the interneuron on the nociceptor is assumed to be inhibitory (hyperpolarizing) and the effect of the non-nociceptor is assumed to be excitatory (depolarizing). This interneuron has an inhibitory synapse in turn with a projection neuron to which the nociceptor and the non-nociceptor are synapsed as well, with both of these synapses now being excitatory. Should the interneuron shown in the Figure be excited, it will act to hyperpolar-ize the projection interneuron, thus inhibiting it from sending its signal to the cortex. However, the projection neuron also is influenced directly by potentials from the C fiber nociceptor and from the A_{alpha} neural afferent, both of which tend to depolarize the projection neuron. In this circuit, both the C fiber and the skin afferent have an effect on the strength of the eventual signal moving through the projection neuron to the spinothalamic tract, either canceling it, weakening it or intensifying it. The glutamate ion and the neuropeptides act as neu-

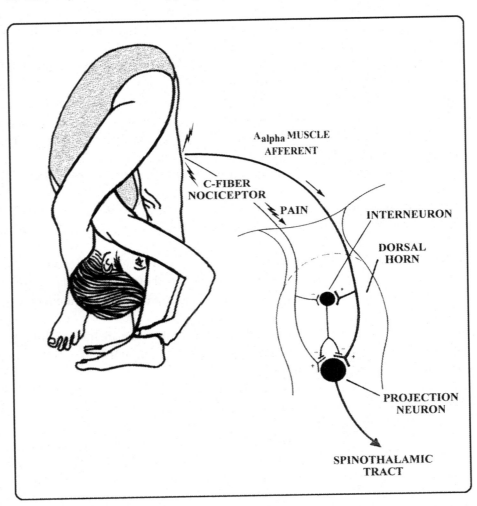

Fig. 10.D-1. The neural connections involved in the gate-control theory of pain. See the text for an explanation of how this mechanism can reduce the intensity of pain coming from the peripheral nerves, as when over-stretching in *ruchikasana*.

rotransmitters (Section 5.D, page 128) in the nociceptor realm.

An alternate scenario [186] also involves the gate-control theory. Here, the ascending nociceptor nerve has two descending nerves by its side, and synapsed to it at several points. Each of these synapses uses either serotonin, norepinephrine or endorphin as the neurotransmitter, and acts as a gate that can either block the pain, lessen the pain or increase the pain, depending upon supra-spinal decisions, mostly subcortical. Thus, in situations of extreme emergency, one might be totally unaware of the pain of one's own injuries, while consumed with the need to help others who are injured. In this situation, the gates for ascending pain signals have been closed by cortical actions that sense a higher priority, *i.e.*, helping others in pain. On the other hand, there is evidence that the sympathetic nervous system can act to intensify pain sensations, just as it sharpens certain other senses in time of danger [186].

Using the gate-control theory, one can rationalize the situation of pain induced by a herniated intervertebral disc, Section 4.C, Intervertebral Discs, page 87. In this case, it is assumed that there are no nociceptor free-nerve endings within the spinal cord, but that the herniated disc exerts pressure on the spinal muscle afferent, and that this pressure impedes the propagation of the action potential along its axon (Section 5.B, Nerve Conduction, page 114). This change in the afferent action potential then influences the potential balance at the projection neuron, Fig. 10.D-1, thereby allowing the pain signal access to the cortex. However, see below for an alternate explanation.

Yoga, Injury, and Pain

Pain is a graded response to injury, and at the lowest end of the pain scale, is expressed as discomfort. Feeling a sense of discomfort in a *yogasana* arises as one chal-lenges the psychological and physiological boundaries of our region of postural comfort. As long as one is comfortable in one's posture, there is no reason to change, no incentive for growth, and a general stagnation (Subsection 7.C, *Proprioception and Yogasana*, page 210). In order to grow and progress in *yogasana* practice, one must learn to push back the boundaries, *i.e.*, to be uncomfortable and to grow in the process. However, it does not follow that there is more growth or more rapid growth if the student will go from discomfort to pain.

As a muscle is stretched in a *yogasana*, many sensations will be sent to the brain for evaluation. At the beginning of the stretch, there is a strong sense of muscle tension from the stretch receptors, and a sense of the changing body position from the proprioceptors. The stretch sensation is a dull, delocalized feeling of discomfort which penetrates to the cortex and so is very present in the consciousness. If the stretch is now taken too far or too fast, the myofascial tissue will tear locally under the stress. In this case, the prostaglandin release will precipitate a sharp and stabbing nociceptive pain signal which is qualitatively and quantitatively very different from that of the stretch discomfort. Needless to say, the sensory goal in *yogasana* practice is to stay within the bounds of discomfort and not cross aggressively into the realm of tearing, pain, and inflammation. This is what Joel Kramer calls "working at the edge", using the breath and the mind to handle the discomfort of going to a new place, all the while honoring *ahimsa* (nonviolence), by remaining conscious of the limits which should not be exceeded. In this context, then, one can speak of "good pain" and "bad pain", depending upon which side of the discomfort-to-pain threshold one is on.

If one is suffering from sciatic pain (referred pain, Subsection 4.A, *Misalignment of the Spine and Deterioration of the*

Vertebral Discs, page 79) which radiates more or less down the leg or legs, then those *yogasanas* that tend to centralize the pain, *i.e.*, make the pain move from a more distant location such as the knee toward the base of the spine, are beneficial, whereas those that extend the pain yet further away from the base of the spine should be avoided [123].

There is another aspect of pain production that may be particularly relevant to the student of *yogasana*. When a muscle is either strongly contracted or over-stretched, there is a mechanical stress on the local musculature which slows the flow of blood into and out of the muscle. In response to this ischemic condition (low or zero blood-flow locally), the stressed cells exude arachidonic acid. In the presence of the enzyme cyclooxygenase, arachidonic acid is oxidized to the prostaglandins and the free nerve endings in the muscle thereby become sensitized to pain [225, 357]. This pain mechanism may be at work when stretching in the *yogasanas*, or afterwards if there is a residual spasm in the muscle in response to stretching. It might also be responsible for the pain of a herniated vertebral disc which presses on spinal muscles in a way that arachidonic acid is released, leading to the production of the prostaglandins (see the work of Sarno [402, 403]). As one might expect, if there are yogic ways to chemically generate pain, there are also yogic ways to chemically eradicate pain (see below, Subsection 10.D, *The Endorphins*).

Regardless of the exact physiological mechanism for pain and its relief, it is a good idea not to directly challenge pain through the *yogasanas*. Thus, for example, if one has a torn hamstring, one should avoid a direct hamstring stretch such as *uttanasana*, but it would be acceptable to work the hamstring peripherally, as in *dandasana*. A timetable for reasonable resting periods following different muscle injuries is given in Table 7.F-1.

If the pain signal stemming from a *yogasana* injury is not too severe, and the site is not inflamed or swollen, a brief but immediate relief of the pain sensation can be had by gently rubbing the affected area or slapping it so that the pain signal is swamped by the signals coming from the touch receptors in the area [366]. Analgesics and balms that cause a slight irritation of the skin also can be used to mask a more internal pain, and it is possible that acupuncture also works in this way to block pain signals to higher centers. Cold also can be effective as a counterirritant in erasing pain.

Yet another aspect of pain control in the yoga sphere involves placebo-like statements by the teacher. In the placebo effect (Subsection 6.F, *The Placebo Effect*, page 164), a person of high authority proclaims a procedure to be physiologically effective in curing a specific problem, and for about 1/3 of the students, there is a beneficial physiological shift on hearing the good news. Thus, receptive students might be reassured by hearing that there is a strong pull on the hamstring of the forward leg of *trikonasana*, and that it is more or less unavoidable in the beginner and is a "good" pain. This positive statement by the teacher would reduce anxiety on the part of the student, and with that, the pain in the forward leg.

Of course, yoga can be used in a deliberate way to reduce pain, rather than generate it. So for example, many stretches are designed to release tension in chronically-tense muscles and so give one a sense of relief from pain and discomfort. Elongations also are used to realign the bones of the body, thereby easing the pain at misaligned joints, *etc.* Mental anguish also can be relieved by *yogasana* practice (Chapter 20, THE EMOTIONS, page 463).

The Endorphins

Not only does the body have its own analgesics against pain (called endogenous opiates), but as will be seen below, these drugs are available on demand to the *yogasana* practitioner. Imagine that a pain signal from an outlying nociceptor travels to the dorsal root of the spinal cord. Normally, at this point, it synapses with a spinal nerve fiber which ascends to the thalamus and beyond to register its painful message in the higher centers (Subsection 4.B, *Neural Connectivity of the Spinal Cord*, page 86).

However, at the level of the dorsal root synapse with the nociceptor, there is a second synapse stemming from a descending neuron from the periaqueductal gray nucleus in the midbrain of the limbic system. The periaqueductal gray area within the brainstem has reciprocal connections to the hypothalamus, and is known to be intimately connected as well to sensations of pleasure and pain. This second synapse uses endorphin, a neuropeptide, as neurotransmitter, and its action when called upon is inhibitory. Thus if a signal is sent downward from or through the periaqueductal gray center to the dorsal horn, its effect will be to lessen or cancel completely the action potential of the ascending pain signal! In this way, the endogenous opiates dull or erase entirely the sensations of pain by effectively changing the threshold for the sensation of pain [225, 357]. This is thought to be the mechanism behind the "runner's high" experienced by distance runners.

Pert [357] also points out that receptors for endorphins are found throughout the central nervous system and that through proper breath control one can achieve control of the release of endorphins from the periaqueductal gray area. These released neurotransmitters diffuse through the cerebrospinal fluid to receptor sites at many places in the central nervous system and in this way inhibit the upward movement of pain signals. It has been shown that acupuncture also stimulates the release of the endorphins into the cerebrospinal fluid [13, 357].

The scheme put forward by Pert would fit with the general experience among students of *yogasana* that the discomfort of a challenging pose can be met by focusing one's attention on the qualities of the breath while keeping it moving in a smooth but deliberate way, or by visualizing each of the exhalations to be through the point of discomfort. It is also known that changes in the rate and depth of the breath release a flood of neuropeptides from the brainstem, and that many of these are endorphins [357].

It also must be said that a large number of pain-relieving neuropeptides have been identified, and that many of them have other functions as well besides that of analgesia. This may explain why there are receptors for these neurotransmitters throughout the body. Moreover, because the important periaqueductal gray area has many reciprocal neural connections with the hypothalamus, the door also is open for the influence of the autonomic nervous system on pain.

SECTION 10.E. DERMATOMES AND REFERRED PAIN

The afferent pain fibers (nociceptors) from the skin show a strong convergence on the dorsal-horn relay cells, often times joining with nerves from a visceral organ. The 31 pairs of segmentally-arranged spinal nerves then lead to a segmental organization of the receptive area of the skin surface into 62 distinct local surfaces, each such surface segment being served by its own spinal-nerve bundle. The area of skin innervated

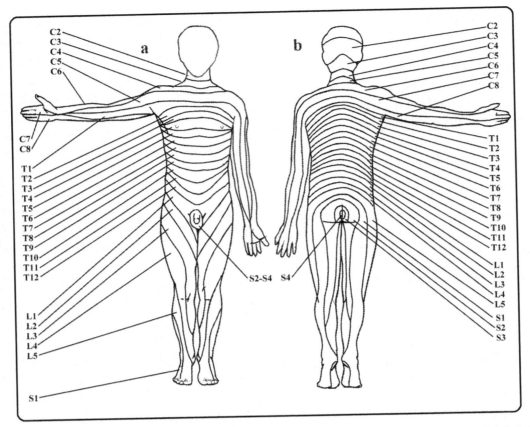

Fig. 10.E-1. The dermatome zones on the front body (**a**) and the back body (**b**), each labeled according to the vertebral designations of its dorsal root, Fig. 4.A-1.

by one spinal nerve is called a dermatome [195, 225, 229, 230, 313]*.

Extensive experimentation has led to the construction of dermatome maps of the sort shown in Figs. 10.E-1 and 10.E-2. Again, each dermatome shown there corresponds to the convergence of all of the superficial nociceptor nerves in that area onto one dorsal root of a spinal nerve. The edges of the dermatomes actually are not as sharply defined as shown here, for in fact, adjacent dermatomes have a large overlap. Table 10.E-1 shows how the nociceptor nerves in various places on the skin join those of the muscles and organs of the body and where they converge on the dorsal roots of the spinal column. One sees that the motor neu-

rons of the muscles closely follow the same nerve bundles as the overlying skin and synapse at about the same place on the spinal cord; in any event, specific spinal nerves receive information from specific body areas.

Interestingly, the visceral organ paired with the skin in a dermatome is not necessarily in close physical proximity to that dermatome. This arises from a lack of correspondence between the position of the skin and the position of the organ due to migration of the organ during both evolutionary development and fetal development (see Box 4.A-1, *Ontogeny Recapitulates Philogeny*, page 69). In the lower animals from which we ascended, the correspon-

*Actually, the first cervical nerve has no dermatome as it has no dorsal root.

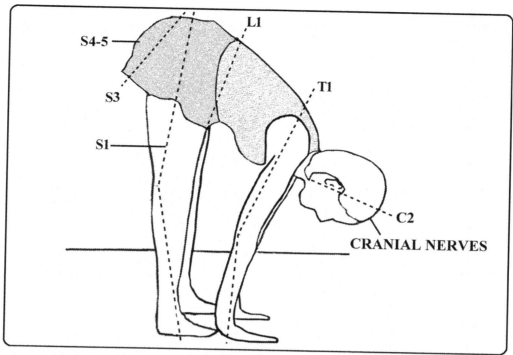

Fig. 10.E-2. The approximate positions of the dermatome boundaries corresponding to a few of the dorsal roots, while in *uttanasana*.

TABLE 10.E-1. CORRELATION OF DERMATOMES WITH SKIN AND ALPHA-MOTOR NEURONS WITH MUSCLES [195]

Dermatome Location	Dorsal Root Location	Muscles or Organ
Neck	C1–C4	Neck
	C3–C5	Diaphragm
Deltoid	C5, C6	Biceps
Radial forearm and thumb	C5–C8	Shoulder joint
Ulnar border of hand and little finger	C7–T1	Heart; Triceps and forearm
	C8, T1	Hands
	T2–T12	Axial musculature, intervertebral, respiration, abdominals
Groin	L1, L2	Thigh flexors
Knee	L2, L3	Quadruceps femoris
Dorsal side of foot and big toe	L5, S1	Gluteals
Lateral side of foot and little toe	S1, S2	Plantar flexor, ankle
Genito-anal	S3–S5	Pelvic floor, bladder, sphincters, genitals

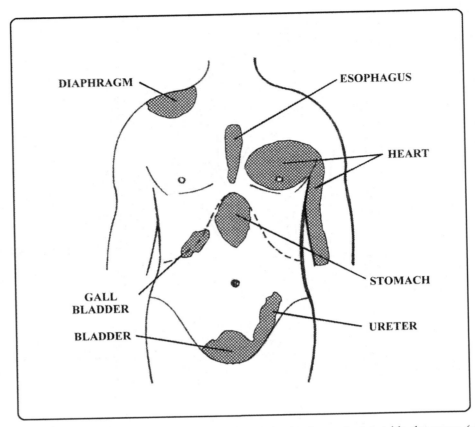

Fig. 10.E-3. Visceral pain can manifest as pain in cutaneous layers just outside the organ (stomach, bladder, *etc.*), or far removed from the site of the organ (heart, diaphragm, *etc.*), depending on the position of the relevant dermatome [195].

dence was more obvious, but evolution has changed this.

The existence of dermatomes which do not necessarily lie over the visceral organs with which they are paired neurally leads to the phenomenon of "referred pain". In this phenomenon, a visceral, deep-tissue afferent pain fiber synapses simultaneously on the spinal cord with other fibers of some superficial-tissue skin dermatome with a significantly different location on the body. The visceral pain signal from the misplaced organ is eventually sensed in the brain and misinterpreted as a pain in the skin rather than in the organ! For example, a heart attack brought on by an inadequate blood supply to the heart often is signaled by pain sensed at the ulnar side of the left arm because the dermatome for cardiac pain is displaced to the left arm (T1, T2); menstrual discomfort appears as lower back pain via L1–L5 [293]; kidney pain may be sensed as pain in the skin at dermatomes T10 and T11, whereas pain from the gallbladder appears in the upper right chest [155] and inflammation of the pleura appears as pain at the tips of the shoulders (C3–C5) [195], Fig. 10.E-3. In all of these cases (and more) the organ in question and the dermatome share a common spinal-cord segment, but the skin in question does not lie exactly over the affected organ, and the brain cannot distinguish the true source of the stimulus. If the nociceptor sensory nerves entering the spinal cord are accidentally pulled free of the cord, pain is then perceived in the corresponding dermatome, much like phantom-limb pain [225].

The dermatome afferent nerves of the facial skin do not pass through one of the segmental spinal nerves, but instead use trigeminal cranial nerve V for access to the central nervous system.

Theoretically, understanding of the dermatomes could be of use in *yogasana* practice, as for example, over-twisting could generate pain in the kidneys which was then referred to dermatome areas T10 and T11 and sensed as pain in the umbilicus. Similarly, the blood supply to the heart could be thwarted in an intense spinal twist, and the discomforting signal of the resulting ischemia could appear in the left shoulder! Severe compression of the right lower abdomen (the area of the appendix), as when performing *parivrtta trikonasana*, could lead to the sensation of referred pain on the center line of the body, close to the solar plexus [308], for this internal organ refers pain to this place; however, if the discomfort were in the peritoneum at the position of the appendix, then the pain would be sensed at the appendix because the point of peritoneum innervation in this case lies just over the appendix [308].

Something resembling the neural confusion inherent in the dermatome maps of the body as organs shift their locations but keep their neural connections appear in other instances. For example, pressure on the rectus muscles of the eyes works to slow the heart beat (Sections 6.D, The Parasympathetic Nervous System, page 150 and 7.D, Reflex Actions, page 211) because the relevant nerves of the rectus muscles of the eyes and the vagus nerve that controls the heart beat are in close proximity. Similarly, bright light often triggers a sneeze (the photic-sneeze reflex) due to the nearness of the optic and nasal nerves. Pain or discomfort along a particular nerve can be eased by scratching or slapping the skin in the area of the discomfort, for this sets up a flood of neural sensations which drown out the pain

signal using the same or nearby neural routes.

SECTION 10.F. GLANDS WITHIN THE SKIN

The Sweat Glands

The sweat glands in the skin of the human body outnumber the receptors by a factor of ten to one (there are 65,000 sweat glands in the palm of the hand and 5 million over the body), though the number of each decreases with age. There are two types of sweat glands in the skin, the apocrine and the eccrine. The first of these exudes a milky fluid in the areas of the armpits, the outer-ear canal, the nipples of the breasts when nursing an infant, the external genitalia and the orifice of the anus. This fluid from that part of the skin covered with hair is rich in fatty acids, whereas the fluid from the second type appears on skin where there is no hair (Fig. 10.B-2) and is much more watery and salty.

The sweat glands within the skin perform several useful functions. First, the fluid expressed by the glands is rich in body wastes. This detoxification is strongest when yoga students sweat, and often is so intense that the air in the yoga room becomes unbreathable after an hour's work. This problem solves itself as the body burns its impurities in the course of the regular practice of *yogasana*. The watery sweat from the eccrine glands also is of great use in cooling the skin surface, as discussed in Section 10.C, Thermal Regulation by Blood Vessels and Sweat Glands in the Skin, page 292).

The Sebaceous Glands

The sebaceous glands in the skin exude a fatty/oily substance (sebum) which helps to lubricate the skin and keep it pliant.

Furthermore, being acidic, the oil from the sebaceous glands is bacteriostatic, and so helps keep the skin healthy. The sebaceous glands are intimately associated with the hair follicles, and use the follicle as a path to the corneal layer of the skin.

The Tear Glands

The tear glands are discussed in Section 14.B, Tears, page 395.

SECTION 10.G. HAIR AND PILOERECTION

Hairs on the body surface are simple extensions of the epidermis, as are the fingernails and toenails. Hairs grow from structures within the skin called follicles; once a hair reaches maturity, it forms a club at the follicle base, which firmly anchors it in the skin, Fig. 10.B-2. When a new hair then begins to grow at the base of the follicle, the old hair drops out. Hair is constantly being shed in this way, at the rate of 50–150 per day. The hairs on our heads grow at 8 to 10 inches per year, and can reach on overall length of 6 to 8 feet. Obviously, such hairs must grow continuously for almost a decade before dropping out.

In emergency situations where the sympathetic nervous system might be activated, smooth muscles at the base of each of the body hairs is activated so that the hairs are brought erect (piloerection) and our body seems much larger to an aggressor [195, 230]. In furry animals, piloerection also seems to trap body heat, but this is not a factor for humans, except for the top of the head. Efferent nerve fibers to the muscles at the base of each hair make it stand on end whenever one is cold or frightened; these are the "goose bumps" we sense in such situations. In practitioners with refined control over the autonomic nervous system, activation of the pilomotor system can be brought under conscious control [282]. In such people, conscious stimulation of the sympathetic nervous system not only raises every hair on the body to an upright position, but also increases heart rate, respiration rate and depth of breathing, as well as pupil diameter and sweating, *i.e.*, the general spectrum of sympathetic responses, Section 6.C, The Sympathetic Nervous System, page 144.

Aside from sexual attraction, hair or the lack of same, seems not to play much of a role in the yogi's practice. Nerve plexi exist at the base of each hair; if and when a hair is moved, an afferent nerve impulse is triggered [229, 230, 473]. These hair receptors are undoubtedly triggered whenever a teacher touches a student's bare skin in order to make an adjustment.

Chemically, hair is composed largely of a piezoelectric fibrous protein called keratin, present as well in animal hooves, nails, horns, fish scales, silk and spider webs. Keratin is a highly elastic protein with a composition very different from that of collagen. The hairs on the heads of Orientals are round in cross section and therefore are straight, while hairs on the heads of African blacks are flat in cross section and therefore are curly, whereas those of Occidentals are elliptic and thus in between. In all cases, hair consists of keratin-filled dead cells, the only live cells being within the follicle embedded in the skin. The nails of the fingers and toes also are made largely of keratin. The growth rate of fingernails is about twice that of toenails.

The amount of body hair is largely determined by genetics, while the texture of the hair changes over a lifetime as the hormonal balances shift: androgens from the kidneys convert fine white hairs into pigmented stiff hairs and also can shift the relative abundances of hair in different areas of the skin [181].

Chapter 11

THE HEART AND THE VASCULAR SYSTEM

According to the ancient yogis, the heart (the *anahata chakra*) is the seat of the soul and the center for compassion. These yogis placed the body's consciousness (*jivatma*) in the heart, just a few inches to the right of the sternum, just where we now know the pacemaker of the heart to be located [399], suggesting that they possibly were conscious of this electrical stimulator.

According to modern medicine, the heart is the center of the circulatory system, pushing blood to every part of the body through its pumping action. The heart together with the various blood vessels that connect it to all the other parts of the body comprise the vascular system. Within the body, not all regions are served equally well by the heart: the primary task of the heart is to maintain the circulation of the blood through the brain, and many areas will be deprived in order to keep the brain well cared for. Of course, the heart itself must be well served by the vascular system if it is to take care of the brain's needs for circulation.

A key tenet of Iyengar's yoga therapy is that the *yogasanas* done properly act first to "squeeze" the blood out of a particular organ or muscle, and then on release of the squeezing, allow the organ or muscle to "soak" in the fresh blood that rushes in. In this way, circulation is brought into dull or sluggish areas and healing commences [407]. Improved circulation in the sick body implies that the body then can work more efficiently, performing the work it needs to

do with the expenditure of the minimum amount of energy. For students who are already in good health, practice of the *yogasanas* will avoid any stagnation of the body fluids, and so will keep them healthy as they age.

Following Schatz [407], assuming a slouched posture day in and day out compresses the multitude of internal organs from the heart to the large intestine as effectively as if they were tied with a tourniquet. In this state, the circulation of blood and lymph (Section 11.G, The Lymphatic System, page 352) is impaired, the channels through which they flow tend to collapse, and the hormones and enzymes produced at various sites in the body are not carried promptly to those places where they can do their work. With poor oxygenation of the muscles due to poor circulation, the muscle metabolism tends to shift toward the production of lactic acid, the presence of which in the body can generate a shift in the autonomic balance toward sympathetic excitation and stress.

In this Chapter, the physiology of circulation and the impact of this on *yogasana* and *vice versa* will be discussed. We will see how the heart pumps blood through the vascular plumbing of the body, how the autonomic nervous system influences this process, and how the internal pressure in the blood vessels is influenced by turning the body more-or-less upside down.

SECTION 11.A. STRUCTURE AND FUNCTION OF THE HEART

The Pumping Chambers of the Heart

Though the heart formally is a single, four-chambered organ, it functions more like two hearts side by side, each with an upper chamber (the atrium) and a lower chamber (the ventricle), Fig. 11.A-1. Let us call them the right heart and the left heart. The function of the right heart is to collect deoxygenated blood from the muscles and organs using the large veins. Contraction of the right ventricle then sends the blood via the pulmonary vein to the lungs for charging with oxygen and stripping of carbon dioxide. Once refreshed, the oxygenated blood first enters the left atrium and then the left ventricle, where a forceful contraction pushes it into the aorta and the arterial system connected to it (Section 11.C, The Vascular System, page 325). The left and right hearts are separated by a common wall, the interventricular septum, and share a common system of nerves which activates the two hearts simultaneously. The circulatory pattern external to the heart is shown somewhat more schematically in Fig. 11.A-2.

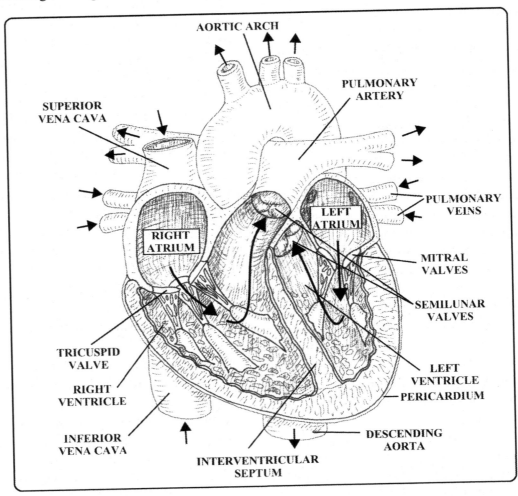

Fig. 11.A-1. Cutaway view of the heart and associated vascular plumbing, as seen from the front.

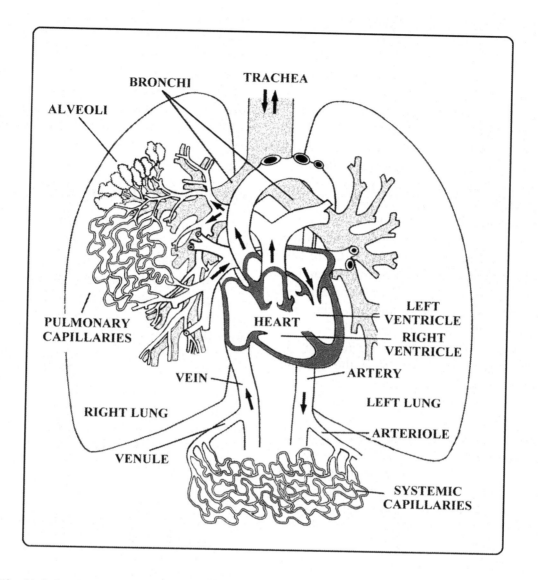

Fig. 11.A-2. Circulation of blood in the body follows a circular path, moving from the right heart to the lungs, back to the left heart and then through the vast network of the body's arteries, arterioles and capillaries, to return to the right heart via the venous network.

The pressure that the blood exerts on the elastic walls of the aorta is highest at the moment of ventricular contraction; this is called the systolic pressure. However, even when the left ventricle is relaxed while filling, the pressure at the aorta is not zero, because the walls of the aorta balloon outward during each pressure stroke, and even in the relaxed state continue to press inward on the blood contained within. This pressure in the relaxed state is called the diastolic pressure, and is nonzero because at the further reaches of the arterial system, the small arteries, called arterioles, offer a high resistance to the peripheral flow of blood and so do not easily allow the pressure to fall to zero.

Your health-care provider measures your blood pressure by putting a pressure cuff on the arm and pressurizing it so that no blood can flow through the artery in the arm. Listening then with a stethoscope, the pressure in the cuff is released until the systolic beating is heard; at that point, the pressure in the cuff is equal to that at systole. Further release of the pressure results eventually in the loss of all sound; at that point, the cuff pressure equals that at diastole.

At systole, the pressure in the aorta as the blood leaves the left ventricle is five to eight times higher than that in the right atrium at the point of entry of the superior vena cava, Fig. 11.A-1. This excess pressurization of the arterioles during the systolic contraction acts both to keep the blood flowing in the arterial system even while the atria are filling for the next power stroke [399], and to keep the pressure in the aorta and arteries significantly above zero long after the contraction of the left ventricle.

Blood pressure at the aorta normally is reported as A/B, where A is the systolic pressure in mm of Hg (millimeters of mercury) and B is the diastolic pressure in the same units. "Normal" pressure is considered to be 120/80, however, see Subsection 11.D, *Vasoconstriction, Vasodilation, and Hypertension*, page 334. Vascular plumbing is torn apart at pressures of 400/200 and blood will not flow through the system at pressures below 60/30 [43].

The volume throughput for the heart (milliliters per contraction cycle) is 5000/HR, where HR is the heart rate in beats per minute; with the heart beating at 50 beats per minute, each cycle delivers about 100 milliliters (about 3 fluid ounces) of fresh blood to the muscles and organs. The heart beats 36 million times a year, delivering about 750,000 gallons of blood in that time.

The diastolic pressure is measured during the passive filling of the atria, and so represents a baseline measure of the vascular pressure within the aorta and large arteries. As we shall see, the diastolic pressure reflects the muscular tone of the arteriole walls and thus the level of arteriole excitation by the nervous system (Section 11.C, The Vascular System, page 325). By contrast, the systolic pressure is more readily interpreted as showing the strength of the heart's contraction. High readings for either the systolic or diastolic phases of the heartbeat cycle mark one as at-risk for heart problems (see Subsection 11.D, *Vasoconstriction, Vasodilation, and Hypertension*, page 334).

The Valves within the Heart

The path of blood flow as driven by the heart is strictly a one-way street: blood enters the heart from the venous system so as to fill the right atrium and ventricle, is pumped to the lungs, then fills the left atrium and ventricle and is pumped into the arterial system, Fig. 11.A-3. The direction of flow is maintained by appropriately placed flap valves in the heart. In these, the flaps point in the direction of blood flow, so that the flaps are pushed open by blood flow in the desired direction, whereas a counterflow will act to close them.

During periods of ventricular contraction, Fig. 11.A-3, the valves between the ventricles and the atria (the tricuspid valve on the right side and the mitral valve on the left side) are closed so as to force the blood flow out of the heart and into the lungs and aorta, respectively. These valves remain open of course during atrial contraction, while the valves in the vessels feeding blood into the atria are closed.

Opening and closing of the appropriate valves at the appropriate times is in part automatic, in the sense that the valve flaps move with the flow as dictated by the contraction of the heart's chambers, and in part is directed by small muscles which are used to pull the flaps into place. If the mitral valve is prolapsed, then the flaps do not close tightly on systole, but billow back into the atrium allowing blood to flow in the upstream direction.

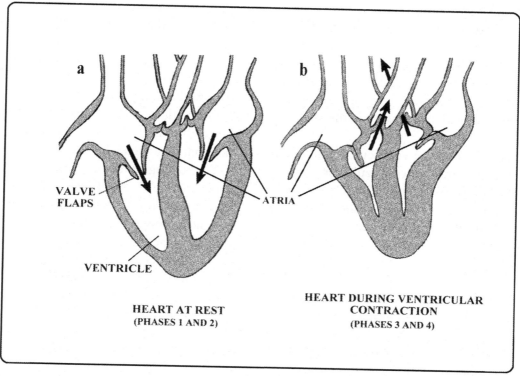

Fig. 11.A-3. (**a**) In the heart at rest, the valves between the atria and the ventricles are open so that the ventricles partially fill with blood. During atrial contraction, the valves within the veins close, but those between the atria and the ventricles remain open so as to more completely fill the ventricles with blood. (**b**) In the ventricular contraction phase, the valves to the atria are closed and blood is vigorously pumped to the lungs by the right ventricle and to the aorta by the left ventricle.

The heartbeat (pulse) that one feels in the body during *yogasana* is due to the ventricular contraction, while the sound one hears through a stethoscope is that of the valve between the atrium and the ventricle opening and closing [473].

The Timing of the Cardiac Contractions and Coordination with Valve Positions

As the actions of the cardiac components are the same on the two sides of the heart, we will discuss that for the left side with the understanding that the situation is the same on the right side. That is to say, both atria contract together, as do both ventricles. Inasmuch as the heart accepts the venous return of exhausted blood, sends it to the lungs for recharging, accepts the recharged blood, and then sends it out to the furthest reaches of the body, it is no surprise that there is some delicate timing involved between the motions of its parts. Consider the cardiac cycle to consist of four phases.

Phase 1. With the heart at rest, blood flows into the left atrium from the lungs via the pulmonary vein, and from the left atrium into the left ventricle. This passive filling is driven by the slight venous pressure in the lungs.

Phase 2. Pumping then begins with the contraction of the left atrium, which acts to close the valves in the pulmonary veins while keeping the valve between the left atrium and its ventricle open. Actually, not much blood is moved in this cycle as most of the filling of the ventricle has already occurred in Phase 1.

Phase 3. Once the ventricular contraction begins, the pressure in that chamber rapidly rises, thus closing the valve between it and the atrium, but at the same time, forcing open the valve to the aorta. About half the blood in the ventricle is forced out in one contraction, and the pressure in the ventricle drops.

Phase 4. Once the ventricular contraction is exhausted and the ventricular pressure is released through the aorta, the closed valve to the atrium again opens while that to the aorta closes. Returning to phase 1, the heart rests while the atrium and ventricle are re-filled passively, awaiting Phase 2 of the next cycle.

It is to be understood at the same time as the four-phase cycle described above for the left heart is playing out, the right heart is going through similar actions with respect to blood received from the superior vena cava and then pumped to the lungs via the pulmonary artery. The total elapsed time for one cycle of the heart-pumping action is about 1–2 seconds, with most of this spent in the resting/filling stage, Phase 1. See Subsection 11.A, *The Electrocardiogram*, page 319, for an experimental display of the relative timing for contraction of the chambers of the heart.

Cardiac Muscle

Note how much thicker and stronger the myocardium (cardiac muscle) is in the ventricular region as compared to the atrial region, Fig. 11.A-1. This is reasonable considering the much more intense work the ventricles must do in pushing blood through the arterioles and capillaries. The muscle fibers of the heart in many ways resemble those of skeletal muscles, but differ from them in several key respects. As with skeletal-muscle fibers, those of the heart also rely upon the actin-myosin interaction for contraction and motion (Subsection 7.A, *Microscopic Muscle Contraction*, page 178), and

are neurally excited, leading to propagating action potentials (Section 5.B, Nerve Conduction, page 114) [230, 473].

However, the list of dissimilarities between skeletal and cardiac muscles is far longer than the list of similarities:

1) The duration of the action potential in the cardiac fiber is about 100 times longer than that in skeletal muscle.

2) The long duration of the action potential in cardiac fiber is followed by an anomalously long refractory period during which time no excitation can take place.

3) Contraction of cardiac muscle is relatively brief, considering that it is followed by a much longer rest period allowing the ventricles to refill for the next cycle.

4) All of the muscle fibers in the atrial section on one side of the heart are interconnected through high-speed gap junctions (Section 5.C, Nerve Connections; Synapses, page 121) such that all fibers are either excited or are at rest. Contraction is like a brief muscle spasm. A similar relationship exists among the cardiac fibers within the ventricles.

5) Unlike skeletal muscle, cardiac muscle is self-exciting. The heart does not need any external neural connections in order to continue beating at a regular pace. However, there are external nerves connected to the heart which influence the heart rate and the strength of the contractions; still, even without these external stimuli, the heart will continue to beat.

6) Skeletal muscle cells are long, slender, multinuclear and shaped to pull on distant bone or tendon, whereas cardiac cells are mononuclear, short and stubby. The cardiac muscle has cross-striations and terminate at "intercalated discs" which act as separations between the bifurcated ends ("Y-shaped" split ends) of adjacent fibers. On contraction, the cardiac fibers essentially pull on one another when they pull on the intercalated discs, the net effect being that the cir-

cumference of the heart shrinks and the internal volumes of either the atria or the ventricles decrease. See Chapter 22, AGING AND LONGEVITY, page 493, for a discussion comparing the enlarged heart of an athlete to the enlarged heart of a hypertensive but inactive person. A further comparison of the properties of skeletal and cardiac muscle appears in Table 11.A-1.

Of course, the heart muscle itself must be served by its own network of arteries and veins in order to keep the muscle fibers oxygenated, fueled and free of wastes. The diameters of these "coronary vessels" are under the control of the autonomic nervous system (Chapter 6, page 133) for the vessel walls carry alpha and beta receptors sensitive to hormonal signals from these systems. Alpha receptors when activated by the sympathetic nervous system promote vasoconstriction (decreasing diameters) of the vessels, whereas with parasympathetic activation, the alpha receptors promote vasodilation (increasing diameters) of the vessels. The beta receptors on the other hand, only promote vasodilation, regardless of whether the stimulation is via the sympathetic or parasympathetic nervous systems [230].

Interestingly, during systole, when the heart is contracted and blood is sent coursing to all of the other parts of the body, the cardiac arteries feeding the heart itself are so compressed that no blood can flow through them; the blood feeding the cardiac muscle passes through the heart during the more passive diastole phase instead.

Innervation of the Heart: the Cardiac Pacemaker

Unlike the situation with skeletal muscle, cardiac-muscle contraction is not driven by a neural impulse from the central nervous system (however, see below). Instead, several cells within the heart are able to launch action potentials without stimulation from the outside and their innate frequency of excitation becomes the essential heartbeat frequency. The first phase of the cardiac excitation begins in the upper right atrium at a spot called the sinoatrial (SA) node. Even in

TABLE 11.A-1. A COMPARISON OF THE PROPERTIES OF SKELETAL AND CARDIAC MUSCLES [299]

Property	Skeletal Muscle	Cardiac Muscle
Striated	Yes	Yes
Electrically coupled	No	Yes
Contraction without nerve input	No	Yes
Duration of contraction equals duration of action potential	No	Yes
Action potential like that of neurons	Yes	No
Ca^{2+} important	No	Yes
Effect of neural input	Excitatory	Excitatory or inhibitory
Nervous system control	Somatic	Autonomic
Neurotransmitter	Acetylcholine	Acetylcholine or norepinephrine
Effect of ion channels	Direct	Indirect

the resting state, tissue in this area has a membrane potential which rises spontaneously to sooner or later initiate a depolarization wave that spreads to other cells in the atria on both the right and the left. This depolarization event is triggered by the influx of Ca^{2+} ions into the cell rather than Na^+ as is the case with skeletal muscle (Section 7.A, page 167). This initial depolarization results in global atrial contraction. See Box 11.A-1 for a brief discussion of the unique character of the cells in the SA node.

A second node within the right atrium called the atroventricular (AV) node senses the excitation from the SA node and then sends its own signals to the Purkinje cells of the ventricles. These cells are poor muscle contractors but excellent conductors of nerve signals. Using gap junctions (Section 5.C, Nerve Connections; Synapses, page 121), the Purkinje cells rapidly and coherently excite all of the other cells in the ventricles to contract sequentially from the bottom of the ventricle to the top. In this case, the ion channels of greatest importance are those for the inward flow of Na^+. The time delay for the signal transmission from the SA to the AV nodes separates atrial and ventricular contractions in time. Neural excitation in the ventricles is a very long process as it is terminated by the slow opening of the K^+ channels allowing this ion to move out of the muscle fiber (repolarization). Depolarization in cardiac fiber lasts approximately 100 times longer than in skeletal fiber, and concomitant with this, the refractory period is also anomalously long. The long refractory period in the heart allows ample time for the heart to refill with blood before the next heartbeat is initiated in the SA node.

For both atrial and ventricular excitation within the heart, it is notable that there is no random firing of muscle units as is common in skeletal muscle which is to be contracted over a long period, but instead all of the contraction possible is called forth in one burst, short-lived but very strong. If, however, the contraction of the ventricles is arrhythmic or the fibers depolarize not as a group but randomly as individuals, then the heart is in fibrillation and a strong DC electrical shock from a defibrillator is necessary to re-establish coherence and rhythm of the contractions. If the ventricular contraction is not stimulated for some reason or its timing is off, the heartbeat can be driven externally by an electronic pacemaker.

BOX 11.A-1: THE CELLS OF THE SA NODE SHARE AN ELECTRICAL BOND

When a heart cell from the SA node is placed in a nutrient solution, it will contract on its own at about 40 times per minute. A second cell placed in this solution, but not touching the first will also beat at this frequency, but there will be no correlation of the times for the contractions of the two cells. That is to say, they will contract independently of one another. If, however, the two cells are able to touch one another, then the contractions immediately fall into synchronicity! A collection of such contacting cells within the right atrium form the SA node and lead to global timing pulses for atrial contraction, wherein all cells are sensibly contracting at the same moment. The SA node continues its electrical output at approximately 40–90 times per minute, without rest, for the entire life of the individual [399].

Inasmuch as the heart has its own pacemaker within it, it is somewhat surprising to find that cardiac muscle is innervated at several places from the outside as well. Cardiac muscle fibers at the SA and AV nodes synapse with the postganglionic neurons from both the sympathetic and parasympathetic nervous systems (Chapter 6, page 133) the neurotransmitter in the former being norepinephrine and acetylcholine in the latter. Activation of the SA and AV nodes by both neural and hormonal routes by the sympathetic channel, either through the fight-or-flight response, through emotional and/or psychic factors or by deliberate conscious action increases the heart rate (by up to 200 beats per minute), its contractile force and stroke volume (by up to 300%), and the blood pressure. If instead, the effect is parasympathetic activation, all of these functions decrease, Table 6.A-2, lowering the heart rate to 30 beats per minute or less and

the volume output by 50% [340]. The parasympathetic signals are carried to the heart by cranial nerve X, the vagus nerve. See Box 11.A-2 for a note on how the vagus nerve can be controlled so as to literally stop the heart for a short time.

The effect of norepinephrine on cardiac muscle is to lower the threshold for production of an action potential by increasing the permeability of the cardiac-cell membranes to the inward flow of Ca^{2+}, which speeds the rise of the resting potential. Sympathetic activation also results in the release into the bloodstream of norepinephrine from the adrenal medulla, however, the stimulation of cardiac muscle by norepinephrine is more importantly by the neural route [195]. The action of acetylcholine is to increase the membrane permeability to the outward flow of K^+, thus making the resting potential more negative and thereby requiring a longer wait for the resting potential to reach

BOX 11.A-2: STOPPING THE HEART BY CONSCIOUS CONTROL OF THE VAGUS NERVE

With constant work on the inner being, adept yoga students are able to gain more and more conscious control over the autonomic nervous system. In doing this, they are then able to perform many seemingly magical feats with their bodies, such as control of their heart rates, breath, blood flow, local temperature, *etc.*

Earlier scientific studies regarding yogi's claims to have "stopped the heart" showed that in these cases there was considerable contraction of the skeletal muscles of the chest and holding of the breath, so that the local contraction closed the venous supply to the heart. With little or no blood being pumped, the heartbeat cannot be heard and there is little or no pulse to be felt, however, the electrocardiograph shows that the heart in these cases was nonetheless beating [481].

In contrast, Swami Rama, *et al.*, [372] present original scientific data from the Menninger Foundation in New York City illustrating some of the Swami's powers over the otherwise automatic processes in his body. As can be seen in Fig. 11.A-4a, over a period of 6 minutes Swami Rama was able to develop and maintain a temperature difference of 10° F between the inner and outer edges of the palm of one hand. One must suppose that in doing this he was able to vasodilate the vessels in one part of the hand so as to warm the skin in that area all the while causing the vessels in the opposite part of the hand to vasoconstrict and hence cool the skin (see Section 10.C, Thermal Regulation by Blood Vessels and Sweat Glands in the Skin, page 292).

To the amazement and horror of the investigating scientists, Swami Rama then caused his heart to stop pumping blood for over 20 seconds, Fig. 11.A-4b, at which point they begged him to resume normal heart action. They found that during the period of zero-blood-flow, the atria were fluttering at a rate of about 300 times per minute, whereas the ventricles had ceased to pump blood. For comparison, compare the electrocardiogram of the Swami for the first 20 seconds with a normal one as in Fig. 11.A-5. In the context of what has been said in this Section, it would appear that he was able to simultaneously drive the atrial flutter using sympathetic excitation and quench the ventricular contraction totally using parasympathetic excitation of the vagus nerve. Amazing!

Other amazing feats of control of the body's inner states have been reported, but the scientific data is not available to substantiate the claims [42, 104, 201, 246].

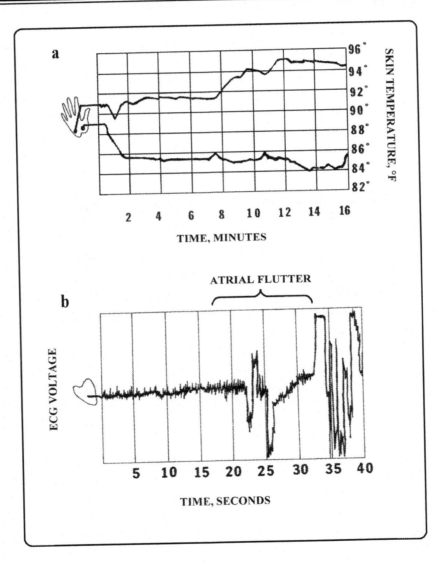

Fig. 11.A-4. (a) Generation of a 10° F temperature differential on the surface of the palm over a 6-minute period by Swami Rama. (b) Electrocardiogram of Swami Rama showing no voluntary ventricular output for over 20 seconds [372].

threshold. Because the heartbeat is controlled in part by the autonomic nervous system through its control of the permeabilities of the cardiac-muscle membrane to Ca^{2+} and K^+ ions, these factors dictate the rate at which the resting potential of the membrane reaches threshold.

There is also a rich innervation of the ventricles directly by the sympathetic nervous system, whereas there is no such direct route to the ventricles for the parasympathetic system.

Interestingly, there is a second pacemaker in the body controlling the rhythmic contraction of muscle. See Subsection 18.A, *Peristalsis*, page 447, for a discussion of the pacemaker driving the rhythmic contractions of the smooth muscle of the gut.

The Electrocardiogram

In a way very much parallel to that in which the brain's electrical activity can be measured using external electrodes on the scalp (Section 3.E, Brainwaves and the Electroencephalogram, page 57), the various phases of the heart action can be followed using external electrodes on the trunk of the body. Called an "electrocardiogram" (ECG or EKG), this recording shows the relative timing of the phases of the cardiac contraction, Fig. 11.A-5. One sees in the Figure that the cardiac cycle begins with a P wave, the electrical signal initiated at the SA node that contracts the atria and fills the ventricles in the diastolic phase. Signals in the Q, R, S regime are initiated in the AV node, and correspond to ventricular contraction appropriate to the systolic phase; the Q wave follows the P wave by about 150 milliseconds. The compressed structure of the Q, R, S region reflects the rapid conductivity of the Purkinje cells in the ventricles. A T wave next appears which serves to reset the voltages on the surfaces of the heart in preparation for the next heartbeat cycle. During the T wave, no further electrical heart action is possible, thus accounting for the long refractory period during which the heart refills with blood for the next heartbeat. Variations in the pattern of cardiac voltages in the ECG are symptomatic for various cardiac malfunctions and are readily diagnosed [230].

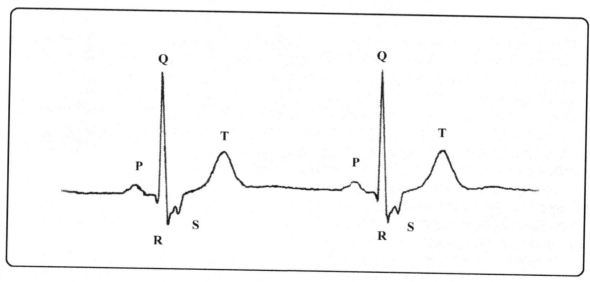

Fig. 11.A-5. The author's EKG recorded in the V5 electrode configuration, showing the P, Q, R, S, and T features. The time between Q pulses was 1000–1200 milliseconds.

TABLE 11.A-2. REDISTRIBUTION OF CARDIAC OUTPUT[a] AS A FUNCTION OF THE LEVEL OF EXERCISE [337]

Tissue	Light Exercise	Moderate Exercise	Maximal Exercise
Abdominal organs	1,100 (12%)	600 (3%)	300 (1%)
Kidneys	900 (10%)	600 (3%)	250 (1%)
Brain	750 (8%)	750 (4%)	750 (3%)
Heart	350 (4%)	750 (4%)	1,000 (4%)
Muscle	4,500 (47%)	12,500 (71%)	22,000 (88%)
Skin	1,500 (15%)	1,900 (12%)	600 (2%)
Total cardiac output[b]	9,500	17,500	25,000

[a] Given as the amount of blood (ml/min) and % cardiac output.

[b] The resting value is 5000 ml/ minute.

Effects of Western Exercise, Yogasana, and the Autonomic Nervous System on the Heart

In general, the body's autonomic response to western exercise (running, tennis, swimming, *etc.*) is just that appropriate for a fight-or-flight situation, *i.e.*, a general tensing of the body and mind in expectation of an attack from outside. The response begins with the hypothalamus signaling the adrenal medullas to release their epinephrine into the blood stream. With respect to the heart, this means a sympathetic excitation which shifts the blood supply away from the viscera and toward the muscles and heart, and an increase of the heart rate, systole strength, and coronary-artery diameters. In this regard, Nieman [337] presents an interesting discussion, Table 11.A-2, quantitatively detailing just how much blood is diverted to and from various body organs as the level of exercise is increased. Thus, at rest, only 15–20% of the cardiac output goes to the large muscles, while at the peak of physical exercise, the cardiac output to the large muscles can increase to 88%. On going from minimal to maximal exercise, the amount of blood in the abdominal organs decreases from 12% to 1%, in the kidneys

from 10% to 1%, in the brain from 8% to 3% and in the skin from 15% to 2%. At the same time, the amount of blood going to the heart muscle remains constant at 4%. All of these changes are just those expected on going to strong sympathetic excitation, Table 6.A-2. The redirection of the blood flow is accomplished by the appropriate vasoconstriction of some blood vessels and the vasodilation of others.

In response to the claims that yoga is not sufficiently aerobic, consider the study of DiCarlo, *et al.*, [119] which compared a 32-minute routine of standing poses in the Iyengar style with a 32-minute treadmill walk at 4 mph. It was found that the yoga routine resulted in a larger increase in heart rate, blood pressure (systolic and diastolic) and rating of perceived exertion than did the treadmill walk, yet showed a lower metabolic demand.

As can be seen from Table 6.A-2, the effects of western exercise on the heart are just those expected for sympathetic excitation of the autonomic nervous system. However, the accomplished student of *yogasana* can control the excitation in the autonomic nervous system, so that when appropriate (in *urdhva dhanurasana* or during *yogasana* jumping, for example) there is sympathetic

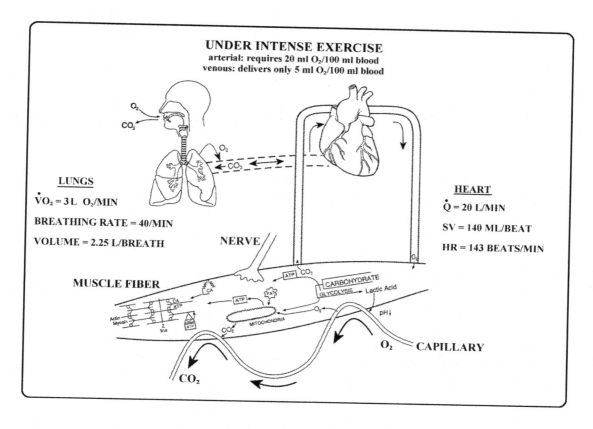

Fig. 11.A-6. The interactions between the respiratory, cardiac and muscle systems of the body during intense exercise. See text for explanation.

excitation and all of its coronary consequences (increased heart rate and strength of systole, with vasodilation of the coronary arteries), but for other poses such as *sarvangasana* and *janu sirsasana*, it is the parasympathetic branch that dominates and the response is one of cardiac relaxation instead.

Large and significant differences were reported in the levels of sympathetic excitation while in the *yogasanas* for two groups of practitioners, those new to the practice and those with 6 months to one year of *yogasana* experience [168]. The steady-state heart-rate-level of the trained group was 11% lower in *sirsasana I*, than that of the novices, and 15% lower in *adho mukha virasana*. Similar indicators of reduced sympathetic excitation in the trained students were

reported for respiratory indicators as well (Subsection 12.B, *Rationalizing the Effects of the Breath*, page 374).

Nieman [337] gives an accounting of the oxygen demand during hard exercise, Fig. 11.A-6. In order to do its work, a muscle may demand 3000 ml of O_2 per minute. With the venous blood containing only 5 ml of O_2 per 100 ml, and the arterial blood containing 20 ml of O_2 per 100 ml, the blood flow can deliver only 15 ml of O_2 per 100 ml. To meet the needs of the exercise, the heart stroke volume (SV) must go up to 140 ml per beat and the heart rate (HR) must increase to 143 beats per minute. At the same time, the respiration rate increases to 40 breaths per minute with 2.25 liters of air inhaled with each breath. Under these conditions, the muscle will be fed the required amount of O_2 via the capillary arteries and will remove from the muscle the corresponding amounts of CO_2 and lactic acid. These parameters of the lungs and heart allow the necessary chemistry (lower part of the Figure) to occur in the muscles doing the work. Note too that exercise not only increases circulation by moving more blood through the vascular system, but actually builds new capillaries as well.

When working the muscles at a high level, the mitochondria are required to produce more ATP. This comes in turn from the phosphorylation of ADP; the energy for this reaction is derived in turn from the oxidation of glucose by oxygen delivered in the bloodstream. As a consequence of this reaction chain, the amount of work that a muscle can do is strictly limited by the amount of oxygen that can be delivered to the mitochondria of its cells by the bloodstream.

As with any muscle in the body, the more the heart is used to pump blood, the larger and stronger (up to a point) it becomes. As a corollary to this, the easing of the load on the muscles, as with bedrest or weightlessness in space quickly leads to atrophy and loss of muscle mass. In fact, it has been found that in prolonged space flight, the human heart shrinks by 15%! Because one might expect approximately the same shrinkage to take effect in the inactive body, it is surprising to see that the weight of the heart on average increases as we age (Fig. 22.A-1).

Because the vascular resistance increases in old age and the diastolic pressure goes up accordingly, the heart must work harder in order to deliver the goods. In response to this extra load, the heart will grow in size; this is bad because unlike the exercise situation, the load on the heart is ever-present, there being no time for cardiac rest and relaxation. This scenario may account for the average weight and volume of the heart increasing as one ages from 20 to 65 years.

In support of this idea, the diastolic blood pressure also rises from age 20 to 65 years, Fig. 22.A-1.

In the course of extended physical exercise, the heart like any other muscle, will grow in size and its wall thickness will increase. These changes in the heart induce an increase in stroke volume with a lower heart rate, an increase in total blood volume and an increase in capillary density which serves to more easily bring O_2, glucose and fatty acids to muscles and carry away waste products. Though there is a large effect of the emotions on the heart rate, chronic exercise tends to decrease heart rate and return it to the resting value more quickly. This suggests that long-term training increases parasympathetic vagal tone. The slower heart rate allows the heart to fill more completely and so to pump more blood per stroke [98]. Through all of this, $\dot{Q}$, the rate of flow, remains unchanged.

The effectiveness of *savasana* as a mode of relaxation has been compared to sitting in a chair or simply lying down, by first stressing the body on a treadmill and then noting the rate of return of the heart rate and blood pressure to initial values when in each of the three modes. Baseline values of these quantities were observed significantly sooner when in *savasana* than when sitting or lying down [37].

SECTION 11.B. BLOOD

Chemistry and Function

Blood is the principal extracellular fluid in the body and serves as the messenger service for a manifold of needs [229, 230, 473]. Acting as the body's active distribution system, the blood not only transports oxygen (O_2) from the lungs to the tissues and cells and then carries the carbon dioxide (CO_2) from these places back to the lungs, it also transports pathogens from everywhere in the body to sites where they can be deactivated, as well as transporting the agents of the immune system to the site of injury. Moreover, the blood also carries vitamins, electrolytes and nutrients from the gut to wherever they are needed, transports hormones from the source to their target organs, and it is the pipeline for moving the metabolic wastes from the muscles to the kidneys.

In the average man, the body contains 5.6 liters of blood, about 8% of the total body weight, while in the average woman, there is 4.5 liters (5.0 liters when pregnant), the difference being due to the man's larger body mass. The heart requires about one minute to pump 5 liters of blood through the vascular system when at rest, but under conditions of heavy exercise [291], this time can be reduced to about 10 seconds! Via the vascular system, blood is sent to within 20 microns or closer of every cell of the body, except for the cornea, bone, cartilage, the inner ear and the testicles.

In addition to transporting the chemical species and discrete cell bodies listed above, blood serves another very important function. In general, the temperature of the core of the body is higher than that of the air surrounding it, so that if the heat of the inner body could be brought to the surface, the body could radiate heat into the air and so cool itself. With control from the autonomic nervous system, warm blood can be transferred from deep inside the body to the outer surfaces, with a subsequent return of the cooled blood back to the inner recesses of the body. Just how this is accomplished is considered in Subsection 11.D, *Vasoconstriction, Vasodilation, and Hypertension*, page 334.

Blood contains both dissolved substances (proteins, salts, organic acids, all in water) forming the blood plasma (55% of the blood volume), and suspended blood cells of vari-

ous sorts and functions. The three major types of blood cells are listed below.

Erythrocytes (Red Blood Cells)

The erythrocytes contain all of the hemoglobin to be found in blood. The structure and function of this important metalloprotein is discussed further in Subsection 12.A, *The Function of Hemoglobin*, page 369. Red blood cells filled with hemoglobin are manufactured largely in the red marrow of bones (in the adult, in the sternum, ribs, vertebrae, skull and pelvis), with the liver and spleen able to generate these cells in an emergency if needed. The bone marrow of the body is a considerably larger organ than one might at first assume, being exceeded in mass only by the liver and the skin. Hemoglobin's sole function is to transport O_2 from the alveoli of the lungs to the tissues and cells (four O_2 molecules per molecule of hemoglobin), and to carry CO_2 away from these sites and back to the lungs. If the partial pressure of O_2 is too low in the air being breathed, then hormones are released which accelerate the production of red blood cells, as will also the direct stimulation of the bone marrow by the sympathetic nervous system, Table 6.A-2.

Consisting of a very flexible sac packed with hemoglobin but lacking a cell nucleus, the red blood cells are able to fold so as to negotiate the tortuous paths of the capillaries in order to serve outlying tissue. Because red blood cells have no nuclei, they are not really "cells" in the conventional sense. Following its birth, the typical red blood cell has a lifetime of about 4 months, during which it will have traversed approximately 1000 miles of vascular pipeline! Once their time is up, tired red blood cells are destroyed by macrophage cells, which then recycle the iron and protein for use in the fabrication of new red blood cells.

The surfaces of the red blood cells are coated with sugar molecules in one of four ways, leading to the four basic blood types (A, B, AB and O). These coding systems on the cells' surfaces are intimately involved with immunity and the identification of foreign cells.

When we bring the sympathetic nervous system into dominance by performing vigorous *yogasanas*, one of the many consequences is that the spleen is prompted to release its store of red blood cells, so that more oxygen can be carried by the bloodstream [319]. Yogic training appears to raise both the hemoglobin content of blood and its hematocrit, all the while lowering its ability to coagulate [63]. *Yogasana* students who have an iron deficiency are anemic and will quickly tire and become breathless during their *yogasana* practice as the low iron levels imply low red blood cell counts and therefore, poor oxygenation of the working tissues.

Platelets

Very large, noncirculating cells in the bone marrow routinely disintegrate, forming platelets by the millions. Having no nuclei or DNA, such platelets are really not cells, but are simply fragments of the larger mother cells; containing serotonin, platelets circulate without effect in the blood until they are called upon to perform their special task. Platelets are responsible for the clotting of the blood when there is an injured blood vessel. Blood in the normal situation does not contact collagen fibers in the body, as the inner layers of the blood vessels are lined with endothelial cells which stand between the blood and the collagen of the blood-vessel walls. However, when there is a cutting of the vascular pipeline, the edges of the cut bring blood into contact with the collagen fibrils of the outer layers. As a consequence of this, the platelets release their serotonin, which then acts to constrict the bleeding vessel while dilating other intact vessels in the area. Most importantly, the

platelets also clump together at the site of the injury, forming a plug for the wound that stops the bleeding [387].

This particular initiating event in the formation of a blood clot, the contact between the platelets and collagen, is of special interest to *yogasana* students. In certain *yogasana* positions, there is a pressing of the muscle against bone which can be so severe that the integrity of the endothelium inner layers of blood vessels caught in the squeeze is compromised. In this case, the contact of the platelets in the blood with the collagen within the wall of the blood vessel can lead to the formation of a blood clot at that point. Further work of the same sort can then act to dislodge the clot, setting the stage for the formation of an embolism further along the circulation route. Such an embolism will lodge in a smaller blood vessel and cause an ischemic attack in the tissues that are normally served by the vessel. See Appendix II, INJURIES INCURRED DURING IMPROPER *YOGASANA* PRACTICE, page 511, for several case histories relating to this problem.

The White Blood Cells

The first line of defense of the body against foreign cells, microbial infections, and toxins is formed by the white blood cells, of which there are a great variety. The first to attack such invaders is the macrophage, which immobilizes them. Neutrophils then attack if necessary, and should this fail, then the monocytes are called into the battle. Functionally, the white blood cells may be divided into those that respond to inflammation and tissue injuries, but are otherwise of a nonspecific nature, and those that are targeted toward specific intruders. Reactions of the first group are innate, whereas those of the second group are acquired through a previous exposure to a particular pathogen. The bones of the skull, spine and ribs produce ten million white blood cells per minute in a healthy adult [43].

Those cells of the immune system [leucocytes (white blood cells), neutrophils, lymphocytes, monocytes, *etc.*] which fight infectious bacteria in the blood stream, their relations to the autonomic nervous system and to *yogasana* practice are discussed further in Chapter 13, THE IMMUNE SYSTEM, page 383.

The Blood-Brain Barrier

The capillaries in most of the body are neither featureless nor continuous pipes, but instead have many small breaks and windows which aid in the mass transfer of materials between the inside and outside of the capillary. Not so in the brain, however, for here the endothelium cells are packed so very tightly that the only way material can pass between the blood and the extracellular fluid is by virtue of the microscopic permeability of the capillary wall. As the capillary walls of the brain are constructed of tightly packed lipids, they are very selective in what chemical species they will let pass from the blood to the brain. In particular, fat-soluble materials in solution find easy passage through the lipid layers, Fig. 5.A-1, whereas materials that are only water soluble cannot penetrate the lipid barrier. The capillary walls thus act as a blood-brain barrier, protecting the neurons of the brain and spinal cord from harm by noxious chemicals and biological substances. Very large molecular species are especially discriminated against, *i.e.*, bacteria, viruses, white blood cells, proteins and parasites can not pass through, whereas small, lipid-soluble species like glucose and small amino acids can. Of course, the blood-brain barrier works as well between the blood and the cerebrospinal fluid, Section 4.D, page 93.

SECTION 11.C. THE VASCULAR SYSTEM

Architecture

The activities and health of all of the body's organs are dependent upon receiving an adequate and timely supply of blood. Thus for example, each muscle fiber is surrounded by a network of capillaries which tend to its needs, supplying fresh blood and carrying away metabolic products.

As described in Section 11.A, page 310, the four-chambered heart is much like two hearts side-by-side, Fig. 11.A-1. The right side of the heart is filled with deoxygenated, depleted blood which it then pumps into the lungs for recharging with oxygen and stripping of carbon dioxide (pulmonary circulation), while the oxygenated blood from the lungs is then pumped by the left side of the heart to the waiting muscles and organs of the body (systemic circulation). The vessels that carry the blood from outlying reaches of the body to the right heart, from the heart to the lungs and back again, and from the left heart to the furthest extremities taken together are known as the vascular system [399].

That part of the vascular system that carries the blood back to the heart is the venous side, while that part that carries blood from the heart to the muscles, the brain and the organs is the arterial side. The artery as it leaves the heart (the aorta) is a very large conduit, but it shortly branches to form smaller arteries which in turn branch further to form arterioles, and these in turn then branch to form capillaries. Blood flow through all of these conduits is driven by the pressure of the left heart's ventricular contractions. The general schematic for the flow of blood through the body is given in Fig. 11.C-1, while the major arteries of the body are shown in Fig. 11.C-2.

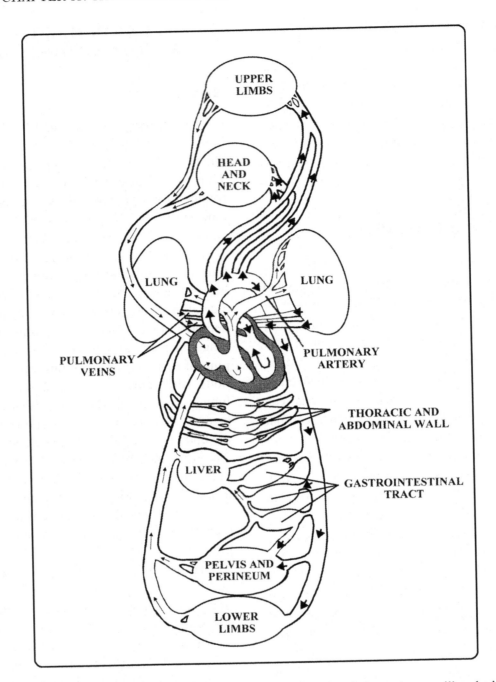

Fig. 11.C-1. Schematic of the general flow pattern of blood through the various capillary beds of the vascular system. The heavy and light arrows represent the directions of blood flow at high pressure (arterial) and low pressure (venous), respectively.

The aorta is a large-diameter, elastic vessel which swells (see Fig. 11.A-1) with each beat of the heart and then shrinks as the subsequent blood flow reduces the pressure within. With increasing distance from the heart, the aorta becomes smaller, less elastic but more muscular. This more distant part of the arterial system distributes blood to the muscles and organs in general, but most importantly, the more muscular the artery is,

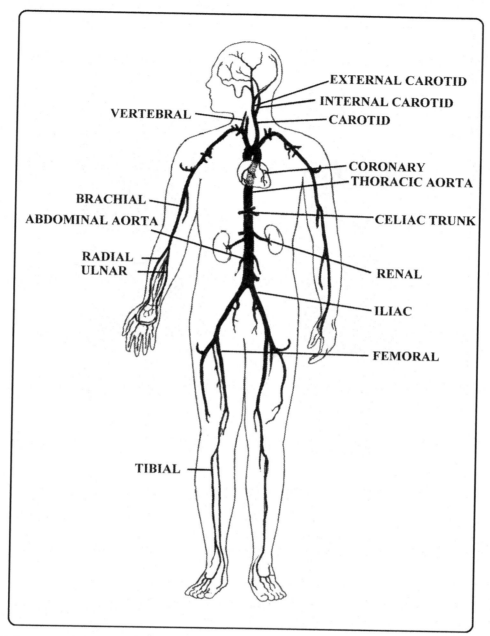

Fig. 11.C-2. The major arteries of the body. Because the veins and arteries in the body are often paired, the Figure also gives a fairly accurate picture as well of the locations of the major veins.

the more its blood flow can be controlled by the nervous system. As can be seen in Fig. 11.C-3a, such an artery is composed of several layers, the middle one of which (layer 3) is a cylindrical muscle which when contracted, acts to narrow the artery's diameter. Contraction of the arterial walls is largely under the control of the sympathetic nerv-

ous system, whereas parasympathetic dominance leads to the dilation of already contracted vessels. It is possible with *yogasana* practice to bring the function of arterial diameter into the conscious realm.

The arterioles are small in diameter (less than 0.5 mm), and are found just at the entrances to the capillary beds. They are

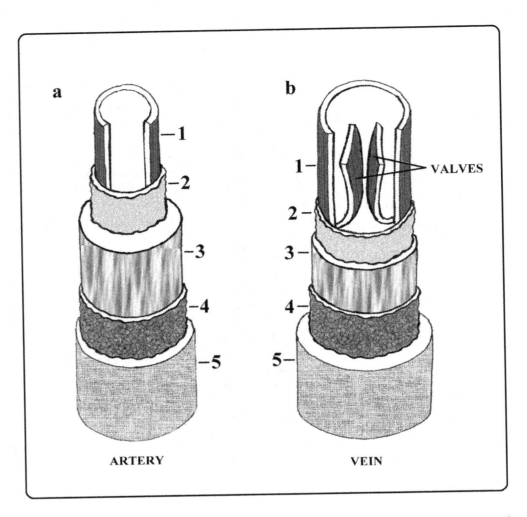

Fig. 11.C-3. Comparison of the multilayer structures of arteries (**a**) and veins (**b**). In an artery, the smooth-muscle layer (**3**) is much thicker and more powerful than in a vein, whereas the latter has directional valves which are absent in the former [229].

sufficiently muscular that they can turn off the local blood supply totally, thus redirecting the blood flow to other organs which need it more.

Arterioles offer the largest resistance to blood flow and therefore the largest pressure drop in the vascular system is across the arterioles, Fig. 11.C-4b.

The capillaries have very thin walls, only a cell diameter or so thick, and it is here that the exchange of gases, metabolites, waste products, *etc.*, between the vascular system and the muscles and organs occurs most easily. The capillary length is about 0.025 cm (1/100 of an inch) but can reach 0.1 cm

in muscles [5]. It is now thought that the straining of the blood through the capillary net within the lungs not only serves to aerate the spent blood, but also to filter out small, mobile blood clots.

On the venous side, the structures corresponding to the artery and arteriole are the vein and the venule. The vein carrying blood from below (the inferior vena cava) and that carrying blood from above (the superior vena cava), empty their loads into the atrium of the right heart, Fig. 11.A-1.

The venous and arterial systems differ greatly in that there is no active, dedicated pump for moving venous blood through the

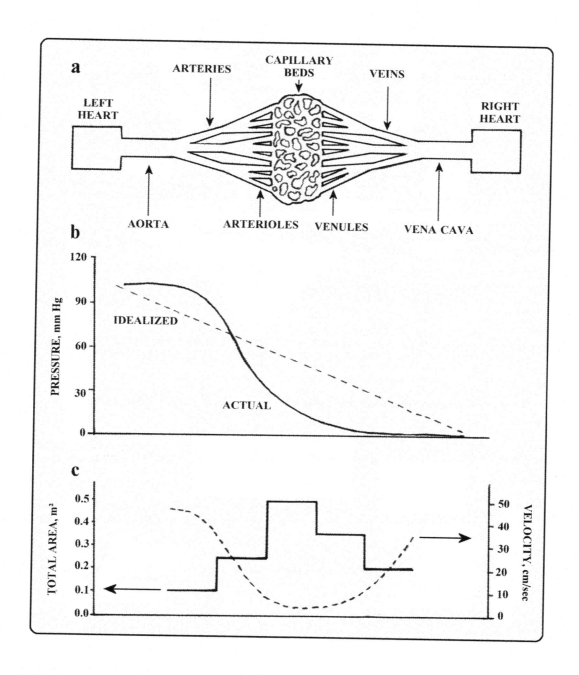

Fig. 11.C-4. (**a**) Schematic display of the branching of the elements within the vascular system, going from the left ventricle to the right atrium. (**b**) The blood pressure at every point in the vascular system assuming that the resistances to blood flow of all of the elements in (**a**) above are equal (idealized, dashed line), and the actual pressure profile across the system (solid line). (**c**) Reciprocal nature of the variation of the cross-sectional areas of each of the vascular elements and the velocity of blood flow through each.

system the way there is for moving arterial blood with the heart. This significant difference is reflected in the internal architecture of these two subsystems. Venous and arterial walls each are composed of five distinct layers of tissue, Fig. 11.C-3, but since the arteries must support a much higher internal pressure*, their middle wall of smooth-muscle cells (layer 3 in the Figure) is much thicker and the walls themselves are much less elastic. The veins, being elastic as they are, can easily swell so as to become blood reservoirs, and as a corollary to this, also can be easily pinched off by any sort of internal pressure (muscle tension, for example) or external pressure (that of the arm against the leg in *maricyasana III*, for example).

Furthermore, the arteries have no valves, whereas the veins below the heart and in the neck have one-way valves which aid in directing deoxygenated blood back to the heart by closing whenever the blood tends to flow backward, *i.e.*, away from the heart. The inner channels of both arteries and veins (layer 1 in Fig. 11.C-3) are lined with endothelium cells which act to separate the collagen of the vessel walls from the blood, which otherwise will clot if it comes into contact with collagen.

The smooth muscle in both the arteries and veins is activated involuntarily, and unlike skeletal and cardiac muscle, can maintain its contraction for very long periods of time. As is discussed below in Subsection 11.D, *Vasoconstriction, Vasodilation, and Hypertension*, page 334, this latter fact is a key to understanding certain aspects of the phenomenon of chronically high blood pressure.

Mechanics of Blood Flow: Blood Pressure

In Table 11.C-1 and Figure 11.C-4, certain parameters of blood flow through the various components of the vascular system are listed. One sees that, as expected, the velocity of flow through the arterial side decreases as the diameter of the carrier decreases. And though capillaries in muscles are generally only about 0.1 cm long, there are so many of them that the total area of the capillary walls is six times larger than that of the wide-diameter arteries. Given that the capillaries are so short, it is a great advantage then that the velocity of blood flow through them is low, for this gives a longer residence time for the diffusive exchange of gases and other cellular materials (see Section 11.B, Blood, page 322) with the outside world. No doubt by design, the diameter of a red-blood cell (7 microns) is just that of the capillary channel (6–7 microns), and so the red-blood cells are just able to squeeze through. If all of the capillaries in the human body were strung together end-to-end, the chain would be 65,000 miles long!

Figure 11.C-4b shows that the largest pressure drop in the vascular system is across the arterioles, and that the venous side of the system supports little or no pressure at all. On the other hand, though blood flow through the capillaries and venules is very slow, blood does not accumulate behind them because there are so many more of them to handle the load.

As there is much overdesign of the vascular system, with many parallel paths to the same end, blockages of the smaller arteries are often of no consequence as other vessels take over. However, in *yogasanas*

---

*The blood pressure at the right ventricle is only 300 mm Hg, whereas that at the left ventricle is 1500 mm Hg.

TABLE 11.C-1. BLOOD FLOW THROUGH VARIOUS COMPONENTS OF THE VASCULAR SYSTEM [230]

Vessel	Velocity, cm/sec	Total area, cm^2
Artery	45	800
Arteriole	10–35	2500
Capillary	5–10	5000
Venule	5–10	3500
Vein	10–35	2000

such as *ustrasana*, in which the neck is strongly flexed backward, the bending at the neck tends to block the large vertebral arteries (Subsection 4.A, *Blood Vessels*, page 81) which are threaded through the cervical vertebrae and serve the hindbrain. This blockage can lead to dizziness, nausea and fainting [92]. Retraction of the scapula down the back toward the waist using the latissimus dorsi muscles relieves this blockage and the symptoms that flow from it.

Blood will flow through a section of the vascular system only if there is a difference of pressure between the two ends of that system. In particular, the rate of "Flow" of blood through a blood vessel will depend directly upon the difference of "Pressure" at the two ends, and inversely on the "Resistance" the blood vessel offers to flow:

Flow = Pressure / Resistance

Blood pressure can be changed by appropriate changes in one or both of the other quantities.

The connections between various components of the vascular system (left heart, aorta, arteries, arterioles, capillary beds, venules, veins, vena cava, right heart) are shown schematically in Fig. 11.C-4a. Imagine for a moment that each of these elements in the vascular loop offers the same resistance to blood flow. In that case, the pressure drop from the high-pressure end of the system (the left heart) to the low-pressure end (the right heart) is shown by the dashed line in Fig. 11.C-4b, *i.e.*, there is a

constant pressure drop of about 15 mm Hg across each segment of the system, and the arterial pressure is between 70 and 85 mm Hg.

In fact, the pressure-drop curve is known to be that of the full curve in Fig. 11.C-4b, which differs from the dashed curve of the idealized situation in that the pressure drop across the arterioles is 60 mm Hg, not 15 mm Hg! This means that there is a disproportionately larger resistance to arteriole flow, with the result that the pressure is anomalously high at their input end (about 100 mm Hg in the aorta and arteries), and anomalously low on the output side (5 to 15 mm Hg in the capillary beds, venules, veins and right heart). It is as if the arterioles are acting like an almost-closed faucet, with high pressure behind, but low pressure beyond, and very little flowing through. The resistance to flow within the arterioles is due to the contraction of the smooth muscles in the arteriole walls which reduces the diameters of the arterioles and so makes blood flow more difficult.

A somewhat similar situation may exist in the arteries themselves. If the arteries are open and unclogged, then little or no pressure difference will be measured between arteries close to the heart and those distant from the heart. Hydrostatic effects will be of no consequence here for reasons discussed in Section 11.F, Blood Pressure in Inverted *Yogasanas*, page 343. If, however, the arteries are blocked by atherosclerotic plaque, then, as with the arterioles, there will be a large pressure drop observable between the ends of an artery, as measured in the arm and at the ankle, for example.

Also shown in the Figure is the reciprocal relationship between the velocity of flow through a vascular section (flow velocity = flow volume/cross-sectional area of the vessel) and the cross-sectional area of that section. Because there are so many capillaries in the capillary bed, its total area is large even though the area of just one of them is small. Correspondingly, the flow velocity is low through the capillaries, whereas in the vena cava and aorta, the total cross-sections are low and the velocity is high.

A further complication of blood flow arises at high heart rates: in this case, the blood flow is turbulent, rather than smooth and laminar, and the net effect of the turbulence is to slow the flow, thereby making the heart work even harder to achieve a certain elevated flow rate.

Venous Flow Against Gravity

When standing upright, how then does the venous blood move from the feet upward to the heart if its pressure is close to zero (Fig. 11.C-4b)? This is especially intriguing considering that if one is upright and motionless, the first reaction to this simple posture is fainting, followed eventually by death*. The answer is that one does not remain motionless, but by contracting the skeletal muscles, the arterial flow is momentarily turned off to the muscle while the venous blood within the muscle is squeezed into the venules, outward and upward. The difference here between blood flow in arteries and veins arises from the fact that, since the arteries are already at high forward pressure and are stiff as well,

contraction of the muscle cannot force arterial blood to flow backward toward the heart, whereas veins being the opposite, are easily deformed so that the venous blood leaves the contracting muscle and overfills nearby venous channels.

Moreover, the veins are outfitted with one-way valves that only allow blood to flow toward the heart, Fig. 11.C-5. The presence of the one-way valves in the veins of the lower body cannot be overemphasized, for without them, the squeezing of the veins would push as much blood away from the heart as toward the heart, making the squeezing totally ineffective. This mechanism works best to pump venous blood when there is a rhythmic contraction and relaxation of the surrounding muscles; in fact, if the muscle is contracted for an extended time, or is "pumped up" by heavy exercise, the resulting congestion impedes blood flow through the muscle. Surprisingly, the two largest veins in the body, the inferior and superior vena cava, have no valves.

The flow of blood through a muscle also can be hindered by the high resting tone (Subsection 7.B, page 204) of the muscle. If there are many muscle fibers contracted for a long period of time, the pressure of the contracting muscles on the blood vessels can effectively pinch them off. Thus, in a sense, muscle tension acts like a tourniquet to impede the flow of both blood and *prana*.

In general, contraction of a muscle lowers the blood flow through it in proportion to the extent of contraction, with blood flow through the contracted muscle being much less in the inner core of the muscle than through the muscle's periphery. On the other hand, stretching a muscle significantly lowers its consumption of O_2 and again

---

*The death that results from crucifixion is in part due to the loss of blood draining from the brain into the legs [473], and in part due to the suffocation that follows from not being able to exhale when hanging from the arms with the hands widely separated [300, 457].

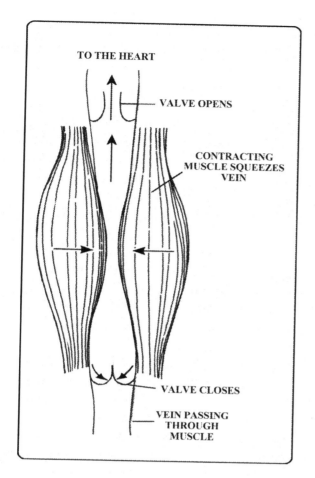

TO THE HEART

VALVE OPENS

CONTRACTING
MUSCLE SQUEEZES
VEIN

VALVE CLOSES

VEIN PASSING
THROUGH
MUSCLE

Fig. 11.C-5. As muscles contract, they press against the veins, pressurizing the blood within. The flap valves within the veins are constructed such that the pressure can be relieved in only one way: flow of the blood toward the heart. A similar drawing is appropriate for the pumping of lymph toward the heart by muscle action.

slows the blood flow, however, on releasing the stretch, blood flow then speeds up considerably [5].

That muscle action of the legs is effective in pumping venous blood from the legs to the heart is shown quantitatively by experiments in which pressure sensors were inserted into the saphenous veins of subjects near their ankles [367]. The average venous ankle pressure when lying down was measured to be 12 mm Hg, but this rose to 56 mm when sitting upright and to 90 mm when standing. However, upon walking, the venous pressure dropped from 90 mm to 22 mm, and then rose again to 90 mm once the subjects stopped walking. Thus the venous pressure in the ankle is reduced by 75% by the simple rhythmic use of the muscles of the leg when walking, as compared with just standing still. A similar type of venous pumping in the *yogasana* standing poses may well be working when one uses the approach of Iyengar [22] wherein one makes ongoing adjustments of the muscles, in essence turning them "on", then "off", repeatedly while in the pose, *i.e.*, his concept of "pose and repose" (see also footnote on page 342).

All of the veins in the torso of the body and in the legs emptying into the inferior vena cava are equipped with the one-way valves, as are the veins in the arms. However, as one is normally upright rather than inverted, the veins from the head leading to the superior vena cava have no valves. This means that when inverted either actively or passively, return of venous blood to the heart against the pull of gravity can be aided only by the rhythmic flexing of muscles in the arms [77, 239].

In the act of respiration, the downward movement of the diaphragm creates a momentary negative pressure above itself (which is sufficient to draw air into the lungs), and a positive pressure below, Section 12.A, Mechanics of the Breath, page 355. In combination, these two pressure effects act to help venous blood from below rise to the level of the heart [407, 443], but only because the venous system of the lower body passes through the thoracic chamber on its way to the heart, and only if the abdominal muscles are relaxed so as to keep the intra-abdominal pressure low. The respiratory pumping of blood works because the inhalation brings blood from the legs to the heart, and because the exhalation allows maximum blood flow through the lungs.

The pumping of venous blood through the action of respiration is strongest when the breathing is deep.

Should the valves in veins of the lower body fail to close properly and thus fail to hold back the venous tide, the veins below the leaky valve will bulge as varicose veins. In a related way, hemorrhoids are blood vessels in the rectum that sag under the pull of gravity when standing erect. As with lymph edema (Section 11.G, The Lymphatic System, page 352), hemorrhoids and venous varicosities are relieved by rhythmic exercises and inverted *yogasanas* which help pump and/or drain body fluids toward the heart. Just as clearly, extended periods of time in poses such as *padmasana*, which impede blood circulation in the legs are contraindicated if one has varicose veins in that region.

Chronic muscle tension that inhibits free-flowing circulation can lead to vasoconstriction of the arteries in the head, leading in turn to headaches (Subsection 3.B, *Headaches*, page 37). When this is the case, relief often can be had by promoting vasodilation using the ocular-vagal heart-slowing reflex, Section 7.D, Reflex Actions, page 211.

Thermoregulation

The body's vascular system is intimately involved with regulating the flow of heat from the core of the body to the skin, with the aim of keeping the core temperature relatively constant (Section 10.C, Thermal Regulation by Blood Vessels and Sweat Glands in the Skin, page 292). That is to say, the core temperature is regulated by shifting more or less of its blood to the skin for cooling by contact with the surrounding air. However, it is known as well that in each of us, the core temperature varies in a regular way throughout the 24-hour light-dark cycle, with a maximum temperature (38.1° C, 100.6° F) in the late afternoon (4:00–5:00 PM, Fig. 21.B-4), and a minimum

(36.3° C, 97.3° F) at about 2:00 AM (Fig. 21.B-2). Because these core temperatures are strongly entrained with the rhythm of the rising and setting sun, they are strongly constrained to a 24-hour cycle. Even when shielded from the sun or when in perpetual sunshine, the "free-running condition", the period of the core-temperature oscillation remains very close to 24 hours in spite of a lack of external visual cues to the contrary or any variations in the sleep-wake cycle [321].

Skin temperature also has its 24-hour cycle when the body is subject to the normal light-dark cycle as provided by the sun. However, when free-running, the period of skin-temperature oscillation can stretch out to 33 hours or even beyond that in some individuals, showing that the body has two or more internal clocks that are kept on 24-hour cycles by the sun but which otherwise run independently of one another when external 24-hour clues are not present (Subsection 21.B, *Circadian Rhythms; Physiological Peaks and Valleys in the 24-Hour Period*, page 476).

The characteristics of the temperature cycling in the human body are only weakly affected by ambient temperature in the range 20–32° C (68–90° F), and exercise raises the body temperature less during the day than during the night. Local temperatures are measured by sensors in the skin, spinal cord, hypothalamus and gut, with all thermal information sent to the posterior hypothalamus for review.

SECTION 11.D. BLOOD PRESSURE

Vasoconstriction, Vasodilation, and Hypertension

The blood vessels of the body are ringed with their own muscular system, Fig. 11.C-

3, which allows them to change their diameters, which in turn controls the blood flow. On signals from the involuntary vasomotor system of the brain, the muscles within the vascular system are contracted or relaxed so as to adjust the local bloodflow, increasing it here, decreasing it there. Moreover, by judicious transfer of warm blood from the inner core of the body to the outer surfaces of the body, again by vasomotor activation, the temperature profile of the body can be regulated (Section 10.C, Thermal Regulation by Blood Vessels and Sweat Glands in the Skin, page 292 and above).

Though the regulation of the overall flow of blood through the vascular system is primarily under the control of the heart, considerable local control can be exerted through the smooth muscles of the blood vessels themselves. Thus the endothelium cells can discharge certain prostaglandin paracrine hormones (see Chapter 15, THE HORMONES, page 399) which vasodilate the vessels, while the sympathetic nervous system can activate the smooth-muscle inner sheaths to cause vasoconstriction [230, 473]. It is also now known that the simple molecule nitric oxide (NO) is very effective in inducing vasodilation, increasing the arterial diameter by up to 15% by disengaging the actin and myosin filaments within the smooth muscles of the arterial wall [10].

Yet another of the body's mechanisms to raise the blood pressure is hormonal. In this case, when the baroreceptor signals to the brain (Section 11.E, Monitoring Blood Pressure with the Baroreceptors, page 339) report a low pressure, the brain directs the kidneys to release renin, which reacts with angiotensinogen circulating in the bloodstream from the liver (Chapter 15, THE HORMONES, page 399). The product of this reaction when acted upon by enzymes in the lungs is angiotensin II, a very powerful vasoconstrictor. Angiotensin II also acts

on the adrenal glands to release aldosterone, a compound that acts on the body's salt and water content to increase the blood volume [77, 86, 461], and thereby raise the pressure.

When the body is gripped by the effects of the fight-or-flight syndrome, the stimulation of certain centers in the hypothalamus directs the sympathetic nervous system to vasodilate the blood vessels to the heart and striated muscles while the blood vessels serving other parts of the body vasoconstrict. However, in this redistribution of the blood supply, more blood vessels are constricted than are dilated, with the result that the *net* effect is vascular constriction. This immediately translates into a higher blood pressure and more work for the heart to do. In Fig. 6.E-2, the interdependence of the various factors that react so as to form the stress response of sympathetic excitation are shown [406a]. Many aspects of this cycle reinforce high blood pressure, both short term and long term. Nonetheless, once the stress has passed, the sympathetic dominance ideally yields to parasympathetic dominance, the peripheral resistance declines as the arterioles return to their net dilated state, and both the blood pressure and heart rate return to normal, as in Fig. 11.E-2.

Many individuals, however, continue to carry the thought of the stressful event in their conscious mind and continue to replay the event over and over again, without understanding that just the thought of the event is enough to trigger the entire sympathetic display, long after the event itself is past. As a consequence of this repeated replaying of the stressful event, there is a long-term vasoconstriction within the vascular system, and a long-term elevation of the blood pressure and heart rate; this is the condition known as "hypertension" [343, 399]. In this condition, the heart is under a constant strain and because the circulatory system then functions at reduced efficiency,

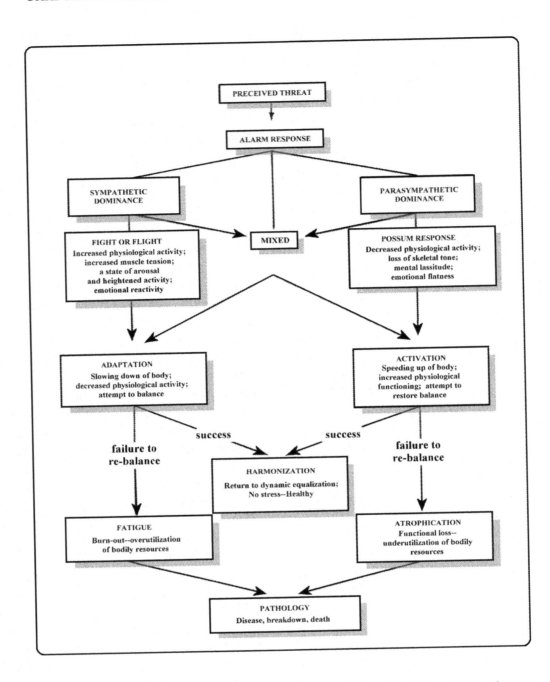

Fig. 11.D-1. The stages of reaction to a perceived threat, involving stimulation of either the sympathetic or parasympathetic nervous systems, and leading eventually to pathology if balance is not achieved.

the organs being served cannot recover readily once they have been used, and so rapidly become exhausted. If the state of high-pressure alarm is maintained for a long time, the baroreceptors will slowly reset the alarm level to a higher value, so that the elevated value then becomes the norm and hypertension then becomes chronic, persistent, and pathological, Fig. 11.D-1.

When hypertensive, the blood vessels are in a constant state of mild constriction, resulting in a heart that has become overworked, enlarged, and eventually weakened. Moreover, the excess pressure on the blood vessels act to produce small tears in the lining of the arteries in the brain, the kidneys and the small vessels of the eyes, thus weakening them with regard to stroke [399].

Of the two numbers given as the blood-pressure reading (Section 11.A, Structure and Function of the Heart, page 310), systolic/diastolic, the first relates to how well the heart is doing, whereas the second is a measure of how well the vascular system is doing, in that a high diastolic reading implies a high pressure even when the heart is in its resting phase, *i.e.*, a high peripheral resistance in the arterioles due to sympathetic vasoconstriction.

Hypertension is an "abnormally high" blood pressure, but the limit is difficult to define. If one accepts as "normal" a systolic/diastolic pressure ratio of 120/80 (Subsection 11.A, *The Pumping Chambers of the Heart*, page 310), then the hypertensive label would apply to those with blood pressures in the range 140/90 and above, in three successive readings. However, blood pressure tends to increase naturally with age [399], with children having a systolic pressure of only 75–90 mm Hg, whereas the elderly clock in at 130–150 mm Hg. Furthermore, "normal" refers to meat-eating subjects in a stressful, high-tech society. Thus blood pressure in the range 140/90 is a much more serious situation for a young person than for an older one, and even a "normal" pressure of 120/80 may be far from ideal considering how unhealthy "normal" might be. External factors also impact on our blood-pressure readings: everyone's pressure rises when they speak, the more so their baseline pressure is elevated, and correspondingly, the pressure drops when we listen [346].

One would expect that as the body goes into a state of hypertension, that the barore-

ceptors would respond to the increased pressure, and thereby moderate the heart and vascular activities so as to reduce the pressure. That this does not happen in the hypertensive person has been traced to a lack of baroreceptor sensitivity [48, 129, 418a]. As this sensitivity is posture dependent, one sees immediately that *yogasana* practice can be of aid in dealing with hypertension.

Eighty percent of hypertension cases, called "essential hypertension," are idiopathic, in that they have no known medical cause, and can be cured only with the help of yoga and meditation [399], though modern drugs too are effective in reducing the symptoms [245].

Assuming that hypertension is rooted in the excessive stimulation of the sympathetic nervous system [245] that one often encounters when living a fast-paced and stressful lifestyle, it is clear why *yogasana* practice is recommended for the hypertensive student. Through the action of *yogasana* on the lungs and its effect on breathing, through the action of *yogasana* on the brain through thought control, and through the action of *yogasana* on the muscles through relaxation, Fig. 6.E-2b, one can reverse the associations that drive high blood pressure. *Yogasanas* performed to reduce the blood pressure at first should be very relaxing and devoid of inversions (see Section 11.F, Blood Pressure in Inverted *Yogasanas*, page 343), with elements of challenge added only as the tension in the vascular system resides [399].

The efficacy of *yogasana* practice toward relieving hypertension has been demonstrated in several medical studies [108, 399, 418a]. Thus following *yogasana* training, heart rate, respiration rate, metabolism rate and blood pressure in the resting state were all decreased while the alpha-wave activity in the EEG increased. All of these changes are consonant with increasing dominance of the parasympathetic nervous system. Of the poses *vajrasana*, *sirsasana*, *sarvangasana*, *viparita karani*, *setu bandhasana* and *savasana*, the last of these was found to be the most effective in lowering the blood pressure. If a student is hypertensive and performs the *yogasanas* with a slight holding of the breath, then parasympathetic balance can be restored by looking down with the eyes [445].

In a study focusing on *savasana* as a treatment for essential hypertension, Datey, *et al.*, [108] found on average that the mean blood pressure (equal to the diastolic blood pressure plus one-third the systolic blood pressure) dropped from 134 mm to 107 mm by daily practice of 30 minutes of *savasana* over several months. For subjects already taking medication for hypertension, *savasana* for several months led to a reduction of their medication by 32% while maintaining a mean pressure of 102 mm. As expected for hypertension driven by atherosclerosis, *yogasanas* had no effect for people having this condition.

Datey, *et al.*, explain that by slow rhythmic breathing, the frequencies of the afferent proprioceptive and enteroceptive signals sent to the hypothalamus decrease, and because of this, the "normal" homeostatic blood pressure level as set by the hypothalamus is reset to a lower level. Similarly encouraging results have been reported for the benefits of relaxation to hypertensive patients in an extensive investigation by Patel and Marmot [352].

In another study of the effects of *yogasana* on essential hypertension, Selvamurthy, *et al.* [418a], conclude that *yogasana* practice works to increase the sensitivity of the baroreceptors and thus amplifies the effects of the baroreceptors on the adrenal hormones as well as on the renin-angiotensin system via the sympathetic nervous system.

In spite of evidence of the sort discussed above, certain practitioners of Western medicine, [179] for example, still feel that alternative techniques "such as relaxation and biofeedback, though appealing in theory, haven't reduced blood pressure significantly in clinical trials," whereas others are becoming more accepting (see, for example, [160]).

It is known that Black Americans suffer a 50% greater rate of death by heart disease than do white Americans, and that this difference is strongly related to differences in hypertension [86]. It appears that both black men and women are deficient in the simple molecule NO which otherwise is very active in dilating the smooth muscles within the blood vessels, thereby lowering the blood pressures within. That is to say, in times of stress, the blood vessels of blacks are less able to relax than those of whites. Social tensions also may be a contributing factor [360a]. In any case, yogic relaxation should be especially valuable. Note however, that there are other theories of hypertension, involving the interactions among proteins in the liver, lungs, and kidneys, which make no mention of NO [86], and the assumed role of the sympathetic nervous system in hypertension has been questioned from several directions by some medical workers [245].

Adults for whom the blood pressure reading is 100/60 or less are termed "hypotensive." Their problem largely is that long-term vasodilation leads to pooling of the blood in the extremities and the abdomen, such that not enough blood is delivered to the brain, and lightheadedness, fainting, nausea, weakness, *etc.*, are common. These symptoms are most often present when standing up from a sitting or lying position, as when recovering from *uttanasana* or *savasana*, for example. Hypotensive students may also display the "possum response", Fig. 11.D-1, demonstrating a parasympathetic (passive) dominance when the situation calls for a sympathetic (energized) response instead.

Hypotension may not be evident at all when measured in a seated position, but then becomes a strong factor when standing upright. In such a situation, a student of *yogasana* may find himself weak and dizzy in the standing poses, but have no such problems when seated or lying down.

SECTION 11.E. MONITORING BLOOD PRESSURE WITH THE BARORECEPTORS

The body's need for homeostasis requires that there be one or more mechanisms available to it for controlling blood pressure within a narrow range. This in turn implies the existence of sensors which can respond

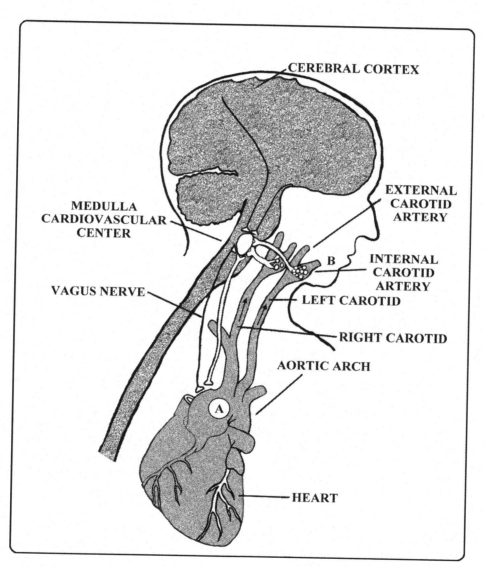

Fig. 11.E-1. Location of the baroreceptors on the aortic arch (**A**) and in the sinus of the left internal carotid artery (**B**). Also shown are the afferent nerves from the baroreceptors to the medulla cardiovascular center in the brainstem, the efferent vagus nerve from the medulla to the heart, and the neural connections to this center from higher centers in the brain.

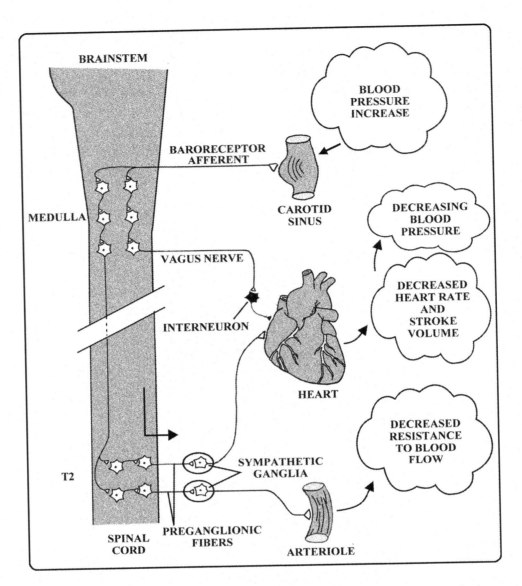

Fig. 11.E-2. The carotid-sinus reflex arc, showing the interneuron, between the sympathetic vagus nerve and the heart, which acts to suppress heart rate (HR), and the inhibition of the ganglionic fibers of the sympathetic nervous system, which acts to lower the heart rate, the force of contraction of the heart (FC), and to dilate the arterioles so as to reduce the peripheral resistance to blood flow. All of these factors acting together lower the blood pressure once the carotid sinus has been pressurized.

to blood pressure changes, together with afferent nerves from these sensors to autonomic control centers in the brain and efferent nerves from there to the various pressure-controlling organs of the body.

The pressure sensors in the cardiovascular system are known as "baroreceptors",

these being a special class of sensor within the larger class of mechanoreceptors sensitive to pressure or mechanical stress, Section 10.B, Sensory Receptors in the Skin, page 285. The baroreceptors responding to blood pressure are located in the aortic arch and in the internal carotid arteries, Fig.

11.E-1. Baroreceptors within the arch use the depressor nerve as afferents, while those in the carotid sinus use the sinus nerve. Neurons from the baroreceptors synapse to the cardiovascular center in the brainstem (the medulla oblongata), with afferent and efferent fibers lying side by side. It appears that the baroreceptors can measure not only the changes in peak and average pressures, but also the time-rate-of-change of pressure and the heart rate as well [230].

Other types of baroreceptors within the heart are sensitive to the degree of filling of the right atrium and to the volume of the blood sent forward by the contraction of the left ventricle.

The Baroreceptor Reflex Arc

In the body's equilibrium resting state, the cardiac baroreceptors output a steady 0.5–2 Hertz modulated electrical signal along the afferent fibers, which synapse at the solitary tract nucleus, a brainstem nucleus prominent in autonomic activity. Suppose then that the blood pressure rises, and that the need for homeostasis then requires an involuntary lowering of the pressure. How can this happen? The answer lies in the baroreceptor reflex arc illustrated in Fig. 11.E-2.

The baroreceptors are embedded in the arterial walls; when the pressure rises, the walls bulge outward somewhat and the baroreceptors sense this increased mechanical stress. In response, they raise the frequencies of the signals launched up the afferent nerves, in proportion to the amount of mechanical strain induced above that in the resting state. On reaching the solitary tract nucleus, the signal is relayed to the nucleus ambiguus [195, 230], which in turn energizes the parasympathetic neurons which inhibit cardiac action by slowing the

heart beat via the vagus nerve. At the same time, there is reduced activity in the sympathetic fibers controlling heart rate (HR), force of contraction (FC) and arteriole diameter. The net result is that the heart rate decreases and the flow resistance in the arterioles decreases* as they dilate, so that the blood pressure drops back into the normal range.

Pressure at the baroreceptors can be raised by tipping the body toward or into an inverted state. As baroreceptor activation requires relatively high over-pressure, it usually does not turn on until the body has been tipped about 50–60° from vertical [77]. The situation involving a posturally-driven increase in blood pressure and the body's response to this are discussed below, Section 11.F, Blood Pressure in Inverted *Yogasanas*, page 343.

If the body is under physical stress so that there is a strong sympathetic activation of the heart calling for more blood flow as with endurance runners, then the heart will enlarge in response to this. A similar enlargement occurs when the source of the stress is nonphysical, but chronic (see Subsection 22.A, *Physical Aging*, page 495). As both the blood pressure and the respiration rate are important factors in delivering O_2 to tissues under stress, their autonomic controls are closely coordinated. Indeed, their simultaneous action must be co-ordinated if the system is to maintain cardiorespiratory homeostasis.

On the other hand, if the pressure becomes too low, the baroreceptor signal frequency drops below 0.5 Hertz and the actions then of the autonomic nervous system are such as to increase the heart rate and constrict the arterioles and veins, thereby resetting the pressure at a higher level. A low blood volume also can give a low-pres-

---

*But not to the brain or to the heart, which cannot afford to have their blood supplies curtailed!

sure signal at the baroreceptors and so stimulate drinking behavior while inhibiting urination [225]; the opposite occurs when inverting (see Box 11.F-3, *Inversion (and Laughing) Can Lead to Urination*, page 351).

With increasing age, the functioning of the baroreceptors normally degrades and so diminishes the body's ability to maintain blood-pressure homeostasis [92]. The situation for yoga students however, may be very different, for they regularly exercise the baroreceptor apparatus through the practice of inversions, and so keep the baroreceptors in working condition.

Cole [79] has observed a rather interesting correlation between baroreceptor stimulation in the carotid sinus and aortic arch with EEG changes signaling sleep or arousal; this is discussed in Section 3.E, Brainwaves and the Electroencephalogram, page 57.

Other Sensors

There are other sensors in the circulatory system which also impact on the return of the blood pressure to its resting value. One such sensor within the cardiac wall of the right atrium measures the fractional volume of blood filling the heart in the diastole phase and adjusts the blood flow accordingly, while another measures stroke volume of

the heart and decreases it when it is too high and increases it when it is too low. According to Cole [77], the atrial baroreceptor is more sensitive than those in the carotid arteries or in the aorta. On the venous side, flow rates in part are controlled by the autonomic nervous system through the diameters of the veins, thus limiting (by vasoconstriction) or enhancing (by vasodilation) the flow of blood to the heart.*

Chemoreceptors sensitive to O_2, CO_2 and pH also reside within the circulatory system, and their inputs to the autonomic-nervous-system centers (again the solitary tract nucleus) are also factors in regulating the heart rate, blood pressure and respiration rate [195]. In particular, carotid bodies in the carotid arteries and aortic bodies in the aortic arch are sensitive to the amounts of O_2 and CO_2 in the arterial blood, and when the amount of O_2 is too low or the amount of CO_2 is too high, these receptors trigger an increase in the breathing rate, using either the vagus nerve (cranial nerve X) from the aortic arch or the glossopharyngeal nerve (cranial nerve IX) from the carotid arteries [340].

The autonomic response to the baroreceptor signals outlined above is subject to control by yet higher centers in the brain. Thus the simple reflex arc of Fig. 11.E-2 can be overridden by deliberately intense

---

*Actually, when the veins in the legs vasoconstrict, there is a momentary surge of blood sent upward to the heart, however, from that point on, there is an increased resistance to venous blood flow through the constricted veins and the flow is therefore diminished. If on the other hand, the muscles of the legs are alternately flexed and then relaxed in a rhythmic way, one has an efficient pump for continuously moving venous blood to the heart against gravity. The importance of muscle action in pumping blood is graphically demonstrated by experiments in which students are leaned against the wall and left in that position *without* any activation of the muscles in their legs; by the end of an hour in this passive position, more than 95% of them will have fainted. Without muscle action in the legs, so much blood will pool in the legs that the atrial baroreceptor will sense an insufficiency of the filling of the right atrium, and will signal the brain to shut down so as to trigger a faint. This reflex then places heart and feet at the same height so that proper filling of the right atrium can again be achieved [77]. See Subsection 11.C, *Venous Flow Against Gravity*, page 332, for further discussion on this point. There are valves in the veins of the limbs and neck, and so muscle action in inverted positions also will pump blood back to the heart [229].

exercise, so that changes in the heart rate, filling volume, blood pressure and blood chemistry rise to anomalous values and stay there for a time in spite of the autonomic tendency toward homeostasis.

SECTION 11.F. BLOOD PRESSURE IN INVERTED *YOGASANAS*

When one goes from an upright position to fully inverted, gravity initially pulls the fluids in the body toward the head rather than toward the feet. This shift of pressure has multiple consequences for the circulatory system and the ultimate blood pressure reached in the head and brain while inverted. The significant factors affecting the blood pressure while inverted are discussed below, whereas the related effects of body orientation on the efficiency of oxygenation of the blood in the lungs are discussed in Section 12.A, Mechanics of the Breath, page 355.

Hydrostatic Pressure

The question of just what happens to one's blood pressure when inverting is a fascinating one. Clearly, there is much more to it than the blood simply rushing to the head, for it is known [77, 443] that a practicing yogi can have a blood pressure in inversions which is *lower* than that when seated! No doubt, there are manifold regulators in the body, the jobs of which are to see that the blood does not just rush into the head where the over-pressure might possibly rupture a vessel, creating a cerebral stroke. In order to understand the situation in regard to the behavior of the blood pressure when inverted, it is useful to first understand the concept of hydrostatic pressure.

The pressure at the bottom of a column of liquid is greater than that at the top because the liquid at the bottom is supporting the weight of all the liquid above it. This pressurization, due to gravity, is called the hydrostatic pressure, and is only dependent on the height of the liquid column involved and

---

BOX 11.F-1: HOW THE GIRAFFE AND THE DINOSAUR GAMBLE WHEN TAKING THEIR FIRST LUNCH

For a giraffe (camelopardus) with its long neck, taking its first drink of water with its head between its long legs can be a risky business, just as it must have been for the long-necked but short-legged dinosaur sampling its first taste of leaves from the top of a tall tree. In both cases, there is an important hydrostatic effect that comes into play that would kill the animal were it not dealt with appropriately.

In the upright giraffe, to the systolic blood pressure at the aorta must be added the hydrostatic pressure of the ten-foot long column of blood that otherwise rests upon the heart. Fortunately for this animal, the material of the arterial walls near the heart is strong enough to withstand this combined pressurization from the systolic heart beat and the hydrostatic effect. Note too that when standing erect, the pressure within the blood vessels in and surrounding the giraffe's brain have no contribution from the hydrostatic effect as they are at the top of the blood column and so are pressurized only to the systolic pressure at the aorta. This is fortunate, for the blood vessels in the brain are much smaller and weaker than is the aorta.

344 CHAPTER 11. THE HEART AND THE VASCULAR SYSTEM

However, when the giraffe bends over to take its first drink, placing its long neck between its long legs, head at ground level, the hydrostatic pressure in the arteries surrounding the brain and the arterial pressure from the contraction of the heart again reinforce one another, but in this case, the resultant over-pressure occurs in the arteries within the brain and is far higher than the blood vessels in this area can withstand. That is to say, the giraffe should suffer a burst artery within the brain the first time it bends over to drink!

That the giraffe does not suffer an anuerysm or stroke is due to two reactions that work to moderate the expected increase in cranial blood pressure when drinking. First, note that the arteries *within* the brain are protected from this over-pressure because they are surrounded by the cerebrospinal fluid which presses inward on the blood vessels, thereby canceling the hydrostatic pressurization by the blood when the animal's head is down. This effect does not come into play, however, for the arteries of the head that are not surrounded by cerebrospinal fluid such as the carotid and vertebral arteries and those within the eyes (see Subsection 11.F, *Inversion and Blood Pressure at the Eyes*, page 349).

The second reaction protects the vessels not otherwise protected by the cerebrospinal fluid: the baroreceptors in the animal's heart and neck sense the rapidly increasing pressure as the animal bends forward, and correspondingly adjust the heart rate downward and enlarge the vascular diameters to allow the pressure in the vicinity of the brain to remain in a safe range.

In the case of the herbivorous dinosaurs, it has been thought that these huge animals with their necks of 30 feet or more in length would eat by grazing the tops of very tall trees. However, this implies a huge hydrostatic pressure at the aorta in addition to the systolic pressure of a column of blood being pumped upward by more than 30 feet. Again, no known biological material is strong enough to stand up to the combined pressures, hydrostatic plus systolic, at the aorta that such a situation implies. In an effort to get around this objection, some have suggested that the dinosaurs had one heart in the chest cavity and then one or more along the length of the neck to act as relay pumping stations, but no evidence for this has been found. It is more likely that these animals had very long necks but never lifted their heads much above their hearts, eating low on the trees and sparing themselves the risk of vascular overpressure at the aorta [446].

Fortunately, we as upright humans do not have the huge hydrostatic forces that an upright dinosaur or a drinking giraffe would have to deal with, but we too have mechanisms that can respond to the increased pressure of yogic inversion, albeit not nearly as rapidly, see below.

its density. Pressurization of the vascular system by the beating of the heart is an independent, but equally important factor. If the pressure within the vascular system at the level of the beating heart is arbitrarily taken to be zero, then the hydrostatic pressure in the feet while in a standing pose will be about 1/10 atmosphere (70 mm Hg, 1.5 pounds per square inch) and that above the heart will be negative. In a person of average height in a fully inverted position, the hydrostatic pressure of the body's blood as experienced in the head will be about 1/7 atmosphere (100 mm Hg, 2 pounds per

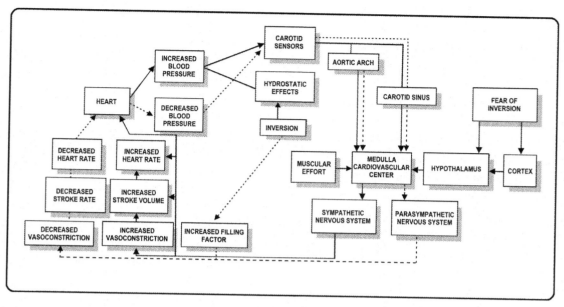

Fig. 11.F-1. The multiple effects of inversion on various circulatory functions. The full lines indicate the paths of sympathetic excitation and the dashed lines indicate the paths for parasympathetic excitation. See text for discussion.

square inch).* This is approximately equal to the normal systolic pressure in the arteries and is about 50% larger than the diastolic pressure. The hydrostatic pressure at the base of a column of liquid such as blood or cerebrospinal fluid which stands L mm high is L/13.6, in units of mm Hg. See Box 11.F-1 for the perilous hydrostatic risks faced by giraffes when drinking and dinosaurs when eating.

As for the effects of hydrostatic pressure while in the inverted *yogasanas*, we consider two possibilities: semi-inversion, where the length of the hydrostatic column is approximately half the body height (as in *halasana* or *uttanasana*, for example), and full inversion where the hydrostatic column height is the full-body height (as in *sarvangasana*, for example). These are discussed below.

General Effects of Inversion on Circulation

In order to illustrate the manifold ways in which inversion can affect the circulatory system, consider the schematic shown in Fig. 11.F-1, imagining it to be appropriate to a beginning student trying *sarvangasana* for the first time. The student's first response to being told that "we will now attempt to stand on the backs of our heads," is one of fear. The fear of inversion will work at both the subconscious level through the hypothalamus and at the conscious level through the cortex. Both of these become inputs to the medulla oblongata housing the cardiovascular center, prompting it to get ready to do battle, *i.e.*, to activate the sympathetic nervous system. If as seems likely, the fear element also results in excess muscular effort when in the posture, this too will

*Actually, in full inversion, the blood drains out of the feet so that the effective height of the hydrostatic blood column is less than the full body height.

become input into the medulla, again promoting an intensified sympathetic response. Finally, fear is known to raise the sensitivity to pain [404], thus increasing the apprehension factor even more.

Once the sympathetic alarm has been rung, the circulatory consequences are a vasoconstriction of the arterioles, an increased cardiac stroke volume and an increased heart rate, all of which act to significantly increase the systolic blood pressure. See Fig. 6.E-2 in this regard.

In addition to the fear reaction, the simple act of inversion leads to two key hydrostatic effects: first, it acts to increase the blood pressure in the head and chest, and this increased pressure is sensed by the carotid sensors in the aortic arch and in the carotid sinuses. Second, Copeland [89] explains that in inverted postures, there is an "easy" return of venous blood to the heart, thus filling it more than otherwise. In response to this larger filling factor for the right atrium, the heart rate tends to drop as more blood is pumped with each contraction.*

To the extent that there is no extra muscular effort or extra demand for oxygen when inverting (*sarvangasana*, for example, performed without undue effort), the extra filling and correspondingly larger stroke volume will activate sensors in the heart for these parameters (Subsection 11.E, *Other Sensors*, page 342), which in turn will be accommodated by a lowering of the heart rate and blood pressure. Indeed, medical students with some experience in doing the inverted *yogasanas* are reported to have had an average heart rate of 67 beats/minute in the supine position, 84 beats/minute upon standing from the supine position, and in

sirsasana I, an average heart rate of only 69 beats/minute [146, 239].

Theoretically, the increased pressure at the baroreceptors in the aorta and carotid arteries will promote a slowing of the heart and a decreased blood pressure in the head upon inversion, however, these receptors may be very slow to act, and so the student's face becomes very red and flushed, and the eyes may even become bloodshot. These effects can be minimized if one goes into the inverted position in steps, and spends time at each step, rather than going too rapidly from upright to inverted [77, 443]. A similar strategy holds for coming out of inversions and not standing up too soon.

Thus we see that there are several opposing factors acting simultaneously, each trying to dictate to the circulatory system, in an effort to coax the autonomic balance in one direction or the other. The various opposing effects of inversion on the blood pressure are summed at the carotid sensors, and the more important will then dictate to the medulla as to the best autonomic balance. The importance of having mechanisms that operate in opposition to one another makes it possible to continuously vary the level of dominance and so prevent a runaway super-excitation of either autonomic branch. Thus, if the sympathetic system is over-excited, then the signal prompting parasympathetic excitation will become dominant, the sympathetic channel will be inhibited and the blood pressure will drop, along with the smooth-muscle tone in the arterioles.

The throttling of the blood supply to the brain can have both positive and negative consequences in inverted *yogasana* practice. For example, in the head-forward positions (flexion), as in *sarvangasana, etc.*,

---

*Actually, Cole [77] reports that the right atrial filling is largest when in a 30° head-down position, and that inversion beyond 30° tends to drain blood away from the heart and toward the head, provided the head is not lifted.

there is generally a slowing of the heart as the baroreceptors in the neck are tricked into reporting a high blood pressure. This is a beneficial effect as it promotes relaxation. On the other hand, when the head is pressed backward (extension) as in *ustrasana*, the

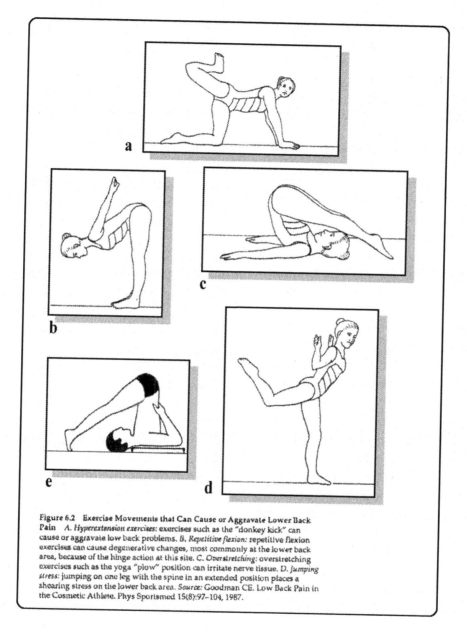

Figure 6.2 **Exercise Movements that Can Cause or Aggravate Lower Back Pain** A. *Hyperextension exercises:* exercises such as the "donkey kick" can cause or aggravate low back problems. B. *Repetitive flexion:* repetitive flexion exercises can cause degenerative changes, most commonly at the lower back area, because of the hinge action at this site. C. *Overstretching:* overstretching exercises such as the yoga "plow" position can irritate nerve tissue. D. *Jumping stress:* jumping on one leg with the spine in an extended position places a shearing stress on the lower back area. *Source: Goodman CE. Low Back Pain in the Cosmetic Athlete. Phys Sportsmed 15(8):97–104, 1987.*

Fig. 11.F-2. (**c**) Demonstration of *halasana* together with a warning about its dangers to the nerves and muscles of the neck and back. If you rotate picture **c**, you will see how closely the illustrated posture resembles full *paschimottanasana*, but with the back rounded/over-stretched and the chin jammed against the chest. (**e**) *Halasana* as it should be practiced, with blankets under the shoulders, the back supported by the arms, and the legs pressed upward so as to protect the neck and back (compare to illustration **c**).

blood flow through the vertebral arteries may be inhibited, with the result that the student feels nauseous and/or dizzy.

As the student's expertise increases in *sarvangasana*, the fear factor and the muscular-effort factor become less important and the ascendance of the parasympathetic channel is more closely approached. Once this happens, *sarvangasana* has been transformed from a fearful, energizing pose into a calm, relaxing one, Fig. 6.E-3.

Blood Pressure in Semi-Inversion

Consider the question of initiating an aneurysm due to increased arterial pressure in the brain by inverting. Lasater [262] has spoken to this point in refuting an earlier claim that *halasana* is dangerous and should not be performed by anyone (see Fig. 11.F-2 for an example of this point of view). In her rebuttal, Lasater points out that on inverting in *halasana*, the hydrostatic pressure of the blood in the brain does increase, tending to push the arterial walls outward. However, with the head lower than the pelvis, there is also the hydrostatic pressure of the cerebrospinal fluid to be considered, for the brain floats in this (Section 4.D, Cerebrospinal Fluid, page 93), and its hydrostatic action is to press inward on the walls of the arteries which it surrounds. Thus the net result of this *halasana* semi-inversion from the hydrostatic point of view is that there is no net increase in the arterial pressure in the brain and spinal cord, for the hydrostatic pressure of the blood is opposed by the hydrostatic pressure of the cerebrospinal fluid. Of course, there is an increase in pressure, but it is borne by the bones of the skull and not by the arterial walls within the brain (however, see *Inversion and Blood Pressure at the Eyes*, below, and Appendix II, INJURIES INDUCED BY IMPROPER *YOGASANA*

PRACTICE, page 511, for an important exception to this statement).

Moreover, with the chin pressed more or less toward the sternum in *halasana*, the baroreceptors of the carotid arteries and the aortic arch will be activated (Section 11.E, Monitoring Blood Pressure with the Baroreceptors, page 339, and Section 7.D, Reflex Actions, page 211). In response to this, the activity in the sympathetic nerves driving the heart beat will be inhibited by the parasympathetic system (Section 6.D, The Parasympathetic Nervous System, page 150), the heart rate will be slowed and the arteries will dilate, thus lowering the blood pressure still further. Nonetheless, *halasana* must be done with the neck soft, so that the blood in the head can move as easily as possible through the neck and back toward the heart. The feedback loop described above and in Fig. 11.F-1 for *halasana* will be more or less active in all of the inversions, especially so in students practicing inversions on a regular basis.

Cole [77] raises another interesting point in regard to inversions. The return of venous blood to the heart from the lower body and the arms is aided by one-way valves in the veins which allow blood to flow only toward the heart (Subsection 11.C, *Venous Flow Against Gravity*, page 332). There are no such valves in the veins of the head as none are needed for the up-right posture which drains the blood back to the heart by gravity flow. However, when inverted, there appears to be nothing to return blood from the head to the heart. Because of this, working the arms vigorously in the inversions is of great benefit as the contraction and relaxation of the muscles of the arms helps to pump venous blood from the arms to the heart against the pull of gravity.

Uttanasana is particularly interesting [77], in that the head is below the heart while the feet are on the floor. In this pose, there is much pooling of the blood in the upright legs while pressure in the carotid arteries promotes a slower heart rate and vasodilation. The problem with this is that on coming back to *tadasana* from *uttanasana*, with the heart rate low, the blood pooling in the legs, and the blood vessels dilated, there is a great rush of blood away from the brain on standing up and the student can feel very faint. This is especially so if *uttanasana* is a new position for the student, or they have a sluggish heart-rate response, or a low blood volume. Similar effects can be experienced on just getting up rapidly from a seated position or getting up to urinate in the morning. This latter voiding is driven by parasympathetic excitation, and so is the decreased heart rate and vasodilation. Even if the student is not feeling faint on coming up from *uttanasana*, doing so rapidly can trigger a too-low signal from the baroreceptors, with consequent racing of the heart and vasoconstriction (but not in the heart and brain!). This too can be avoided by coming up slowly. Should a person faint from lack of blood to the brain, the situation is self-correcting: in the prone and supine positions, the blood pressure quickly equalizes head to toe.

In *viparita karani*, the pelvis is positioned so that the abdomen is more or less horizontal, forming a lake into which the blood of the legs can drain [215a]. Done in this way, there is no rise in the pressure in the head, while the blood and lymph in the legs have the advantage of a free ride downhill to the abdominal pool. In this way the blood does not rest on the heart but only gently spills over in that direction.

Full-Body Inversions

In full-body inversions such as *sirsasana* or *adho mukha vrksasana*, the column of cerebrospinal fluid is only about half as long as that of the column of blood, and so its pressure acts to counter only about half of the hydrostatic pressure of the blood in the arterioles of the brain. Still, the carotid baroreceptors do their all to reduce pressure by reducing heart rate and by vasodilation, Fig. 11.E-1. Again, active use of the muscles of the arms in these poses will aid the return of venous blood to the heart, which in turn will act to reduce the heart rate and blood pressure, but the muscular effort expended in the poses also will act to increase the heart rate in opposition to the effect of the baroreceptors.

Benefits of full-body inversion include improved drainage of body fluids from the legs toward the heart and a different flow of blood through the heart. Regular practice of inversions within a balanced *yogasana* program are said to correct general fatigue or lack of vitality, headache and migraine, loss of or graying hair, bad facial complexion, eye, nose and throat ailments, indigestion, constipation and diabetes, prolapse of internal organs, sexual malfunction, varicose veins and hemorrhoids, rheumatism, depression, tension and anxiety, insomnia, and general psychological problems [215a, 400].

Inversion and Blood Pressure at the Eyes

In the discussions above, the hydrostatic pressure of the cerebrospinal fluid was described as countering the hydrostatic-pressure rise in the arterioles of the brain and spinal cord when semi-inverted. This counter pressure is effective because the cerebrospinal fluid completely surrounds the brain and spinal cord. Like the brain, each of the optic nerves and most of each eyeball is surrounded by the dura mater and pia-arachnoid sheaths, and so is continuous with the meningeal spaces around the brain. However, because the cerebrospinal fluid does not completely surround the arterioles of the eyes, any increase in the hydrostatic pressure of the blood in the skull, as when inverting, is transmitted hydrostatically to

---

BOX 11.F-2: TURNING RED DURING AND AFTER INVERSIONS

When one temporarily deprives a muscle of its blood supply, the muscle cells nonetheless continue their metabolizing, with the consequent accumulation of CO_2 and acidic products. These metabolites act as local vasodilators, such that when circulation is once again restored, there is a strong surge of fresh blood into the dilated blood vessels in an attempt to restore normalcy as quickly as possible. This effect is readily observed by hanging head down in an inversion swing for about 5 minutes. Lack of blood to the feet first cools them and the veins dilate in expectation of a return of the blood supply. Once out of the swing and on your feet, see how red and warm the feet become as they suck up blood like a dry sponge. Once the metabolites are flushed from the feet, circulation returns to normal, as does the color and temperature of the feet.

One often notes a reddening of the face when a student is in *sarvangasana*. In this case, there is a collapse of the jugular veins draining blood from the head and neck due to too sharp an angle at the throat. This condition is relieved by opening this angle using more blankets under the shoulders [258], and by leaning backward so that the weight is heavier on the elbows and lighter on the back of the skull.

---

these arterioles without a compensating balance from the cerebrospinal fluid. This excess pressure on inverting may lead to complications for individuals with a disposition toward bloodshot eyes, glaucoma or detached retina [77, 443].

The general anxiety felt by many students in inversions moreover leads to a general sympathetic response which increases arterial and intraocular pressures in the eye. Though the arterial pressure in general is sufficient to bring blood to the eye, the compensating pressure of the cerebrospinal fluid can impede the drainage of both lymph and blood from the retina, and so encourage hypertensive retinopathy. This mechanism is exactly parallel to that faced by the uterus during inversions in menstruating women (Section 19.A, page 453), and so argues against such inverted poses in the hypertensive student or in students with eye problems.

For students who experience deep reddening of the face and pressure behind bloodshot eyes in *sirsasana*, this can be reduced by first resting the weight of the head on the forehead on the floor in *adho mukha virasana* for 5 minutes and then going inverted without lifting the head off the floor. This action activates the vagal heart-slowing reflex which reduces the blood pressure before going up (Section 7.D, Reflex Actions, page 211). At the other end of the body, in the fully-extended inversions, the arterial pressure in the feet will rapidly fall to zero as the heart is not strong enough to pump blood successfully to the feet against gravity [77, 264, 443] (see Box 11.F-2). This lack of circulation in the full inversions leads to very cold feet after many minutes of being inverted.

Inversions and Hypertension

The above descriptions apply to the average student with average blood pressure. If the student is hypertensive, then one cannot depend upon the compensating factors to do their job immediately. In this case, mild inversions can be introduced slowly, with great attention paid to their outward effects on the blood pressure. For both normal and hypertensive students, there is great value in doing the appropriate inversions or variations of them, for in doing so, the baroreceptors are thought to eventually reset at a lower level, thus keeping the blood pressure on a long-term basis within a lower range of values [264, 443]. However, the inverted *yogasanas* should not be performed by hypertensive students if the blood pressure rises in the course of their performance [445].

Inversions can be approached rationally by breaking them up into stages, and then performing each of the successive stages as a complete asana. If one then rests in each stage to allow the body to accommodate to the partial inversion, the fully inverted position may eventually be achieved. For example, first work on *sirsasana* with the knees on the ground. When this can be done without a significant rise in pressure, then start straightening the legs in order to elevate the pelvis. Once this is accomplished without a significant rise in pressure, elevate the legs slightly with the legs straight, and in time, work toward having the legs straight and supported at chair height. Continue working in this way so that students can slowly work toward inversion without risking a precipitous rise in their blood pressure. The idea here is that by performing the intermediate steps in the inversion, the blood pressure will slowly lower, and so not be too much out of range when the final inverted position is attempted.

The elderly often show "postural hypotension" (Subsection 11.D, *Vasoconstriction, Vasodilation, and Hypertension*, page 334), where cardiac baroreceptors and the volume receptor fail to induce proper vagal stimulation and/or reflexive sympathetic action (speed the heart and constrict the blood vessels). This leads to a fainting feeling when standing erect [195].

Benefits of Inversions

It is thought that by doing inversions which temporarily raise the blood pressure, but learning to relax while doing them, the baroreceptors react by resetting their trigger levels in the downward direction. This means that following an inversion, one's blood pressure should be lower thereafter, even when sitting passively [443]. This does not mean that inversions are appropriate work for students who are hypertensive! Their blood pressure can be brought down through the use of inversions, but to do it safely, one must introduce the inversions slowly, and slowly work toward attaining the fully inverted position.

Lymph flows easily from the feet to the heart in inversions, and so inversions can be very helpful in relieving edemous conditions in the legs*. Inversions also help sluggish venous blood flow at the end of a long day on one's feet, when blood and lymph tend to pool in the lower extremities. Inversions are the standard *yogasana* approach to relieving the pressure in varicose veins and hemorrhoids, and also are effective in relieving constipation [216] and promoting urination, Box 11.F-3, page 352.

As discussed more fully in Section 8.G, Osteoporosis, page 269, exercise helps to strengthen those bones which bear weight, thus protecting them from osteoporosis. Only yoga offers the opportunity to safely bear weight on the head and so strengthen both the muscles of the neck and the vertebrae in that area.

---

*In edema, there is a localized fluid retention in the legs which can be relieved by performing *viparita karani*. In this, the gravitational pull leads blood and lymph more easily to the heart, and as a result, the brain then dilates the blood vessels in the kidneys which results ultimately in a diuretic-like effect in an effort to lower blood volume in the body [77]. See Box 11.F-3, page 352.

BOX 11.F-3: INVERSION (AND LAUGHING) CAN LEAD TO URINATION

Whenever we go inverted, the volume sensors in the atria of the heart sense the increased blood volume and the reflexive reaction to this is for the brain to dilate the blood vessels in the kidneys, thus processing more blood into extracellular fluid and urine and so promoting urination. By urinating, the blood volume and hence blood pressure are reduced, bringing the body back to a homeostatic condition appropriate to an inverted posture. Of course, once on your feet again, having urinated, the blood pressure and blood volume will then be momentarily low, and long-term homeostasis in the upright posture can then be restored only by the in-take of fluids.

It also can happen that if one rises in the middle of the night to urinate, the simultaneous flow of blood away from the heart toward the feet coupled with the parasympathetic action that slows the heart, dilates the blood vessels, and releases the urinary sphincter are sufficient to cause one to faint while urinating. Being related to parasympathetic relaxation, urination is begun on an exhalation.

On the other hand, laughing also dilates the blood vessels and so lowers the blood pressure. This parasympathetic response might explain in part why we tend to pee in our pants when laughing too hard, for urination is also driven by the parasympathetic system, Table 6.A-2. See also Subsection 7.D, *Other Reflex Actions*, page 220, for an account of the effects of laughter on muscle tone.

Of course, how the blood pressure changes in inversions also can reflect the performer's emotional attitude and fears about being turned up-side-down, and these psychological effects can compete successfully with the purely physiological ones discussed above. The imagined danger of being in such a precarious position is as potent as any real threat from any source, and will be sufficient to excite the sympathetic fight-or-flight response. Further, anticipation can be more stressful than the real thing.

SECTION 11.G. THE LYMPHATIC SYSTEM

Structure and Function

At the level of the capillaries of the blood's vascular system, the capillaries are often at a distance from the cells which they serve, and thanks to the arteriole pressure applied to their near ends, they tend to leak fluid into the extracellular space surrounding these cells. This fluid, called lymph, and the channels which transport it form the lymphatic system. Like the vascular system, the lymphatic channels interconnect so as to form larger and larger conduits for their fluids. However, the lymphatic system is not a closed loop like the vascular system, being open ended at the level of the smallest channels. Lymph flows toward the heart in the same direction as venous blood [319].

The lymph system serving more superficial tissues is rather independent of and disconnected from that part of the system serving the deeper tissues [106, 291]. The largest of the lymphatic vessels drain their contents into the thoracic and right lymph ducts in the vicinity of the upper chest. The lymphatic system does not extend into the brain, spinal cord, bone marrow or avascular structures such as cartilage and epidermis. Surprisingly, the lymphatic system is an active part of the digestive system (Chapter 18, THE GASTROINTESTINAL TRACT AND DIGESTION, page 441), for it serves to carry emulsified fats from the small intestine into the blood stream. The lymphatic system processes 2 to 4 liters of lymph per day, whereas the heart pumps 5 liters of blood every minute.

The composition of lymph is very much like that of the blood plasma from which it is derived, except for the near absence of blood proteins such as serum albumin, which are too large molecularly to diffuse through the capillary walls. Lymph contains many large fragments of cell debris [239] as well as bacteria, *etc*. In healthy, active muscle tissue, the weight percent of the lymphatic fluid bathing the cells is about 15% [109].

As the gravitational effects on the body are minimal when the body is horizontal, the lymph in the body is minimal and evenly distributed when we get out of bed in the morning, however, in the course of a day spent on our feet or just sitting, the gravitational pull toward the feet is sufficient to promote leakage of lymph preferentially in the lower limbs, and so the legs tend to swell. At this time, the volume of blood is depleted by the amount converted into lymph, and so the low blood volume may promote a faster heart rate in compensation.

In order to prevent swelling of the tissue, it is necessary to somehow pump lymph back to the heart where it will again join the blood supply in the vascular system. The mechanism for moving lymph to the heart is much like that for moving venous blood: the larger lymph vessels contain one-way valves, so that on compression of the vessels by the action of the surrounding muscles, the low-pressure fluid is pumped in one direction only toward the heart, Fig. 11.C-5. If the lymph system breaks down or a limb is injured or one simply is too passive

physically, the lymph accumulates in that limb and edemic swelling of the tissue ensues. On the other hand, in the case of a blood hemorrhage, the vascular system can draw on the lymphatic system for fluid, as the lymph is re-absorbed into the capillaries.

As the capillaries offer a significant resistance to blood flow, they support in part the blood-pressure surge on cardiac systole. This periodic pressurization of a relatively weak structure leads to a pulsation of the capillary diameter, which then serves to pump nearby lymph toward the heart [473]. Some of the smaller lymph vessels drain directly into small veins and so contribute to relieving the lymphatic pressure.

It is generally agreed that exercise and inversion are important factors in keeping lymph in circulation. As a corollary to this, lymphatic swelling results when a limb is positioned below the heart and is physically inactive. However, the yoga practitioner must use caution in prescribing lymph-activating *yogasanas* for relief of edema in certain situations, for the lymphatic system also can be the pathway for the spread of cancer cells. As similar caution is in order for students having sinus infections, for inversions can help spread the infection to other sites [239].

As with the venous supply to the heart, the motion of the diaphragm when breathing will act to pump lymph from the feet toward the heart, this being strongest when breathing deeply [407]. As for using upright *yogasanas* to improve lymph circulation, repetitive motions are better than static holdings [293]. *Yogasanas* recommended for promoting lymph drainage are given by Schatz [407] and by MacMullen [293].

Lymph Nodes

Though the lymph channels closely resemble the venous system in form and function, they do differ in one very significant way. The lymph vessels at several points contain structures (nodes) the size of small beans, the purpose of which is to filter the lymph fluid on its way to the heart. Lymph nodes are most prominent on the underside of the jaw (cervical lymph nodes), in the arm pits (axillary lymph nodes) and in the groins (inguinal lymph nodes). The lymphatic nodal system is a very important part of the body's defense system as it contains macrophage cells which intercept and kill foreign bacteria, and lymphocytes which manufacture antibodies in order to control foreign microorganisms. By our practice of *yogasanas*, we promote the more rapid circulation of the lymph through the nodes, and so are performing acts of blood purification in doing so.

In modern man, lymph nodes are colored blue/black due to filtered particles of carbon and dust [319]. The swelling of one of these nodes is obvious whenever the node begins rapid manufacture of lymphocytes in response to an infection. If and when lymph nodes are removed surgically as for breast cancer, lymph edema often occurs in the arm or leg closest to the site of removal.

Two organs in the body are lymph-node-like in their function, the spleen and the thymus gland. The spleen produces lymphocytes and is a storehouse for red blood cells, while the thymus gland lies just behind the upper part of the sternum and contains several lymphatic nodules, however, these are of marginal value in the adult.

Chapter 12

RESPIRATION

SECTION 12.A. MECHANICS OF THE BREATH

For over 5000 years, mystics and Eastern medical practitioners have argued that control of the breath and/or modification of the breath could have profound impact on the health and well being of an individual. Today, medical researchers are confirming these ancient views with studies that show the relation between the way we breathe and our cardiovascular functioning, the circulation to the brain, metabolic and endocrine activities, muscular, visceral, and vascular tones, lymph drainage, arteriole blood flow, blood pH and autonomic homeostasis [315]. Respiration has been coupled to the spinal cord physiologically and psychologically in several ways, and so cannot be considered separately from these connections. In particular, the breath directs the movement of the ribs, dictates the intra-thoracic and intra-abdominal pressures, the cyclic change of the spinal muscle tone on inhalation and exhalation, the balance in the autonomic nervous system, the emotions, the heart rate and the respiratory sinus arhythmia.

The breath is of the utmost significance to our *yogasana* practice and to our health and well being. Outside of the yoga community, it is little appreciated in general that control of the breath is possible, and that with control of the breath, there follows control of our mental and somatic states. The first step in controlling the nervous system is modifying the respiration pattern, for the respiration is the most easily modified of the vital functions [377]. The link between breathing and the other autonomic functions involves strong interactions between the cortex, the brainstem and certain hormones.

Control of the body through *yogasana* and control of the breath through *pranayama* form the doorway to higher levels of meditation. Furthermore, the yogic preference for breathing through the nose rather than the mouth, is given credence by the work of Wernitz [389], who showed that the EEG patterns of nasal and oral breathing were quite different.

The Ayurvedic approach to understanding the functioning of the body divides breathing phenomena into two catagories called "*langhana*" and "*brmhana*", meaning "to fast" (as when one goes without eating) and "to expand," respectively. Miller [315] gives a long list, which is presented here in an abbreviated form in Table 12.A-1, demonstrating how these two qualities or principles differ. Note that this Table is not unlike Table 1.A-1, describing the two World Views given in the Introduction. According to Table 12.A-1, the two ways of breathing, abdominal-diaphragmatic (*langhana*) and thoracic (*brmhana*), correlate with many aspects of the autonomic nervous system. Some authors consider other modes of breathing to be more basic and so there is no unanimity as to the "basic" forms, but the differences are not large. The two types of Ayurvedic breathing will be discussed in this Chapter along with a few other related types. But first, we must consider the anatomy of the breathing apparatus.

TABLE 12.A-1. COMPARISON OF THE *LANGHANA* AND *BRMHANA* PRINCIPLES OF AYURVEDIC MEDICINE [315]

Langhana	*Brmhana*
Contraction/exhalation	Expansion/inhalation
Abdominal-diaphragmatic breathing	Thoracic breathing
Left-nostril dominance	Right-nostril dominance
Right cerebral dominance	Left cerebral dominance
Apana moves upward	*Prana* moves downward
Located in colon and pelvis	Located in chest and stomach
Forward bends and twisting	Backbends
Catabolic	Anabolic
Female	Male
Parasympathetic	Sympathetic
Afferent nerves	Efferent nerves
Activated by darker colors (brown, violet, *etc.*)	Activated by lighter colors (red, yellow, *etc.*)
Positive feelings of love and compassion	Positive feelings of activity and intelligence

Journey into the Lungs

The respiratory passage begins its downward journey at the nasal cavity (Subsection 12.C, *Internal Structure of the Nose*, page 375), moving then through the pharynx and larynx within the throat, and on to the trachea, which is open as well to any food swallowed by the oral cavity, Fig. 12.A-1. Though both air and food travel through the pharynx, however, the epiglottis just below the pharynx then is either closed to route food down the esophagus or open to route air down the larynx. When the epiglottis is open, air passing downward through the larynx can enter the trachea, a pipe of smooth muscle and cartilage [230]. As the trachea descends to enter the chest, it branches into two limbs, here called the bronchi, at the level of vertebra T4, with each limb going to its respective lung on the left or the right, Fig. 12.A-2a.

The inner surfaces of the trachea and bronchi are covered with epithelial cells bearing hairlike appendages which in turn are covered by a thin mucus film that traps any debris in the inspired air (Chapter 14, EXTERNAL SECRETIONS, page 393). In addition to trapping foreign particles in the upwardly mobile mucus film, the passage of incoming air through the nose and the trachea warms the air on cold days using heat from underlying blood vessels, and also raises the humidity of the air before it enters the lungs [229]. On hot days, the nasal heat exchanger can work to reduce the temperature of the blood in the head. These nasal blood vessels are close to the surface and have only a very thin layer of skin between them and the outside air for obvious reasons of efficient heat transfer; however, one must be careful when putting anything up the nose as it can easily tear the thin layer and cause a nosebleed.

The right lung is sculpted into three distinct lobes, whereas the left is separated only into two. Within each lung, the bronchi again bifurcate, first forming secondary bronchi, and then the bronchioles, which continue to branch until the level of the alveolar sacs is reached, Fig. 12.A-2b. These sacs at the terminal edges of the

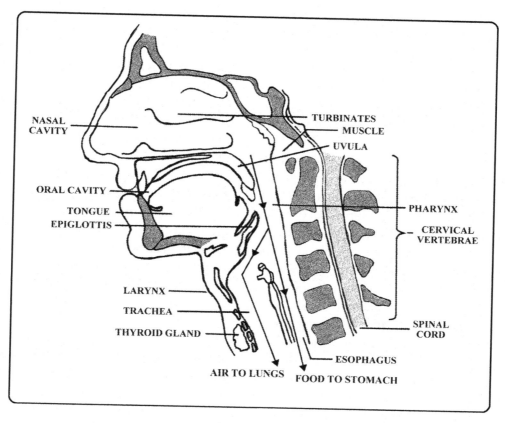

Fig. 12.A-1. Medial section through the head showing the common path of the nasal and oral cavities down to the epiglottis, at which point they separate, with air going down the larynx and trachea, and food going down the esophagus [229].

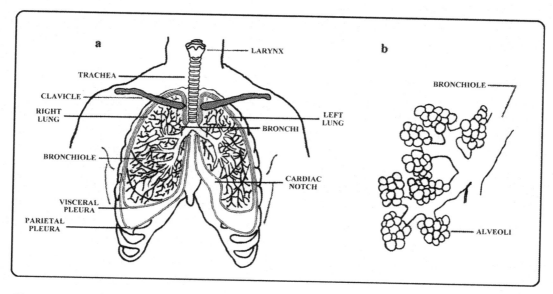

Fig. 12.A-2. (**a**) As the trachea descends, it bifurcates first to form the left and right bronchi, and each of these further branches repeatedly, leading eventually to the grapelike alveoli shown in (**b**). The empty space depicted as the cardiac notch in fact is occupied by the heart, not shown here [229].

bronchial tree appear like clusters of grapes, each "grape" being a sac of approximately 0.03-cm diameter. If we assume that such sacs half fill the lung volume of 6000 cm^3 (6 liters) when expanded, then the total number of alveoli in the lungs comes to 300 million, a number which implies 28 successive bifurcations! Being as finely divided as they are, the alveoli within the lungs if spread flat would have an area approximately equal to that of half a tennis court.

Each of the alveoli is surrounded by a capillary system with which it is in close contact. Venous, deoxygenated blood from the right side of the heart (the right ventricle, Fig. 11.A-1) is pumped through the lung capillary system where it absorbs fresh oxygen from the alveoli and releases carbon dioxide into the alveoli. Blood refreshed in this way is sent back to the left side of the heart (the left atrium, Fig. 11.A-1) and then pumped through the left ventricle and the aorta into the arterial system. The gas exchange across the walls of both the alveoli and the capillaries is diffusional but rapid because the cells in this area are very thin and the distances involved are very short [230]. Moreover, because the resistance to flow in the pulmonary venules and in the capillary nets of the lungs is so small, a pulmonary pressure of only one seventh that at the aorta is necessary to drive blood through the lungs. This small pressure drop from one end of the capillaries to the other within the lungs translates into a long residence time for the venous blood in the lungs, and correspondingly, an increased opportunity for the venous blood to exchange its burden of carbon dioxide for oxygen. Occasionally, the blood pressure in the lungs is unusually high, leading to pulmonary hypertension, a condition in which oxygenation of the blood is poor and the person suffers fatigue and breathlessness.

Over 50% of the lung volume is occupied by blood and the blood vessels [229]. It is the large surface area defining the interface between the air in the lungs and the blood in the lungs that makes breathing so efficient that little or no reserves of oxygen are necessary in the body. If the overall area of the alveoli is reduced or if the alveoli lose their elasticity, as when a person has emphysema, then breathing becomes substantially more difficult.

Though the lungs are partially filled with the alveoli and the capillary systems intertwined with them, the effect of gravity is to bring the larger portion of the pulmonary blood to the lower regions of the lungs when the person is upright, as in *tadasana*. Because of the pooling of the blood in the lower regions of the lungs, there is less room for air in those lower regions, whereas at the top of the lungs, there is an excess of air and too little blood to take advantage of it. Only in the middle third of the lung tissue is there a more equal volume of blood and air, and it is here that the most efficient transfer of gases between air and blood takes place [77, 374]. If one were inverted, as in *sirsasana*, then gravity would carry the oxygen-poor blood to just the upper parts of the lungs, forcing the air out of this region and into the lower regions. Again, the optimum ratio of air volume to blood volume (called the ventilation-to-perfusion ratio) would be found in the middle third of the lungs. In order to work the other portions of the lungs adequately, one has to tip the ribcage through various angles as in *trikonasana* so that the portion of the lung volume having a ventilation-to-perfusion ratio near one occupies different parts of the lungs, and then one must breathe while in these tipped positions for a significant time. Respiration in the lying position is more efficient than when standing because there is a more complete mixing of the blood and the air in the prone position [273].

Resistance to the flow of breath is governed in part by the diameters of the airways, with the small airways offering more resistance to breathing than do the large airways. The bronchial diameters are controlled by the smooth muscles within their walls, which in turn respond to signals from the autonomic nervous system: in times of crisis, the smooth muscles are relaxed by norepinephrine, the bronchi dilate, and the breath flows more easily, whereas in a more calm environment, it is the acetylcholine of the parasympathetic nervous system that keeps them somewhat contracted (Section 5.D, The Neurotransmitters, page 128).

Should the airways go into bronchospasm, *i.e.*, swelling from the inside and constricting from the outside, the airflow is severely restricted and an asthma attack is underway. In general, the bronchospasm is either initiated by a high sensitivity to allergens such as pollen or cat hair, or by nonallergenic situations such as breathing cigarette smoke or overexercising. The excitability of the airways due to vagal stimulation can be reversed through a *yogasana* practice which emphasizes the *langhana* aspect of the breath [330], and in cases of mild asthma, *pranayama* also can be an effective cure [431].

The heart lies between the lungs, more so on the left side, where there is a cardiac notch in the left lung to accommodate it, Fig. 12.A-2a. One sees from the Figure that there is less weight pressing on the heart when resting on the right side than when on the left and so suggests why we turn to the right side when recovering from *savasana* (however, see Subsection 12.C, *The Conscious Development and Shift of Nasal Laterality*, page 378, for another reason to come out of this pose by turning onto the right side).

The lungs rest on the diaphragm, Fig. 12.A-3, which itself forms a dome over the stomach, liver, and spleen, separating these viscera physically from the heart and lungs. This dome rises higher on the right-hand

side in order to accommodate the liver [215]. In fact, the lower surfaces of the lungs are attached to the upper surface of the diaphragm, which in turn is pierced by three openings to allow passage of the esophagus, the descending aorta, and the inferior vena cava.

Notice that though the lungs are totally involved in the strong muscular action of the breath, there is very little muscle tissue to be found in the lungs, just that within the components forming the vascular web. The lungs are largely passive organs, the functioning of which is totally dependent upon a complicated mechanism of external musculature and bony levers.

The Ribs

The ribs are part of a bony cage which not only offers protection to the lungs and heart, but is an active participant in the breathing process. As seen in Fig. 12.A-4, there are twelve pairs of ribs, connected by hinge joints to vertebrae T1 through T12, the top ten of which are hinged as well in the front body. The volume enclosed by the ribs and their junctures defines the thoracic cavity; the floor of this cavity is the muscular sheet known as the diaphragm.

The upper ten ribs are joined in the front body at the sternum via the sternocostal joints, whereas all twelve pairs of ribs are joined to the vertebral column in the back body through the costovertebral joints. That is to say, the lowest two ribs are joined to the vertebrae, but float unconnected in the vicinity of the sternum.

Additionally, each of the ribs is bound to its neighboring ribs through a pair of muscle sheets, the external and internal costal muscles. Contraction of the external costal muscles pulls the outer surfaces of the ribs toward one another, thereby flaring the ribs outward, whereas contraction of the internal costal muscles pulls the ribs more toward the centerline of the thoracic cylinder; the

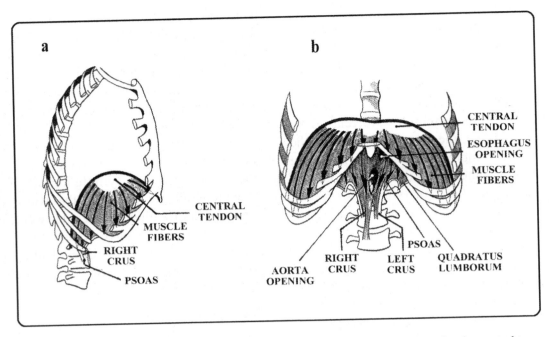

Fig. 12.A-3. (a) A lateral view of the diaphragm within the thoracic cavity, showing its central tendon, the radially-aligned muscle fibers, attachments to the anterior sides of the lower vertebrae, and the direction of the tension (arrows) when the diaphragm is contracted. (b) The anterior view of the diaphragm within the thoracic cavity, showing more clearly its attachments to the lumbar vertebrae. Also shown are the openings through which the aorta and the esophagus pass [228].

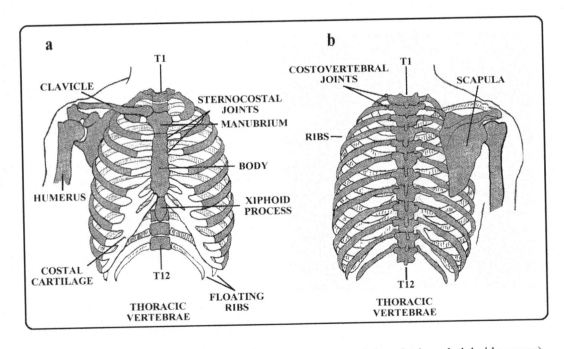

Fig. 12.A-4. (a) The attachment of the ribs to the sternum (manubrium, body and xiphoid process) via the sternocostal joints and the costal cartilage, as seen from the front. (b) The attachment of the ribs to the twelve thoracic vertebrae via the costovertebral joints, as seen from the back.

internal and external costal muscles cross one another at 90°. The ribs, together with their joints front and back, and the muscles between the ribs, collectively form the ribcage. It is the motions of the walls of the ribcage, the abdomen, and the diaphragm that work to pump air in and out of the lungs.

Each rib is joined to the thoracic vertebral column by two synovial joints, one each to adjacent vertebrae, except for the uppermost and lowermost ribs which, respectively, are connected to vertebrae T1 or T12 only (see Section 8.E, The Joints, page 260); the joint couple so formed is reinforced by many strong ligaments. Motion of a particular rib then is restricted to rotation about the line connecting the two points of attachment on the vertebral column. In the lowest ribs, the line connecting the two points of attachment of a rib is more or less horizontal front-to-back, so that were these ribs to be lifted, the ribs on each side would swing up like the handle of a bucket so as to increase the side-to-side diameter of the thorax. On the other hand, in the upper chest, the orientation of the line of attachment of the ribs to the thoracic spine is more or less horizontal left to right, such that lifting the ribcage results in an increase of the front-to-back diameter. Intermediate ribs show some of each of the motions of the extremes [54]. Thus it is seen that lifting of the ribs through the action of the external costals acts to increase the thoracic volume, and in doing so, aids inspiration, whereas relaxation of the ribs involves lowering of the ribcage, with more or less help from the internal costals, as on expiration [228] (see below). The ability to inhale and exhale fully will depend in part upon the strength and flexibility of the costal muscles and their mutual inhibition, and in part on the quality of the *yogasana* and *pranayama* practices.

The sternum itself consists of three sections: 1) the manubrium, which forms the joints for the ribs attached to T1 and for the clavicles, 2) the body of the sternum, consisting of a series of fused bones in adults much like the sacrum and coccyx, and joined to ribs connected in turn to vertebrae T2–T7, and 3) the xyphoid process, Fig. 12.A-4a. Rib pairs issuing from T8–T10 have fibrocartilaginous joints attached to the sternocostal joint of T7, whereas the ribs connected to T11 and T12 are not connected at the sternum, and so are said to be floating ribs; they terminate in the muscles of the abdominal wall. Contraction of the abdominal muscles thus acts to pull the anterior rib cage toward the pelvis and to round the lumbar spine, changing its curvature from slightly concave to convex.

Unlike the thoracic spine which has the potential to bend and twist at each vertebra, the sternum in young students has such a potential only at two points, where the manubrium attaches to the body of the sternum and where the body of the sternum attaches to the xyphoid process, Fig. 12.A-4a. Like the intervertebral discs in the spine, the cartilage of the sternum also can ossify with age [473]. Hopefully, with *yogasana* chest opening and *pranayama* deep breathing, the cartilage of the sternum can be kept supple, allowing the chest to expand fully on inhalation. Lacking this, the manubrium and the body of the sternum fuse together in adulthood, and the xiphoid process ossifies by age 40 in the general population [476].

The thoracic spine in a skeleton is far more mobile when it is disconnected from the ribcage, showing that though the ribs do offer protection to the organs contained within and are essential for breathing, they also inhibit spinal movement. This resistance to motion in the thoracic spine is less apparent in the young, but much more obvious in the elderly for whom the costal cartilage has ossified [228]. Just as with the intervertebral discs, it is likely that bending the spine as when doing backbends will also work to keep the joints within the sternum from freezing.

Using the Diaphragm and the Ribs to Breathe

Air that makes its way into the alveoli rapidly would become stagnant were it not replaced forcefully and frequently by fresh air from the outside. This important task falls to the muscles and bones surrounding the lungs, which act in such a way as to repeatedly fill and empty the otherwise passive lungs of their air. A prime mover among these muscles is the diaphragm, a muscle unique to mammals [319].

The diaphragm is a large, horizontal, sheetlike muscle which effectively separates the abdomen from the thorax. As shown in Fig. 12.A-3b, the diaphragm is anchored to the lowest ribs and to the anterior side of the lumbar and sacral spine, and is domed upward in the relaxed position. The apex of the dome is the so-called "central tendon," which in this case is not connected directly to a second bone forming a joint, but rather, is a tendonous island surrounded by the radially-aligned muscle fibers of the diaphragm. As the muscle fibers run radially from the outer edges of the diaphragm to the central tendon, the diaphragm area shrinks when contracted, the sheet is pulled downward by 1–2 cm, and the thoracic volume correspondingly increases. This action of expansion momentarily causes a reduction of the air pressure within the lungs as compared to that outside the lungs and so air flows into the lungs, *i.e.*, one has inhaled. Viewed somewhat differently, the diaphragm acts like a piston, drawing air into the lungs on the down stroke (diaphragmatic contraction) and releasing the air in the lungs on the up stroke (diaphragmatic expansion).

When one is at rest, the volume of the inhalation amounts to about 0.5 liters, followed by an exhalation of the same volume. The terms "inhalation" and "exhalation" are synonymous with "inspiration" and "expiration," respectively, and are used here interchangeably. With practice of the control of the breath (Section 12.D, *Pranayama*, page 381), the volume of air inhaled with each breath can be increased from 0.5 to 6 liters [215]. As the lungs are pressed pneumatically against the ribcage but are separated from it by the well-lubricated pleural membranes (Fig. 12.A-2a), they are able to move against the ribs without friction.

When resting, exhalation of the inhaled air is a more passive action, as one merely relaxes the breathing muscles and the lungs then exhale 0.5 liters of air as the diaphragm expands and rises, and the thoracic volume returns to the initial value. Even when one takes a slow inhalation, there is nonetheless a significant pressure difference between the lungs and the atmospheric pressure outside the lungs which continues to drive the expansion of the lungs, as the flow resistance in the medium-size bronchioles only allows these pressure quantities to equalize slowly. As the inhalation is a muscular action whereas the exhalation is more passive (in many senses of the word), it is not surprising that in those who do not practice breath control, the exhalation can require an almost 50% longer time than does inhalation [387].

Were the diaphragm the sole driving force to the inhalation, then the contraction of the diaphragm on inhalation would act to pull the lowest ribs in toward the center of the body. A moment's investigation will show the reader that in fact it is just the opposite: on an inhalation, the diaphragm attached to the lowest ribs is pulled downward, but at the same time, these lowest ribs to which the diaphragm is attached are moved outward and upward rather than downward and inward! This seemingly contrary action is shown schematically in Fig. 12.A-5, and comes about through the agency of the abdominal muscles and the external costal muscles which bind each rib to its neighbors. In the course of an inhalation, the diaphragm initially is pulled downward, but very quickly is pressing down upon the abdominal contents, which are incompressible if the abdominal muscles are toned. At the same time, the external costals contract and in doing so, pull the ribs upward and outward in order to increase the thoracic volume which otherwise is being expanded by the diaphragm; it is estimated that the external costals contribute 10 to 25% to the work necessary to inflate the lungs [230], the more so the deeper the breath taken.

To recapitulate, when breathing in a restful way, the central tendon of the diaphragm descends 1–2 cm and the external costal muscles weakly flair the lowest ribs up and to the sides. Exhalation is completely passive, with the diaphragm rising as it relaxes and the ribs falling in at the same time as the external costals release. If, however, the breathing is more forceful, then the central tendon of the diaphragm can descend by up to 10 cm, and the exhalation also can become a more active process as the antagonist muscles to the external costals, the internal costals and the abdominal muscles come into play, pulling the lowest ribs down and inward.

Note the important role the abdominal muscles play in the breathing process. The strength and rigidity of the abdominal muscles give strength and stability to the central tendon. When the central tendon is pulled down, it presses upon the viscera below it, however, the residual contraction of the abdominal muscles at this point acts to stop the downward motion of the diaphragm.

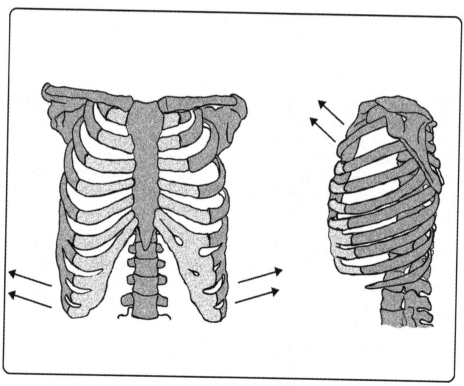

Fig. 12.A-5. Motions of the ribs and sternum upon inspiration while breathing in the thoracic mode.

Because the diaphragm at this stage is still above the lowest ribs but cannot move down any further, the effect of continued diaphragmatic contraction is to lift the lowest ribs up! Thus the actions of the diaphragm and the abdominal muscles are both antagonistic (Subsection 7.A, *Reciprocal Inhibition and Agonist/Antagonist Pairs*, page 193) in that there is a general cross inhibition of the diaphragmatic and abdominal muscles, yet they are synergistic in that abdominal-muscle tone helps inspiration lift the ribcage [25, 228].

When one coughs or spits, it is the reflexive contraction of the abdominal and internal costal muscles that makes the action possible. It is usually assumed that in the act of vomiting, the stomach contracts and forces its load in the upward direction. In fact, during this act, the abdominal muscles and the diaphragm contract simultaneously and so put external pressure on the stomach to release its contents upward [313]. The actions occurring during a sneeze are described in Subsection 12.B, *Factors Affecting the Breath*, page 373.

Exhalation of the breath is based on the lungs assuming their initial volume once the force that fills them is released. Experiments show that about one-third of the contractile force tending to collapse the lungs does come from the elasticity of the lung tissue, but that two thirds comes from the special material with which the alveoli are bathed. Called a "surfactant", this fluid material acts to increase the surface tension of the alveolar tissue, thereby encouraging it to have the smallest possible surface area, *i.e.*, to contract [230].

When we inhale, the brain moves forward and conversely, when we exhale the brain moves backward. When we hold our breath in the *yogasanas*, the brain is immobilized and its function is impaired [211]. In *savasana* especially, we allow the brain to relax and fall to the back of the skull. The

breathing cycle also has an impact on the heart rate and blood pressure [68]. As the chest expands on an inhalation, blood pools in the lungs and the blood pressure drops. In compensation for this, excitation along the vagus nerve relaxes and the heart rate accelerates. As the chest is compressed on exhalation, blood is squeezed out of the lungs, the blood pressure rises, as does the parasympathetic signal from the vagus nerve to the heart, and the heart rate decelerates.

Given that the exhalation is the breath of relaxation and calm, we use the exhalation as a doorway to enter into each of the *yogasanas*. For example, starting on hands and knees, we exhale as we lift the body into *adho mukha svanasana*, and we lean into *trikonasana* on an exhalation. However, though the *yogasanas* are to be entered on the exhalation, the chest should not be allowed to fall toward the pelvis in the process, even in forward bends.

Not all of the air inspired acts to oxygenate blood in the alveoli. Thus 30% of the inhaled air remains in the trachea and upper airway passages as dead air, and does not make it into the alveoli for gas transfer during the breathing cycle. Assuming that the inspired and expired volumes are the same, the "minute volume" of gas moved is defined as the volume inspired through the nose in one breath (the tidal volume), corrected for the part that is nonfunctional in gas transfer (the dead volume), times the number of breaths taken in a minute. At ten breaths per minute, the minute volume would be 10 X (1−0.3) X 0.5 liters = 3.5 liters. As discussed in Box 12.A-1, the unavoidable reduction in the effective volume of the breath due to the dead volume can be of tremendous importance to undersea divers, and perhaps to *yogasana* students as well.

In working with *yogasana* students, teachers have the opportunity to monitor and direct not only the mechanics of the stu-

BOX 12.A-1: DIVERS AND *YOGASANA* STUDENTS MUST BE AWARE OF THE DEAD VOLUME

Imagine a diver in her diving suit at the bottom of the ocean, connected to the source of fresh air by a long hose. Ideally, movement of her lungs would be able to expel 0.5 liters of deoxygenated air and to inspire 0.5 liters of oxygenated air to replace it. However, in the normal breathing situation, less than 0.35 liters of air (less than 70% of 0.5 liters) is truly fresh air, having come from outside the breathing apparatus, with the remaining 0.15 or more liters being deoxygenated air within the dead volume of the lungs, the trachea, and the hose. Moreover, if the dead volume of the system, lungs plus trachea plus hose, is larger than 0.5 liters, then the inhalation only succeeds in filling the lungs with the deoxygenated air left in the dead volume by the previous exhalation, and the diver soon suffocates! That is to say, the volume of air moved in an inspiration must be larger than the dead volume in the system if breathing is to be efficient and long lasting. Furthermore, even in the best of situations, the "fresh" air being breathed is always contaminated with 30% or more of the deoxygenated air exhaled in the previous breathing cycle, but remaining in the dead volume.

To say it differently, following an expiration, the first 0.15 liters of air inspired into the lungs is stale, useless air left in the airways by the previous expiration; if one is to inhale enough oxygen to survive, the amount of air inspired must be much larger than that of the dead volume. As this was not realized in the early days of diving, many deaths by suffocation occurred even though the air line to the surface was not blocked. The problem today is solved by having the diver exhale directly into the water through a check valve in the diving helmet, thus reducing the effective dead volume of the apparatus.

Though no one has died from suffocation in the *yogasanas* (however, see [91]), somewhat the same principle applies. In a pose such as *ardha navasana*, the strong contraction of the abdominal muscles reduces the effective tidal volume of the lungs so that it approaches the dead volume of the respiratory system, about 0.15 liters regardless of circumstances. Were the tidal volume and the dead volume equal, breathing would involve pushing the same air back and forth within the dead volume without its ever being refreshed by oxygenated air from the outside, and one would tire quickly. Similar results are expected in other poses in which the breath's tidal volume is strongly restricted by abdominal contraction, as in *ardha navasana*, by compression of the abdomen as in poses where one lies belly-down on the floor (*dhanurasana*, for example), or by compression of the chest itself, as in *maricyasana III, virabhadrasana 1, urdhva dhanurasana, etc*. In these cases, the tidal volume is diminished but the dead volume remains constant, leading to the situation in which the air being breathed has both a smaller volume and contains a lower percentage of oxygen than when breathing freely. Consequently, breathing in these poses will be rapid but shallow, and the duration of the pose will be shorter than normal. Because deep breathing can raise the tidal volume to as much as 6 liters, whereas the dead volume remains constant at 0.15 liters, deep breathing can be very beneficial in overcoming the dead-volume penalty during *yogasana* practice.

dent's breath, but the odor as well. This can be important because the odor of the breath often can be diagnostic for certain aspects of ill health, as outlined in Table 12.A-2.

Innervation and Control of the Breathing Centers

The breath is unique in that it alone can be controlled equally well by both voluntary and involuntary processes. On the voluntary side, the cerebral cortex has direct neural connections (the corticospinal nerve tracts, Section 5.B, Nerve Conduction, page 114) to both the muscles of inspiration and of expiration (the costal muscles, the abdominal muscles, and the diaphragm), and these can be controlled at will as when one plays the clarinet. The muscles of inspiration and expiration are interconnected through inhibitory interneurons such that when one type is active, the other is inhibited. The efferent nerve effecting contraction of the diaphragm is the phrenic nerve, derived from cranial nerves V and VI (Section 6.A, Introduction to the Autonomic Nervous System, page 133).

When breathing in the involuntary mode, there would seem to be a natural pacemaker for inspiration, running at about 15 full-breathing cycles per minute, but this is dependent upon many external factors. There does not seem to be any pacemaker for expiration, for these signals are simply keyed to those of inspiration through other neurons. The exhalation should be slightly longer than the inhalation, and if this is not so, then one is over-breathing (hyperventilating).

Involuntary breathing is controlled by brainstem centers in the vicinity of the pons and medulla, Subsection 3.A, *The Spinal Cord and Brainstem*, page 29. The respiration rate when breathing quietly is controlled by nuclei in the medulla. Fewer than 50 cells in the medulla are thought to be involved in the control of the breath. When signaled to do so by the medulla, the diaphragm and costal muscles contract, drawing air into the lungs; when this neural signal is turned off, the expiration phase begins without any further neural input. However, other control systems also can be activated. For example, during exercise, there are heavier demands made on the breath. In this case, another center in the medulla drives the inhalation and a neural center in the pons then drives the exhalation.

A chemoreceptor in the medulla which is sensitive to CO_2 in the blood is able to speed respiration if it senses that the level of CO_2 is too high [340]. Other receptors receive signals from various chemoreceptors in regard to pH, pO_2 and pCO_2 and which

TABLE 12.A-2. ASSOCIATION OF THE ODOR OF THE BREATH TO STATES OF ILLNESS

Odor	Illness
Sour	Gingivitis, sinus, chest or tonsil infection, lung disease
Ketonic (nail-polish remover)	Diabetes, anorexia
Fruity, sweet	Oral thrush
Metallic	Ulcers
Ammonia or fishy	Kidney disease
Musty	Severe liver disease

then either increase the rate of inspiration or decrease it, depending upon what is appropriate to the situation*. Thus, if the intense work of the *yogasanas* increases the metabolism so that more CO_2 is released into the blood, there is an immediate increase of the H^+ and bicarbonate ion concentrations in the cerebrospinal fluid which stimulates receptors for H^+ in the medulla, and the medulla in turn speeds ventilation [340]. In a similar way, if pO_2 is too large, sensors within the aorta and carotid arteries sense this and promote more rapid ventilation and increased blood pressure by stimulating the release of dopamine into the bloodstream from the carotid glands. In general, the regulation of the breath is more strongly affected by changes in the levels of CO_2 than by changes in the levels of O_2 [273, 473].

When a muscle or nerve is compressed so that the flow of blood through it is hindered, the muscle or nerve suffers an ischemic condition known as hypoxia. In this case, the ventilation rate and cardiac output will increase reflexively in an attempt to raise the O_2 level, and over time, a new set of capillaries also may develop in order to try and overcome the blockage.

Just as with the muscles (Section 7.B, Muscle Sensors; The Mechanoreceptors, page 198), there are stretch receptors in the walls of the lungs, the purpose of which is to see that lung expansion does not proceed too far. Should the amount of inspired air exceed 1 liter, the stretch receptors are activated, the warning signal travels to the pons via the vagus nerve, and the inspiration is then reflexively switched to expiration, unless the conscious will intervenes.

All of the above are essentially subcortical control processes, but as the practice of *pranayama* so clearly shows (Section 12.D,

Pranayama, page 381), control of the breath can be assumed by the intelligence of the cortex so that it can control the breath, starting and stopping it or otherwise modulating it to suit the needs of the cortex. In this case, the cortical signal bypasses the medulla and pons, and using the corticospinal tract, goes directly to the respiratory muscles.

The lessening of the thoracic pressure on inspiration acts not only to inflate the lungs, but momentarily over-pressures venous blood in the lower regions of the body and pumps it toward the heart, thanks to the actions of the valves within the veins. Thus venous return to the right atrium (Section 11.A, Structure and Function of the Heart, page 310) would seem to be accelerated by inspiration, resulting in a larger stroke volume and a lower heart rate, however, other avenues of sympathetic excitation overcome this effect (Subsection 12.B, *Abdominal Breathing*, page 370), so that the heart rate actually increases by about 20% on inspiration [67].

Given that the inspirational breath is energizing and sympathetic, whereas the expirational breath is calming and parasympathetic, it is no surprise that the heart rate is higher during the former than during the latter. Going into somewhat more detail, as the lungs expand on an inspiration, there is a slight pooling of blood in the lungs, and a consequent lack of blood entering the heart. In response to this, the parasympathetic excitation in the vagus nerves decreases and the heart rate therefore increases. On the other hand, on expiration, the excess blood is squeezed out of the lungs, the vagal tone increases and the heart rate slows as there is blood enough to fill the heart's left ventricle [68].

---

*The symbol "p" is used by chemists to refer to the negative logarithm of the concentration of the chemical species that follows it. For the purposes of this Handbook, the combination "pX" may be taken qualitatively as chemical shorthand meaning the reciprocal of the concentration of X, *i.e.*, a large value of pX means a low concentration of X, and *vice versa*.

The difference in heart rate during the inspirational and expirational phases of the breathing cycle is called the "Respiratory Sinus Arrhythmia" or RSA [67, 315]. Because a nonzero RSA implies a responsive autonomic nervous system, having a large RSA is a general sign of good health, whereas a low or zero RSA suggests a manifold of health problems, including depression and cardiac conditions. A high RSA correlates with a generally high parasympathetic tone to the nervous system, and is promoted by deep, slow, rhythmic breathing as per the abdominal and diaphragmatic modes (Section 12.B, The Three Modes of Breathing, page 370). If one emphasizes the exhalation in poses that are meant to be relaxing, then the RSA will lengthen the cardiac-deceleration phase of the breath [80].

A study comparing the autonomic excitation in a group of trained *yogasana* students *versus* that in a similar group of untrained students [167] showed that the respiration rate in the steady state of several elementary poses was approximately 50% lower in the trained group, while at the same time, the respiration volume was much larger in all poses. Clearly, *yogasana* training can lower the level of sympathetic excitation generated when practicing *yogasana*, as compared to the situation with beginners.

It is known that on taking a deep breath, the eyes tend to look up and the cervical and lumbar curves tend to flatten, whereas when exhaling, the opposite tendencies prevail. Experiments show that beginners practicing *uttanasana* more closely approach the floor with their hands when they exhale and look downward as they go into the pose [5].

The Effects of Exercise and Emotion on Respiration

The effects of exercise (long term and short term) on the respiration are interesting. Consider first the short-term effects of exercise. The lungs do appreciable work in moving O_2 into the body and CO_2 out: when working at one's maximum, 10% of the total energy is expended in the lungs. In general, systolic blood pressure increases with aerobic exercise while the diastolic pressure remains constant. However, in isometric exercise such as that found in *yogasana*, both the systolic and diastolic pressures can show large increases.

As the cardiac output $\dot{Q}$ increases with work, the arterial blood vessels dilate and so reduce the resistance to the flow of blood to the muscles. Increased work leads to increases in the production of lactic acid, and in response to this, the pH of the blood drops from 7.4 to 7.0. Again, all of these changes are those signaling momentary sympathetic excitation, Table 6.A-1.

The heart rate increases in proportion to the short-term work load (intensity of exercise). With increasing load in standing poses, the stroke volume goes up to a certain point and then levels off, while the cardiac output $\dot{Q}$ = stroke volume X heart rate) increases from about 5 liters/minute to about 30 liters/minute at maximum workload. As expected, the venous blood is much poorer in O_2 than is the arterial blood; during work, the concentration of O_2 in the arteries is 3–4 times larger than that in the veins. As the work load increases, so does $\dot{V}O_2$ up to $\dot{V}O_{2max}$. Following heavy work, there is a remaining O_2 debt. The amount of air breathed per minute is equal to the amount of air breathed in a single inhalation (the tidal volume) times the respiration rate. As the tidal volume is fixed, the increased ventilation is due almost totally to increasing respiration rate.

When the student goes from lying to standing, the stroke volume decreases due to the less efficient filling of the right ventricle due to gravity, but the heart rate increases in order to maintain some constancy of $\dot{Q}$, the cardiac output. That is to say, when a *yogasana* is performed with the body in the horizontal plane, the stroke volume is larger and the heart rate smaller than when the same *yogasana* is performed with the body in the vertical plane.

The Function of Hemoglobin

With each inspiration, the oxygen that we breath into our lungs dissolves in the blood that flows through those organs. Eventually, this oxygen is brought to the mitochondria within the body's cells and is used then to oxidize the body's fuels (carbohydrates, sugars, fats, *etc.*) in a chemical chain reaction that leads to the eventual formation of adenosine triphosphate, ATP. It is this high-energy molecule that drives the body's energy-demanding processes (see Subsection 7.A, *Muscle Chemistry and Energy*, page 182). A key material in this chain leading from inspired air to ATP is hemoglobin, an iron-containing protein found in the red blood cells.

Oxygen inhaled into the alveolar depths of the lungs crosses the thin layers of cells separating the alveolar and capillary tissues and tends then to dissolve in the blood. Were the blood free of hemoglobin, the dissolved oxygen would rise to the level of 0.3% within the plasma, however, with a normal amount of hemoglobin in place, the value rises to over 20%. This increase of almost a factor of 70 in the oxygen-carrying capacity of the blood is directly related to the molecular structure of the hemoglobin molecule within the red blood cells, Fig. 12.A-6.

Within the hemoglobin molecule, there are four molecular subunits as indicated by the four types of shading in the Figure, and each subunit contains a nonprotein heme group having a central divalent iron ion capable of binding oxygen. Each of the heme groups in turn is surrounded by a polypeptide web. The blood issuing from the aorta has oxygen bound to virtually all (97%) of the iron at the heme sites, whereas in the oxygen-depleted blood in the pulmonary vein, many of these sites (75% in the course of intense physical exercise) have been stripped of their oxygen, and the hemoglobin molecules carry a derivative of carbon dioxide instead.

Studies of the chemistry of hemoglobin show that the strength of the attraction of a heme site for oxygen and conversely, how easily such a site will give up its oxygen when it is needed, depend upon how many sites in the hemoglobin molecule are occupied. Thus the binding and unbinding of oxygen to hemoglobin is a cooperative process, and works best when there are four heme units participating in the binding, for in this case the binding is substantial, yet not so firm that there is any difficulty in removing the oxygen when needed.

The situation for carbon dioxide is rather different from that of oxygen in that carbon dioxide is very soluble in water without the aid of hemoglobin; when dissolved in water, carbon dioxide first forms carbonic acid (H_2CO_3), which then dissociates to form H^+ cations and bicarbonate anions (HCO_3-).

The red blood cells containing hemoglobin are manufactured largely within the marrow of the bones (Section 11.B, Blood, page 322), however, some are produced by the liver and spleen as well. The bones of the sternum are cancellous and contain red marrow and so are part of the red-blood-cell factory of the adult body.

Yoga students with an iron deficiency will have a low red-blood-cell count and consequently will quickly become breathless in their *yogasana* practice due to the low level of oxygen in the blood. Similarly, the carbon monoxide in cigarette smoke combines strongly with the heme sites in hemoglobin and so blocks them from carrying oxygen. It requires eight hours for the

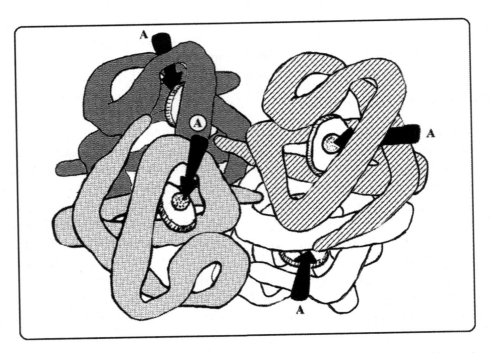

Fig. 12.A-6. The molecular structure of the four subunits forming the hemoglobin molecule. Within each subunit, there is a disc-like heme group having an iron atom at its center (arrows labeled **A**), with a surrounding web of polypeptide. Oxygen is adsorbed onto and released from the iron atom within each heme [230].

carbon monoxide from one cigarette to clear the bloodstream.

SECTION 12.B. THE THREE MODES OF BREATHING

To this point, we have seen that there are three main muscle groups involved in drawing a breath, *i.e.*, the abdominal muscles, the diaphragm, and the intercostal muscles. Though there are many, many ways of breathing, it is logical to divide the breathing types on the basis of which of the three muscle groups is most strongly involved in the breath. This is the approach taken here, based on the earlier work of others [97, 135, 315].

The intimate connection between the breathing pattern and the patterns of sympathetic-parasympathetic switching of the autonomic dominance suggests that any idiosyncracy in the breathing pattern will have repercussions on the nervous system, and *vice versa*.

Abdominal Breathing

The mechanics of abdominal breathing are shown in Fig. 12.B-1a; in this case, as the diaphragm descends, there is little or no resistance from the abdomen, which simply pushes forward in response to the diaphragmatic pressure. There is little or no involvement of the ribcage in abdominal breathing, and though it strongly involves motion of the abdomen, the abdominal muscles remain relaxed throughout the breath, with the diaphragm driving the action. Being the breath of minimal muscular involvement overall, the abdominal breath is a relaxing breath, appropriate to *savasana*, *viparita karani*, and relaxing poses of that sort.

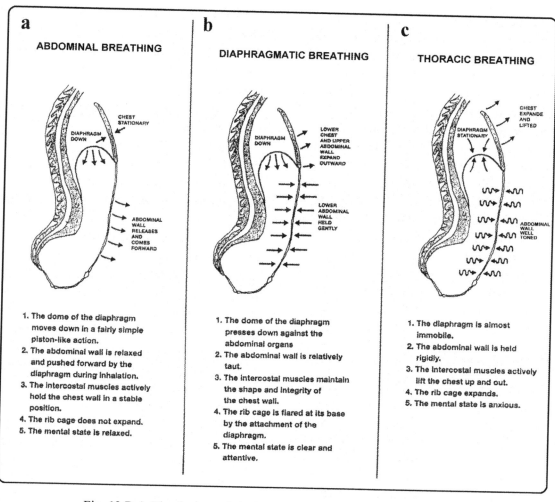

a

ABDOMINAL BREATHING

1. The dome of the diaphragm moves down in a fairly simple piston-like action.
2. The abdominal wall is relaxed and pushed forward by the diaphragm during inhalation.
3. The intercostal muscles actively hold the chest wall in a stable position.
4. The rib cage does not expand.
5. The mental state is relaxed.

b

DIAPHRAGMATIC BREATHING

1. The dome of the diaphragm presses down against the abdominal organs
2. The abdominal wall is relatively taut.
3. The intercostal muscles maintain the shape and integrity of the chest wall.
4. The rib cage is flared at its base by the attachment of the diaphragm.
5. The mental state is clear and attentive.

c

THORACIC BREATHING

1. The diaphragm is almost immobile.
2. The abdominal wall is held rigidly.
3. The intercostal muscles actively lift the chest up and out.
4. The rib cage expands.
5. The mental state is anxious.

Fig. 12.B-1. The three modes of inhalation, according to Coulter [97].

Abdominal breathing directly influences the visceral organs lying below. That is to say, on inspiration, the visceral organs below the diaphragm are compressed as the diaphragm descends, and conversely on expiration, the diaphragm rises and so releases the pressure on the viscera. In this way, the breathing action massages the internal organs, promotes blood flow through them, and some say, acts to promote peristalsis [25, 315], Subsection 18.A, page 447. It also has been proposed that the rhythmic rise and fall of the chest while breathing acts to massage the heart and the right and left vagal nerves as they pass through the tho-rax, and so helps in some unspecified way to control the heart rate [343].

Diaphragmatic Breathing

In diaphragmatic breathing, Fig. 12.B-1b, the movement is largely that of the diaphragm moving down on inhalation and up on exhalation. However, in this case there also is a specific involvement of the abdominal muscle wall which results in a lift and expansion of the lower ribcage on inhalation because the taut abdominals confine the viscera as the diaphragm descends. It is the involvement of the muscles of the abdomen (and the external intercostals) which flare the lower ribs on inhalation that distinguishes the diaphragmatic breath from the abdominal breath. The effect of the diaphragmatic breath is a stimulation of the parasympathetic system, *i.e.*, a general calming and cooling of the body's autonomic systems in accord with Table 6.A-2, and the mental effect is that of clarity and attentiveness. This is clearly the appropriate breath for most of the *yogasanas*, and has been recommended as the breathing approach to use when an asthma attack is about to begin [177]. Through breath control, one often can achieve the same physiological effect, *i.e.*, an opening of the airways, as when using bronchodilator medication. However, an intense *yogasana* practice also can precipitate an asthma attack if the air is cold and dry [177].

Thoracic Breathing

In this style of breathing, the action is opposite to that of diaphragmatic breathing, *i.e.*, the upper ribs and upper chest expand maximally on inhalation, with a minimum of diaphragmatic involvement, and the abdominal wall is tightly held [97], Fig. 12.B-1c. The effect of such a vigorous breathing style, called chest breathing in the Figure, is stimulation of the sympathetic nervous system and a general arousal of the body's autonomic functions in accord with Table 6.A-2 [343]. Accordingly, the mental state associated with thoracic breathing is arousal and anxiety, as appropriate for an emergency situation, however, thoracic breathing can be a source of ongoing stress if allowed to continue once the emergency has passed.

If the diaphragm is tense for whatever reason, as it is in thoracic breathing, then the inspiration is less than adequate to supply the normal demand for oxygen, and the body reciprocates by breathing more rapidly than normal (16 to 20 breaths per minute versus 6 to 8 in the case of diaphragmatic breathing). As a result, one experiences a sense of breathlessness during thoracic breathing, which is acted upon by breathing faster yet. This rapid breathing is called hyperventilation [65, 135, 343]; you are hyperventilating if your breathing rate is significantly above 14 breaths per minute while resting.

Regardless of the manner in which we breath, the demands of the body for oxygen are rather constant, and will be met by regulation of the breathing rate; if the oxygenation is low per breath, then the rate will be high in compensation. It is interesting then that, when breathing in the thoracic mode, the hyperventilation associated with this mode requires up to 50% more energy than does diaphragmatic breathing [343]. The energetic inefficiency of thoracic breathing is a consequence of the fact that, when upright, gravity pulls the blood in the alveoli into the lower halves of the lungs, whereas in thoracic breathing, the inspired air is held in the upper two-thirds of the lung volume. In contrast, during diaphragmatic breathing, the newly inspired fresh air is sent more to the lower halves of the lungs for maximum efficiency in gas exchange [343].

When the parasympathetic nervous system is ascendant, we breathe diaphragmatically, whereas when we are involved in a challenging *yogasana* practice, we switch to sympathetic thoracic breathing in order to satisfy the demand for more oxygen. Normally, the rise in the body's level of energy is controlled by the demands of the exercise, however, if the sympathetic system is activated when there is no need for it, as when breathing in the thoracic mode while at rest, then the result again is hyperventilation and lightheadedness. By continuous thoracic breathing, we establish a constant state of sympathetic arousal characterized by a high oxygen level, anxiety, lightheadedness, and hyperventilation [374].

The direct physiological consequence of hyperventilation, as when performing thoracic breathing, is a drop in the level of CO_2 in the blood, and a shift toward alkalinity, which in turn has many ramifications. When the CO_2 level is depressed, the arteries to the brain and to the muscles contract (producing headache and cold hands and feet), muscles imbibe too much calcium and become hyperactive (producing muscle tension), the nervous system becomes far more excitable (producing rushed and inappropriate responses, and overreaction to minor problems), and the hemoglobin is reluctant to exchange its oxygen with tissues (producing yet more breathlessness) [135]. All of the consequences of hyperventilation as listed above are opposite to those of the parasympathetic action of diaphragmatic breathing, and so most likely have a general sympathetic excitation as their source.

It is also possible to breath by expanding the chest and contracting the abdominal muscles simultaneously. Termed "reverse" breathing, this mode is pathological, and has its cause in emotional responses to external events [374].

Factors Affecting the Breath

As infants and young children, we strongly tend to breath abdominally, for the diaphragm is the only muscle available for the task, whereas in adults, women tend to breath more in the upper chest (and more rapidly) and men tend to breath more in a mixed diaphragm-upper chest mode (and more slowly) [228]. Once we are aged, the accentuated curvature of the thoracic spine, the ossification of the cartilage in the ribcage, and flabby abdominal muscles all work to make the inspiration more shallow and more abdominal/diaphragmatic, so that eventually we will be breathing again as a child, unless we are able to keep the spine in alignment, the cartilage of the ribs supple, and the muscles of the abdomen toned. Thus

we come to see another benefit of *yogasana* practice: the muscles of the body are conditioned so as to support healthier modes of breathing into old age.

When lying on one's back, the abdominal viscera press on the diaphragm and make inhalation difficult. Further, when lying on one's side, the lower lung becomes less efficient, and it may develop circulatory problems. The problem of the viscera pressing upon the diaphragm should be yet more important when one becomes inverted, for in this case, one must lift the viscera with each diaphragmatic contraction. Note however, as stated above, that in the prone position, there is a more efficient mixing of air and blood in the lungs, which will act to slow the heart and the respiration.

Should an allergen or a foreign particle of some sort become lodged in the nose, then a reflexive sneeze may be in order to rid the body of this irritant. Irritants in the nasal tract signal their presence to the medulla which then acts to raise the volume of inspired air to 2 to 2.5 liters [387]. This is the "aaahhhh" of "aaahhhhchooo". With the lungs filled with air, the glottis closes, and as it does so, the diameter of the trachea collapses. In order to "chooo", the medulla instructs the abdominal muscles and the internal costals to contract so as to compress the air in the lungs, the glottis opens rapidly and the compressed air is blown through the narrowed trachea at almost the speed of sound (Mach 0.85). During this nasal explosion, the eyes close to avoid being sprayed with germs and the muscles of the middle ear contract so as to lessen the impact of the loud noise on the auditory sensors (see Box 17.A-1, *Relaxing the Muscles of the Middle Ear*, page 435). Strangely, there is a well-known photic-sneeze reflex, in which brief exposure to intense light will trigger a sneeze [387].

Some reflex actions (Section 7.D, Reflex Actions, page 211) are strictly spinal and so remain active during sleep, whereas those that go as high as the brainstem are turned off during sleep. Sneezing is one of the latter reflexes, and so there is no reflexive sneezing during sleep.

Rationalizing the Effects of the Breath

With the above exposition of how the lungs, ribs, diaphragm and associated muscles work together in order to drive the breath, one can then rationalize the Ayurvedic description of the breath as being either *langhana* or *brmhana* in the following way. When breathing in the *langhana* mode, the muscle action on inhalation is largely diaphragmatic, the breathing is shallow, and the effect is stimulating to the parasympathetic nervous system. The exhalation when in *langhana* is rather passive, relying on the elastic energy stored in the cartilage of the ribs and on alveolar surface tension to return the ribcage to its initial position. The characteristics of *langhana*, Table 12.A-1, are most obvious when breathing in the abdominal or diaphragmatic modes.

In contrast, when breathing in the *brmhana* mode, the diaphragm is pulled down more forcefully so as to be resisted by the muscle tone in the abdomen, and at the same time, the external costal muscles contract so as the lift the ribs upward. This lift of the ribs acts to increase the three diameters of the thorax, and the volume increase fills the lungs with inspired air. The effect of the muscular action on the nervous system is to stimulate the sympathetic nerves. In the case of *brmhana*, exhalation can be more active, with the contractions of the internal costal muscles and those of the abdomen driving the air from the lungs. The thoracic breath is *brmhana*.

Physiologically, the effect of diaphragmatic breathing is to drive the level of CO_2 in the blood upward, thereby making the body acidic [315]. In response to this hyper-

acidity, there is a decreasing cardiopulmonary stress as the heart rate and blood flow decrease, metabolic activity decreases, as do blood sugar and lactate levels, muscle tone and skin conductivity. Further, this type of breath promotes oxygenation of the heart and brain as it promotes blood flow to these areas, and it increases the ease with which hemoglobin can transfer oxygen from the blood to the tissues. In contrast to the above, thoracic breathing promotes the increase of the O_2 level, with physiological results just opposite to those quoted above for diaphragmatic breathing [315].

Several psychological effects are reported which also serve to distinguish *langhana* from *brmhana* breathing. Slow, even, deep diaphragmatic breathing increases emotional stability, calmness, and greater self confidence while reducing anxiety, whereas thoracic breathing results in the opposite effects [315]. It is also thought that the turbulence of the breath as it passes through the nasal cavity is more or less stimulating to sensors in the mucosal linings of the nose which connect to the sympathetic nervous system, and that the neural effects of this turbulence can have profound changes elsewhere in the body (See Section 19.A, Menstruation, page 453, and Subsection 11.A, *Cardiac Muscle*, page 314), providing one is breathing through the nose rather than the mouth. It is known that the EEG shows demonstrable changes when one switches between nasal and oral breathing (Section 3.D, Cerebral Hemispheric Laterality, page 49).

SECTION 12.C. NASAL LATERALITY

For over a thousand years, the *Swara* yogis (*Swara* means breath) have been aware of a natural left-to-right rhythm of the breath and the subtle psychological and physiological changes that this lateral oscillation promotes. The effect, called nasal laterality, involves breathing predominantly through one nostril for an extended time (an hour or more) and then slowly shifting to breath predominantly through the other nostril. A second shift back to the original nostril completes a "nasal cycle". This lateral oscillation of the breath between the two nostrils occurs without any deliberate effort, as if driven by an internal clock. In the past 100 years, Western science has gone on to confirm the observations of the *Swara* yogis and to quantitatively expand on them [24, 26, 66, 70, 128, 147, 148, 203, 204, 374]. In order to understand this phenomenon, we will first undertake a brief exploration of the structure and function of the nose.

Internal Structure of the Nose

For our purposes, we can consider the nose to consist of two chambers side-by-side, separated by the nasal septum [374]. The side wall on each side opposite the septum carries three structures known collectively as the "turbinates" or "conchae", Fig. 12.A-1, which work to exchange heat and moisture with the in-coming and out-going air. The innermost tissues of the nose covering the septum and the turbinates exude a continuous layer of mucus which acts to adsorb all those airborne particles which otherwise might prove deleterious if allowed into the alveoli of the lungs. This blanket of mucus is actually in motion, the mucus and its embedded particles being transported to the throat, eventually to be digested by the acid in the stomach.

Because the nose is designed to both filter dirt from inspired air, and to warm and humidify it, whereas the mouth is designed instead for eating, we practice *yogasana* only while breathing through the nose, not the mouth. Moreover, there are nerve plexi in the mucus lining of the nose which are connected to the sympathetic nervous system and which are stimulated when breath-

ing through the nose, but not when breathing through the mouth [208]. Yet another reason for preferring nasal to oral breathing lies in the fact that the brain generates a large amount of heat in the process of burning glucose, and this excess body heat is carried from the brain to the nose by the venous blood. Once the hot blood enters the nose, its heat burden is relieved by exchange with the cooler in-coming air, but only if the breathing is nasal. If the brain is allowed to overheat, the risk of stroke becomes significant.

Just below the mucus-secreting tissue of the internal nose lies a much thicker layer of tissue, innervated and heavily vascularized. This is erectile tissue which when stimulated, can become so engorged with blood that the nasal passage is totally blocked. Nasal laterality results when the erectile tissue on just one side of the nose is engorged, while that on the opposite side remains flaccid. Air flow is then redirected when the passive tissue expands while the active tissue of the other side shrinks.

Interestingly, the erectile tissue within the nose responsible for the laterality is closely related to the erectile tissue in the genitals and the nipples of the breast; thus sexual stimulation of these latter areas readily causes nasal congestion and difficulty in breathing [26, 374]. This connection led Sigmund Freud to consider the sexual/nasal interplay, and techniques were later developed to successfully ease certain PMS symptoms by treating the nerves in the erectile tissue of the nose!

Periodicity of Nasal Laterality

Recent studies of nasal lateralization show that nostril dominance switches every 1–6 hours depending upon the individual, is more regular in the morning than at the end of the day, is often incomplete in some subjects, while being much more complete in others over the course of a day, and can be

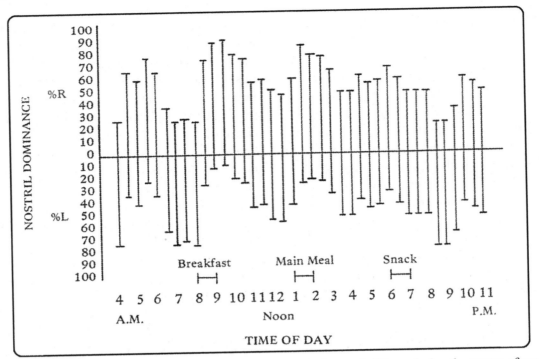

Fig. 12.C-1. Oscillation of nostril dominance as measured every half hour during the course of one day, expressed as the percentage of each nostril that is active [147].

more complete on one side than the other. In some cases, there seems to be little constancy of the left-right pattern from one day to the next, but averaging the nasal openings as measured at half-hour intervals over a month clearly reveals the lateral oscillation, Fig. 12.C-1. In contrast, the subject in Fig. 12.C-2 showed nasal lateralization which was constant with respect to the time of day, over a period of 3 days [128]. In both cases, the period of the oscillations was very nearly 5 hours. It is noted as well that the oscillation is most obvious in adolescents and fades with age, and has been reported as well in rabbits, rats, and pigs [148]. Even when the nasal cycle is in full swing, it is found that both nostrils are simultaneously open about 10% of the time [148]. This opening is the case as well during orgasm [454], *samadhi* and a sneeze. The significance of this will be discussed below (Section 12.D, *Pranayama*, page 381).

The periodicity of the nasal laterality is reflected as well in the secretory activity of

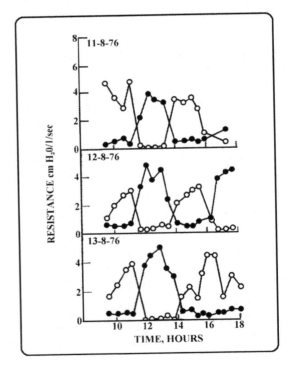

Fig. 12.C-2. Changes in the nasal conductance for air flow through the left nostril (-○-) and through the right nostril (-●-) of a subject for three consecutive days [128].

the nasal mucosa. As this is under the control of the parasympathetic nervous system, it is likely that the laterality and mucus production go hand in hand and are controlled by a central hypothalamic region [128]. Comparison of Tables 12.C-1 and 6.A-2 supports the conclusion that the symptoms attending the oscillating dominance of the nasal breath follow the shifting dominance of the sympathetic and parasympathetic nervous systems (see Section 6.A, Introduction to the Autonomic Nervous System, page 133).

Physiological and Psychological Effects of Nasal Laterality

Our interest in the oddity of nasal laterality stems from the fact that there are distinct psychological and physiological consequences of breathing through either the left nostril or the right. As tabulated in Table 12.C-1, breathing through the right nostril is energizing, making a person outwardly directed, somewhat aggressive and prepared for vigorous physical activity, all the while sharpening mental acuity. In contrast, breathing through the left nostril leaves one more quiet, physically passive and introspective, and tending toward depression. Breathing through the open right nostril promotes digestion of solids, increases body temperature and blood pressure, whereas breathing through the open left nostril promotes digestion of liquids and lowers the heat of the body. The wide range of physiological rhythms tied more or less strongly to the nasal laterality of the breath is presented in Subsection 21.B, *Ultradian Rhythms*, page 474.

Yet other effects of nasal laterality have been mentioned without specifying a left-right correlate: pupil diameter, congestion

TABLE 12.C-1. EFFECTS OF NASAL LATERALITY*

Left open/right closed	Right open/left closed	References
1) More quiet, receptive mood, introspective	1) Outwardly directed aggressive attitude	[66, 147]
2) Passive	2) Vigorous activity	[26, 147]
3) Promotes digestion of liquids	3) Promotes eating and digestion of solids	[26, 66, 147, 374]
4) Reduces body heat	4) Creates body heat	[66, 374]
5) *Decreases blood pressure*	5) Increases blood pressure	[24]
6) Induces depression	6) *Relieves depression*	[24]
7) *Diffuse mental state*	7) Improved mental analysis	[66]
8) Stronger right-hemisphere EEG activity	8) Stronger left-hemisphere EEG activity	[389]
9) Parasympathetic activation	9) Sympathetic activation	[66, 389]
10) Imaginative pursuits	10) Intellectual pursuits	[203]
11) Intuitive, holistic thinking	11) Deductive, rational reasoning	[203]
12) Subjective decisions	12) Attention to detail	[203]
13) Playing music, singing	13) Hunting and fighting	[203]
14) Expend energy in slow, sustained way	14) Expend energy in a vigorous way	[203]

* Entries in italics are not reported, but have been interpolated by the author.

TABLE 12.C-2. NASAL LATERALITY EFFECTS NOT SPECIFIED IN REGARD LEFT AND RIGHT NOSTRILS

Effect On	Reference
1) Pupil diameter	[24, 389]
2) Congestion of blood vessels in middle ear	[24]
3) Body tone	[148]
4) Left to right shift on drinking coffee	[66]
5) Higher cortical functions	[389]

of the blood vessels of the middle ear, body tone and higher cortical functions, Table 12.C-2. Assuming a one-to-one correspondence between sympathetic and parasympathetic activity on the one hand, and right-nostril and left-nostril breathing on the other, one can guess that enlarged pupils and increased body tone and mental functioning, as sympathetic system attributes, are promoted by right-nostril breathing, and that engorgement of the middle ear is promoted by parasympathetic stimulation, *i.e.*, breathing through the left nostril.

Returning to the observations of the *Swara* yogis, the oscillation of the nasal cycle was taken by them as a sign of good health, whereas little or no oscillation on a long-term basis presaged illness. At those times when the left and right nostrils are equally open, it is recommended that one turn away from one's more mundane pursuits, and focus instead on spiritual matters, self-study and meditation [204].

A most unexpected consequence of nasal laterality is reported by Shannahoff Khalsa, *et al.* [424], who found that unilateral breathing when purposely closing off one nostril resulted in different concentrations of the catecholamines in the blood coursing through the two arms! This implies that if one is breathing through one nostril, one of the adrenal medullas is stimulated more that the other, so that the blood on one side of

the body is richer in the hormones expressed by that medulla.

As for a possible mechanism for the laterality of the nasal breath, consider the following: different portions of the hypothalamus regulate the vascular tone in the two hemispheres of the brain (Table 6.B-1) and so control the flow of blood preferentially into one hemisphere or the other. The dominant, blood-rich hemisphere then dictates to the contralateral side of the body, giving sympathetic (left hemisphere dominant) or parasympathetic (right hemisphere dominant) control to all physiological functions that are bilateral, including nasal congestion.

The Conscious Development and Shift of Nasal Laterality

Making precise and repeatable measurements on nasal laterality has proven to be problematic because the laterality seems to vary greatly from one person to the next, and can be switched by relatively small events, either internal (thoughts, emotions, *etc.*), or external (thirst, movement, reading, *etc.*). On the other hand, this sensitivity means that one can easily arrange to breathe through a specific nostril at will, provided one is inwardly centered and free from external and internal perturbations.

It is reported that deliberate switching of the breathing nostril can change the location and intensity of a headache or can change a sense of pain into warmth. *Swara* yogis deliberately open that nostril appropriate for digestion before eating, and when going to sleep, first turn onto their left sides to warm the body (Table 12.C-1) and then onto their right sides in order to relax into sleep. In line with this, getting up from *savasana* by turning onto the right side will leave the student in a more relaxed state than getting up from the left side. As expected for a stimulant, drinking coffee promotes opening of the right nostril [66].

It has been found [148, 374] that if you lie on your right (left) side for 5 minutes or so, the right (left) nostril will close and the left (right) will open, the mechanism again involving preferential engorgement of the turbinate on the right (left) side. However, the effect is not one of gravity as one might at first believe, but rather when the right (left) axilla (armpit) is pressed, there is a reflex reaction closing the right (left) nostril and opening the left (right). This is suggested by the fact that merely tilting the head does not induce nasal laterality, but walking with a crutch (*danda*) under one armpit does, as one so often sees holy men in India doing for the purpose of switching the nostril dominance [315]. One imagines that performing *yogadandasana* would have the same effect on the nostril dominance, and if so, performance of this *yogasana* on the left and right sides should result in rather different mental states.

There is a specific *yogasana* called *padadirasana* which is most effective in switching nasal laterality [421]. In *padadirasana*, one begins by sitting in *vajrasana*, crossing the arms so as to place each hand in the opposite armpit, thumbs resting on the armpit chest. When only the right hand is so placed in the left armpit, then the right nostril will open and the left will close after a few minutes. The opposite situation obtains when the left hand is placed in the right armpit, the right hand resting on the thigh. The use of *yogasana* to direct the laterality of the breath is discussed further in Subsection 3.D, *Using Cerebral Hemispheric Laterality in Yoga*, page 55.

It is difficult to see how axillary pressure can affect the swelling of the turbinates so as to cause nasal laterality. The most prominent structures in the axilla are sets of lymph nodes (Subsection 11.G, page 353), which largely serve lymph vessels from the arms and the thorax. Axillary pressure would block lymph flow from these lower points to the ducts in the region of the clavicle. Though there are lymphatic channels within the tissue of the nose, it is hard to see any connection to those in the axilla. One possible connection is that the first eight cervical nerves join to form the brachial nerve plexus, this being a bundle of nerves that passes behind the clavicle on each side, to the armpit and down each arm to the fingers [257]. Cranial nerve I is involved with the nose in olfaction, and so may be the connection between nasal laterality, the armpit, and cerebral laterality. The mechanism connecting axillary pressure to nasal laterality is a fine example of a well-known yogic phenomenon waiting for an explanation from Western medicine.

It has been shown repeatedly that one nostril can be blocked with the thumb so that the nasal laterality is forced, and that the physiological asymmetries are still present if the breathing is continued for about 30 minutes. Thus, under forced nasal laterality, the blood glucose level rises or falls, intraocular pressure falls or rises, eye-blink rate falls or rises, and heart rate decreases or increases depending on whether it is the right or the left nostril, respectively, that is blocked [422]. Moreover, forced nostril breathing through the left nostril has been found to enhance the performance of spatial tasks (a speciality of the right cerebral hemisphere), whereas forced breathing through the right nostril enhances verbal tasks (a speciality of the left cerebral hemisphere [218]. At the level of the emotions, forced breathing through the left nostril correlates with the production of negative emotions in the right cerebral hemisphere, whereas forced breathing through the right nostril correlates with the production of positive emotions in the left cerebral hemisphere [218]. It is but a logical extension of this work to suggest that a simple nose clip designed to close one nostril or the other could shift the autonomic dominance in various *yogasanas*, in support of their natural tendencies (see also Subsection 16.D, *Yoga in Colored Lights: A Proposal*, page 428, for a related approach to controlling autonomic dominance).

Given the firm connection of nasal laterality to the laterality of so many other physiological functions, it would seem highly unlikely that nasal laterality is not connected as well to the performance of lateral *yogasanas*, and unlikely as well that they do not strongly influence one another. I can find only one paper in the literature on what I feel should be one of the most important aspects of *yogasana* practice: taking advantage of the mutual influence of lateral breathing and lateral bending in the *yogasana* postures in order to raise or lower the energy level of the body/mind.

In a highly thought-provoking paper, Sandra Anderson [8] gives detailed guidance as she takes the student through the series *tadasana*, *trikonasana* right and left, *tadasana*, *parsvakonasana* right and left, and *tadasana* with the emphasis on keeping the breath calm and stable, and on thinking of the breath moving in a lateral way. I strongly recommend this paper to any student or teacher who wants to connect their *yogasana* practice to the finer aspects of their breath so as to attain sympathetic/parasympathetic balance.

The practice of nasal laterality while in the *yogasanas* should lead one to the state where both nostrils are fully open at the same time. In this state of balance, the body's energy will flow up the *sushumna*, the mind's awareness will turn inward, and the pose becomes meditative.

In addition to the paper of Anderson [8] on developing nasal laterality while in the *yogasana* poses, Sovik [440] gives instructions on how to develop nasal laterality when in a meditative sitting position. Note that there is no real reason to focus especially on nasal laterality as the key to unleashing other lateralities; it is just that it is the easiest portal through which to go when in search of the other manifestations of laterality.

Relation of Laterality to Other Aspects of the Breath

The close connection between the dynamics of the breath and the regulation of body functions discussed above relates directly to *pranayama*. In fact, it is claimed that the *pranayama* practice of *nadi shodana* (alternate nostril breathing) not only heightens one's sensitivity to the flow of the breath (Section 12.D, *Pranayama*, page 381), but when practiced without sound or turbulence, can promote a more regular rhythm to the normal left-right nasal cycle, thus furthering overall good health.

It is amazing how closely the laterality of the breath description follows the ancient description of the flow of *prana* through *ida* and *pingala nadis* to terminate at the left and right nostrils (left = *ida* = *chandra*; right = *pingala* = *surya*), Section 4.F, *Nadis, Chakras,* and *Prana*, page 100. If we complete the correspondence, then *ida* corresponds to parasympathetic activation whereas *pingala* is sympathetic. When flow of *prana* is balanced through *ida* and *pingala* and is rapid, then *kundalini* starts to rise through *sushumna* and the mind ascends to a higher meditative level.

Though the nasal laterality of the breath is a sign of good health and is to be encouraged, the more meditative states that can be reached in yoga are achieved when the breath is in the intermediate, balanced state [204, 375]. That is to say, one wants a balanced autonomic nervous system free of any disturbing fluctuations or colorations in order to achieve higher internal levels of consciousness. This level of nasal balance is achieved by diaphragmatic breathing, and occurs most naturally in the hours just before sunrise and just after sunset [204]. Note that these times are just those at which the parasympathetic dominance shifts to sympathetic (5:00 AM to 8:00 AM), and the sympathetic shifts to parasympathetic (6:00 PM to 7:00 PM), Subsection 21.B, *Circadian Rhythms; Physiological Peaks and Valleys in the 24-Hour Period*, page 476.

Connection to Cerebral Hemispheric Laterality

Study of the nasal laterality has recently taken on a new meaning with the discovery that this laterality is driven in synchronicity with the oscillating dominance of the cerebral hemispheres, Section 3.D, Cerebral Hemispheric Laterality, page 49. See Table 3.D-1 for the attributes of cerebral laterality, and see how nicely they compare with the data in Table 12.C-1 concerning nasal laterality, with due regard for decussation.

SECTION 12.D. *PRANAYAMA*

As several long discourses on the subject of *pranayama* are available to the reader, [215, 216, 374], and it is only of tangential interest to our work on *yogasana* for beginning students, only a brief overview will be presented here. In this, we are largely following the discussion of Swami Rama and his coworkers [374, 375, 376, 440]. Our focus will be on how the practice of *pranayama* impacts on the autonomic nervous system, and thence onto bodily functions.

Pranayama is important because in the 8-step hierarchy of yoga it is the lowest level to explore the conscious control of the autonomic nervous system (as viewed from the Western perspective), or (as viewed from the Eastern perspective) to control the fluctuations of the mind by cleansing the energy channels of the body, and to control the flow of the vital force through these energy channels. From either perspective, it is the control of the breath that eventually leads to the desired control of more subtle bodily functions. As such, *pranayama* consists of breathing exercises done with an inner awareness, and done in ways that deliberately harness the breath to the autonomic system. Through practiced control of the breath (*pranayama*), one slowly brings all other aspects of the autonomic system under control. *Pranayama* practice demonstrably eases stress when performed correctly [341].

As concentration on the breath is so easily disturbed by external factors, it is important that the body be strong and free of discomfort for the long periods of time during which the breath is being refined. This level of inner strength and quietude is provided by the practice of the *yogasanas*. In what follows, we will briefly discuss a few of the *pranayama* practices which impact directly on our understanding of the autonomic nervous system.

All agree that there are three basic functions one can perform with the breath: 1) inhalation (*puraka*), 2) exhalation (*rechaka*), and 3) holding the breath (*kumbhaka*) after either 1) or 2). These functions can be exercised rapidly or slowly, using one nostril or both. Simultaneous consideration of these factors in all their permutations and combinations leads to a vast array of possible breathing patterns, the totality of which is called "*pranayama*", *i.e.*, control of the life force. Those breathing patterns that stress exhalation over inhalation with very little holding of the breath are relaxing, whereas those for which the inhalation and exhalation are equally important, but with holding of the breath after the inhalation are energizing [361].

In his detailed book on *pranayama* [215], Iyengar ignores the abdominal breath, but states that one can breathe into either the lower ribcage, the middle ribcage, or the upper ribcage, and that the breath appropriate to *pranayama* practice is all three of these. In this breath, the abdominal muscles are quite active, but they are not allowed to press forward on inhalation as they do in the abdominal breath of Fig. 12.B-1a. In the upper-ribcage phase of the *pranayama* breath, the lifting of the ribs is aided by the contraction of many accessory muscles in the neck, shoulders and back. In terms of the diagrams in Fig. 12.B-1, the Iyengar breath would be closest to the diaphragmatic breath, but with the involvement of the entire chest rather than just the lower few ribs.

There are several lateral-breathing protocols within *pranayama* which promote either *langhana* or *brmhana* in the Ayurvedic sense: in every case, one can rationalize the effect as either heating or cooling (sympathetic or parasympathetic excitation) based upon right-nostril inspiration being very heating, right-nostril expiration being somewhat heating, left-nostril inspiration being somewhat cooling, and left-nostril expiration being very cooling. Taken largely from references [315] and [215], several of these breathing techniques are described briefly below.

Chandra Bhedana: In this technique, one inhales through the left nostril and exhales through the right nostril. This has a calming and cooling effect on the body, and so is stimulating to the *langhana* side of our nature, *i.e.*, is stimulating to the parasympathetic nervous system. Apparently the left-side inhalation has a stronger effect than the right-side exhalation.

Surya Bhedana: This technique in a sense is the opposite of that given above, involving an inhalation through the right nostril and exhalation through the left nostril. As expected, practice of this technique has a stimulating and energizing effect on the body, and so it is stimulating to the *brmhana* side of our nature, *i.e.*, is stimulating to the sympathetic nervous system.

Nadi Shodana: Because this technique uses inhalation and exhalation through both sides of the nostrils alternately, it is a balanced breathing exercise. In this, one first exhales through the left nostril, inhales through the left nostril, then exhales through the right nostril and finally inhales through the right nostril to complete the cycle. Balance of the body's basic elements (*Vata*, *Pitta*, and *Kapha*) which is so necessary for good health is achieved through this practice.

Bhastrika: In this breathing protocol, called the bellows breath, the shallow breath is driven rapidly in and out by the forceful contraction of the external costal muscles and the forceful contraction of the abdominal muscles, respectively. This forceful action raises the breathing rate into the range of the heart rate (approximately 110 beats/minute), dramatically increases the need for oxygen, and proves to be generally stimulating to the sympathetic nervous system [169, 202].

Copeland [87] considers the possibility that the holding of the breath following inhalation (*kumbhaka*) in the course of *pranayama* practice acts to increase the level of CO_2 in the blood, which depresses cortical actions, and so quiets the mind.

Chapter 13

THE IMMUNE SYSTEM

The human immune system is a wonderfully complex mechanism whereby the body recognizes foreign proteins, microorganisms from viruses to fungi, as well as parasites, tumors, foreign tissues and allergens, and once having recognized them as foreign, sets about to neutralize them by killing them. The cells responsible for such actions, the white blood cells, are called leucocytes, and are found in the blood, tissue, lymph, and lymphoid structures, but are most often manufactured in the bone marrow. It is only relatively recently that scientists have promoted the immune system to the level of one of the body's major regulatory systems, a co-equal with the autonomic and endocrine systems [389].

In regard to immunity, there are two basic types, innate and acquired. The first of these offers a general nonspecific first line of defense against all foreign cells and toxins, and is found for example in the antimicrobial action of the skin and among the digestive enzymes of the stomach. The leucocytes that make up the innate system are cells of large size which function as phages, encountering foreign bodies, enveloping them, digesting them and then displaying the protein coat of the invader on its outer surface. This trophy display then summons a second immune subsystem into action (the acquired immune system); though not as rapidly acting as the first line of defense, the second line has a memory of the particulars of each invader derived originally from the protein coat of the phagocyte that first encountered it, and becomes more potent in defense with each new exposure to the invader.

In order to function properly, the acquired-immunity system must distinguish between cells of its own body (self) and those of any foreign invader (nonself) by sensing the molecular pattern of proteins on the surface of the cell in question. Because cells of each particular type of invader have a pattern that is characteristic of that invader (much like a fingerprint among humans) but different from that on cells that are of the body, the cell-mediated immune system is species specific. As this is an acquired immunity, it grows with increasing repetitive exposure to the pathogen, *i.e.*, it is a weak defense on first meeting a particular pathogen, but is much stronger should that pathogen be met again.

Other less-obvious systems are also at work in defense of the body against bacterial invasion. For example, there is a small protein called the endogenous pyrogen, the job of which is to pull iron out of the bloodstream and to deposit it in the liver, so that it is not available to invading bacteria [43].

SECTION 13.A. LYMPHOCYTES AND LEUCOCYTES

Though there are many varieties of white blood cells, we are interested in the neutrophils and the monocytes, which are the active components in the innate defense system, and in the lymphocytes. The neutrophils (45 to 75% of the white blood cell count) attack and destroy foreign cells in the blood, and the monocytes grow into huge single cells (macrophages) capable of enveloping and destroying invaders within the body tissue. Because the neutrophils are in circulation, they are able to move rapidly to the site of an infection and fight it so as to try to keep it from spreading throughout the body. Those white blood cells that die in the service of our bodies appear as pus at the site of the infection. In addition to the phagocytes, the innate system uses the structural barrier of the skin and various chemical means to defend the body [292].

Because the efficiency of the immune system in defending the body is so dependent upon the patterns of circulation, the work inherent in doing the *yogasanas* has an immediate positive effect on the efficiency of the immune system, since it acts to dramatically increase circulation to all parts of the body.

The lymphocytes (15–45% of the white cell blood count), which are found largely in the lymph fluid where they act to destroy invading bacteria, *etc.*, are subclasses of the more general white blood cells so important to the defense of the body against foreign cells. Though the lymphocytes form the backbone of the acquired immune system, they are activated by the actions of the innate system, and only then spring into action. There are two general classes of lymphocytes, the B lymphocytes and the T lymphocytes, as discussed below.

The B Lymphocytes

The B lymphocytes ("B" for bone) are born in the bone marrow, circulate briefly in the blood, and come to collect in the lymph nodes of the body and the spleen [153, 230, 292, 389]. Through interaction with the innate immune system, each of the mature lymphocytes is coded to be responsive to a particular invading bacteria, fungus, parasite, cancer cell, *etc.*, that may be circulating

in the lymphatic fluid. Each of the invading cells is covered in a specific protein or polysaccharide coating that is termed the antigen, and it is by the chemical nature of the cell's antigen that it is recognized by the B cells as self or nonself. When a B cell is contacted by a foreign antigen, its response to it is to generate and release into circulation a particular antibody which is effective in killing the invader and others of its kind once it binds to the antigen. The antibody is a proteinaceous material called an immunoglobulin (Ig), of which there are five general types. The B lymphocytes not only attack foreign invaders, but also are responsible for allergic reactions.

However, not all B cells act as described above, for certain of them, called memory cells, are content to simply record the invader's antigen surface data and then wait for a second invasion of cells bearing that particular antigen. Should that then take place within one's lifetime, the memory cells are able to immediately release the relevant antibody in great quantities, thus making a second attack by the foreign cell even less effective. Thus, when we are vaccinated with dead cells of a foreign invader, the memory cells become charged so that if and when we were to meet the live organism later on, our antibodies would be primed for maximum defense.

The T Lymphocytes

The T lymphocytes also battle foreign invaders [153, 230] or abnormal but nonforeign cells such as those within the body which are responsible for tumors and cancer. Like the B cells, the T cells are first born in the bone marrow as stem cells, but then migrate to the thymus gland ("T" for thymus) where they mature into one of three major types of T cell. The helper T cells identify the intruder cell and signal the killer T cells to attack. In this case, the killer T cells directly bind to the foreign cells and inject toxins that kill the foreign cell. Once the attack of the killer T cells is finished, the suppressor T cells then call a halt to the killer T cell activities. The circulating killer T cells are effective in attacking viruses, tumors, cancer cells, parasites, and bacteria [408], while the braking actions between helper and suppressor T cells keeps the immune system in homeostatic balance. The memory T and memory B cells circulate for years, always on the alert for a new invasion. Though the acquired immune system is relatively slow to come into play, requiring several days for full effectiveness, the B-cell and T-cell arms of the immune system are closely coupled to one another, and work together to eventually fight off attacks on the body.

Immunotransmitters

Among the great variety of T cells are those with the abilities to support or suppress the immune reactions of other types of cells. These T cells are readily influenced by our state of mind [389], and so form the basis of a hypothalamic-immunity axis. Both B and T cells have superficial receptors to specific chemicals called immunotransmitters (cytokines) which allow such cells to turn one another on or off and to otherwise direct and influence their behavior in regard to immunity. As such, the immunotransmitters of the immune system function like the neurotransmitters of the nervous system and the hormones of the endocrine system [389]. In fact, the immune system is sensitive to input from the neural and hormonal systems, and *vice versa* [408], and so can vary its response with due consideration of factors such as exercise, diet, levels of stress, attitudes, relationships with others, *etc.* As an example of this interdependence, Schatz [408] explains that when a macrophage does battle with a virus, it signals hormonally to the brain to raise the body temperature, as a higher temperature

increases the efficiency of the macrophage assault while decreasing the vitality of the virus. Cells infected by virus are tagged by the viral protein coat and then killed by the T cells before the virus can multiply and spread.

Strangely, when T cells are activated by the presence of a foreign body, they produce an immunotransmitter that also activates the osteoclasts in the bones, Section 8.G, Osteoporosis, page 269. Once activated, the osteoclasts work to thin the bones, resulting eventually in osteoporosis.

Steroids such as cortisol tend to increase the amounts of immunotransmitters in circulation in the body and when these bind to cell surfaces, they diminish the ability of the cells to fight invading cells. It also appears that endorphins suppress the immune system, implying that exercise taken to the limit where endorphins (and cortisol for that matter) become prominent may not be healthy for the immune system.

It is the immunotransmitters such as ACTH (Section 6.B, The Hypothalamus, page 140) that allow the immune system to influence the body's other regulatory systems. For example, the inability to cope with stress leads the hypothalamus to promote release of ACTH from the pituitary gland, which in turn forces the adrenal glands to release corticosteroids such as cortisol which inhibit the immune response. If the release of the corticosteroids is prolonged, the thymus gland, prominent in the armamentarium of the immune system, shrivels and eventually the entire organism dies of an irreversible pathology.

The B cells and T cells work in tandem during an invasion, and the numbers of such immune cells are readily increased when one thinks positively about an immediate challenge, whereas negative thinking in the same context can reduce their numbers [389]. If, however, the invading virus is AIDS, then the helper T cells are killed by the virus, and the body is then laid open to infection by other opportunistic viruses or bacteria which ultimately can prove fatal. The AIDS virus itself actually hides within the infected T cells and can be detected only indirectly through the antibody that may be formed in response to its presence.

SECTION 13.B. THE AUTONOMIC NERVOUS SYSTEM AND IMMUNITY

The autonomic nervous system plays an important role in the functioning of the immune response. In fact, the three structures of the immune system, the thymus, the lymph nodes and the spleen are all innervated by branches of the autonomic nervous system. Thus, when there is a sympathetic activation of the adrenal cortex so as to release cortisol, the immune response is weakened, but at the same time, norepinephrine and epinephrine are released by the adrenal medulla, and these promote the formation of lymphocytes, and so strengthen the immune system. Though the adrenal medulla also releases other mineralocorticoids which work to inhibit the suppressive action of the corticosteroids, it now appears that epinephrine and norepinephrine not only stimulate the release of lymphocytes, but also promote the growth of disease-producing bacteria in culture [32]! Thus there are several channels of both suppression and intensification of the immune system, modulated by autonomic factors, and working simultaneously to keep the immune system in dynamic balance. Activation of the parasympathetic nervous system also releases acetylcholine which strengthens the immune system. These hormonal paths are activated by exercise that drives $\dot{V}O_2$ to within 60% or more of $\dot{V}O_{2max}$. As appropriate for a function with strong parasympathetic character, the immune system is strongest at about 2:00 AM, Fig. 21.B-2, the time of parasympathetic dominance.

Among song birds, it is found that the healthiest males immunologically, have the largest spleens, the largest repertoire of songs and are the most successful at mating [15]. That the immune system of songbirds could have any relevance to the health of humans in the 21st Century at first seems farfetched. However, it recently has become very clear that we humans share a common immune system not just with songbirds, but with species as far distant as plants, for it seems that an ancient immune system has been passed down to both plants and animals from a common ancestor [173]. Thus, for example, plants and animals use nearly identical systems to resist common pathogens. This clear link between the immune systems of such seemingly diverse species is less surprising when one reads of the large numbers of genes in bacteria, plants, worms, flies, mice, tree shrews, zebras and chimpanzees that are found as well to be functioning in humans [72].

Once the links between the autonomic system, the body's hormones, and the immune system are established, it is easy to see how mental attitudes can affect one's resistance to infection and disease. The more a body resides in the sympathetic mode, the stronger the inhibition of the immune system, which would appear to be a long-term factor whereas the sympathetic response is a short-term event. On the other hand, parasympathetic excitation as when in *savasana*, *etc.*, promotes a strengthening of the immune system [408]. Inasmuch as the autonomic balance is so very much dependent upon psycho-social interactions and events, it is no surprise that moods, attitudes, life's gains and losses, *etc.*, can have an eventual impact on the immune system and hence on one's health. Tingunait [463] discusses this depression of the immune system from the point of view of depression of the heart *chakra* (*anahata*, Subsection 4.F, *Relation of Chakras to Anatomical Features*, page 105), saying that repressing the heart center works to dull the effectiveness of the lymphocytes residing not only in the thymus gland, but also in bone marrow, the spleen and the lymph nodes. See also Table 13.D-1 below.

SECTION 13.C. MALFUNCTIONS OF THE IMMUNE SYSTEM

It appears that stress is a necessary but not sufficient factor in many diseases. Thus, for example in peptic ulcer, it known that there are three essential ingredients: a high level of pepsinogen in the digestive tract, a dependent personality and a high level of stress. A person having any two of these will not have such an ulcer, but someone with all three is at very high risk for this condition. In general, the immune system collapses under stress (probably due to chronically high levels of cortisol), whether it is physical stress or mental stress, and this when coupled to other problems can generate illness. As another example, consider trench mouth, an infection of the mouth and gums often occurring in college students just before final exams. In this case, there is an ever-present colony of the relevant bacteria living in the mouth, but under control of the immunoglobulin IgA in the saliva. At the time of stress, however, the level of IgA in the saliva drops markedly, and the infection then proceeds at a rapid pace. Similarly, the herpes virus is kept under control by T cells, until that time that stress lowers the effectiveness of the T cells, and a herpes episode soon follows.

The immune system can malfunction in three general ways: it can be underactive, it can be overactive and it can be misdirected [389]. We consider four examples of well known diseases that are now considered to be immune related.

Cancer

Cancer cells are known to be present at all stages of the growth and development of the human body, but they normally do not grow into recognizable tumors, thanks to the quick and efficient responses of the B and T cells. Cancer as a disease becomes significant to an individual when the immune response is underactive and so does not control the wild proliferation of cancer cells. To date, many of the successful cancer therapies depend upon chemical or radiological poisoning of the tumor with consequent suppression of the immune system, however, there is increasing evidence that learning how to cope with stress can be an important component of this treatment. Thus experiencing events that lead to the production of corticosteroids (Section 6.C, The Sympathetic Nervous System, page 144) and thence to conditions of anxiety, depression and low ego strength all act to further depress the immune system and so interfere with its abilities to fight cancer. Actually, it is not the experiencing of certain events in life that leads to negative consequences, as much as it is not being able to cope with them; not everyone reacts negatively to events that may cause depression, *etc.*, in others.

Allergic Reactions and Autoimmunity

In contrast to the underactive condition of the immune system which can be a factor leading to cancer, an overactive and/or misdirected immune system can lead to asthma and allergies [16, 389]. In the case of allergies, innocuous proteins introduced into the body sensitize it so that, when introduced a second time, there is a meaningless and destructive mobilization of the acquired immune system, and one has an allergic reaction to an otherwise innocuous but foreign protein. Once again, the hypothalamus has been found to be a prominent player in either softening or exacerbating the effects of allergic reactions, for the sympathetic nervous system promotes the release of histamine which heightens allergic reactions, whereas parasympathetic stimulation inhibits histamine release.

The basic idea behind the functioning of the immune system is the identification of cells that are a part of the self, and the identification of cells that are foreign. Once this identification is accomplished, the cell in question can be ignored or attacked depending upon whether it is home-grown or foreign. When this identification process breaks down so that the immune system attacks its own cells, then one has an autoimmune condition. This appears to be the case in rheumatoid arthritis (Subsection 8.E, *Joint Lubrication and Arthritis*, page 265), where the joints of the body slowly become painful, stiff and swollen in response to the attacks of both B and T cells on the synovial cartilage of the joint capsules. Negative emotions are a factor in promoting rheumatoid arthritis through the hypothalamus-pituitary axis. It is possible that though the problem in rheumatoid arthritis would appear to be overly active T killer cells, it may come about instead, because the T suppressor cells are underactive and so fail to keep the immune system in balance. Interestingly, as we age and the immune system becomes less effective in doing its job, the severity of autoimmune attacks lessens.

Fever

When there is a superficial, local injury to the skin, the body's response is inflammation, *i.e.*, a local swelling and a local rise in temperature (Subsection 10.D, *The Physiology of Pain*, page 296). If, instead, the insult to the body is more global, as with an infection by a pathogenic organism, then the body's core temperature rises to produce a fever. As the monocytes go into action, immunotransmitters are produced which then trigger the release of prostaglandins in the brain. In response to this, the hypothalamus increases the metabolic rate, the core temperature rises, and one has a fever.

By raising the core temperature, the replication of the invading organism is slowed, while at the same time, the T-cell efficiency increases as they work best at 100.4 to 104° F (38 to 40° C). When feverish, the body also withdraws the circulating iron in the blood so that it is not available to the pathogens for reproduction. When infected, the body's response is not only to heat up, but to otherwise slow down, thereby speeding recovery.

AIDS

In the situation involving AIDS, it is not that the immune system is a causitive factor in the illness, but that the immune system itself is under viral attack. In this case, the AIDS virus infects the T4 helper cells and disables them so that they are no longer effective in helping to combat other diseases that otherwise are normally overcome. Once the T4 cells of the lymphatic system are under attack, the lymph glands first swell, and should they become sufficiently incapacitated, an AIDS patient then becomes vulnerable to certain lung infections and skin cancers. AIDS most often is acquired through contact with infected blood, and is not spread by ordinary social contact.

The Brain's Immune System

Thanks to the blood-brain barrier (Subsection 11.B, page 325), the innate immune system of the brain is isolated from that of the rest of the body, and consists primarily of the microglial cells. Much as macrophages function in the rest of the body, the microglial cells of the brain detect faulty cells, kill them with toxins and then engulf and destroy the remains. Should the microglial cells malfunction and attack healthy brain cells as well, then the result is a gradual loss of brain function and a descent into Alzheimer's disease [221].

SECTION 13.D. YOGA, THE IMMUNE SYSTEM, AND ILLNESS

The field of exercise immunology is a rapidly changing one, with conflicting reports, unsubstantiated findings, and new ideas appearing with great frequency. Our work reports on a few of the more general points in this field, especially as they relate to the *yogasana* student.

Fatigue has long been known to be a significant factor in the susceptibility to infectious disease, either due to intense manual labor or to intense physical training [292]. Thus endurance athletes who train intensely are known to have an increased susceptibility to infectious illness, especially to upper respiratory tract infection. It is doubtful that *yogasana* students work at the level of intensity for this effect to manifest. In fact, there is considerable evidence that moderate exercise of the sort performed in *yogasana* practice infers a small but measurable increase of the immunity over that of the inactive person, possibly because the *yogasana* practitioner is adept at optimizing circulation and at replenishing the body's storehouse on a regular basis through efficient relaxation and through *pranayama*.

The mechanism whereby moderate exercise such as *yogasana* practice can stimulate the immune system would appear to be as follows: during exercise, there is a sympathetic release of epinephrine which promotes an increase in the numbers of circulating neutrophils and lymphocytes, followed by a delayed increase in circulating cortisol, which acts to promote yet higher levels of neutrophils but depresses the lymphocytes. Normal levels of the leucocytes return within 24 hours of exercise. The application of *yogasana* practice to the stimulation of the immune system involves many poses that are supported backbends, so as to open the chest [215a]. Though it is often said that these actions serve to stimulate the thymus gland, it should be noted that in the adult, the thymus gland has degenerated to a yellow, fatty blob of questionable function in the health of the immune system.

According to Nieman [337], exercise done at the level of runners who run for two to three hours nonstop has the effect of sharply reducing the immune function, for times lasting as long as 72 hours. Heavy training, day in and day out, appears linked to a depression of the neutrophil function (to meet bacteria at the site of infection and kill them), whereas more moderate training can increase the strength of the immune system. Thus, in contrast to the immunosuppression found in the dedicated runners mentioned above, those who are over 40 years old and walk only 40 to 45 minutes per day, cut the incidence of colds by 50% thanks to an increased immune response to this moderate exercise. In regard to the immune system, it appears that moderate physical activity is better than no activity, but that too much activity is worse than no activity!

The timing of exercise with respect to exposure to an infection is of great importance [292]. Thus, experiments show that moderate exercise done before an intentionally initiated infection can infer resistance to the infection, whereas intense exercise done at the time of infection increases the chance of illness. For example, the severity of paralysis from polio correlates strongly with the exercise pattern of the patient at the time of the appearance of symptoms, with those who exercised moderately before infection showing only mild paralysis, and those who exercised with high intensity during and after the symptoms appeared suffering a much more severe paralysis.

Yogasana is known to bolster the immune system, for it promotes the formation of both red and white blood cells [408, 410]. Perhaps the largest effect of *yogasana* on the immune system is the effect of such work on the circulation. It is clear that a large part of the immune response is the transport of the infectious agents to the sites of lymphocyte action. If this circulation is brisk, then the maximum immunological response can be expected, however, if the flow of body fluids is sluggish, then so will be the immune response of the body [408]. Through our practice of the *yogasanas*, we maintain an optimum circulation of the body fluids, thereby ensuring that every last drop of fluid is promptly processed by the elements of the immune system, and that all parts of the body are visited regularly by the mobile components of the immune system. Yet a second factor in regard circulation is the idea that many of the immune factors are stuck to the cell walls in times of poor circulation, however, as *yogasana* work demands more oxygen and circulation accelerates, so too does the number of circulating corpuscles increase [16].

Yogasana practice not only speeds the delivery of disease-fighting cells to the sites of infection, but the exercise also works to build high levels of the immune components. Done the correct way, *yogasana* practice will also lead to a more positive parasympathetic response at the expense of the sympathetic response, and this too will bolster the immune system. In addition, neutrophils are thought to clear muscle-tissue damage incurred through intense exercise.

Though there is no evidence that *yogasana* practice can either cure or prevent a serious problem such as AIDS, it is clear

that it nonetheless can be of use in reducing anxiety, managing stress, and can be a form of exercise which is readily adjusted to the exerciser's limits on strength and energy. Similar statements can be made for other serious diseases [408].

Nieman [337] gives some simple rules for exercising while not feeling well, and these would apply to *yogasana* students as well. If your symptoms are above the neck, which is to say, only nasal, try a simple, undemanding practice. If there are signs of infection, avoid inversions that might encourage it to spread. If the symptoms are below the neck and flu-like (fever, swollen lymph glands, fatigue, sore muscles, aching joints), then the best approach is total rest. When the symptoms are below the neck and one insists on working, then the door opens wide for much more serious problems.

Schatz [408] presents an interesting Table listing common behaviors and attitudes and how they impact on the immune system, either bolstering or suppressing immunity. As can be seen in Table 13.D-1, the yogic ideals of moderate activity, high spirits and a calm demeanor all work to keep us healthy.

Though psychoimmunology is a very new field, it is already known that older people who are physically and mentally active and healthy have unusually strong immune systems [460], and *vice versa*. To the extent that our *yogasana* work keeps us physically and mentally healthy, we can expect to be free of the more common diseases of old age. The lack of immunocompetence in the elderly is largely due to inactivity; the positive effects of *yogasana* practice on the immune systems of the young should work as well for the elderly.

Unfortunately, there appears to be a second side to the above argument. As we age and T-cell production and activity begin to wane, the thymus gland degenerates, and the overall strength of the immune system slackens.

One of the problems of extended space flight is that the immune system is compromised in a weightless environment [482]. This immediately brings to mind the situa- tion in regard to weightlessness (and bed- rest) leading to soft bones and flabby mus- cles, and suggests an intimate connection between the immune and the musculo- skeletal systems.

TABLE 13.D-1. HEALTH PRACTICES AND ATTITUDE AS FACTORS IN THE STRENGTH OF THE IMMUNE SYSTEM [408]

ENHANCES IMMUNE FUNCTION	DEPRESSES IMMUNE FUNCTION
HEALTH PRACTICES	
Good nutrition	Poor diet (poor quality, improper quantity)
Proper exercise	Lack of exercise
Adequate sleep	Insomnia, somnolence
Relaxation, meditation	Constant stress
Breathing practice	Smoking
Low alcohol consumption	Heavy alcohol consumption
ATTITUDES	
Active approach to illness	Resigned, helpless approach to illness
Optimistic	Pessimistic
Sees change as challenge	Sees change as threat
Controlled from within	Controlled from without
Inner stability, equanimity	Agitated, volatile
Appropriately self confident	Self confidence out of balance
Sense of purpose, commitment	Apathy
Social support system	In isolation
Involvement	Alienation
Warm relationship with parents	Poor communication with parents

Chapter 14

EXTERNAL SECRETIONS

This Chapter considers all of the important external bodily secretions (saliva, mucus, tears, sweat, and body wastes); because the hormones of the endocrine system are secreted internally, they are considered instead in Chapter 15, page 399. These secretions, external and internal, are largely under the control of the autonomic nervous system, but as discussed below, there can be a strong conscious component to the secretion process. As is the case with most subsystems under the control of the autonomic nervous system, release of the secreted substances is often dictated by a circadian rhythm, Subsection 21.B, page 476.

SECTION 14.A. SALIVA AND MUCUS

The salivary glands are under the control of both the sympathetic and the parasympathetic nervous systems [230], however, in this case, the parasympathetic system stimulates the production of one type of saliva, and the sympathetic system stimulates the production of a second type. Efferent signals in the salivary branch of the parasympathetic system originate in the salivary nuclei within the brainstem, and stimulate the secretion of a thin, watery saliva (saliva consists of water, protein and salts) from the parotid glands via ducts in the mid cheeks on both sides. The parasympathetically-produced saliva is present when food is placed into the mouth or when one simply thinks of food. The parotid secretions are important as they are bacterial suppressants of tooth decay. Rising levels of nasal mucus and the release of tears are driven by the same parasympathetic branch that is responsible for parotid salivation [225].

On the other hand, sympathetic stimulation releases a thick, mucoid saliva which is high in amylase (an enzyme important for the digestion of carbohydrates) from glands at the edge of and beneath the tongue. Because the amylase in our saliva turns carbohydrates into sugars, bread tastes sweet as we chew it. The protein in saliva makes it both stickier and a better lubricant for swallowing. Strangely, the same lubricating protein is secreted in the vagina during sexual arousal [43]. Of the 1.5 to 2 liters of saliva produced each day, by far the larger part is produced by the glands driven by parasympathetic excitation.

In a situation that is fearful, exciting, or otherwise stressful as when we have to speak publicly (see Box 14.A-1), the sympathetic dominance of salivation leads to a mouth that feels dry, whereas during a relaxing *savasana*, the parasympathetic system takes over and the result is a mouth that can be wet to overflowing. Cranial nerves VII and IX are involved in these glandular secretions.

Salivation has its own circadian cycle, being more copious in the morning and least in the afternoon. The quantity of saliva released is also dependent upon posture, being larger when standing up or lying down, and less so when sitting [225].

Compounds called N-nitrosamines are known to be powerful carcinogens in the stomach, and are to be avoided at all costs. In order to reduce the chances of forming N-nitrosamines in the gut, large efforts recently were made to reduce the amounts of nitrates and nitrites in our food (particularly in cured meats), as it was felt these compounds could lead to the formation of the N-nitrosamines in the digestive tract. However, it is now known that there are common bacteria in saliva whose job it is to convert nitrate into nitrite before swallowing, and in the absence of sufficient nitrate, the saliva itself will supply the deficit! Once the nitrite in the swallowed saliva reaches the strong acid of the stomach, it is converted into nitric oxide, a gas which is poisonous to salmonella, E. coli, and other harmful bacteria. The same gas is found in the sinuses of the forehead where it acts to prevent the growth of bacteria in these dark, moist cavities.

The inner surfaces of the trachea and bronchi are covered with epithelial cells bearing hairlike appendages which in turn are covered by a thin mucus film. Any particulate matter breathed through the nose or mouth is trapped in the turbulent swirl of air in the trachea and bronchi, is deposited in the mucus film, which is continuously moving upward, eventually to be swallowed when it reaches the level of the esophagus (Subsection 12.C, *Internal Structure of the Nose*, page 375). Mucus is also produced by the linings of the sinus cavities in the regions of the forehead and cheekbones. When the orifices of the cavities are blocked so that mucus cannot flow outward, then one has sinus congestion. Inversions can be of great help in relieving this congestion [215a].

The discharge of nasal mucus is increased by parasympathetic excitation and decreased by sympathetic excitation, Table 6.A-2. Given that *sarvangasana* is a cooling/relaxing *yogasana*, one concludes that when done in the proper way and for a sufficient duration [209], it leads to parasympathetic dominance. This leads one to expect that the performance of *sarvangasana* will bring relief to stuffy, clogged sinuses in spite of the fact that when inverted, the drainage is upward, against the pull of gravity. *Sirsasana* and its variations also will be effective in relieving clogged sinuses [209] if done so that the parasympathetic system remains dominant, however, these poses are

---

BOX 14.A-1: USING THE SALIVARY GLANDS AS LIE DETECTORS

The fact that the stress and nervousness that usually accompany lying lead to sympathetic arousal and a dry mouth was used in ancient times as a lie detector. Thus among the ancient Bedouins of the Arabian peninsula, a suspected liar was made to lick a red-hot poker; if the suspect's tongue burned, that was taken as proof that his/her mouth was dry and that therefore he/she must have been lying. Similarly, the suspect in China is made to chew a mouthful of rice powder and then spit it out. If the powder comes out dry, this was considered proof of lying. Among the British, the rice powder was replaced by a large wad of bread and cheese. If the suspect could not wet it enough to swallow it, it could only be because he or she was a liar. Clearly, these tests were very unforgiving for those with dry mouths due to a fear of test taking or a distaste of bread and cheese. The modern-day polygraph (lie detector) tries to smooth over these irrelevant responses, but can be beat by a yogi in control of his/her autonomic nervous system (see Box 6.E-1, *Yogis Can Beat the Lie Detector*, page 160).

counterindicated if one has a sinus infection that might be spread by inverting.

Structure and Function of the Eyes, page 411.

SECTION 14.B. TEARS

The lachrimal glands, located in the upper-outer corners of the eyes, exude tears onto the eyeballs through the lachrimal ducts, in order to keep the surfaces of the eyeballs clean and wet. Drainage ducts for the tears are positioned at the lower-inner corners of the eyes, and drain the used tears into the nose and throat. However, the size of the drainage ducts is often inadequate, and excess tears may spill onto the cheeks.

The parasympathetic fibers of cranial nerve VII divide so as to innervate both the lachrimal and salivary glands. Excitations along these fibers produce copious amounts of tears and saliva, respectively. Of course, the lachrimal and salivary responses usually are stronger for emotional stress than for physical stress, but the physical work of *yogasanas* may bring emotional factors to the surface. It is no surprise then that students in *savasana*, a pose with strong parasympathetic action, may need to swallow often and perhaps even cry. Tears are squeezed from the lachrimal glands in part by muscle contraction.

Tears are a complex mixture, containing oil to lubricate the motion of the lids over the corneas of the eyeballs, salts, sugar proteins which serve as wetting agents, and enzymes which are effective in digesting bacteria [387]. When we blink, the action of the eyelid is to pull tears from the lachrimal glands, sweep the tears across the eyeball and tunnel it into the tear ducts. As this process works even when we are inverted, tears still drain into the throat, and so do not run down the cheeks when we do long-lasting *sirasanas*. The physiological and psychological effects associated with tears and blinking are discussed in Section 16.A,

SECTION 14.C. SWEAT

Sweat glands are found all over the body, but are at their highest concentrations in the palms of the hands, on the soles of the feet, and in the armpits (axilla). As discussed more fully in Section 10.C, Thermal Regulation by Blood Vessels and Sweat Glands in the Skin, page 292, the sweat glands are involved in cooling the body through evaporation using the eccrine sweat glands, and ridding the body of toxic wastes using the apocrine sweat glands. Sweat produced through the eccrine glands is watery and is a useful tool in regulating the body's temperature, whereas sweat produced by the apocrine glands (armpits, pubic, and anal areas) is activated not by heat or exercise, but by stress, anxiety, and fear.

When we are hot and exercised, the skin sweats in order to produce an evaporative cooling while blood at the surface of the skin radiates heat to the surrounding air. In contrast, when the sympathetic nervous system is aroused, the sweating is cold and clammy and the blood is pulled away from the surface of the body to better serve the muscles.

The dirty smell of the air in a closed room after a beginner's *yogasana* class is in part due to the detoxification of their systems through the work of *yogasana* via the apocrine sweat glands and in part due to bacterial action in the hairy parts of the skin. On the other hand, performing the standing *yogasanas* on a hot day can be difficult because of the excessive sweat appearing on the soles of the feet via the eccrine sweat glands. The sweating reflex originates within the medulla in the brainstem, Subsection 3.A, *The Spinal Cord and Brainstem*, page 29.

Yet another secretion appears on the skin, for at the base of every hair on the body, there is a small gland secreting an oily substance called sebum. Excessive output from the sebaceous glands leads to a heavy case of oily, greasy hair.

SECTION 14.D.
BODY WASTES

Urination

The urinary bladder is a simple organ, being a muscular sac with the ability to hold up to a pint of urine for hours on end if necessary. As the bladder fills, it expands, and when full, stretch receptors in the bladder walls signal the brain as to the full condition. Sphincters at the two ends of the urethra, the internal and the external sphincters, control the flow of urine out of the bladder. The action of the parasympathetic system during filling and distension of the bladder walls is to contract the bladder muscles and open the internal sphincter. During filling, this parasympathetic tendency is momentarily inhibited by the sympathetic nervous system, and no urine passes. However, once the bladder distension reaches a high level, the sympathetic inhibition is turned off by supraspinal centers, parasympathetic domination reasserts itself and urination commences with both sphincters open and the bladder walls contracting. In the young, all of the above is just spinal reflex, but in adults, the control is supraspinal and conscious [225].

At night, the urinary bladder fills so as to stretch to paper thinness. When in this state, the bladder signals spinal centers to contract the muscles of the bladder, and to open the internal sphincter so as to release the pressure. However, when asleep, the external sphincter, controlled by the brainstem nuclei, is closed tightly. Only upon awakening does the conscious need to urinate

become apparent. That urination action usually cannot be begun without releasing the breath is an indication of its parasympathetic nature. When in a tense situation in the presence of others, the external sphincter in men can tighten so that one cannot urinate even if there is a strong need to do so [43]. When arousal of the sexual apparatus involves the sympathetic nervous system and so inhibits the contraction of the bladder, then urination is inhibited. This is a natural reflex.

Because of the large size of the uterus in women, there is correspondingly less volume for the urinary bladder, all of which can lead to frequent trips to the bathroom. When this occurs during a *yogasana* class, one should honor the urge and not try to suppress it, as the bladder should be empty for *yogasana* practice. Inversions and poses that squeeze the abdomen will promote the need to urinate, especially in women. See Box 11.F-3, *Inversion (and Laughing) Can Lead to Urination*, page 351 for a further discussion of this topic.

When the water level in the extracellular fluid becomes too low, the hypothalamus stimulates the pituitary gland to release antidiuretic hormone (ADH) into the bloodstream. This hormone then acts upon the kidneys, forcing them to retain urine. Somewhat the opposite reaction occurs during inversion. When in an upright stance, there is an insufficiency of blood returning to the heart and the volume receptors in the atrial chambers (Section 11.E, Monitoring Blood Pressure with the Baroreceptors, page 339) report a low blood volume. However, upon inverting, the blood and lymph otherwise pooled in the legs now fill the atria and the volume receptors in the atria then report an excess of extracellular fluid. Once the extracellular fluid is sensed to be in excess, the body reflexively rids itself of the extra fluid through urination. One understands from this the need to urinate after performing inversions of long duration, or even when thinking about them. This mechanism works only during the day, being nonfunctional at night when the body is horizontal [321].

The voiding of urine frees the body of excess water and of several salt components, and as might have been expected, the body does this in a regular way by the clock (Chapter 21, TIME AND BODY RHYTHMS, page 473). Thus, the urination prompted by inversion rids the body of Na^+ and K^+ in addition to water, and the amounts lost daily are largest in early afternoon. Similarly, when we lie down at the end of the day and so remove the gravitational stress from the skeleton, the bones begin to demineralize as with osteoporosis (Section 8.G, page 269), and Ca^{2+} leaves the bones and enters the extracellular fluid, to be released the following afternoon in the urine if not reabsorbed. The acidity of urine is higher at night and less during the day.

When devoid of 24-hour cues, the body's salt and water excretion become free running, with periods of either 24.8 or 33.5 hours or both, Fig. 21.B-2. As shown there, the release of Na^+ and K^+ in the urine adhere to the 24.8-hour cycle with little or no release at 33.5 hours, whereas for Ca^{2+}, there is a prominent 33.5-hour periodicity, with little release at 24.8 hours. The volume of urinary water released during free running peaks significantly at both 24.8 and 33.5 hours, as does the core temperature [321].

Defecation

The processing of food by the gastrointestinal tract up to the point that the digested mass enters the colon is described in Chapter 18, THE GASTROINTESTINAL ORGANS AND DIGESTION, page 441. The ascending and transverse sections of the colon function mainly to remove water from the stool and give it solidity, whereas the descending and sigmoid sections, Fig. 18.A-1, serve largely as storage for the fecal matter prior to the opening of the anal sphincters and defecation. At the colonic end of the gastrointestinal tract, the control of the muscles is again shared by the enteric plexus and by the parasympathetic nervous system, with strong input from higher centers. Peristaltic-like contractions in the descending and sigmoid sections of the bowel compact the fecal matter in the rectum, distending it. Sensed by stretch receptors in the rectum, the distension leads to a reflexive contraction of the rectum, together with the opening of the internal anal sphincter. The nerve supply to the anus and rectum is largely sympathetic, and provides a great many sensors on the anal skin [31].

Release of the external anal sphincter and the act of defecation is triggered by pressure in the terminal part of the colon, as governed by the parasympathetic nervous system. When this mechanism is active, there is a feeling of relief and relaxation throughout the body. In fact, defecation is medically advised for people suffering from paroxysmal tachicardia in order to bring their heart rate back to normal!

Suppression of the natural defecation reflex by keeping the external anal sphincter closed using the higher centers in the adult central nervous system is the unspoken cornerstone of our civilization, for it is only through the intervention of these higher centers that defecation can be postponed to a more socially convenient and private time.

The effects of diet on the stool and on constipation are discussed in Subsection 18.A, *The Colon*, page 446. The lack of effective peristalsis that characterizes constipation may be due in part to a sluggish blood supply to the abdominal area [31] and in part to gravitational compression [239]. It is understandable then that the *yogasana* cure for constipation consists of inversions that release the compression due to gravity and *yogasanas* such as *adho mukha padmasana* [31] in which the pressure of the heels against the colon massage it and so induce peristaltic movement. Similarly, Mehta, *et al.*, [306] recommend *pindasana* in *sirsasana* or in *sarvangasana* for constipation, in which the legs are first put into *padmasana* and the heels then pulled against the abdomen while inverted.

Chapter 15

THE HORMONES

SECTION 15.A. GENERAL FEATURES OF HORMONAL SYSTEMS

As primitive organisms became larger and more complex, cell functions became more specialized and spatially separated from one another. In order to coordinate the functions of such specialized but widely separated groups of cells, two paths of communication evolved, both using chemical messengers: the neural pathway and the hormonal pathway. It was long held that the neural and the hormonal systems of the body were rigidly separate, but with more study, this is seen to be less and less true. Thus, for example, stimulation of the adrenal glands by the hypothalamus is now known to occur both neurally on a short time scale and hormonally on a long time scale. Moreover, a classical hormone such as insulin known to originate in the pancreas is now known also to be produced by some cells in the brain. The modes of action in conventional neural conduction and in hormonal signaling involving the hypothalamus are compared in Fig. 15.A-1.

Hormones are chemical messengers connecting glands in one part of the body with receptive cells in far distant places within the body. In this scheme, the hormone is released into the blood stream by the relevant endocrine gland, and is carried to the receptor site by the circulation of the blood. Receptor sites might be other endocrine glands which are stimulated to release other hormones in turn or they might be organs within the body. Once the hormone is bound to the receptor site, physiological changes are initiated as the hormone is a modulator of the cell's potential function. Though the same molecule can serve in the human body as both a messenger in the hormonal system and a neurotransmitter in the neural system, the functions triggered by the molecule in the two systems will not be the same [438]. Note that not all glands within the body are endocrine glands, *i.e.*, the sweat glands, for example.

Initial stimulation of an endocrine gland begins with afferent neural signals that originate in the visceral organs and go first to the nuclei of the solitary tract, which in turn either stimulate the hypothalamus to release hormones that release other hormones, or stimulate the brainstem nuclei, ending in an autonomic neural output that stimulates an end organ. When these two modes (neural and endocrine) function simultaneously, the result is a neuroendocrine function.

As compared with the direct link between the originating cell and the target cell in the neural network, the action in the hormonal system is more indirect, for in the latter, the general action is a release of the messenger molecules into the bloodstream for distribution throughout the body. Reflecting the different modes of deployment, the neural effects are apparent in times of a few milliseconds, whereas for hormonal deployment, times of hours may be required before the effect is apparent. Though hormonal stimulation is a much slower process than neural stimulation, it can last for a much longer time, however, both modes operate on the basis of transmitter molecules binding sooner or later to receptor sites on distant cells, and thereby activating the cells to a specific function.

Stimulation of the afferent visceral nerves promotes sympathetic responses, most likely via endocrine stimulation within the hypothalamus. As many *yogasanas* could easily stimulate these visceral nerves, they easily could result in endocrine shifts [86a]. Almost all glands are controlled by brain structures such as the hypothalamus and pituitary.

From the yogic point of view, the glands and their excretions are held to be of the highest importance, and though there is little or no scientific evidence to support the idea, it is generally held that the stimulating effects of *yogasanas* on a specific hormone is gained through increased vascular circulation in the area of its gland [483]. However, there is no medical evidence to support the common yogic point of view that apply-

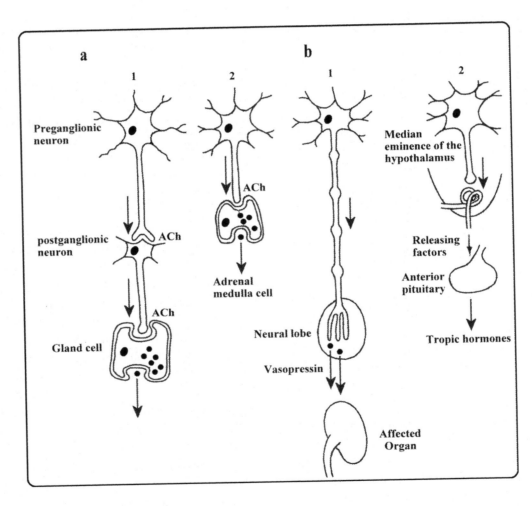

Fig. 15.A-1. (**a**) In the conventional autonomic system, acetylcholine (ACh) serves as the neurotransmitter, inducing the release of hormones (1 and 2). (**b**) The two modes of neuroendocrine release in the hypothalamus, 1) the direct release of hormone from the neural lobe of a neural cell, and 2) the hypothalamus stimulates the hormonal release into the anterior pituitary which then releases the specific hormone into the general circulation.

ing external pressure to an endocrine gland will stimulate it to release its hormonal load, unless the pressure is so extreme that the glandular cells are ruptured. In this regard, the endocrine glands differ from the eccrine glands (see below).

Types of Glands and Hormones

There are two general types of glandular structure. In an eccrine gland, there is a well defined duct which leads the secretion from some reservoir to its target cells, Chapter 14, EXTERNAL SECRETIONS, page 393. For example, the eccrine sweat glands and sebaceous glands deliver their messengers to the skin surface through distinct ducts as do the eccrine tear ducts which carry tears to the surface of the eye; similarly, the bile within the gallbladder is delivered to the small intestine through such a duct as well. In the case of the gallbladder, stimulation of the parasympathetic vagus nerve to the liver simultaneously releases the sphincter to the gallbladder and contracts the muscles of the gallbladder walls so that the bile that is stored in the bladder is expelled into the small intestine [57]. These however, are not endocrine glands.

On the other hand, in the endocrine glands of the human body, there is no such duct evident, and the hormones are simply released into the extracellular fluid surrounding the local capillaries, and these then absorb the hormone and distribute it widely through the circulatory system. In one sense, the hormonal release mechanism in the case of endocrine glands closely resembles that of the neurotransmitters (Fig. 5.C-1), for the hormones are stored in vesicles, and when needed, the vesicles migrate to the outer surface of the gland, fuse with the membrane, and there open to release their hormonal loads into the neighboring area, to eventually find a receptor site [57]. The positions of these endocrine glands in the body are shown in Fig. 15.A-2.

Even within the class of endocrine glands, there is a subclass of glands within organs which largely serve just that organ hormonally. This is so for the hypothalamus, the liver, the thymus, the heart, the kidney, the stomach and for the duodenum [230].

Chemically, there are two general types of hormones, the peptides and the steroids. The peptides are composed of long chains of amino acids, as is the case with insulin and gastrin, for example. The steroidal hormones have chemical structures which are based upon that of cholesterol, and include cortisol, corticosterone, aldosterone, progesterone, testosterone and estrogen. As discussed in Subsection 3.C, *Teaching Yogasana*, page 48, hormones also can play an active role in memory and learning.

Rhythmic Release of Hormones

The release of the endocrine hormones in the body follows the 24-hour circadian clock (Section 21.B, page 476), but with a 1–2 hour ultradian rhythm superposed. Thus at the time in the 24-hour cycle of a hormone's maximum release, there will be a release of several spurts of hormone, with a delay of 1–2 hours between spurts. Rapid fall of the hormone levels is a consequence of the rapid clearing of hormones from the receptor sites through metabolic processes. The times of maximum and minimum release of various hormones are listed in Table 15.A-1, and the periodic release of specific hormones is discussed in more detail in Section 15.B, page 403.

The hormones CRF and ACTH involved in the hypothalamus-pituitary axis (Section 6.B, The Hypothalamus, page 140) also have plasma concentrations that are tied to the circadian clock. Though the corticosteroids in humans peak just as the day begins, and then fall to a minimum in the evening, it is just the reverse in nocturnal animals.

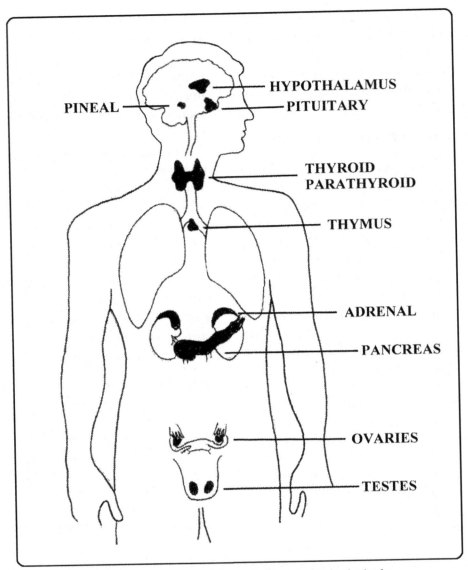

Fig. 15.A-2. Placement of the endocrine glands in the body.

TABLE 15.A-1. TIMES OF MAXIMUM AND MINIMUM CONCENTRATIONS OF HORMONES IN BLOOD PLASMA [321]

Hormone	Time for Maximum	Time for Minimum
Cortisol	4:00 AM	10:00 PM
Growth hormone	10:00 PM	All day
Aldosterone	4:00 AM	All day
Prolactin	4:00 AM	All day
Testosterone	2:00 AM	6:00 PM
Luteinizing hormone, male	No peak	No peak
Follicle stimulating hormone, male	No peak	No peak
Thyrotropin	10:00 PM	All day

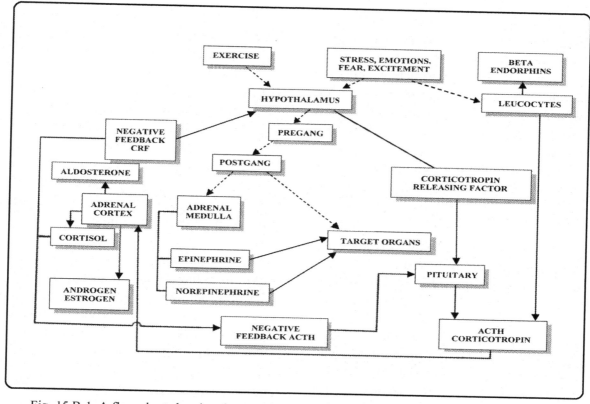

Fig. 15.B-1. A flow chart showing the neural (dashed arrows) and hormonal consequences (full-line arrows) of stress and exercise on the body, and the interactions between neural and hormonal processes.

SECTION 15.B. SPECIFIC GLANDS AND THEIR HORMONES

The Hypothalamus

Located just above the pineal and the pituitary glands, Fig. 15.A-2, the hypothalamus integrates neurological information from other nerve centers and chemical information from the bloodstream into a coherent course of action for the other glands. Through the release of its hormones, it regulates not only the hormone production of the pituitary, but of the adrenal glands as well. The functioning of this gland is described in detail in Section 6.B, The Hypothalamus, page 140, and in Fig. 15.B-1. All three hormones involved in the interactions along the hypothalamus-pituitary-adrenal cortex axis shown in Fig. 15.B-1 follow circadian rhythms dictated by the suprachiasmatic nucleus, which in turn is keyed to the light-dark cycle of the sun as sensed by the eyes (Subsection 21.B, *The Sleep/Wake Cycle and Relaxation*, page 488).

Many hypothalamic hormones are first released into the duct going directly to the anterior and posterior lobes of the pituitary, which then releases hormones into the general circulation which eventually find their target organs in the ovaries, testes, thyroid, bones, skin, kidneys and the breasts. The intended action at the target organ then releases yet another hormone which acts in an inhibitory way with the hypothalamus so as to regulate its actions through feedback [229]. Among many others, the hypothalamus releases the following hormones directly to the pituitary gland: a) gonadotropin releasing factor, which promotes the subsequent release from the pituitary of luteinizing hormone and the follicle stimulating hormone, b) corticotropin releasing factor, which promotes the release of corticotropin from the pituitary, eventually to influence the adrenal cortex, and c) thyrotropin, which releases thyroid stimulating hormone from the pituitary [230, 438].

The Pituitary Gland

This endocrine gland is widely known as the master gland, however, it is activated by hormonal secretions of the hypothalamus just above it in the midbrain. Hormonal action of the pituitary gland is readily divided into that governed by the anterior portion of the gland and that governed by the posterior portion. Secretions from the anterior pituitary include growth hormone, ACTH, prolactin, gonadotropin releasing hormone, and thyroid stimulating hormone, whereas secretions from the posterior pituitary include oxytocin and vasopressin.

The sex hormones that are active at the onset of puberty and throughout the adult reproductive period also originate with signals at the hypothalamus and pituitary glands [230, 438, 461]. On command from the hypothalamus, the pituitary will release follicle simulating hormone to stimulate the growth of follicles in the ovaries, luteinizing hormone to convert a follicle in the ovary to a corpus luteum, and corticotropin (ACTH) to the adrenal cortex in order to promote the release of cortisol. The release of oxytocin is responsible for the contractions of the uterus both during labor and lactation thereafter. The pituitary is also the source of vasopressin (also known as antidiuretic hormone, ADH), a very powerful hormone which not only acts on the kidneys to retain water, but constricts the vascular system to raise the blood pressure, and works on the liver to break down glycogen, a polymeric form of glucose.

Vasopressin serves as a messenger in both the neural and hormonal circuits. As a hormone, vasopressin is released by cells in the posterior pituitary, and acts both to constrict blood vessels and to hold water within the body. Release of vasopressin acts to raise the blood pressure, especially at times of heavy blood loss. As a neurotransmitter, vasopressin is found in the synapses of the brain, and is assumed to play some role in memory [101, 438].

Massive amounts of oxytocin are released from the uterus both during the labor of a pregnant woman and during orgasm. Because oxytocin tends to produce amnesia, many mothers have little or no memory of having given birth to a child [389]. At much lower concentrations, oxytocin promotes and regulates social memory and social relationships, and is an integral part of the memory process when sexual or maternal bonds are being formed [75]. Both vasopressin and oxytocin are released during copulation. In contrast, many autistic individuals have low levels of oxytocin, as do many women who have life-long troubles with close relationships.

The Pineal Gland

Located deep in the brain, the pineal gland is at about the level of the eyes. In the dark, the pineal gland secretes melatonin, a natural antidepressant and a factor in setting the biological clock (Subsection 21.B, *Circadian Rhythms: Peaks and Valleys in the 24-Hour Period*, page 476). The pineal gland is not only photosensitive, but psychosensitive, for it also releases melatonin during meditation (and presumably during yogic relaxation); evidence suggests that melatonin is an active agent in fighting prostate and breast cancers [76].

The Thyroid Gland

The thyroid gland is located at the base of the throat, and its hormones are regulators of human growth and metabolism. The thyroid hormones triiodothyronine and thyroxine generate heat in the body through the regulation of the body's rate of metabolism and promotion of protein synthesis. These hormones also act to increase heart action and the brain's excitability [45, 230]. Circulation in the vicinity of the thyroid would be promoted by inverted *yogasanas* such as *sarvangasana* and *halasana*.

The hormone calcitonin is also released by the thyroid when the level of Ca^{2+} in the blood rises too high. Calcitonin serves to lower the level of Ca^{2+} in the blood by encouraging the osteoblasts to incorporate Ca^{2+} in bone formation and simultaneously discouraging the release of Ca^{2+} from the bones by the osteoclasts [45, 230] (Subsection 8.B, *Hormonal Control of Ca^{2+} in the Body Fluids*, page 242).

The Parathyroid Gland

A hormone from the parathyroid regulates the Ca^{2+} and PO_4^{3-} levels in the blood (Subsection 8.B, *Hormonal Control of Ca^{2+} in the Body Fluids*, page 242). In order to increase the level of Ca^{2+} in the body fluids, parathyroid hormone stimulates the osteoclasts to dissolve bone, thus setting the Ca^{2+} free. When the proper level of Ca^{2+} in the body fluids is reached, the parathyroid ceases to release its hormone. Through the release of parathyroid hormone, the synthesis of vitamin D is activated.

The Thymus Gland

Being located just behind the heart, the thymus gland is the center of the heart chakra (*anahata*). Its only function appears to be its association with the immune system, for it appears to be a depot for the storage of the T cells of the immune system [230], Chapter 13, page 383. Though the thymus is formally a part of the lymphatic system, its activity wanes considerably after puberty, becoming yellow, fibrous tissue in the adult. *Yogasana* exercises designed to stimulate the adult immune system by virtue of increased circulation to the thymus would seem to have minimal value in view of this early degeneration [229].

The Adrenal Glands

Atop each kidney, there is a cluster of glands that play a huge role in the body's response to stresses of various kinds. This glandular complex is divided into a central part, the adrenal medulla, and a wrapping about the medulla, the adrenal cortex. Though side by side, the medulla and cortex as glands differ in their structures, embryonic origin, the hormones they release, and the hormones to which they respond [230, 438, 461]. The adrenal cortex is the origin of the hormones known as the corticosteroids, and the adrenal medulla is the origin of the hormones known as the catecholamines (Subsection 5.D, page 129).

The adrenal cortex is further divisible into three zones. In the innermost zone, the sex steroids, the androgens and estrogen are released in small amounts. The middle zone is responsible for the release of cortisol, a hormone which is very important in resisting stress, and which increases the glucose supply for the brain and heart in times of stress. The outer zone of the cortex releases the hormone aldosterone, which acts within the kidney to regulate the concentration of Na^+ and K^+ ions in the body fluids, increasing the former and reducing the latter. It is released only in cases of dire emergency involving loss of blood or blood pressure. As seen in Table 15.A-1, other than for emergencies, the peak release of aldosterone is almost coincident with the time of general early-morning arousal of the entire body (4:00 AM).

The adrenal hormone cortisol is one of great interest to the teacher of *yogasana*. Under heavy exercise, the hypothalamus triggers a cascade of hormonal events that end with the release of cortisol from the adrenal cortex, Fig. 15.B-1. The best known action of cortisol is to increase the levels of glucose in the blood and at the same time inhibit the uptake of glucose by the muscles in order to insure adequate fuel supplies for the brain and heart under conditions of stress. Ideally, too high a level of cortisol will turn off the initiating event in the hypothalamus. For a given level of stress, the largest stress-stimulated release of cortisol occurs at times of lowest ambient cortisol level (10:00 PM, Table 15.A-1), and is least when the level of ambient cortisol is highest (4:00 AM). Accordingly, the amount of cortisol generated by *yogasana* practice will be least for a morning practice and largest for an evening practice. The circadian rhythm describing the early-morning release of cortisol is very strongly tied to the rising and setting of the sun, even in blind people, and is very resistant to perturbation from the outside.

When the source of the stress is chronic, so too is the elevation of the cortisol level in the blood. In this case, the middle zone of the adrenal cortex becomes hypertrophied, and one faces the increased risks of stomach ulcers, loss of immunity due to shrinkage of the lymph glands, hypertension and other vascular disorders, excess sugar in the blood, heart disease and upper respiratory infection.

In an interesting experimental study, Brainard, *et al.* [49], measured the amounts of cortisol in the blood of three groups of subjects, a group of beginning *yogasana* students, a group of experienced *yogasana* students and a control group. The first two groups were to perform their asana practice while the control group was to sit and read. Cortisol measurements were made before and after a one-hour *yogasana* practice, and it was found that the control group showed a slight cortisol drop between 11:00 AM and 12:00 noon, as is normal for the circadian rhythm. On the other hand, the beginners showed a much more substantial drop in cortisol, and the more experienced students showed even more of a drop. The authors concluded tentatively that *yogasana* practice could be an antidote to the many stressful scenarios which otherwise raise the levels of this stress hormone. However, as seen in Fig. 21.B-8, the spurting nature of the cortisol release means that one must measure cortisol at time intervals much shorter than 1 hour if one wants to accurately assess the effects of *yogasana* practice on plasma cortisol.

The effects of cortisol extend to the moment of birth: when the baby is ready to be born, the baby's adrenal cortex releases cortisol into the common bloodstream of mother and baby. With increased cortisol in the blood, the mother's progesterone level falls while estrogen remains high. Uterine contractions then begin, and a baby is delivered who is alert, charged with life, and ready to meet life's challenges [473]. The circadian release of cortisol does not develop until the age of 2–3 years.

In contrast to the situation with the adrenal cortex, the adrenal medulla only can be activated neurally. Under stress, the medulla is signaled by the sympathetic nervous system to release the catecholamines, epinephrine and norepinephrine (earlier known as adrenaline and noradrenaline) into the bloodstream, typically in the proportions 80% to 20% [230]. Epinephrine is targeted toward tissues carrying beta receptors, whereas norepinephrine targets tissues with alpha receptors. Thus epinephrine acts on the beta receptors of the heart causing increased pumping rate and a more forceful contraction, and on the beta receptors of the smooth muscles of the bronchioles to relax and so dilate them. Epinephrine also promotes the breakdown of glycogen and fat to glucose for use as fuel.

The alpha receptors of the visceral blood vessels are stimulated by norepinephrine to contract the vessels, thereby rerouting blood from viscera to the large muscles, raising the blood pressure; this effect is stronger yet in the presence of cortisol. The alpha receptors in the heart react toward norepinephrine to stimulate contraction, and also work to increase the strength of contraction of the muscles in the arms and legs [438, 461]. In keeping with the fight-or-flight syndrome, the sympathetic release of the catecholamines raises the levels of alertness and excitability in the brain. The catecholamines are the short-term response to stress. Simultaneous with the release of the catecholamines, cortisol also can be released, and this has a long-term effect in response to stress.

Epinephrine is dumped from the adrenal medulla into the bloodstream when triggered to do so by the opening of K^+ channels; the triggering level is highly variable between species and between individuals within a species. It is hypothesized [414a] that among thrill seekers, for whom ordinary life is too boring without the excitement of risking life and limb, the trigger level is set extraordinarily high, so that one must be close to death in order to feel the epinephrine rush. Though epinephrine cannot pass from the bloodstream into the brain, its presence in the blood leads to the release of dopamine in the brain, always a pleasurable sensation. The epinephrine rush can be triggered by physical, emotional or intellectual means.

The synapse between the sympathetic preganglionic fiber and the adrenal gland itself is cholinergic, otherwise were the synapse adrenergic, the initial release of the

catecholamines would stimulate the further release of yet more catecholamines in a runaway fashion. The stimulation of the sympathetic nervous system and the release of the catecholamines requires about 20 minutes to wear off, the time it takes for these hormones to clear the system [473]. This fact suggests that 20 minutes is a reasonable time for performing *savasana*, and that ambient catecholamine levels can change dramatically in less than a half hour.

Yet another hormone excreted by the kidneys when prodded to do so by the sympathetic nervous system is renin. As described in Subsection 6.C, page 150, renin acts indirectly to produce angiotensin II, which causes blood vessels to constrict and also promotes aldosterone release in order to increase the blood volume, all of which act to raise the blood pressure [57, 77, 321, 461].

The Pancreas and Gastrointestinal Glands

The pancreas contains both eccrine and endocrine glands, the former of which release digestive enzymes into the digestive tract. The endocrine cells are of two types, the alpha cells which release the hormone glucagon into the blood, and the beta cells which release insulin instead. Insulin is very important because it allows the glucose in the blood to cross a cell's outer membrane and so become fuel within the cell. If for some reason there is too little insulin or it is unable to enter the cell, the result is one form or another of diabetes.

Insulin is packaged within the beta cells in vesicles which migrate to the cell membrane, fuse with it and thus release their hormonal burden to the extracellular fluid outside. Release of insulin can be triggered either neurologically or hormonally [461], however, more than half of the insulin released by the pancreas is scavenged by the liver before it can be of any use to distant cells. Glucagon is also involved with blood sugar, as it acts in the liver, converting glycogen into glucose [461].

The pancreas is innervated by both the sympathetic and parasympathetic nervous systems, with the former inhibiting the release of insulin and the latter promoting its release. On this basis, one would guess that *yogasanas* leading to parasympathetic dominance might be curative in those cases where there is a insufficiency of insulin, and though there are several reports of the efficacy of yoga in regard to diabetes, there is as yet no firm evidence that *yogasanas* can affect insulin production [139, 318].

Several small glands are scattered about in the stomach, small intestine and liver, releasing hormones to the digestive system. Thus the hormones gastrin and somatostatin when released into the stomach respectively promote and inhibit the secretion of stomach acid, and the presence of enkephalins in the intestines controls peristalsis [39a].

The Gonads

The glands in question here are the ovaries in women and the testes in men, in both cases being responsible for the growth and development of the reproductive organs and for sexual behavior. The ovaries release estrogen, progesterone, and relaxin (the female steroids), while the testes release the androgens (the male steroids), including testosterone.

Men and women produce both estrogen and testosterone, but in differing amounts. In men, estrogen has a key function in the regulation of sperm production, and estrogen-like compounds in the environment are a real threat to men's fertility. The testosterone normally produced in the woman's body by the adrenal cortex is only 1/12 to 1/16 that normally found in men, but women appear to be much more sensitive to low concentrations of the hormone than are men. The sex hormones also exert actions on nonsexual organs such as the muscles and skin [461].

Normal concentrations of testosterone act to sharpen one's focus and concentration on a particular subject, but lessens one's ability to do several things at once, for example, to press out through the big toe, straighten the leg, lift the inner thigh, lift the ribs, pull the shoulder blades down and lift the chest, *etc.* Testosterone levels are low in vegetarians, and it is believed that *yogasana* practice also works to lower testosterone levels.

In maturing young women, estrogen and progesterone from the ovaries spur the development of breasts, the uterus, fallopian tubes and the vagina, while at the same time, they slow the growth of the long bones, regulate the muscle tone in the urinary tract, control bone density, and regulate fluid retention [45]. The ovaries also produce inhibin, a hormone that acts on the pituitary and hypothalamus to restrict the production of gonadotropin releasing factor and of follicle stimulating hormone. The hormonal paths by which the brain and the female reproductive apparatus influence one another is shown in Fig. 15.B-2.

The "estrogens" are really a family of closely related hormones. Before menopause, the key actor is estradiol, a hormone that helps the reproductive system to mature. At menopause, there is a shift of relative importance, with estrone then becoming important; it is the loss of estradiol that brings about hot flashes, *etc.* The testosterone level in women also falls at menopause, but the sex drive can remain high as long as the ovaries remain intact (see also Section 19.C, Menopause, page 459).

In the male, the secretion of testosterone by the testes increases strongly at puberty. As a result, the facial and other hair thicken, the voice becomes deeper, and long bones grow rapidly, then stop. At this time, the body loses fat and becomes stronger and more muscular, and the generation of sperm

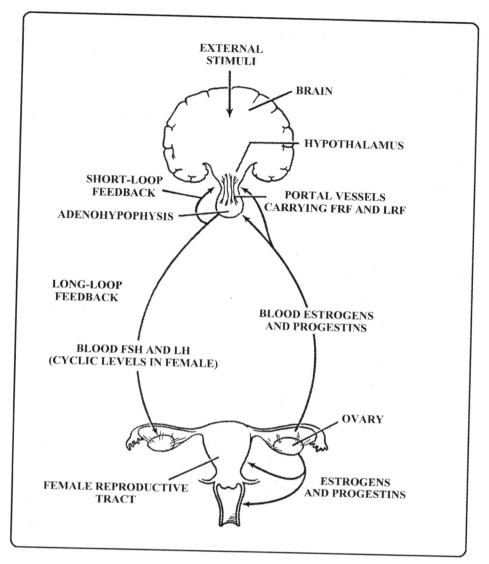

Fig. 15.B-2. Hormonal paths by which the brain and the female reproductive tract influence one another. The abbreviations are as follows: FSH is follicle stimulating hormone; LH is luteinizing hormone; FRF is follicle stimulating hormone-releasing factor; and LRF is luteinizing hormone releasing factor.

is begun [461]. Androgen production remains relatively constant in the male into the seventh or eighth decade, especially as compared with the swings of the sex hormones in mature women. Testosterone levels in males fall by only 50% on going from 40 years old to age 70. As the hormone levels shift in older men and women, they tend to move toward one another, so that in old age, men and women become more alike from the hormonal point of view.

Excess testosterone *in utero*, either from the mother or the embryo, is known to temporarily inhibit left-cerebral hemisphere development, so that an overly developed right hemisphere and correspondingly underdeveloped left hemisphere can result. As an adult, such asymmetric cerebral development can lead to autism, homosexuality, left handedness, dyslexia, the ring finger of the right hand being significantly longer than the index finger of that hand, and enhanced musical ability [59, 328]. Correspondingly, if estrogen were present in too large amounts in the womb, the opposite cerebral asymmetry results and the child can have an index finger much longer than the ring finger, a feminine personality, and a higher-than-normal tendency toward breast cancer.

It is strange but interesting that when a gonad is removed in either a male or female, the intraocular pressure in the opposite eye is significantly lowered [370]. If both gonads are removed, then the intraocular pressure drops in both eyes. This is an example of "pure nervous feedback from an endocrine organ". Intraocular pressure also can be lowered by meditation and yogic relaxation.

Chapter 16

THE EYES AND VISION

SECTION 16.A. STRUCTURE AND FUNCTION OF THE EYES

"Eyes are the windows to the soul," said Shakespeare, but he was only half right; what he neglected to mention is that not only do we look into the windows of the eyes to see the soul, but we also look out of the windows of the eyes to see the world, for fully 80% of the information that comes into our brain passes through the eyes! In response to this flood of visual information, between one third and one half of the brain's huge capacity is involved with processing visual signals in thirty separate areas dedicated to visual aspects such as form, color, movement, texture, identification of hands, identification of faces, *etc.* Needless to say, we would be overwhelmed if all of the visual information received by our eyes were to appear in our consciousness.

Inasmuch as the eyes are so much a contributor to our awareness, it hardly seems possible that the eyes are not in some way involved with our practice of the *yogasanas* as well. Moreover, being strongly innervated by the autonomic nervous system, the eyes also reflect the levels of physical and emotional tension within the body, and so are useful indicators of overall stress when practicing *yogasana*. In periods of stress, the sympathetic nervous system is dominant and the eyes become more tightly focused toward the nose so as to ignore any peripheral disturbances. On the other hand, as

pointed out by Ruiz [393], in order to relax the brain and fall asleep, we must close our eyes and so block the otherwise constant stream of visual information. This blocking of the visual pathway then allows the parasympathetic nervous system to assert itself, and sleep follows. As many of us are chronically tense visually, the prime consideration of *yogasana* for such students as regards the eyes is relaxation, whereas for the mentally depressed, it will be important to keep the eyes open and alert. The eyes also can be used to advantage with an active sympathetic nervous system when one is involved in *yogasana* balancing poses, as discussed in Subsection IV.D, *Vision and Balance*, page 533.

External Structure of the Eye

The structure of the eye can be divided nicely into those components within the eyeball itself and those components that are essentially outside the eyeball but still closely related to its function. The six muscles external to the eye which work to position the eyeball in its socket are innervated by cranial nerves (Subsection 2.C, page 17) largely within the control of the autonomic nervous system. Each eyeball is pointed in space using these six muscles as shown in Fig. 16.A-1a and 1b. As can be seen there, four of the muscles are set at the cardinal points so as to give motion in the up, down, left, and right directions, whereas two others serve to rotate the eyeball about the optic axis. However, virtually any movement of the eyeball is complex, in that it involves

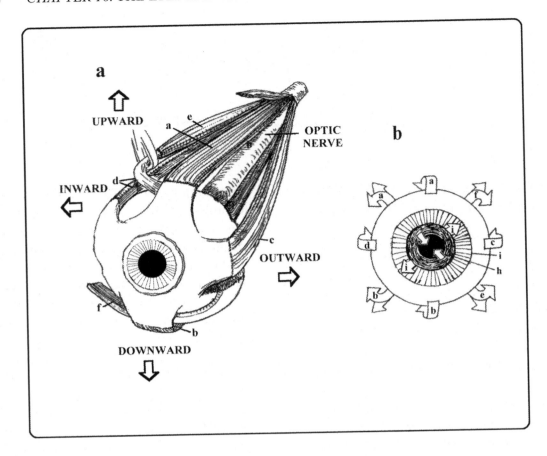

Fig. 16.A-1. (**a**) The extrinsic muscles of the left eye, labeled *a* to *f* (*a* = superior rectus, *b* = inferior rectus, *c* = lateral rectus, *d* = medial rectus, *e* = superior oblique and *f* = inferior oblique). (**b**) The directions in which the muscles *a* to *f* rotate the eyeball. The intrinsic muscles surrounding the pupil are labeled *h* (sphincter pupillae) and *i* (dilator pupillae) [229].

several or all of the six extrinsic muscles simultaneously [229].

As the volume of the eyeball is only 6.5 cm^3, whereas that of the eye socket is 29 cm^3 [43], there is considerable room for movement of the eyeball forward and backward in the socket. Still, the eyeball does not rattle around in the spaciousness of the eye socket because there is a constant tension in the external muscles that keeps the eyeball relatively immobile, though changes in the pattern of tension among the muscles can move the eyeball significantly. Indeed, the position of the front of the eyeball in the eyesocket is a reflection of tension in the eyes and facial features, with tension pressing the eyes forward. As we age, the body part that grows the least is the eye; though the adult's body volume is 20 times that of the infant, the volume of the adult eye is only 3.5 times that of the infant's.

Strangely, the extrinsic muscles of the eyes are outfitted with muscle spindles (Section 7.B, page 198) which are capable of monitoring possible over-stretching of skeletal muscle, yet these muscles of the eye are never harnessed to an external load and therefore can not be over-stretched, nor are they part of any known stretch reflex. Perhaps they are used instead as proprioceptive sensors rather than as stretch-limiting safety switches.

The external muscles of the eyes have two other important mechanical functions other than the important function of aiming the gaze: blinking and scanning the visual scene. When our eyes blink, they are being washed down by the upper eyelids in order to keep the corneal surface hydrated and free of grime (Section 14.B, Tears, page 395). In persons who are 20 years or older, the eyes blink in a reflexive action about 24 times per minute, however, the rate is dependent upon one's mood; when we are angry, stressed out, or talk to a stranger, the blink rate increases [171, 387]. Infants on the other hand, blink less than once per minute. When we blink, the eyes are closed for a significant fraction of a second (400 milliseconds), and in that time all processing of visual information stops in the brain, however, the brain smooths over these blank spots to present a seamless picture of visual events to the consciousness. What is even more remarkable, is that the cessation of visual processing begins about 50 milliseconds before the eyelids even begin to move!

Blinking is driven by the superior tarsal muscle, the job of which is to lift the upper eyelid; only the upper eyelid moves when we blink or squint. Interestingly, this muscle is innervated by the sympathetic nervous system, thus accounting for the correlation between blink rate and the level of stress [154]. Though the blink rate rises when we are under stress, when concentrating intensely as when in the *yogasanas*, the blink rate drops significantly, and the corneas will tend to dry out.

Rapid external motions of the eyes called "saccadic motions" are used to scan the visual scene for important details, and these areas of importance are then given special attention. Such saccadic motion is known to be essential for the visual process, as described below in the discussion of the retina, Subsection 16.A, *Vision and Neuroanatomy of the Eye*, page 415.

Internal Structure of the Eye

Of the five functions of the eye that are controlled by the autonomic system, three of them involve intrinsic muscle actions which change the eye's optical parameters, *i.e.*, they change the focal length of the lens, open the pupil of the eye, and close the pupil of the eye, Fig. 16.A-2a.

Light incident on the eye first passes through the transparent cornea and is then focused by the lens in a left-to-right (reversed), top-to-bottom (inverted) fashion onto the retina. The focusing of the image on the retina is accomplished in part by changing the curvature of the lens using the ciliary muscles, as shown in Figs. 16.A-2b and 2c. This process is called accommodation. The ciliary smooth muscle attaches to the outer rim of the lens and is normally in a state of tension which acts to flatten the lens, Fig. 16.A-2b, thereby increasing its focal length as appropriate for far-field vision. This muscle is innervated by cranial nerve III of the parasympathetic system, originating at the oculomotor complex within the hypothalamus. Upon activation of cranial nerve III, tension on the ciliary muscle is released, allowing the lens to assume a more spherical shape, thereby shortening its focal length, as appropriate for vision in the near field, Fig. 16.A-2c. There are no nerve fibers to the ciliary muscle from the sympathetic nervous system. Contrary to popular opinion, the lens is not the only structure that determines the effective focal length of the eye, for strong focusing also is obtained at the interface between the cornea and the air outside the eye [171].

As we age, the center of the lens begins to accumulate dead cells and the lens stiffens and becomes more resistant to changing its shape. Accommodation of the eyes by age 40 years, then must be accomplished with the aid of glasses. However, it would not be surprising that the generally limber-

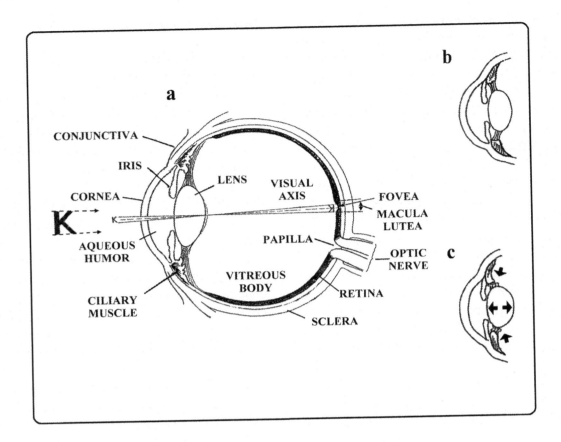

Fig. 16.A-2. (**a**) The inner structure of the eye. Note how the lens works to invert and reverse the image at the retina. (**b**) Curvature of the lens with the ciliary muscle toned and (**c**) increased curvature of the lens with the ciliary muscle relaxed.

ing effects of yoga applied to the eyes could keep the lenses supple enough to not require glasses in middle age.

The cornea and the sclera (the white part of the eye surrounding the iris) differ in their optical properties because the sclera is filled with loosely packed collagen fibrils (Subsection 9.A, page 273) and so scatters light and appears opaque, whereas the collagen in the cornea is much more tightly packed, does not scatter the incident light, and so is transparent. In old age, the collagen bundles in the cornea tend to become less tightly packaged and more like scleral tissue, and light-scattering cataracts are so formed.

Because the cornea has no blood supply and is nourished by the aqueous humour (the fluid between the cornea and the lens, Fig, 16.A-2), it is virtually isolated from the rest of the body. The lens, too, is free of vascular plumbing. Though the cornea is free of blood vessels, it is richly supplied with nerve endings that signal irritation and pain. If a gritty particle settles on the cornea, a reflex action is activated that leads to blinking and the secretion of tears (Section 14.B, page 395).

Between the cornea and the lens is the iris, consisting of two circular sets of pigmented muscles forming an opening (the pupil) to the inner eye. Cranial nerve III innervates one of these, the sphincter pupillae (also called the constrictor pupillae), with muscle fibers running tangentially to the inner rim of the iris, Fig. 16.A-1b. Reflexive excitation of this parasympathetic system contracts the muscle fibers so as to decrease the pupil diameter, as when the light incident on the eye is too bright [473]. As agonist to the sphincter pupillae (Subsection 7.A, *Reciprocal Inhibition and Agonist/Antagonist Pairs*, page 193), there is the second set of muscles, the dilator pupillae, just outside the sphincter pupillae and having its muscle fibers running radially rather than tangentially, Fig. 16.A-1b. Contraction of the dilator pupillae muscle fibers via the sympathetic nerve originating at the uppermost paravertebral ganglion (Chapter 6, THE AUTONOMIC NERVOUS SYSTEM, page 133) acts reflexively to increase the diameter of the pupil, as when the light level is too low to see clearly. This response of the dilator pupillae is also present when the adrenal medulla releases catecholamines into the blood stream as when under stress. Returning to the idea that sympathetic stimulation would be in aid of the fight-or-flight response (Section 6.C, The Sympathetic Nervous System, page 144), it can be argued that having a larger pupil diameter increases one's peripheral vision and so adds to the security against peripheral attack, all the while sacrificing spatial resolution. In the battle for dominance of the pupillary diameter, the parasympathetic system generally is the stronger source of excitation.

The diameter of the pupil also controls the amount of light reaching the foveal spot on the retina. In bright light, the pupil diameter reflexively narrows to 2 mm, however, when the sympathetic signal is activated, the diameter of the pupil increases to as much as 8 mm, allowing up to 16 times as much light to enter. The limbic system also has its effect on the pupil's diameter as the diameter reflexively tends to increase dramatically whenever we look at someone that we love or admire.

Though Western medicine considers the deterioration of one's vision with increasing age and needing glasses to see properly as "natural", it is not true that nothing can be done to impede one's failing eyesight. With increasing age, the number of receptors and synapses used in vision decreases, thus impairing sight and ocular reflexes generally [92]. This, however, may not be the case for those who do yogic eye exercises [150, 288, 317, 373, 464]. Indeed, in many cases, simple yogic eye exercises can be very effective in keeping the eyes in fine condition into old age.

Vision and Neuroanatomy of the Eye

The intrinsic muscles of the eye adjust its optics so that a focused image falls upon the retinal layer containing the visual receptors, the so-called rods and cones, Fig. 16.A-3. The rods are useful for sensing a black-and-white visual pattern in dim light, whereas the cones operate at higher light levels and are color sensitive, coming in three varieties: red-light sensitive, green-light sensitive, and blue-light sensitive. The rods are most prominent on the periphery of the retina, whereas the cones are tightly clustered about the fovea, Fig. 16.A-2a. Rods are quite sensitive to motion as appropriate for detecting a predator moving toward one from the periphery at sunset, whereas the cones offer a high-resolution color scan of a panoramic view in bright light. Signals from the rods often initiate reflexive actions and rods are twenty times more numerous than cones.

Each of the three types of cone shows color sensitivity largely in its particular color band, as displayed in Fig. 16.A-4. The optic signal containing the color-encoded images from the three types of cones travels then from the retina to the occipital lobes,

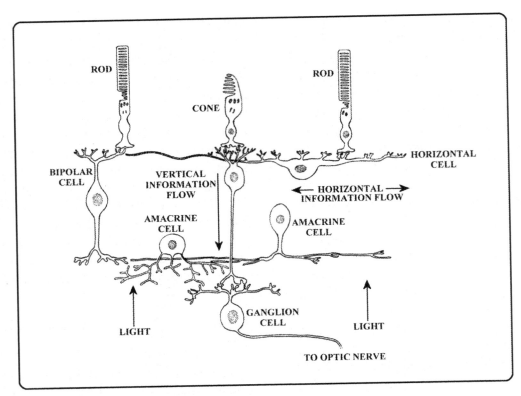

Fig. 16.A-3. The cellular structure of the retina. Note that light must penetrate several layers of nerve tissue before reaching the photosensitive rods and cones. The nerve tissue of the retina functions much like brain tissue, in that it too shows a strong neural convergence, with many rods and cones sharing a common ganglion cell.

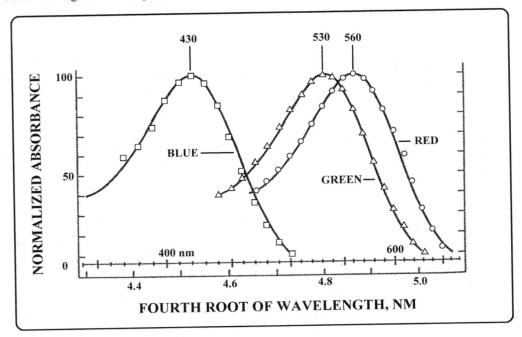

Fig. 16.A-4. Normalized absorption spectra of the blue-, green-, and red-sensitive cones of the retina. There is little or no sensitivity at wavelengths below about 380 nm, the ultraviolet region, except in persons with very blonde hair and light-blue eye color.

among other places. In contrast, the signals from the rods have no such direct route to the cortex and travel much more slowly into our consciousness.

Visual resolution (the ability to see two nearby features as distinct) is at its highest at the spot on the retina called the fovea, whereas no sensing can be done at the papilla (the blind spot), where the various nerves from the retinal cells and the arteries and veins to these cells coalesce to form the optic-nerve bundle. One would logically expect that the part of the image at the papilla would be sensed as a black spot within the visual scene, however, the brain smooths it over with information borrowed from adjacent areas, so that the blind spot is automatically erased. Though there are 125 million receptors in the retina of each eye, each with its own neural fiber, these are combined before entering the optic nerve, which only contains about 1 million fibers. This convergence of the neural fibers results in a smaller, more flexible optic nerve, which in turn moves more easily when the eyeball moves.

It is striking that light incident on the rods and cones of mammals must first pass through three layers of nerve cells before reaching the sensory cells of the retina, Fig. 16.A-3. The outermost layer of the retinal neural cells consists of the retinal ganglia. Though every neural fiber originating at a sensory cell (rod or cone receptor) in the retina finds its way to the layer of ganglion cells, there are only 1/125 as many such ganglion cells as there are receptor cells. Thus there is a strong neural convergence at this point in the visual pathway, with each retinal ganglion being connected to between 100 and 1000 adjacent receptor cells. Any cluster of receptor rods and cones in the retina having neurons that converge on a common ganglion is called a "receptive field". The smallest receptive fields, and therefore

the areas of highest visual acuity are found in the foveal spot.

Studies of the functions of individual receptive fields show that they can be very specific sensors for certain geometric features in the vision pattern. For example, it is known that such a field may be sensitive to sensing straight lines inclined at a specific angle, and that if the angle is turned by 10 degrees or so, then the sensation activates a different receptive field. Other receptive fields are sensitive to the motions of edges or lines in the visual field, and yet others respond only when the motion is in a specific direction. It is my hypothesis that these motion-sensitive/angle-sensitive receptive fields in the retina are of great use in the process of yogic balancing with the eyes open as they can easily sense when a straight line in the field of view begins to rotate as the body starts to fall. On the other hand, trying to balance with the eyes in an environment free of cues as to where the horizon lies or with the eyes closed can be very difficult (Subsection IV.D, *Vision and Balance*, page 533).

The density of cones is very high in the area of the fovea (1 mm X 1 mm), and this is the site of high-resolution vision in the retina at moderate or high light levels. However, the area of the fovea is only a small percentage of the total area of the retina available for imaging. In fact, the eyeball executes a constant series of small but jerky motions so that the fovea successively but momentarily inspects small areas of the total scene, moving several times per second. Studies of these "saccadic" motions show that the attention will be strongest on certain features of the scene, the eyes and mouth of a face for example, and that the visual process is turned off while the eyeball is in motion so that the integrated image is not blurred. Those aspects of a scene picked for more intense scrutiny during the saccades are largely out of our conscious control.

Moreover, even in that stationary state when a small area of the scene is brought to the fovea and held there, microsaccades then take place. Because the pigments in the retina are very rapidly adapting (Subsection 10.B, *Receptor Adaptation*, page 285), the image tends to fade quickly (lifetime about 1 second) if the image is static on the retina, and the shifts inherent in the microsaccades thus act to constantly refresh the picture. This is reminiscent of the pose-and-repose action of Iyengar in the *yogasanas* [22], which acts to refresh the proprioceptive picture of the body.

Strangely, there is a significant dark current from the retinal receptors, and on being illuminated, the cells hyperpolarize [207] rather than depolarize, and the amount of neurotransmitter released is decreased (Section 5.D, The Neurotransmitters, page 128). Thus the visual signal is measured as a decreasing dark current and a lowering of the excitation frequency in the optic nerve! Needless to say, this is completely the reverse of normal nerve action (Subsection 5.C, *Excitation versus Inhibition*, page 123).

Because the neural tissues of the eye are directly traceable to corresponding tissues in the brain, one might rightfully consider the retina to be an extension of the brain. Indeed, it is abundantly clear [207] that the neural layers of the retina are both inhibitory and excitatory in about equal proportions, just as with the brain. Furthermore, in support of this idea, many brain tissues and structures exit the brain and are continued down the optic nerve (channels for cerebrospinal fluid, for example) and even penetrate into the eyeball itself [195]. For example, the white part of the eyeball, the sclera, is just a continuation of the dura mater, the outer covering of the brain [142]. In agreement with the idea of the eyes being extensions of the brain, it is observed that animals with very complex eyes have sim-

ple brains and *vice versa* [171]. *Vis-a-vis* human beings, we have relatively simple eyes and very complex brains.

The Ocular-Vestibular Connection

The inner ear contains specialized sensors, the vestibular organs, which contain proprioceptors that are important in both static and dynamic balancing, both upright and inverted (Section 17.B, page 437 and Appendix IV, BALANCING, page 525). Among these organs are the semicircular canals, which monitor the sense of rotation and speed of rotation of the head as when falling. Interestingly, there are neural interconnections between the vestibular nuclei serving the semicircular canals and the oculomotor nuclei in the brainstem. These interconnections reflexively integrate the actions of the lateral and medial recti muscles of the eyes with head rotation, such that when the head turns, the eyes rotate oppositely but at a rate so as to keep the fovea fixed on an external point [225]. This is the reflex that keeps the page you are reading in focus as you slowly move your head to the left and right. Though the reflex is nominally controlled by centers in the midbrain of the brainstem, it can be overcome by deliberate actions originating at higher centers of consciousness.

The existence of the vestibular-ocularmotor reflex leads one to think that balance could be affected by and through the eyes. Indeed, yogic practice shows that the use of the eyes in balancing can be very stabilizing and can work at a level higher than that of the reflexes (see Box IV.D-1, *Using Your Eyes to Balance*, page 534). Thus, it is likely that in moving from *virhabdrasana I* to *virhabdrasana III* and from there to *ardha chandrasana*, for example, the vestibular-ocularmotor reflex would be of great use in maintaining one's balance during the in-motion phases of the *yogasanas*. As discussed more fully in Appendix IV, BAL-

ANCING, page 525, it is very stabilizing while in stationary balances to fix the eyes on a stationary spot on the wall. Thanks to the vestibular-ocularmotor reflex, it is also possible to keep one's vision fixed on a stationary point even though the body is in motion; this helps keep one balanced while moving, just as it does when one is not in motion.

SECTION 16.B. STRESS, VISION, AND YOGA

The picture painted above assigns the intrinsic muscles of the eye to making accommodations for optimum focusing and light level, whereas the extrinsic muscles are innervated by the cranial nerves and serve to steer the gaze in space. Bates [28], however, finds that imbalance among the six extrinsic muscles can prevent the intrinsic ones from functioning properly. Hence, yogic eye exercises [61, 150, 373, 393, 464], which both stretch and release tension in the extrinsic muscles, can indirectly lead to better accommodation by the intrinsic muscles and improved vision.

Stress and Vision

Chronic stress, anxiety, and emotional reactions lead to refractive changes in the eye and often to blurred vision. Thus, for example, eyes that are 20/20 become nearsighted (myopic) whenever a lie is told [150], and seeing an attractive person tends to dilate the pupils, signaling arousal of the sympathetic nervous system.

Though the visual field spans 200° in an angular sense, the size of the fovea is only 1° [225]. According to Bates [28], the proper function of the eye is to detect details in the small visual field of the fovea (less than 1 mm square) and then rapidly switch (at a rate of 70 times per second) to another small field of the overall image. In this way, the visual image is scanned over the fovea (the spot of highest visual acuity), and a high-resolution global image then is reconstructed by the brain. That part of the image not scanned by the fovea becomes the peripheral visual field. Bates calls this motion of the eyeball "central fixation and shifting", whereas others call it "saccadic motion" [225]. However, stress, fear, and anxiety trigger sympathetic signals according to Bates, which result in transfer of the optic neural signal away from the striate cortex to the frontal cortex, with dilation of the pupils. In this case, one has a myopic stare, with the eye attempting to see all areas in sharp detail simultaneously, even though this is not possible because of the small size of the fovea.

Yogic Relaxation for Visual Stress

The attempt to view a panoramic image (resulting from sympathetic excitation in an effort to form a large pupil diameter) with the high-resolution but very small fovea leads to eye strain, pain, frowning, holding of the breath, increased heart rate, tense neck and jaw, shoulders and jaw rotated forward, depressed chest, tension in the mid and lower back, and stiff legs! Moreover, when the stress is habitual, the sympathetic arousal threshold is lowered and the effects then last longer. These symptoms correlate with the fear that without special exertion, one cannot hold one's world together, a fear that is said to be common in nearsighted people [287]. As people who are extremely nearsighted are at high risk for retinal detachment [483], yoga students with this condition should avoid extended and/or challenging inversions.

As fine as one's vision may be, it is still the case that what we "see" in our consciousness often is a reflection of our expectations and is strongly colored by our past experiences [142, 191]. Studies show that our vision habits are related to our personalities, and that changing our vision profile can change our personality [287].

To avoid tensing the eyes, one must learn to relax the gaze, breathe deeply, maintain elasticity of gaze, and not give in to tunnel vision. One must be more global in one's vision and awareness. If one can do this, the eyes will accommodate in a relaxed way to the large diameter of the pupils and not add yet more stress. As applied to the *yogasana* student, this suggests that our aim should be to keep the gaze broad, soft, and fuzzy, with a global awareness which is the opposite of tunnel vision [194]. To this end, one should work the *yogasanas* in a position where other objects in the surround are not so close that the eyes will be drawn to them and become nearsighted.

Yogis have found that a general state of tension in the body can lead to a pull on the eyeballs, pointing them in toward the nose, as is appropriate for sharp focus of nearby objects, and that the body can be relaxed by consciously turning the eyes to look toward the outer corners instead. This relaxation probably involves parasympathetic excitation of cranial nerve III (Table 3.B-1). It is this connection between the extrinsic muscles of the eye (the inferior recti muscles, Fig. 16.A-1a, and Subsection 7.D, *A Reflection on the Cervical Flexion Reflex*, page 218), the parasympathetic nervous system, and the state of body tension that makes this relaxation possible.

Actually, though the muscles of the eyes easily function to force the eyes to cross inward, this is not so for the outward-uncrossing motion, and so the best one can hope for

here is to allow the eyes to return to their straight-ahead orientation on relaxation.

If it is accepted that the relaxed position for the eyes has them pointing downward and outward to the sides, then the eyes turned upward and inward must be a position of high stress. Interestingly, it is the ease of attaining this position of the eyes that hypnotists have used to judge the hypnotizability of subjects, with those who can easily turn their eyes in this way making the most easily hypnotized subjects. This position is the gateway into the hypnotic state as it promotes a strong dissociation of the mind from the body in those who can do it well [279]. While this body-mind dissociation may be appropriate for the more meditative states of yoga practice, it is counter to the aim of the beginning student who is working to reconnect mind and body. Indeed, the connection of eye rolling to hypnotizability has been challenged by Hilgard [199].

It is interesting that in *savasana*, there is often considerable random eye movement, reminding one of the REM phase of sleep (Subsection 21.B, *The Sleep/Wake Cycle and Relaxation*, page 488). This movement weakens as the relaxing effects of the parasympathetic system take hold. Lacking that, tension in the eyes can be relieved by wrapping the head with a bandage or using an eyebag placed briefly over the eyes when in the supine position.

If students with high blood pressure are working hard in the *yogasanas* while slightly holding the breath, they must look down to relax [445], but students with low blood pressure or depression should look up as long as their eyes do not pull inward toward

*As mentioned above, looking upward toward the pineal gland (the "third eye" above the brow) by forcefully turning the eyes upward and inward can lead to a mental state in which one senses that the consciousness has left the body, *i.e.*, dissociation. Apparently, this involves interactions within the reticular formation, Subsection 3.A, *The Limbic System*, page 33. This eye-rolling action is possibly a factor in *sarvangasana* while looking at the feet or in *urdhva dhanurasana* when looking at the floor, and is probably desirable in very advanced students, but would be counterproductive in beginning and intermediate students.

the bridge of the nose. The eyes-up position is a strong indicator of mental activity and is usually inappropriate for *yogasana*.*

The intraocular pressure of the vitreous humour of the eye serves to keep the eyeball round, however this pressure can become chronically high when drainage is impeded. In this case, the added pressure on the optic nerve degrades its function, and the result is a condition known as glaucoma. Relaxing so that the parasympathetic nervous system becomes dominant is effective in lowering intraocular pressure. Certain *yogasanas* such as *urdhva dhanurasana*, *sarvangasana*, and *sirsasana* are not recommended for those inclined toward glaucoma due to the risk they pose for such students. Specifics of these situations as they have been reported in the medical literature are summarized in Appendix II, INJURIES INCURRED DURING IMPROPER *YOGASANA* PRACTICE, page 511, and specific cautions are given for these poses in Iyengar's book [215a].

Inverted *yogasanas* also can act adversely on the eye by increasing the pressure of the cerebrospinal fluid (Section 4.D, page 93) on the veins of the eyes, leading to papilledema, and by over-pressurizing the veins and arteries within the retinal layer, leading to hypertensive retinopathy [195].

In the act of "seeing", the visual pigments of the retina are temporarily bleached and deactivated, leading to a chemical stress within the eyes which can be released by periodic closing of the eyes, which allows the pigments to return to their active forms [393].

Clearly, when the mind is alert, the eyes are wide open in every sense, and when the mind is relaxed, the eyes close. Indeed, when light enters the eyes, there is an activation of the reticular formation (Subsection 3.A, page 31) and unavoidable arousal which would be appropriate in active *yogasanas* such as *trikonasana*, but not in *savasana*. The standard yogic way of quieting the brain is to quiet the eyes by wrapping them with a soft bandage, thus stilling their motion and blocking the light. Should the extrinsic muscles of the eyes be overworked and stressed out, they can be profitably exercised using a yogic approach [194, 373, 393]. Practice of the yogic eye exercises leads to an increased ability to relax and to release into sleep, as progressive relaxation of the extrinsic muscles of the eyes leads to reduced mental activity. This will be true for relaxing the mind in *savasana* as well.

The relaxed watchfulness of *savasana* with the eyes closed generates alpha waves in the EEG (Section 3.E, Brainwaves and the Electroencephalogram, page 57) of the occipital region, a region of the brain which is dedicated to processing visual information. It has been shown that with training, the alpha-wave pattern can be maintained even though the eyes are opened, if the gaze is defocused [194]. This defocussing of the gaze is important when working to develop the alpha-wave relaxation of *savasana* in all of the more demanding *yogasanas*.

The Eyes Set the Body's Clock

The general effect of *yogasana* practice is a slowing of the body's clock, with fast-twitch muscle fibers (types 2 and 3) and their rapidly conducting nerves being converted into slow-twitch fibers (type 1) with slower nerves (Subsection 7.A, *Types of Muscle Fiber*, page 189), and the ascendancy of the body's parasympathetic nervous system. However, it also has been shown that with practice of the *yogasanas* and associated techniques, both the visual and the auditory response times are shortened [294], and visual perceptual accuracy increases [219]. This suggests that though *yogasana* training slows skeletal-muscle action, it does speed certain other neural responses.

Many physiological processes in the human body are controlled by a 24-hour clock (Subsection 21.B, *Circadian Rhythms; Physiological Peaks and Valleys in the 24-Hour Period*, page 476). The timing of these circadian rhythms is set by dawn and dusk signals sensed by photopigments in the inner retinal layer, whereas vision involves photopigments in the outer retinal layer [468].

As a sensory organ, the eye is paramount as it produces over 80% of the sensory information going to the brain, and it must play a large role in the fight-or-flight response originating in the hypothalamus. It is no surprise then that the sensory information from the retina is sent as well to the suprachiasmatic nucleus within the hypothalamus, where it is processed for eventual response by the autonomic nervous system [195]. Specifically, the circadian rhythms (Subsection 21.B, page 476) have a 24-hour period tied to the light/dark cycle of the earth and sun. This arises because there are separate neural channels linking the retina of each eye directly to the superchiasmatic nuclei in the hypothalamus, Fig. 6.B-1 [387]. These nuclei are the internal clocks that regulate the entire endocrine system. Most interestingly, the nature of the autonomic response triggered by the eyes is dictated by the color of the image presented to the retina! For examples, see Subsection 16.D, *Color Therapy*, page 426.

Yet another connection exists between the eyes and the passage of time. As we go from normal illumination to dim light and the visual sensors switch from the cones to the rods, the time that it takes the visual signal to travel from the retina to the cortex lengthens appreciably [190, 196]. Because of this slowing of the reaction time in dim light, it is more difficult to balance in the *yogasanas* in dim light (Subsection IV.D, *Vision and Balance*, page 533) and especially difficult in total darkness (or with the eyes closed).

SECTION 16.C. VISION AND CEREBRAL LATERALITY

In several of the earlier Chapters (especially 3 and 12), it was explained that many body functions that appear on one side of the body or the other have neural connections that connect the function on that side of the body to the cerebral cortex on the opposite (contralateral) side of the brain. For example, breathing through the left nostril produces a mental state that is characteristic of the excitation of the right cerebral hemisphere (Section 12.C, Nasal Laterality, page 374), and the conscious stiffening of the right arm in *vasisthasana*, for example, involves the motor cortex in the left cerebral hemisphere. Because the sympathetic and parasympathetic aspects of the autonomic nervous system also are strongly lateral as well, their relative dominance can be shifted by either breathing through one nostril, or accenting the muscular action on one side of the body. This neural crossover usually occurs at the level of the spinal cord or brainstem.

As will be explained below, there are several aspects of vision (anatomical, physiological, and psychological) which lead one to believe that there also are specific neural connections between each of the eyes and the contralateral cerebral hemisphere, and that these hemispheres can be selectively activated through the eyes in order to alter the balance within the autonomic nervous system. Following this, we then go on in Section 16.D, page 426, to a discussion of how this phenomenon might impact on *yogasana* practice.

Crossover of the Optic Nerve

The phenomenon of stereo-optical images that leads to depth perception requires

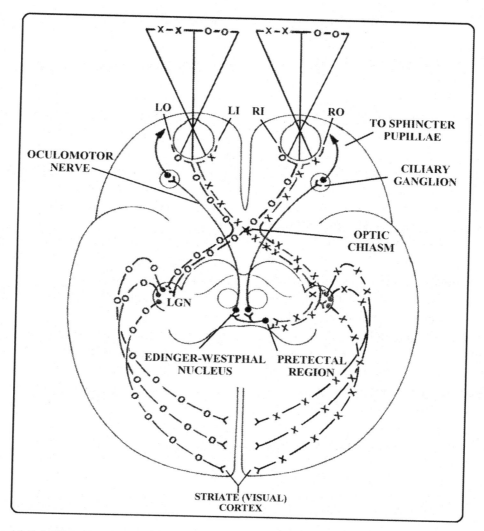

Fig. 16.C-1. The neural pathways from the retinal hemifields to the striate cortex showing the crossing over of the optic nerves at the optic chiasm [195]. Note that the right part of the image (-o-o-) is sensed by the LO and the RI hemifields and eventually appears as sensation in the left cerebral hemisphere, whereas the left part of the image (-x-x-) is sensed by the LI and RO hemifields and appears as sensation in the right cerebral hemisphere. The striate cortex is not in any way the final picture screen, but rather is just an early stage in the visual processing [206].

that the images received by the two eyes be kept separate on their way to higher centers in the brain, and then compared for differences. This is performed by having separate neural tracts for the left and right eyes and synaptic neural connections at equivalent sites in the left and right cerebral hemispheres, as shown in Fig. 16.C-1. But the story is much more interesting than that.

The retina in each eye is divided into two hemifields, with one half of the retina being closer to the nose and the other closer to the temple. Call those hemifields in the right eye RI and RO for right inner and right outer, and similarly LI and LO for the left eye. Because the lens of the eye inverts and reverses the image on bringing it to a focus on the retina (see Fig. 16.A-2a), light coming from the right side of the visual field will illuminate the LO and RI hemifields, whereas light coming from the left will illuminate the RO and LI hemifields. As shown in Fig. 16.C-1, each of the four hemifields has its own dedicated neural branch, and as the coding in the Figure reveals, the inner hemifield neurons cross over at the optic chiasm, a point just below the suprachiasmatic nucleus within the hypothalamus. Once past the optic chiasm, the inner hemifield nerves continue on to the cerebral hemisphere on the opposite side of the brain, whereas the outer hemifield neurons do not cross to opposite sides. Thus, the LO and RI neural signals come from the left half of the visual field and will synapse in the right cerebral hemisphere, whereas the LI and RO neural signals will come from the right half of the visual field and will synapse in the left cerebral hemisphere. Notice, too, that each eye nonetheless has direct input to *both* of the cerebral hemispheres. This split-retina-with-crossover has several interesting consequences (see for example, Box 3.D-1, *Determining Your Lateral Preference for Vision*, page 52).

Light falling on the LI and RO hemifields of the retinas generate signals that synapse first at the lateral geniculate nucleus (abbreviated LGN in Fig. 16.C-1), then at the peritectal region, and finally at the parasympathetic center, the Edinger-Westphal nucleus. A reflex arc is completed by innervation of the ciliary ganglion by neurons from the Edinger-Westphal nucleus in order to drive the sphincter pupillae. The reflex arc is such that with bright light entering either eye, the pupils of both eyes will be reduced in diameter. Because there is no equivalent arc originating at the LO and RI hemifields, the pupillary diameter is controlled by the parasympathetic center within the right cerebral hemisphere in the first approximation, but transfer of information between the hemispheres is possible via the corpus callosum, Section 3.A, Structure and Function of the Brain, page 21. Also see Box 3.D-1, *Determining Your Lateral Preference for Vision*, page 52, for more on the reciprocal effects of mood and visual laterality on one another.

The Higher Visual Centers

It is especially relevant that the center of highest spatial resolution, the fovea of each eye, can be in the nasal hemifield, and so is subject to hemispherical crossover of the neural signal, whereas the peripheral rods are more in the temporal hemifields and would not cross over. Once past the chiasm, the signals from the nasal hemifields retain their left-right character and are deposited in the lateral geniculate nuclei (LGN in Fig. 16.C-1) as alternating slabs of R-L-R-L-L-R information together with the information from the temporal hemifields, but without crossover in this case. Two of the slabs in the LGN contain the information about the shape of the visual image and four of the slabs contain information about its color.

From the LGN, the visual information is projected backward to the striate cortex in the occipital lobes (Fig. 16.C-1). The regular deposition of visual information in the striate cortex results in a map of the visual receptor fields of the retina projected onto the striate cortex, much like the inputs of the sensory modes and the outputs of the somatic modes are mapped onto the cortex as homunculi, Fig. 3.A-5. In blind people, the visual cortex receives no retinal signals, and so is used instead to process auditory information.

It is at the level of the striate cortex that complementary cells in the receptor fields of the left and right eyes may interact to form centers of binocular action. These centers in turn may show binocular dominance, with one hemifield dominating the other. In this way, visual sensations may find their ways preferentially into one cerebral hemisphere or the other.

Visual processing occurs at many other centers beyond the striate cortex, as described in the excellent book by Hubel

[207], but his text goes far beyond our needs as *yogasana* teachers.

Memory and Visual Laterality

It is surprising to find that extrinsic eye movements can be correlated with how people store and retrieve information from memory. As studied by neurolinguistic programming (NLP), it has been shown that people, in trying to remember certain sensory events, often use a specific eye movement, Fig. 16.C-2, to promote easier access to the memory [281]. For a right-handed person with a "normally organized" brain, *i.e.*, sympathetic hemisphere on the left and parasympathetic on the right (Section 3.D, Cerebral Hemispheric Laterality, page 49), and referring to Fig. 16.C-2, one finds the following:

1) When asked to remember (R) a previous visual image (V), the eyes shift upward and leftward (V^R)

2) When asked to construct (C) a new visual image (V), as for example, imagine Albert Einstein with orange hair in *ardha chandrasana*, the eyes move upward and rightward (V^C)

3) When asked to remember a previous auditory memory (A), for example, to hum a few bars of one's favorite song, the eyes move laterally to the left (A^R)

4) When the auditory memory involves constructing an auditory scenario, say, the sound of a violin played under water, the eyes move laterally, but to the right (A^C)

5) Kinaesthetic images (K) including those of taste and smell, are remembered by first looking downward and to the right.

That the directions in which the eyes turn are reversed for people who are left handed would seem to be evidence for the lateralization of these memory functions in the brain, as handedness and hemispheric laterality are very strongly correlated (Section III.D, Handedness, page 523).

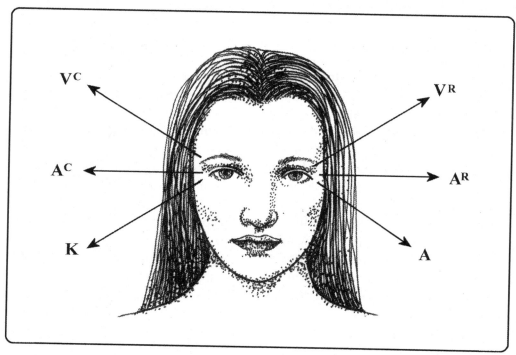

Fig. 16.C-2. Directions in which the eyes turn when asked to remember a visual thought (V^R), an auditory thought (A^R), or a kinaesthetic thought (K). Alternatively, on being asked to think of a visual construction (V^C) or an auditory construction (A^C), the eyes turn as indicated.

As might have been expected, searching the brain for visual information involves motion of the eyes upward. In contrast, auditory memory involves only a lateral shift, and kinaesthetic feelings will involve motion which is downward and to the right. Deliberate side-to-side motion of the eyes has been used to access traumatic experiences in a subject's life, as have bilateral acoustic tones; the result is an "emotional detoxification" that comes with the surfacing of emotions and their reprocessing.

The strong connection between mental processes and extrinsic eye movement is easily demonstrated, for it is readily seen that when one is thinking in a logical mode, the eyes tend to shift to the right, as if searching the left hemisphere, whereas when thinking analogically, the eyes tend to shift to the left as if searching the right hemisphere [389]. On the other hand, when one is asked an emotional question about oneself, or is thinking in an emotional, non-linear way, the eyes look to the left consistently, suggesting that the right cerebral hemisphere plays a special role in emotions [120]. These observations imply that there is a connection between the extrinsic muscles of the eyes turning them left and right (largely the medial and lateral recti muscles in Fig. 16.A-1) and the choice of neural branches used for transducing the thoughts.

In Box 3.D-1 (*Determining Your Lateral Preference for Vision*, page 52), a simple test was introduced to expose any visual dominance. However, just as with the *yogasanas* where we delegate extra work to the side that is the weaker in order to achieve a more balanced situation in the body, so too must we work to lessen the dominance of the stronger eye. If one eye is dominant, one can then wear a patch over the stronger eye for short periods in order to restore visual balance and hence release the tension that comes from imbalance and lack of fusion of the images of the two eyes

[166]. The laterality of visual effects are discussed as well in Section 3.D, Cerebral Hemispheric Laterality, page 49.

The totality of the evidence presented above strongly supports the notion that the unquestioned laterality of brain functions extends to the eyes as well, even though it is not clear just how this comes about. Nonetheless, regardless of the details of the possible mechanism, one can go on to explore the possible relationships between the color of the light entering the eyes, eye/brain laterality, and the their effects on the practice of the *yogasanas*, as shown below.

SECTION 16.D. COLOR THERAPY AND YOGA

Color Therapy

The use of color as a therapy appears to have begun more than 5,000 years ago in India with the Ayurvedic physicians. More recently (1933), Ghadiali [281] proposed that there is a color specific to the activation of every organ, and another for its deactivation, which immediately brings the sympathetic/parasympathetic dichotomy to mind. As color therapy has changed little through the millennia, we look at the color effects as first put forth by the ancients [232, 252, 281, 444], Table 16.D-1. Indeed, one sees from the Table that the colors red and yellow evoke physiological and emotional responses that are understandable in terms of sympathetic arousal, whereas blue and violet act to stimulate parasympathetic responses. Green is held to be a more neutral, balancing color. Though most human eyes do not sense ultraviolet wavelengths below about 380 nm, there is considerable evidence showing the role of ultraviolet light in good health [253, 347]. Note however, that the traditional visual pathway from the retina to the striate cortex, Fig.

TABLE 16.D-1. PHYSIOLOGIC AND PSYCHOLOGIC RESPONSES TO COLOR [1, 154, 232, 252, 414, 444]

Color	Response
Red	Heating, stimulating, promotes circulation and vitality, energizes will power and nervous system
Orange	Warming, builds sexual energy and high levels of emotional and mental energies; alkaline, relieves congestion
Yellow	Heals, cleanses, purifies digestion; stimulates understanding, intelligence
Green	Balances heart, blood pressure and body temperature; neutral, harmonizing, soothing, cooling, sedative, refreshing, alleviates headaches, lifts depression
Blue	Cool, soothing, contracting, calming, sedating; works mostly on mouth and throat, removes burning sensation
Violet	Sedating, sexual inhibitor, increases mental awareness, lightness in body, opens doors of perception

16.C-1, is generally held to be devoid of any emotional content [427].

Scientific evidence is available in support of the idea that viewing specific colors can change the balance of sympathetic/parasympathetic activation in the body [427]. In an extended study, Gerard [154] investigated the effects of red and blue light on the physiology of a group of college students. He found that viewing red light raised the respiration rate 2.5%, but that blue light lowered it by 3%. Systolic blood pressure was raised 2.3% by red light, but was decreased by 1% in blue light. Heart rate, palmar conductance, and eyeblink rate were all significantly higher in red light than in blue. On the other hand, viewing red light significantly lowered the percentage of the relaxing alpha waves in the EEG as compared with the percentage when viewing blue light. Also, though red is energizing, viewing pink is sedating, but only for 20 minutes

or so, after which it becomes strongly agitating [281, 347]. Extended viewing of colored lights also has been found effective in relieving PMS in some women (Subsection 19.A, *Premenstrual Syndromes*, page 454).

When colored placebo tablets (Subsection 6.F, *The Placebo Effect*, page 164) are offered to subjects who either are in need of sedation or who are depressed, it is found that the placebo effect is strongest when the depressed subjects are given small yellow sugar tablets, and is strongest for patients suffering from anxiety and needing sedation when they are given large blue ones [346]. Similar results as regards sympathetic versus parasympathetic exhaltation were obtained when hypnotized subjects were told to visualize the colors and report their feelings/sensations [1].

Gerard [154] also studied affective responses and found red light to promote unpleasant thoughts, nervous tension, irritation and annoyance, discomfort, anxiety, heat, and alertness. In contrast, viewing blue light led to responses of comfort, happiness, relaxation, well-being, calm, and pleasant thoughts. The physiologic and psychologic results of this study are totally in accord with a red-light stimulation of the sympathetic nervous system and a blue-light stimulation of the parasympathetic nervous system. Presumably, these responses to the colored lights originate in the left and right cerebral hemispheres, respectively, though there is no mention of any uneven illumination of the retinas.

In regard the above, note that it has been said [414] that one need not really have to look at the colors, since just thinking about them can lead to the same autonomic activation [1, 281, 405]. If this effect is real, it must involve the deliberate activation of higher brain centers to control what otherwise are involuntary responses.

How is it possible that viewing colored lights evenly through the two eyes can change the physiology and psychology of the viewer? Assume first that the two hemispheres of the brain are involved separately in driving either the sympathetic or parasympathetic branches of the autonomic nervous system, with the left hemisphere directing sympathetic action and the right hemisphere directing parasympathetic action (Section 3.D, Cerebral Hemispheric Laterality, page 49). It is as if blue light is excitatory to the right cerebral hemisphere and so produces parasympathetic relaxation whereas red light is excitatory to the left cerebral hemisphere and so produces sympathetic arousal; but how can this be? For a possible answer, return to Fig. 16.C-1. Suppose that the LI and RO hemifields of the retinas are richer in blue-sensitive cones while the LO and RI hemifields are richer in red-sensitive cones. In that case, when both eyes are illuminated with blue light, the LO and RI hemifields are excited preferentially,

leading to left-hemisphere excitation and the sympathetic response, whereas with red light incident on both eyes, the LI and RO hemifields will be preferentially excited, leading to right-hemisphere excitation and the parasympathetic response. The green cones, lying as they do between the responses of the red and blue cones, Fig. 16.A-4, would be neutral in regard hemispheric activity, as observed, Section 4.F, *Nadis, Chakras,* and *Prana,* page 100.

The explanation given above is based upon the red-sensitive cones being placed in one area of the retina, and the blue-sensitive cones being placed in another. If, in fact, these cones prove not to be geometrically segregated, then perhaps something can be made of the fact that the sensation of "red" is known to appear in the consciousness more quickly than the sensation of "blue" [427], *i.e.,* perhaps the effects of color on the autonomic nervous system involve kinetic rate factors rather than geometric factors. In any case, there is good reason for thinking that the asymmetric routes of the optic nerves into the cerebral hemispheres (Fig. 16.C-1) in some way is at the root of the mechanism behind the selective actions of differently colored lights on the autonomic response within the body/mind. Yet other examples of this strange connection between color and physiology are given in Box 16.D-1, *The Effects of Colors and the Emotions on Muscle Strength,* page 429.

Yoga in Colored Lights: A Proposal

In the Subsection above dealing with the mechanism of color vision, observations were quoted for the physical and emotional effects of colored lights, and possible mechanisms were put forth to explain this. Even if the true mechanism is far from those advanced above, the fact remains that lights of different colors can activate either the sympathetic or parasympathetic responses,

BOX 16.D-1: THE EFFECTS OF COLORS AND THE EMOTIONS ON MUSCLE STRENGTH

The suggestion that certain colors and/or emotions can promote a shift of autonomic dominance in regard muscle strength can be readily shown without any scientific apparatus, *etc.* In the first case, have a person hold their arms out horizontally, and ask someone of approximately the same strength to try pulling their arms down, qualitatively noting the level of resistance to their effort. Then have the person being tested stare at a large square of pink cardboard or construction paper placed about 15 inches in front of the eyes for about 30 seconds. On testing the arm strength in the same way, it will now be found that the arms are less resistant to being pulled down to the waist! To restore the arm strength, stare at a blue piece of cardboard placed similarly and for a comparable length of time. It is also said that weakness is induced by wearing a wristwatch or wearing clothing made of synthetic blends. Though it is difficult to imagine how this might work, it may be that we will perform the *yogasanas* with more strength if we avoid these energy-sapping objects.

The color pink has been shown to be quite effective in calming aggressive and potentially violent people, but only if the exposure to the color is of the order of ten minutes or so, for if the stimulation extends beyond a half hour, the opposite emotional response results. Thus the color pink must be used judiciously in the *yogasana* studio, if at all.

With respect to the arm-strength test described above, Schauss [405] reports that the effect of staring at a pink square of cardboard is evident in less than 3 seconds, that it works as well with colorblind subjects, and that accomplished athletes and martial-arts practitioners cannot resist the effect, no matter how consciously they try. He invokes the endocrine system in the effect, but otherwise offers no further explanation.

The same decrease and restoration of the arm strength can be demonstrated using the emotions rather than colored cardboard [354]. In this case, it will be found that the arms are more easily pulled down if the person being tested is thinking of something very sad at the time of the test, but that arm strength is restored upon thinking of something very happy.

In both of the cases cited above, it would appear that both the color pink (a shade that results from mixing red with white) and sad thoughts stimulate the parasympathetic nervous system, resulting in a relaxation of the muscles and a consequent relative isometric weakness (Subsection 7.A, *Types of Muscle Contraction*, page 187), whereas happy thoughts and the color blue erase the parasympathetic dominance and restore the isometric strength. These observations are odd, for blue, in general, is a parasympathetic stimulant, and red is a sympathetic stimulant [154], yet in these experiments, the opposite correlation is suggested.

Perhaps the answer lies in the visual stimulation involving a left-right neural crossover at the optic chiasm, whereas thinking of positive or negative emotional situations is localized in one hemisphere or the other, but there is no crossover. Moreover, pink is not red, and though blue often may be sedating, it can be relatively energizing with respect to pink. Another possibility is that the effects of the colors are not directly on the muscle strength, but on the motivational system within the emotional limbic area of the brain (Section 2.B, The Central Nervous System, page 16) for this controls the tendency to want to use the muscles.

shifting the balance between them. As the sympathetic and parasympathetic nervous systems are very active in the changes wrought by *yogasanas* (Chapter 6, THE AUTONOMIC NERVOUS SYSTEM, page 133), it is immediately interesting to ask if the physiologic and psychologic effects of *yogasanas* can be modulated by performing them in colored lights.

It is my thesis that energizing *yogasanas* such as *urdhva dhanurasana* when performed in red light will be even more energizing, especially when the light is incident on the student's face from the right so as to excite the left cerebral hemisphere, whereas illumination with blue light from the left will act to stimulate the right hemisphere and so lower the excitation level of the same pose! Similarly, if the *yogasana* is inherently cooling and relaxing, say *sarvangasana*, then the same effects mentioned above still will be expected, *i.e.*, blue-light illumination will be more calming still and red-light illumination will add a component of arousal. Changes of autonomic excitation could be measured using what are by now standard means (blood pressure, heart rate, blink rate, palmar conductance, *etc.*).

The yogic counterpart to the arm-strength test described in Box 16.D-1 might be performing the plank position or standing in *tadasana* with the arms extended forward or to the side while staring at either a pink or a blue card. In the case of the pink card, one expects a shortening of the duration that the pose can be held comfortably, and the reverse effect when the color of the card is switched to blue.

In chromatic *yogasana* experiments such as those described above, one wants minimum overlap of the two test wavelengths, but high retinal sensitivity at each; from the data in Fig. 16.A-4, it is clear that wavelengths of 570 nm (red) and 390 nm (blue) would do nicely. More interesting yet is the possible effect of blinking the colored lights

at the various rhythms of the brain waves (Table 3.E-1), *i.e.*, blinking the red light at 25 cycles per second in order to promote the alertness of the sympathetic beta-wave state or the blue light at 4 cycles per second to stimulate the drowsiness of the parasympathetic delta-wave state. Additionally, as described in Subsection 12.C, *The Conscious Development and Shift of Nasal Laterality*, page 378, simply blocking one nostril or the other also is effective in triggering a shift of cerebral dominance, and would make an interesting addition to the study of the color effects on *yogasana* practice. These experiments soon will be under way.

Though the external manipulation of the autonomic nervous system through the use of blinking colored lights does not sound very yogic, perhaps one can accept it more readily if it is thought of as just another prop, like a bolster or a belt. As such, it can help lead one more quickly to experience the full spectrum of the effects of a particular *yogasana* on the body/mind, but it is to be done with the attitude of eventually working without the prop. Most importantly, the benefits of enhancing the effects of a *yogasana* through the use of colored lights could be profound in those cases where yoga is being practiced as therapy for a condition involving imbalance within the autonomic nervous system.

With the regular white lights on in the *yogasana* room, the colors entering the students' eyes will be those of the paint on the walls and the props nearby. These colors should be chosen with due regard for the physiological and psychological effects desired by the teacher.

White-Light Starvation

In the Arctic Circle, there is near or complete darkness throughout the winter days, 24 hours a day. In response to this lack of light in the winter months, the population becomes depressed and the suicide rate soars. In more normal situations, the short days of winter still deprive office workers and shut-ins of their optimum dose of natural light, and seasonal affective disorder (SAD) sets in [253]. Whereas SAD affects only 9% of the winter population of Sarasota, Florida, the corresponding figure for the more northern city, Nashua, New Hampshire is 30%. Women are far more likely to be affected by the lack of natural sunshine in the winter months than are men.

SAD is largely an emotional disorder, with symptoms that include strong mood swings, low energy, depression, overeating, low sex drive, social withdrawal, continued sleepiness, and lowered immune function. These symptoms appear with the winter months and disappear once spring arrives [82, 252]. It is interesting to note that the symptoms for SAD closely match those reported for atypical depression, Subsection 20.A, *Symptoms of Depression*, page 464. Indeed, just as there is an atypical depression, there is also a summertime SAD, with symptoms opposite to those stated above for wintertime SAD [253].

Patients with SAD are easily treated by exposure to full-spectrum lights, which exposure drives down the melatonin in the blood (Subsection 15.B, *The Pineal Gland*, page 404) and erases all SAD symptoms in a few days [280]. It is possible that the energizing *yogasanas* performed in red light, incident from the left and blinking at 25 Hz also would be of use in dispelling SAD symptoms, as *yogasanas* are already known to be effective against depression (Section 20.A, page 467). Bright-light therapy is also known to be effective against bulimia and premenstrual depression [253], and a switch to pulsed colored lights may enhance these therapies as well.

Chapter 17

SOUND, HEARING, AND BALANCE

SECTION 17.A. THE MIDDLE EAR

The Mechanics of Hearing

Hearing is another of our sensory organs in which the primary sensor is a hair cell sensitive to the motions of the medium in which it is immersed. The outer ear functions as a funnel, steering sound into the external auditory canal and down onto the tympanic membrane of the middle ear, Fig. 17.A-1. The sound waves, being alternate compressions and expansions of the air carrying the acoustic energy, beat upon the tympanic membrane and set it into motion. If the sound is pitched high, the membrane will oscillate at a high frequency and if the sound is at a low pitch, the frequency of the membrane vibration will be correspondingly low.

The inner surface of the tympanic membrane is connected to the first of three small bones in the middle ear (the malleus, the incus, and the stapes), Fig. 17.A-1, which together function as a mechanical amplifier, increasing the amplitude of the mechanical vibration by a factor of almost 20 [195, 225]. The stapes in turn is connected to the oval window, which is the thin membrane covering the entrance to the endolymph-filled cochlea. As its name implies, the cochlea is a spirally-wound tube resembling a cockle shell; down the center of this tube there is a basilar membrane of decreasing thickness and decreasing tension which bears the motion-sensitive hair cells.

Incoming sound waves that beat upon the oval window set up standing acoustical waves in the cochlea to be sensed by the motions of the hairs protruding from the sensor cells. The position of largest disturbance along the basilar membrane is dependent upon the frequency of the sound at that moment. High-frequency sound will excite hairs close to the oval window while lower frequencies will produce disturbance further from the window. There are no blood vessels serving the basilar membrane, for if there were, the beating within the arteries would be deafening [171].

As seems to be the case with all hair cells in the body, those of the cochlea also transduce their bending under a mechanical stimulus (sound in this case) into a modulated electrical wave, the neural frequency of which reflects the intensity of the sound wave at the particular acoustic frequency for which the hair cell is sensitive. Moreover, the nerves that synapse with the hair cells also are strongly frequency-tuned, so that each hair-cell/nerve combination is very frequency selective and can phase lock to a pure tone.

The auditory nerve fibers (cranial nerve VIII) deliver the acoustic signal to the cochlear nucleus, and this signal then ascends from there to eventually reach the superior temporal gyrus in the cortex, where the sound finally makes its impression on the conscious mind. The signals from each of the ears have neural connections to both cerebral hemispheres, but the stronger connection is to the contralateral hemisphere

[157, 243]. Interestingly, there are several sites in the brainstem at which the auditory signal can crossover in order to terminate at the contralateral cerebral hemisphere [340]. Specific nuclei in the brain receive signals from both ears, compare their timing and then compute a direction and distance for the sound source, thereby allowing the brain to compose a sound map of the environment.

Inasmuch as the left cerebral hemisphere is more effective at speech processes in right-handed people, the contralateral right ear is more effective at receiving and interpreting speech messages in such people [225], whereas pure tones are heard equally well by the two ears [243]. On the other hand, the left ear is the superior one for music, as it activates the right cerebral hemisphere [120].

Considering the two ears as antennae, their peak sensitivity will be at an acoustic wavelength equal to the ear-to-ear distance [473]. For humans, this distance corresponds to a frequency of about 2000 Hz; for the squeaking mouse, it will be at much higher frequency, and for the rumbling elephant much lower. This law relating the ear-to-ear distance and the frequency of highest sensitivity is obeyed by the ears of all mammals.

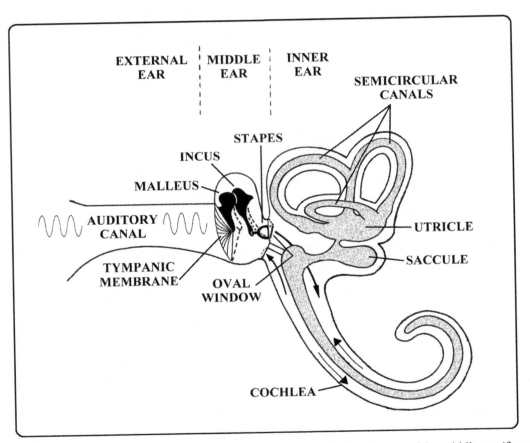

Fig. 17.A-1. Structures of the middle and inner ears [195]. The three bones of the middle ear (from left to right, the malleus, the incus, and the stapes) stop growing in infancy and so are the smallest bones in the adult body. Their positions are shown as dashed lines when the tympanic membrane is pushed inward by a sound wave traveling from left to right. In order to more clearly show its internal structure, the cochlea has been drawn partially uncoiled. The arrows show the direction of the sound waves in the cochlea.

Yoga and the Middle Ear

There are several notable facts about the clever mechanical system within the middle ear. First, the two end bones of the middle ear (the malleus and the stapes) are connected to muscles which, when contracted, restrict the motion of the bones and so lower the amplification factor for sound traveling through the middle ear. This is used in the middle-ear reflex [195, 473], wherein the muscles tighten in response to loud sounds, and so restrict the motion of the bones whenever the acoustic intensity becomes too high.

The muscles of the middle ear are skeletal muscles, just as the biceps and quadriceps are skeletal muscles. However, whereas the latter can be activated when we will them to be so, that is not the case with those of the middle ear. These muscles can be activated only reflexively in response to a loud noise or in expectation of a loud noise [155], however, they can be relaxed voluntarily as discussed in Box 17.A-1.

The auditory muscles of the middle ear have a significant muscle tone in the normal, everyday situation, but during relaxation, the parasympathetic branch of the autonomic nervous system is activated

BOX 17.A-1. RELAXING THE MUSCLES OF THE MIDDLE EAR

When a bat screeches for echo-locating flying insects, the muscles in its middle ear become very taut, thereby decreasing the bat's aural sensitivity. This guarantees that the loud screech does not flood the sound sensors; however, immediately afterward, the same muscles relax totally and the sensitive ears then listen for the tell-tale echo of the bat's next meal [486]. In humans, something of the same sort happens, for as we sneeze, the muscles of the middle ear are drawn tight so as to lower the auditory sensitivity to the roar of the barely subsonic explosion of gas from the lungs through the nose (see Subsection 12.B, *Factors Affecting the Breath*, page 373).

The muscular mechanism protecting the inner ear from acoustic overload is analogous in a way to that of the iris of the eye, which contracts under conditions of bright light thus protecting the retina from sensory overload, but which dilates in dim light to raise the sensory-signal level (Chapter 16, THE EYES AND VISION, page 411).

You too can experience directly the effects of relaxing the muscles of the middle ear in the following way. First set the volume control of your radio so low that it is barely audible or just inaudible when placed next to your mat. Then lie down in *savasana*; immediately upon relaxing, note how much louder the radio volume seems to become as relaxation of the muscles of the middle ears increases the ears' sensitivity. Keep this increased aural sensitivity in mind when you bring your students out of *savasana*.

The opposite response of the ears' sensitivity is also easily experienced. In this case, set the radio volume so that it is just audible, and then lay back over an exercise ball, so as to be in a passive, supported backbend. The radio's message will fade within a minute after beginning the backbend, and full auditory sensitivity will be restored immediately in healthy students on becoming upright. This loss of hearing on inversion has been reported in the medical literature [365], and has been attributed to high pressure in the middle ear which stretches the ligament attached to the stapes footplate, and so stiffens the ear's response. Anoxia also may be a factor in this effect.

{trigeminal nucleus (cranial nerve V) for the malleus, and the facial nucleus (cranial nerve VII) for the stapes}, and the muscles relax, thereby greatly increasing the ears' sensitivity. Thus, when in *savasana* with the body very relaxed, the ears become very sensitive and a modest noise can be very startling [473]. The muscles of the middle ear are very active during the REM phase of sleep (Subsection 21.B, *Circadian Rhythms; Physiological Peaks and Valleys in the 24-Hour Period*, page 476), along with the movement of the eyes in this phase [225]. On the other hand, the muscles of the outer ear are vestigial, and are no longer of any use, except to amuse children.

In the human ear, even with no sound incident on the tympanic membrane, there is a 100–300 Hz hum coming from the resting hair cells in the cochlea [236], this being a frequency well within the auditory range. Consequently, when one's meditation is deep and oriented toward hearing the inner sound, the resting signal of the hair cells can be heard loud and clear as "*nada*", the sound current [236, 143]. As one ascends the ladder of yoga, the *nada* current becomes the inner focus of the practices from *pratyahara* to *samadhi*. From the perspective of kundalini yoga, the *nada* is sensed as the kundalini passes through the *anahata* (heart) *chakra*, and is heard in the right ear [453].

The yoga texts are filled with the reports of sensing the sound of the universe as the all-permeating "Om" [144] when in deeply meditative states. Is it possible that this has any connection to two recent scientific discoveries? It is recently reported that the earth undergoes free oscillations with a period of between 150 and 500 seconds as determined from an analysis of seismic data [85, 451]. The most probable force driving this bell-like ringing of the earth arises from variations in atmospheric pressure alternately pressing inward and outward on the earth's surface. Note that though we speak of this ringing of the earth as a "sound", it is at far too low a frequency (a few milliHz) to be heard by the middle ear.

In an independent and totally unrelated study, it is reported that very small pressure changes of the order of 1/1000 of the total atmospheric pressure having periods of about 15 to 90 seconds are sensed subconsciously by human beings as witnessed by their clear effects on mental activity and test-taking [475]. Perhaps in the altered consciousness of the meditator, the effects of the low-frequency pressure changes and the earth's constant low-frequency hum are brought into the conscious realm and interpreted as sound within the normal acoustic range.

The earth's hum is now known to rise and fall in intensity, peaking in December-February and again in June-August; one would predict the same for the volume of the "Om" sound if it is really related to the earth's oscillation! If so, then the "sound" is truly global if not universal. It is also possible that the earth's ringing relates in some way to the sense that many animals have of an impending earthquake.

Students performing *sirsasana I* on the bare floor occasionally report hearing clicking sounds within the head during the first few minutes. Donohue [124] attributes this to rapid contractions of the muscles in the middle ear or the palate, whereas von Hippel [473] attributes it instead to electrical stimulation of the inner ear in some unspecified way. Referring to it as a form of tinnitus, Donohue points out that it can be erased by muscle relaxants or surgery.

It is known that there are both efferent and afferent nerve fibers to and from the cochlear hair cells. The former are a puzzle, as other hair-cell sensors in the body are not supplied with efferents (however, see Section 10.G, Hair and Piloerection, page 308). On the other hand, other hair cells are not frequency sensitive as these are intended to be; perhaps the efferent nerve stimulates muscles at the base of the hair cell and in some way helps to fine-tune the stiffness of the hair so as to adjust its frequency response. If so, then its action would be somewhat like that of the contractile tissue at the ends of the muscle spindles (Subsection 7.B, *Structure of Muscle Spindles*, page 199).

For the general population, the numbers of receptors and synapses in the auditory channel decrease with increasing age, and so the ability to hear is degraded with time [92]. However, as inversions such as *sirsasana* and *sarvangasana* bring fresh blood to the head, it may be that for the aging students who do these inverted *yogasanas* regularly, the loss of hearing is slowed.

Input from the auditory nerve into the reticular formation has a strong effect on the arousal, attention and wakefulness of the listener, depending upon the quality and intensity of the sound. When we are asleep, the muscles of the middle ear are relaxed, and so the ear has maximum sensitivity to extraneous noises. Moreover, there are collateral neural tracts from the middle ear directly to the reticular formation in the pons (Subsection 3.A, page 31), this being the wakefulness center. If and when there is a threatening noise while we sleep, the reticular formation will receive the message and immediately awaken both the central nervous system and the muscles for defensive action.

The connection of sound to other body/mind processes is well known. For example, it is known that by playing soft music before surgery, 50–60% less anaesthetic is required, and that the nausea of chemotherapy can be reduced also by such soft music [56]. In a technique called "toning", singing the vowel "e" is stimulating, bright and awakening, while the same song sung with "ah", resembles the sound of exhalation and brings on the full relaxation response [56]. Yogis will recognize this effect when chanting "OM".

SECTION 17.B. THE VESTIBULAR ORGANS OF BALANCE

Structure and Function of the Inner Ear

In addition to the middle ears so essential for hearing, all vertebrate animals have inner ears (vestibular organs) which serve as organs of balance [473]. Unlike our other senses such as vision, taste, temperature, *etc.*, the sensations of the balancing organs of the vestibule are not at all bright in our consciousness, being more obvious only when we become dizzy or nauseous. The sensory signals from the three types of vestibular organs (called the utricle, the saccule, and the semicircular canals), together with those from the eyes (Subsection 16.A, *The Ocular-Vestibular Connection*, page 418) and the body's proprioceptors (Section 7.C, page 208) work together to maintain posture and balance.

The otolith organs within the inner ear, the utricle and the saccule (Fig. 17.B-1), are largely responsible for sensing either the static orientation of the head in the gravitational field (see Appendix V, GRAVITY, page 553) or the direction of linear accelerated or decelerated motion of the head, whereas the three nearby semicircular canals in each inner ear (Fig. 17.B-1) are sensitive to the dynamic forces generated by accelerating or decelerating rotational motions of the head [195, 225, 230, 473]. The vestibular organs on the two sides of the head work together, so that those in one inner ear may reflexively excite extensor muscles on its side of the body, for example, whereas those on the other side inhibit the corresponding extensors on the contralater-

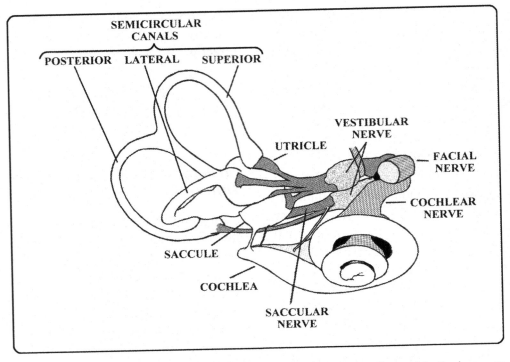

Fig. 17.B-1. Details of the vestibular organs and associated nerve bundles within the inner ear, as would be seen if viewed through the right temple [195].

al side of the body. The entire inner-ear structure is surrounded by a sack of perilymph which serves to isolate it acoustically from extraneous bone-conducting vibrations and from the sounds of the blood flowing through the skull [473]. The actions of the vestibular organs in maintaining balance in various asanas are described in Appendix IV, BALANCING, page 525 and in Subsection 16.A, *The Ocular-Vestibular Connection*, page 418.

The semicircular canals are responsible for the nausea of seasickness and motion sickness. With each lurch to the side, the semicircular canals signal the brain to turn the eyes, to squeeze the internal organs and to shift weight in order to regain balance. However, just as this is accomplished, the body is tossed in the opposite direction, and a new compensating strategy is set into play. It is this effort to compensate for this back-and-forth motion that quickly upsets our brain and our digestion.

Sensors for the Static Position of the Head

The utricle, Fig. 17.B-1, is a small closed sac containing both a lymph-like fluid and a gelatinous mass in which are embedded microcrystals (otoliths) of calcium carbonate. It contains as well a horizontal swathe of very specialized hair cells, each of which is in truth a bundle of yet smaller hairs. In this bundle, there is one special hair called the kinocilium, which resides on the outermost surface of the bundle. If, for some reason, the hair bundle were bent toward its kinocilium, this then induces a permeability change in the wall of the hair cell allowing potassium ions (K^+) to flow through the membrane with the development of a depolarization voltage. If, on the other hand, the bending were opposite, then the transmembrane voltage across the wall of the hair cell becomes hyperpolarized, indicating that the K^+ ions flow in the opposite direction.

It is the tipping of the head, causing the gelatinous matrix to press obliquely on the hair bundles, that bends the hairs of the utricle. The mechanism by which the hair cells of the vestibular apparatus sense an external force (gravitational or one of accelerating or decelerating motion) resembles that used by the Pacinian cells (Section 10.B, Sensory Receptors in the Skin, page 285) to sense pressure on the skin. However, the skin sensors have no directional sense and use changes in Na^+ permeability rather than K^+.

The kinocilium is always found on the side of its hair bundle, but not on the same side in all bundles. Thus a force on the plane of bundles, as when tilting the head, will bend some kinocilia in a direction leading to hyperpolarization and others in a direction leading to depolarization. It is this directionality of the hair cells' sensitivity and their ability to both hyperpolarize and depolarize that allow the brain to deduce both the magnitude and the direction of the displacement force. This ability of the vestibular sensors is rather unique, for most peripheral sensors (such as the Pacinian organs, Subsection 10.B, *Deep Pressure*, page 290) only depolarize or only hyperpolarize (the retinal cells of the eyes, for example, Section 16.A, page 411). Note too, that the Ruffini corpuscles (Subsection 7.B, page 208) are sensitive to both the pressure applied to the skin and to the direction from which the pressure comes.

As with the other mechanoreceptors, the membrane potentials of the hair cells in the inner ear are transduced into frequencies; when the head is held horizontally, the static hair-cell output has a constant frequency of 100–300 Hz, which then is increased or decreased as the hair cells are bent either toward or away from the kinocilium. Quite possibly, this resting frequency of the vestibular apparatus can be heard when meditating on the inner sound (*nada yoga*, see Subsection 17.A, *Yoga and the Middle Ear*, page 435) [236]. Since the different cilia are tuned to different frequencies, shifting between them can give rise to a variety of sounds, as observed in *nada yoga*.

The saccule seems to be much like the utricle, with two exceptions. First, it is exposed to external sound waves whereas the utricle is not, and second, its swathe of hair cells is oriented vertically rather than horizontally. It is thought to function in a way parallel to the utricle, but sensing tilt away from verticality. The saccule does appear to have an auditory sensitivity in the 50–1000 Hz acoustical range, and with direct connections to the hypothalamus, may be responsible for the pleasure derived from chanting and listening to music [298].

Sensors for the Dynamic Movement of the Head

The semicircular canals are composed of three half-circle tubes oriented with their planes mutually perpendicular so as to be sensitive to rotation about any or all of the three axes of the head. Each such canal has a filling of viscous fluid and a pad of hair cells (which act just as those described above for the utricle) behind an elastic membrane. However, in the case of the canals, it is accelerating or decelerating rotation of the head that stimulates the hair cells, with the canals moving more rapidly than the fluid inside of them due to the inertia of the latter. The inertial drag on the cells by the enclosed fluid then bends the hair bundles and so alters the rate of firing of the hair cells, with those on one side of the head having an increased rate and those on the opposite side decreasing in rate. The signals output by the semicircular canals travel to the medial and superior vestibular nuclei. The information on the speed and direction of head rotation no doubt complements that from the joint receptors monitoring the kinesthetic stimuli as the limbs move (Section 8.E, The Joints, page 260).

If the head rolls in one or more planes simultaneously, the hyperexcitation of the semicircular canals can lead to motion sickness. This can be cured with anticholinergic drugs [309], but then the vestibular input to the central nervous system is blocked and one is disoriented and has blurred vision. The semicircular canals also are important in the reflex action which keeps the eyes turning left, for example, while the head is turning right, thus allowing the eyes to stay focused on a single point in space as the head turns. This reflex involves the neural interaction between the medial nucleus and the oculomotor nucleus in the brainstem (Subsection 16.A, *The Ocular-Vestibular Connection*, page 418). Other, more indirect connections between the balancing organs and vision must exist, as those *yogasana* students can attest who have tried to balance with their eyes closed (Appendix IV, BALANCING, page 525).

Innervation of the Vestibular Tract

The afferent nerves from the vestibular balancing organs form a part of cranial nerve VIII, are myelinated, and synapse with the four vestibular nuclei in the lateral parts of the brainstem, just below the fourth ventricle. The vestibular nuclear complex is large, occupying a substantial part of the medulla. Descending fibers from the medial and inferior nuclei of the vestibular tract go only to the upper part of the spinal cord, and are concerned with head and neck movements in response to vestibular excitation. The afferent nerves from the utricle input to the lateral nucleus while the alpha- and gamma-motor neuron efferents from this point are facilitory for extensor-motor neurons and inhibitory for flexor-motor neurons. Neurons from the cerebellum and spinal-cord proprioceptors also converge on the lateral vestibular nucleus (Fig. 3.A-8). From its mode of action, it is deduced that the utricle in conjunction with other peripheral sensors can be an important proprioceptor in standing postures.

Neural connections are also made from the four vestibular nuclei to the cerebellum and back again, supposedly for fine tuning of balance reflexes. There is evidence as well that connections also are made between the vestibular nuclei and higher centers, all the way up to the cortex. If so, this would allow a conscious sensing of static and dynamic head position in space.

The initial sensing mechanism in the vestibular organs is seen to be a mechanical shift of a viscous fluid as the head is tilted. As such, it is inherently slower than balancing signals sent upward by the eyes or the proprioceptors, and so would be most useful in sensing slow motions, such as the rocking of the boat, or the swaying of the bus, and would be less useful when balancing in the *yogasanas*.

Chapter 18

THE GASTROINTESTINAL ORGANS AND DIGESTION

SECTION 18.A. STRUCTURE AND FUNCTION

As has been pointed out many times, all human beings are hollow. Each of us has an open tube over 30 feet in length, running through us from mouth to anus. The inner surface of this tube is just a continuation of our outer-surface skin; without a seam, the skin of the face becomes the skin of the inside of the mouth, and this continues inward and downward to become the surface of the throat, the stomach, the small and large intestines, the skin of the anus and the skin of the buttocks (Section 10.A, Structure of the Skin, page 283). Actually, closer inspection of the cells and their functions in the various parts of the gastrointestinal tract reveals how very special each of these parts is and the special role each plays. This inner "empty" space as defined by the walls of the gut, expresses our hollowness and technically is known as the lumen.

In contrast to the situation with skeletal muscles (Chapter 7, page 167), the smooth muscles of the internal organs (the viscera) consist of long cylindrical cells with no cross striations, and are found in the walls of organs having cavities such as the urinary, reproductive, respiratory, gastrointestinal, and vascular organs. The job of the smooth muscles is to move material (urine, air, blood, *etc.*) through the cavities using slow, sustained, rhythmic movements. These smooth-muscle contractions are generally not under voluntary control, but are responsive to both neural and hormonal stimulation. Smooth muscle as found in the gastrointestinal tract can contract for very long periods of time as compared with most skeletal muscle which quickly suffers ischemia and fatigue when contracted. Furthermore, smooth muscle can still contract after being stretched 500% [230]. The lengths of the gastrointestinal tracts in various animal species depends upon their diets. Vegetarian animals have relatively long tracts, carnivores have relatively short tracts, and omnivores such as humans have tracts of intermediate length.

It is known that different tissues have different responses to stimulation. In the case of the gastrointestinal tract, there are no pain sensations from the gut if it is manipulated, cut extensively or even burned, but pain is sensed if it is stretched or distended excessively, or is in spasm [308].

Through the hunger center, the hypothalamus is able to sense a low level of glucose in the blood, and in response to this, alerts the cortex to act to find food. Through conscious action, the cortex can ignore the hypothalamic request for about 12 hours before insistent hunger pangs set in. Once our sensors for the sight of food, or its smell or taste are activated, the sensations are recorded in the cortex of the brain. From there, cortical messages are sent to the medulla, the upper terminus of the parasympathetic vagus nerve, which in turn has branches innervating the stomach. Activation of the vagus nerve results in the release of hydrochloric acid (more than a quart each day) and other digestive enzymes into the stomach, and the process of digestion is underway. Other routes to the same end also exist: stretch receptors in the walls of the stomach will be activated as the stomach fills, sending their signals to the medulla via an afferent branch of the vagus nerve, consequently turning on the digestion process via an efferent branch of the vagus nerve. As the stomach fills, the hunger center is turned off and the satiety center turned on, until the next time the glucose level drops too low and food again must be found. Chewing and swallowing also act to stimulate the flow of the digestive juices.

Local reflexes are also at work so that digestion can be started or stimulated without any signal going beyond the spinal cord. The sensation of hunger persists even in persons having no stomach, for it is the centers in the hypothalamus that control the sensations of hunger and satiety [321].

Note again that the vagal stimulation of the digestive process is driven by the parasympathetic side of the autonomic nervous system; in times of crisis, when the sympathetic nervous system is dominant, blood is pulled away from the viscera, and digestion stops until the crisis is weathered and parasympathetic balance can assert itself again.

Neurologically, the central nervous system is able to control muscular action from the mouth to the pyloric sphincter of the stomach and from the colon to the rectum, however, in the intermediate regions of the intestines, it is the enteric nervous system that dictates both the muscular and glandular instructions [155].

In what follows, let us look at the physiological processes that take place sequentially in the gastrointestinal tract, Fig. 18.A-1, once eating commences. As will be seen, these processes are not without impact on the student practicing *yogasana*.

The Mouth and Esophagus

The mouth is the first station for digestion of food. Mechanically, food is processed into a form suitable for swallowing by the actions (both voluntary and involuntary) of the mouth, lips, teeth and tongue. At the same time, glands in the mouth secrete enzymes, lubricants, and adhesives to further prepare the bolus formed by chewing for transport through the esophagus to the stomach, Figs. 12.A-1 and 18.A-1. One of the enzymes released into the mouth during chewing is lysozyme, an antibacterial disinfectant; its presence in saliva is why animals lick their wounds and why people with a persistently dry mouth suffer abnormally high tooth decay [473]. Simultaneously with chewing, the taste buds are activated, as is the olfactory sense of smell, both using the cranial nerves (Subsection 2.C, page 17). The sensation of "taste" is really a combination of tasting using the tastebuds in the tongue and smelling the odor of the food using the receptors in the nose. As the nose's sense of smell is so much more discriminating than the tongue's sense of taste, it is the former that adds so much pleasure to the gourmand's palate.

When swallowing food that has been chewed, the epiglottis closes the path to the lungs, and the uvula (adenoids) close the path of the food bolus to the nose, leaving the esophagus as the only open path, Fig. 12.A-1. Because the food or liquid in the swallowed mass is propelled toward the stomach by muscular action, we can swallow upward in inverted poses such as *sirsasana* and *sarvangasana*; were it otherwise, as it is with birds, we would have to be sitting or standing upright and tip our heads back in order to swallow.

At the two extreme ends of the gastrointestinal tract, the conscious and reflexive actions are mixed and present simultaneously, whereas between these points, the action

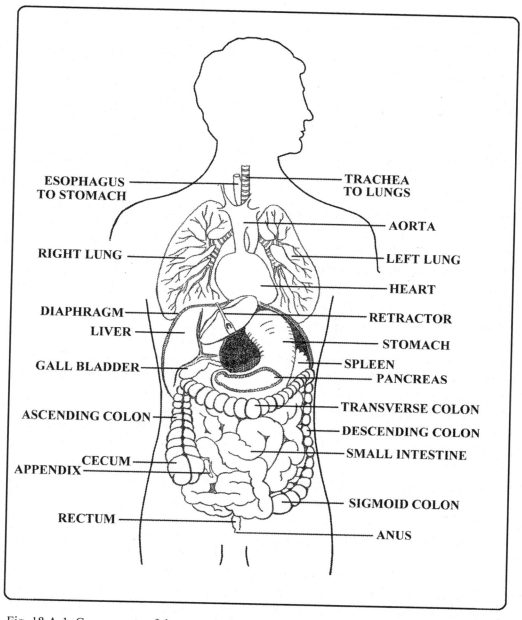

Fig. 18.A-1. Components of the gastrointestinal tract and its accessory organs. The retractor pulls a portion of the liver out of the way so that more of the stomach can be seen.

is totally reflexive, involving the parasympathetic and enteric nervous systems. Swallowing is a reflexive action driven by the medulla, however, the intervention of the higher cerebral centers can impact this innocent act and so cause a "choking up" for emotional reasons originating in the limbic region.

The stomach has a special coating which renders it inert to the strong acid involved in digestion, however, should the stomach contents reflux and so enter the esophagus, then the lack of a similar protective coating in the esophagus leads to the sharp, burning sensation of heartburn. Digestive strength can be increased by performing those *yog-*

asanas (spinal twists, supported forward bends, *etc.*) that increase the blood supply to the digestive system [215a, 305].

The Stomach

Using digestive enzymes and strong acid produced by the cells lining the gut, the stomach is the primary site for the digestion of food, though there is very little absorption that takes place here. The enzyme pepsin is expressed in the stomach, and is used for converting protein into smaller peptide fragments. Inasmuch as all cells have a large protein component, it is at first sight strange that the cells lining the stomach excrete protein-digesting enzyme, but are not themselves digested by this enzyme. Nature solves this problem by storing the pepsin within the cells in the form of inactive pepsinogen, which then becomes active pepsin only when it is outside of the cell and in the presence of strong hydrochloric acid. This strong acid not only activates pepsin, but is effective in killing many bacteria. In this regard, see Section 14.A, Saliva and Mucus, page 393.

There are many signals that precipitate a release of hydrochloric acid: in order of increasing effectiveness, thinking about food, smelling food, chewing food, swallowing food, and having food press against the lumen of the stomach all are effective in releasing stomach acid. In the absence of these triggering events, there is no release of pepsinogen or acid.

The stomach is important not only in digestion, but thanks to its structure, it is also a holding vessel, capable of expanding manyfold to accommodate excessively large meals without an increase in internal pressure. Because there is no excess pressure even when one has eaten excessively, digested food (chyme) is not forced backward from the stomach into the esophagus, however, stretching of the stomach inhibits food intake [321].

The residence time of food in the stomach will depend upon just how digestible it is; a heavy meal containing a high proportion of fatty meat may require up to 6 hours digestion in the stomach before it is ready to be passed through the pyloric valve to the small intestine, whereas a light meal of carbohydrates may be ready in just two hours, and a meal of lean meat will have an intermediate residence time [421, 473]. Water, on the other hand, is rapidly absorbed from the stomach. See Subsection 18.B, *Yogasana Practice and the Digestive Process*, page 449, for the relevance of the residence time to *yogasana* practice.

Generation and Containment of Stomach Acid

The contents of the stomach when in action are just as easily capable of digesting the cells that line the stomach as they are of digesting beefsteak. That the cells of the stomach wall are not appreciably attacked is due to an alkaline mucus gel coating that separates the cell surfaces from the potent brew contained within. In keeping with the rough neighborhood in which the intestinal cells live and though they are coated with an alkaline mucus, even then, they must be replaced every three days [387, 155]. Preventing access of the stomach acid to the other structures in the gastrointestinal tract (the esophagus, for example) which are not so protected is the function of stout valves at the entrance and exit to the stomach, which normally are closed, and which open only when absolutely necessary. Should any stomach acid work its way past the upper sphincter and enter the unprotected esophagus, the result is heartburn.

The cells of the stomach that produce the hydrochloric acid necessary for digestion are called parietal cells; cells that sense the degree of acidity in the stomach and so signal for a greater or lesser release of acid are called G cells. The cell walls of the parietal cells facing the lumen are able to absorb K^+ ions from the stomach contents and in return pump H^+ ions into the lumen. It is this H^+ that is the acid component of hydrochloric acid (HCl). The brew of concentrated acid and active pepsin in the stomach is highly effective in dissolving not only the proteins of animal muscle, but also the protein of most microbes, parasites, worms, *etc.*, that may be in the food. Any such bacteria that are strong enough to survive the digestive brew in the stomach then go on to colonize the colon (see below).

The absorption of K^+ from the lumen and its replacement with H^+ on a large scale is a process that is very energy intensive. The energy needed for this ion pumping is derived from ATP within mitochondria feeding on glucose and oxygen (Subsection 11.B, *Blood Chemistry and Function*, page 322). The parietal cells are stocked with many large mitochondrial centers; when these are called upon to generate up to a quart and a half of concentrated hydrochloric acid per day, they make a large energy demand on the body, as large as that made by the skeletal muscles. During the digestion of proteins, the oxygen consumption of the body may go up by 25% in order to feed the gastric fire that produces hydrochloric acid [115].

The amount of hydrochloric acid required for digestion depends upon what one eats; those who eat large amounts of meat and its associated fat will require much larger amounts of hydrochloric acid, pepsin, oxygen, and energy to digest a meal than will the same person eating a meat-free, carbohydrate-loaded meal [421].

Should a parietal cell of the stomach wall die and disintegrate, the door is then open for seepage of strong acid (pH 1) and enzyme into unprotected places and the possibility of forming an ulcer (self-digestion) in the lining of the stomach. However, this does not happen very often because when a parietal cell dies, prostaglandins are released in the area, and this stimulates neighboring cells to immediately expand into the opening, thus keeping the parietal layer intact.

Acid production by the parietal cells is triggered chemically by the gastrin released by the G cells, which in turn acts on parietal cells sensitized by their absorption of histamine released by mast cells. This absorption of the sensitizer histamine can be blocked chemically by drugs that compete successfully on the parietal-cell surface for the receptor sites which normally accept histamine molecules. Such "H2 blockers" in this way are able to turn off acid production for many hours at a time. Parietal cells also can be excited to generate hydrochloric acid by both the enteric and central nervous systems. Thus one needs only to think of "food" and the acid will immediately begin to flow into the stomach. This neural system is activated much more quickly than the chemically activated one.

The Small Intestine

The initial step of digestion begun in the stomach is completed in the small intestine. With the aid of the enzymes and alkaline buffering provided by the pancreas, the small intestine is able to handle small aliquots of the highly acidic chyme from the stomach, by neutralizing its acidity (returning it to pH 7–8) and digesting the larger molecular fragments (fats, proteins and starches) down to their ultimate molecular components. The smaller amino acids and saccharides that result from this digestive process are then absorbed through the walls of the small intestine directly into the blood stream. Any emulsified fat at this stage is absorbed instead into the lymph and then dumped into the venous bloodstream near the neck.

Absorption of the nutrients in the lumen of the small intestine is efficient due to the huge area of the intestinal walls. The walls of the small intestine are multiply folded so that the structure has the largest surface area through which nutrients can pass while occupying the smallest volume. Were the small intestine opened up lengthwise and stretched taut, it would cover three tennis courts! As described below, the slurried mass of digested food (chyme) is moved along the ten-foot length of the small intestine by the reflexive muscular action of peristalsis. Peristalsis in the small intestine is a one-way-street, moving the contents only in the mouth-to-anus direction. Once the fluid mass has been propelled downward to the end of the small intestine, usually a trip of one or two hours, it is ready then for processing by the colon.

Ninety percent of the nutrients in the food we eat are absorbed in the small intestine, with the other ten percent divided between absorption in the stomach and the colon [345].

The Colon

The primary functions of the colon (also called the large intestine) are to first absorb up to 99% of the water and salts in the fluid mass sent to it; if this water is not recovered (2 quarts per day), the result is diarrhea and a dangerous dehydration of the body. With the water and salts removed, the stool becomes a semisolid mass consisting largely of the indigestible remains of the earlier meals, and of refuse from the liver's purification of the blood. Second, the colon is home to a wide variety of microbes, some beneficial and some not. Every stool contains a significant amount of bacterial debris.

If the meal in question contained a sufficient amount of fruits, raw vegetables and whole grains, then the resultant stool will be high in indigestible cellulosic fibers, will be firm and bulky, and will press strongly against the walls of the colon. The pressure that such a stool generates at the walls is the stimulus for the peristalsis that carries it along from the small intestine to the anus for easy expulsion. Because it requires much more effort to move a solid stool through the colon than a fluid slurry through the small intestine, it is understandable that the muscles encircling the colon are larger and stronger than those about the small intestine, Fig. 18.A-1. Though the colon is less than half the length of the small intestine, the passage of the solid stool through the former may take more than 10 hours, compared to only 2 hours for the fluid chyme in the latter.

If the diet is low in fiber, then the stool in the colon is greasy and small, does not press enough on the walls of the intestine to elicit a strong peristaltic reflex, and is expelled only with great effort and abdominal strain. Many years of a low-fiber diet will result in a colon that is weak and flabby from lack of exercise.

Though very little gas is generated in the small intestine, between 7 and 10 liters of gas (largely carbon dioxide, hydrogen, and methane) are generated each day in the colon, however, most of this is reabsorbed by the cells lining the intestinal walls [322].

The small intestine is essentially a sterile place, whereas the colon is filled with bacteria. The two contrasting environments are kept apart by the ileocecal valve [230], which allows transport of refuse only from the small intestine to the colon. Several strains of bacteria in the colon are able to synthesize important vitamins which are absorbed by the colon for general use throughout the body, whereas several other strains of bacteria in the colon are pathogenic. In a healthy colon, the populations of the various bacterial strains compete so as to keep one another in check; in the process of fighting an infection, antibiotics or even a change of diet can upset this balance and so lead to other problems. When there is a bacterial imbalance or a new strain of bacteria is introduced into the colon, immune cells in the lining of the intestine may be called upon to re-establish equilibrium.

Pressure in the anus can be varied in both the positive and negative directions through voluntary control by the *yogasana* student, even though the student has done no work otherwise aimed at controlling the anal sphincters [52]. This may be of relevance to the performance of *uddiyana bandha* in the *yogasanas*.

Peristalsis

When there is an internal pressure that presses outward against the intestinal wall, a rhythmic action of the intestine is triggered reflexively that pushes the intestinal contents from the oral toward the anal end. This is the peristaltic reflex. Interestingly, if all of the parasympathetic vagal nerves (cranial nerve X) from the brain's medulla to the intestine are severed in a live animal (including man), the peristaltic reflex remains active. Like the heart beat (Subsection 11.A, *Innervation of the Heart: The Cardiac Pacemaker*, page 315), peristalsis of the intestine is self-stimulating, yet subject to limited control by the autonomic nervous system as well. Further, a loop of intestine totally cut out of the animal continues to show this reflex! It is as if the intestine has a nervous system (and brain) of its own and can function without direction from the autonomic nervous system [155]. This so-called "enteric nervous system" consists of a very dense web of neural tissue wedged between two layers of muscle that encircle the gut. The pacemaker that drives the peristaltic action is contained within cells in the enteric system [11], the peristaltic frequency being 3 contractions per minute in the stomach and 12 per minute in the small intestine. The enteric system also has its own sensors, and these too, do not synapse with the autonomic nervous system. Whereas this enteric sys-

tem is able to drive the peristaltic action, the acts of swallowing and defecation do require direction from the autonomic and central nervous systems.

Within the walls of the intestine, there are two layers (three in the stomach) of directionally-oriented, smooth-muscle fibers. The innermost layer has radially directed fibers, which on contraction act to pinch off the gut so that its contents can not move backward if further squeezed. The second outermost layer then squeezes with muscle fibers oriented in the longitudinal direction, so that the digested mass is pushed forward, toward the anus. To be effective, these two muscle actions must be coordinated by the enteric nervous system as the peristaltic wave moves in one direction only along the gastrointestinal tract [473]. If the swallowed food is in some way defective or toxic, a reverse peristalsis is also possible, in which case the food is vomited in the direction from which it came.

Accessory Organs of Digestion

There are several organs in the abdominal cavity that are not part of the gastrointestinal tract as such, yet supply important enzymes to it in aid of digestion. Prime among these is the pancreas, which is able to supply enzymes to the small intestine in wide enough variety as to digest almost anything that can be swallowed, including bacteria, protozoa, and intestinal worms. The pancreas performs two other essential duties: it supplies insulin to the bloodstream so as to regulate sugar levels in the blood, and it is able to add an alkaline solution of bicarbonate ion to the small intestine to counter the high acidity of the chyme entering the small intestine from the stomach. This latter buffering against acid is essential, as the small intestine is not able otherwise to protect itself against the high acidity of the stomach juices, and also because many of the digestive enzymes such as pancreatic enzyme that function in the small intestine will not do so at high acidity. The neutralization of acid is keyed to the flow from the stomach; as a small dose of acidic chyme is added to the small intestine via opening of the pyloric valve, it is neutralized by the bicarbonate solution so as to bring the pH back to 7–8. At this point another small aliquot of the chyme is moved into the small intestine and the bicarbonate brought on again for pH neutralization. This stepwise neutralization of the stomach acid continues until the entire contents of the stomach have been moved down and neutralized.

The liver is the largest internal organ in the body, and is located just behind the right ribs, Fig. 18.A-1. This organ is constructed with a high degree of redundancy, *i.e.*, one can lose 80% of the liver and still function without any symptoms, and the organ also has a very high degree of regeneration. All of the blood vessels that absorb nutrients from the gastrointestinal tract join to become the portal vein to the liver. This vein carries the sugars, vitamins, amino acids, drugs, bile salts, and toxins absorbed from the gastrointestinal system to the liver for purification [276]. Toxins absorbed from the gut are solublized in the liver and then excreted in the feces and urine. It is generally held by yogis that toxins are wrung from the liver and are forced into the body fluids by spinal twists, however, I could find no scientific evidence either for or against this idea.

The liver stores bile and bile salts in the gall bladder until that time when chyme enters the small intestine. The addition of the bile to the chyme occurs only when fat is sensed in the chyme, and acts to emulsify any fat so as to make it water soluble. Whereas the digestion products of proteins and carbohydrates are pulled from the small intestine directly into the bloodstream, emulsified fat is pulled instead into the lymph (Section 11.G, The Lymphatic System, page 352), eventually to be dumped into the venous bloodstream near the neck.

It appears generally true that bodily secretions are driven by the parasympathetic branch of the autonomic nervous system, as opposed to the sympathetic branch, which favors muscle contraction instead. This is true as well in the gut where it is known that gastric secretions are driven by the parasympathetic branch [195], or possibly by the enteric nervous system [155].

Pain signals from distressed internal organs often use the same afferent neurons used to signal pain in the skin close to the affected organ. Due to this common neural path, the brain often interprets pain signals from the visceral organs as coming from the associated dermatome, or skin area (Section 10.E, Dermatomes and Referred Pain, page 303). However, in the course of human evolution, the organs and their associated dermatomes have drifted apart, so that real pain in the gall bladder may be manifest in the brain as a pain in the skin of the right shoulder, for example, Fig. 10.E-3.

The Effects of Stress on the Gastrointestinal Tract

If the vagus nerve is intact, then it has a certain neural control over the digestive system, as does the enteric nervous system. It is no surprise that these two entities through their common ground in the gut can influence one another as well. Thus, as the central and/or the sympathetic nervous systems send their signals to the peripheral effectors in the abdominal area, the enteric system can intercept these and either inhibit them totally or else modulate them in some way [155].

It was long believed that, as a result of emotional stress, there was a strong vagal excitation that led to the delivery of excess hydrochloric acid and pepsin to the stomach, and that this excess was able to eat into the lining of the stomach, producing an ulcer. It is now believed that this can happen only under the most extreme stress, and that the normal sort of everyday stress is not a factor here. Instead, many ulcers can be traced to a bacterial infection (Helicobacter pylori) of the stomach which is able to promote high acidity [155].

When the body is under stress, the sympathetic nervous system exerts its dominance over the digestive tract. At such times, the blood flow to the small intestine is severely curtailed as the blood is shunted instead to the large muscles of the body. Consequently, digestion and peristalsis in the small intestine slow, and the absorption of nutrients from the small intestine into the intestinal vascular system comes to a halt, while in the upper digestive tract, acidity increases, leading to indigestion and heartburn. If the stress is chronic, one craves complex carbohydrates (pasta, bread, *etc.*) as these foods trigger the release in the brain of the calming neurotransmitter serotonin. Eventually, through chronic stress, one can become addicted to the calming effect of serotonin release and pay for it with a corresponding increase in weight. As the unfortunate set of gastric circumstances comprised of indigestion, hyperacidity, and heartburn are triggered by stresses which activate the sympathetic nervous system, the symptoms can be countered by *yogasanas* such as *savasana* and supported forward bends which promote parasympathetic rebalancing.

SECTION 18.B. DIGESTION AND METABOLISM

Yogasana Practice and the Digestive Process

As discussed above, the production of hydrochloric acid in the amounts and concentrations necessary for digestion requires a great expenditure of energy. Following a meal, the gut demands considerable oxygen, glucose and ATP in order to drive acid production. Because these materials are also in demand when doing the physical work of the *yogasanas*, it is not a good idea to try to perform *yogasana* and digestion simultaneously. Thus, you should not eat anything requiring a large amount of acid for digestion in the hours preceding your *yogasana* practice; Geeta Iyengar [216] recommends a period of between one and four hours between eating and practice, depending upon how large the meal. If this rule is followed, then one can avoid the unnecessary competition between the gut and the skeletal muscles for energy resources.

Note too that the digestive juices are set flowing not only by the presence of food in the mouth and the act of swallowing, but that the smell of food will start the digestive process going, and even just the thought of food is enough to begin acid production! Thus the *yogasana* practice space should be free of the smells of food preparation, and the student should not dwell mentally on the meal to come, hungry though he/she may be.

With the stomach filled with acid during the digestion process, it would seem foolhardy to attempt any sort of inversion, for this would seem to spill corrosive acid into the throat. However, the acid-containing stomach is well sealed off from the upper and lower regions of the tract connected to it by the upper and lower sphincter valves that restrict flow out of the stomach in both the upright and inverted positions. Once having eaten a meal, the digestion process can be speeded along by activating pressure points in the instep of the foot and lower leg [149], as when doing *yogasanas* that press this portion of the anatomy to the floor, *i.e.*, *vajrasana* or more ideally, *supta virasana* [216].

At the other end of the gastrointestinal tract, stool in the colon can be expelled only if peristalsis is strong enough to move it into the descending or sigmoid sections of the gut (Subsection 14.D, *Defecation*, page 397). This peristalsis is most naturally achieved through the reflex action of the intestinal walls responding to the pressure of the stool on the walls. If this pressure is insufficient, the peristalsis is weak, and the result is constipation.

Note that any pressurization of the wall from the outside toward the inside as with the wringing action of *maricyasana III* (see Fig. 4.A-7), for example, does not activate the stretch receptors in the intestinal wall, and so will not promote peristalsis. The yogic approach to overcoming constipation is to perform *inversions* of long duration such as *sirsasana I*, *halasana*, and *sarvangasana*, and their variations [216]. Perhaps this can be understood in the following way. When in the upright position, moving stool from the ileocecal valve through the ascending colon is uphill with respect to gravity (Fig. 18.A-1) and so may prove to be difficult, whereas when inverted, this step is moving with gravity, rather than against it. Moreover, it is the pressing of the stool against the intestinal walls that gets it moving; perhaps when inverted, the pressure on the walls is applied to a more sensitive spot, thus stimulating a stronger peristalsis. Variations on *pindasana* are also useful in relieving constipation.

The hiccup would seem to be a reflex action without a purpose, unlike sneezing, blinking or coughing, all of which are protective in one way or another. It appears that the hiccup is due to a twitch of the diaphragm when the nerves that drive its contraction are irritated. Thus when the filled stomach pushes against the diaphragm and irritates the phrenic nerve when in *sarvangasana*, and especially when in *karnapidasana*, the result many times is a case of hiccups [387]. With less frequency, the same result may be had when in *sirsasana I*.

Irritation of the vagus nerve also can trigger a case of hiccups. Because hiccups are a strongly rhythmical phenomena, anything that will serve to break the rhythm can serve as a cure.

Metabolism

The chemical products resulting from the digestion of our food yields high-energy materials that can then be used to perform work. However, 80% of the calories so derived from our food are used just to maintain a body temperature of 98.6° F. Maintaining this temperature within narrow limits is important, for many of the body's enzymes have been tailored to work best at this temperature.

Using the chemical potential of our ingested and digested food implies that the glucose so formed from our food intake is readily absorbed from the blood stream into the cells that will eventually do the work based on that chemical potential. In fact, the critical step of absorption from the blood into the cell is dependent upon the presence in the blood of the hormone insulin, produced by the pancreas. When the pancreatic source of the insulin is subject to an autoimmune disease, the body becomes deficient in that hormone, and the result is type I diabetes; when the insulin levels are adequate, however, the cell receptors which allow glucose into the cells still may not respond to the insulin. In this case, the result is type II diabetes. In both types of diabetes, the blood sugar levels reach very high values (hyperglycemia), but on correction, may fall to very low levels (hypoglycemia). In either case, these are serious diseases, and are potentially fatal (see Subsection 15.B, *The Pancreas and Gastrointestinal Glands*, page 407, for a further discussion of diabetes and *yogasana*).

The application of *yogasana* practice to the control of type I diabetes is described by Cook [84], who found that a vigorous practice combining both sympathetic and parasympathetic stimulations was very effective provided it was done on a regular daily schedule. Similarly, it is known that type II diabetes responds well to moderate exercise; again, *yogasana* practice of about an hour a day is sufficient to reactivate the receptors and allow glucose to flow into the cells.

With respect to the autonomic nervous system, the beta cells of the pancreas that produce the insulin are stimulated by the parasympathetic action of the right vagus nerve (cranial nerve X), and inhibited by sympathetic action [318]. Thus the cooling poses of *yogasana* would be of help in type I diabetes as they would promote increased insulin production. In addition to the strong effects of insulin, glucose levels in the blood are also strongly affected by other hormones such as epinephrine, norepinephrine and cortisol, each of which in turn is more or less susceptible to control through stress reduction using *yogasana* principles (Section 6.E, Autonomic Balance: Stress and *Yogasana*, page 153).

Chapter 19

SEXUAL FUNCTION, GYNECOLOGY, AND PREGNANCY

SECTION 19.A. MENSTRUATION

The Menstrual Cycle

The view is presented by Sparrowe [442] that the menstrual flow is purifying, and that one should feel that through this process the body has rid itself of many impurities, both physical and mental. In order for the purification to work, one must eat properly, exercise moderately, and rest during the first few days, in order to give the body every opportunity to do its work.

The menstrual cycle in women consists of the expulsion from the uterus of blood and tissue every 28 days, the flow lasting for 3 to 7 days; day 1 of the cycle is taken as the first day of menstrual flow. The cycle itself begins approximately 14 days previous to the time of first menstrual flow when the hypothalamus releases two hormones into the ducts leading to the anterior part of the pituitary gland just below it, Fig. 3.A-2. Called the follicle releasing hormone (FRH) and the luteinizing releasing hormone (LRH), these two substances then promote the release into the bloodstream of the gonadotropic hormones FSH (follicular stimulating hormone) and LH (luteinizing hormone) which have the woman's ovaries as their destination and site of action. Once in the ovaries, the FHS and LH stimulate one of the follicles in the ovaries to prepare for fertilization, by releasing an egg (ovum) from the follicle into one of the fallopian tubes. After this ovulation phase, there fol-

lows 14 days of estrogen and progesterone production by the FHS and LH, respectively, aimed at turning off the flow of FHS and LH from the pituitary, and preparing the lining of the uterus to receive the descending egg. At this second stage, known as the luteinizing phase, the ovum is called the corpus luteum. In the luteinizing phase, estrogen acts to build up a thick but unstable layer in the uterus, and progesterone then acts to stabilize this layer and prepare it further for the corpus luteum [442]. The blood flow to the uterine lining (the endometrium) is increased in the luteinizing phase, as is its thickness.

If, by the 28th day, the corpus luteum has not been fertilized by sperm, the endometrium (seedbed) of the uterus collapses, tissues disintegrate, and another menstrual flow begins. At the same time, estrogen and progesterone levels return to their low values characteristic of day 1. If instead, the egg is fertilized, then progesterone stays high as estrogen levels fall. As for what happens next, see Section 19.B, Pregnancy, page 456.

The relative constancy of a regular menstrual cycle implies some sort of pacemaker within the body that controls the timing of the process, and it has been postulated that the regulator lies within the pineal gland [442], already known to regulate hormones within a 24-hour sleep/wake cycle (Subsection 21.B, page 488).

Detectable levels of both FHS and LS can be found in the male body as well as in the female, however, in the female, there is a strong 28-day cycle of peak concentrations, whereas in the male, there is no detectable fluctuation of these hormonal levels over time. The changes in a young girl's body at puberty, *i.e.*, the appearance of breasts, pubic hair, a feminine voice and broader hips, are all driven by the appearance of estrogen in the body at the time of first menstruation.

Menstruation occurs only when there is sufficient body fat in the woman's body to support both her needs and that of the fetus, if there is to be one. Thus, menstruation will shut down in the female superathlete who has too little body fat, and menarche, the time of first menstruation, can be 4 years later for undernourished young girls in poor countries as compared with that for well-fed girls in the more developed countries [43].

Premenstrual Syndromes

The complexities of the menstrual cycle and the delicate balance involved between powerful hormonal forces imply a multitude of ways that the cycle can go wrong. In addition to the specific problems of lack of ovulation, too little or too much bleeding, endometriosis, fibroids, and ovarian cysts, there is a less specific broad class of menstrual-related symptoms collectively called the premenstrual syndrome (PMS). It is said that there are at least 150 different symptoms associated with PMS [99], relating primarily to an imbalance of the estrogen/ progesterone levels or to a sluggish liver which is unable to handle the efficient removal of toxins generated by the menstrual process.

For the sake of specificity, consider the approach taken by Rychner [396] based on an earlier classification scheme of PMS symptoms. She assigned such symptoms to one of four categories: type A (anxiety, irritability, mood swings), type C (craving, fatigue, headache), type D (depression, confusion, memory loss) and type H (water retention, bloating, weight gain, breast tenderness). Mixed-type symptoms are seen, and the pattern is not necessarily constant from one month to the next.

The *yogasanas* recommended for type-A PMS symptoms are *savasana*, downward-facing *savasana*, and child's pose (*balasana*), all of which are consistent with the idea that type-A anxiety involves a predominant excitation of the sympathetic nervous system, and that parasympathetic balance can be restored by such relaxing poses (Section 20.C, Anxiety, page 470). Note too that the universal antidote for mood swings is regular exercise [99].

At the other extreme, type-D PMS symptoms signal the need for more sympathetic energy in the autonomic nervous system, and so it is no surprise that the recommended poses focus on backbending: *urdhva mukha svanasana*, *setu bandhasana*, and *dhanurasana*, specifically (Section 20.A, Depression, page 464). More intense backbending would be appropriate only for those with considerable experience in *yogasana*, as the universal recommendation during menstruation is to take it easy.

Interestingly, the symptoms of Seasonal Affective Disorder (SAD, Subsection 16.D, *White-Light Starvation*, page 430) are said to be much like those of PMS, and in some women, phototherapy has been found to be effective in relieving PMS symptoms [297]. As SAD phototherapy involves a rebalancing along the sympathetic-parasympathetic axis, the effects of phototherapy in erasing the SAD-like symptoms of type-D PMS would be understandable.

Rychner explains that in type-C PMS, the craving for sugar or chocolate is driven by the hyperactivity of the body's insulin at this time and its need for glucose as a substrate (Subsection 18.B, *Metabolism*, page 450). The cravings are eased by promoting blood flow to the abdominal and pelvic areas using poses such as *dhanurasana* and *setu bandhasana*.

Given that type-H PMS symptoms involve water retention and bloating primarily, it is at first logical that the *yogasana* antidotes are inversions, *i.e.*, *upavistha konasana* against the wall, wall *padasana*, and *ardha halasana*. Indeed, as mentioned in Box 11.F-3, inversions do promote urination. However, full inversions at this time are a controversial subject (see Section below), and even *ardha halasana* may have crossed over the line of permissibility in some teacher's eyes.

Many recent studies [337] have focused on the effects of exercise on the menstrual cycle and have found significant effects. Women who exercise regularly and vigorously have two to four times the rates of oligomenorrhea (scanty periods) or amenorrhea (no periods) than do otherwise sedentary women. Moreover, the oligomenorrhea is accompanied by significant bone loss, with estrogen levels depressed and cortisol levels elevated (see Section 8.G, Osteoporosis, page 269, and Section 6.C, The Sympathetic Nervous System, page 144). Amenorrheic women athletes at age 25 can have the spinal bone mineralization characteristic of women of age 57 due to their low estrogen levels. However, oligomenorrhea is rapidly reversible when a young woman returns to a less demanding exercise schedule. For women who are having menstrual difficulties due to intense overtraining in their athletic specialty, the introduction of a *yogasana* practice can be an acceptable mode of restoration and recovery.

Inversions at That Time of the Month

Long before the menstruation process was understood scientifically, the ancient yogic texts explained that during menstruation there is a strong downward flow of *apana* energy, and that this natural direction

of flow is upset by inversion. Today, there is general agreement among yoga teachers [216, 217, 293, 406, 413] that full inversions are contraindicated during the menstrual period. By "full inversions", we mean *sirsasana*, *sarvangasana*, *halasana*, all manner of hand balances and all of their variations. Only MacMullen [293] demurs from outright prohibition of inversions during menstruation, saying that up-to-date (1990) data is not available on this question. Geeta Iyengar holds that inversions can arrest the menstrual flow as they dry up the uterus. She does open the door somewhat however, in saying that such an action actually may be beneficial if the flow is of an overly long duration or occurs at a time out-of-sync with the normal flow [217].

As for why inversions are forbidden at this time, Schatz first pointed out that the ligaments from which the uterus is suspended carry both the thin-walled veins transporting blood out of the uterus and the stout-walled arteries which carry blood into the uterus [406, 413]. Upon inversion, gravitational stresses in the ligaments of the uterus act to stretch them and so reduce blood flow through the collapsible veins, but not through the arteries. As a result, the uterus becomes engorged with blood, leading to increased menstrual flow. This argument seems reasonable, but its conclusion is opposite to that of Geeta Iyengar who states that the flow is retarded by inversions. Lasater [269] argues that inversion blocks the flow of blood to the uterus, thus decreasing or even stopping the flow, but that heavy bleeding then may begin a few hours after the flow has slowed. Clennell [71a] points out that inversion at the time of menstruation promotes holding of the unwanted material within the body and then its absorption, rather than expulsion.

The older ideas that inversions during menstruation act to promote endometriosis and/or pelvic infection have been convincingly countered by Schatz [412], who shows them to be misconceptions in light of newer data. However, she does recommend strongly that women do not invert at this time, as it would be working against the self-understanding (svadhyaya [209]) toward which we strive in yogasana practice.

During menstruation, there is tissue damage and therefore the release of prostaglandins locally (Section 10.D, Pain, page 294) [293]. These hormones not only sensitize the free nerve endings that signal "pain" to the higher cerebral centers, but also act to seal off the bleeding area. In doing so, they vasoconstrict the arteries so strongly that the arteries can go into spasm, thereby generating the feeling of menstrual cramps. Inasmuch as aspirin works to reduce prostaglandin production, it can be effective in reducing these menstrual symptoms, just as it can help reduce the arterial spasms of a migraine headache. Lower-back pain felt during menstruation is said to be referred pain (Section 10.E, Dermatomes and Referred Pain, page 303) from the uterus [293].

Rolf [386] mentions another point relevant to doing sirsasana in or around the menstrual period. She reports that some women experience pain elicited by pressure on a circular area about 1 inch in diameter at the very crown of the head, and assigns this to a menstrual disturbance of fascia in the congested region which propagates to fascial tissue at the top of the head. Right or wrong, it is a factor to keep in mind when women want to do sirsasana during menstruation.

SECTION 19.B. PREGNANCY

The main focus of the practicing yogasana student who becomes pregnant must shift from meeting the challenges of their practice to doing what is most protective of the baby. With this in mind, one does not work so as to become tired or fatigued, and

one does not work so hard that one is distressed during pregnancy. That is to say, the pregnant student's yogasana practice will have to be ratcheted down a few notches, as she now has something even more important to focus on: the successful outcome of her pregnancy. At this time, she would be wise to continue what she is doing, but at a less vigorous level, and to not start anything new.

During the nine months of pregnancy, the most critical period is the first three months, the time during which the embryo implants in the uterus. Women who have a history of miscarriage or of cervical insufficiency should not start yoga during this period, and experienced students who are in this category should do no unsupported standing poses during this time. Yoshikawa [483] recommends no inversions for a pregnant woman in her second and third trimesters, however she allows that this will depend upon the woman's experience and condition.

The general effects of pregnancy on the body of interest to yogasana students involve changes of numerous hormonal levels, all acting to prepare the body for delivery of a healthy baby, and the effects of the growing pressure within the thorax as the baby and the uterus increase in size. As discussed in Subsection 19.A, The Menstrual Cycle, page 453, the level of estrogen is low at the time of conception, whereas that of progesterone is high. These factors are discussed below.

The Balance Between Estrogen and Progesterone

The condition of the female reproductive apparatus is dictated in part by the relative amounts of circulating estrogen and progesterone, two steroid hormones of closely similar molecular structures, but with rather opposite effects. As regards pregnancy, estrogen will work to contract the uterus and expel the fetus, whereas progesterone works against this tendency. Early in the pregnancy, progesterone rules the physiology, but with time, estrogen gains the upper hand, and with that, the delivery process (parturition) is set in motion [435].

In the early stages of pregnancy, the uterus is a relaxed bag of disconnected smooth-muscle cells separated by collagenous tissue, and closed at its cervical neck by a ring of tough collagen fibers. As delivery draws near and the estrogen from the placenta begins to exert itself by rising in concentration, the uterus synthesizes a protein called connexin that acts to connect the muscle cells electrically such that, when called upon, they can all contract simultaneously, much as the cells in the atrial chambers or in the ventricles of the heart contract in unison (Section 11.A, Structure and Function of the Heart, page 310).

Additionally, under the influence of estrogen, the uterus becomes outfitted with receptors for the brain hormone oxytocin, which increases the force of uterine contractions, induces delivery, and also produces prostaglandins which work to unravel the collagenous ring in the cervix, allowing it to dilate. The hormone oxytocin also acts on the breasts of the new mother, encouraging the flow of milk.

The hormonal systems of the fetus are active as well at this time, with the adrenal glands producing cortisol which acts to eventually inflate the fetal lungs by removing the amniotic fluid that otherwise fills them. As the fetal brain develops, it also begins to release CRH to its pituitary, which in turn releases ACTH in order to promote cortisol release from the fetal adrenal glands. The fetal cortisol in turn stimulates the placenta to produce yet more CRH, but on the maternal side. This CRH then acts on the fetal adrenal glands, making them manufacture estrogen! It is the concentration of maternal CRH that controls the fetal estrogen production, which then dictates when the delivery process will begin [435].

Many of the hormones involved in the birthing process are involved as well in the stress-related hormonal shift following excitation of the sympathetic nervous system (Section 6.B, The Hypothalamus, page 140), but in that case, there is of course no fetal component and no delivery. On the other hand, there is evidence [259] that excessive muscle tension (sympathetic excitation) in the last few weeks of pregnancy can lead to breech presentation upon delivery, but that in many cases, purposeful relaxation (parasympathetic excitation) can turn the fetus into the more normal head-first presentation for delivery. *Yogasana* practice directed toward relaxation of the muscles and the breath would thus be of great value where a breech birth and caesarian section otherwise might be the case.

If the birth is by caesarian section, light stretching for the incised area may start in two weeks because the abdominal area is highly vascularized and heals quickly, whereas for more weakly vascularized areas following surgery, no stretching should be done for at least three weeks [256].

It is interesting that there are both annual and circadian rhythms to the birthing process in humans. Giving birth at a time of the year that enhances survivability of the baby is achieved by the circadian monitors of the brain which detect the length of the days and so promote fertility at a time 9 months previous to the best delivery date. Furthermore, most deliveries occur between 3:00–4:00 AM, just a few hours previous to the daily arousal boost (Section 21.B, Periodicity of Body Rhythms, page 474).

Muscles, Joints, Ligaments, and Tendons During Pregnancy

The general structures of joints and their associated substructures are discussed in Section 8.E, The Joints, page 260. Special mention must be made here of these structures as they can change considerably when the *yogasana* practitioner becomes pregnant. In preparation for the delivery of the baby, the body produces a hormone called relaxin [256]; as its name implies, relaxin has a relaxing effect on the entire musculoskeletal system, but especially so on the ligaments binding the pubic symphysis together, Fig. 4.F-2. *Yogasanas* such as *malasana*, done with support and with the feet wide apart, also can be used to help open this joint.

The action of relaxin on the pubic symphysis is easy to understand, for this joint must be able to open considerably in order for the baby to pass to the outside, however, relaxin's similar effect on all the other joints of the body can make problems for the *yogasana* student. As the tension within the ligaments binds the joints together, the pregnant student must be careful not to overstretch, or she runs the risk of destabilizing the joints so opened. The arches of the feet are held up by a spring-like ligament, the plantar calcaneonavicular ligament (Fig. 8.D-4), the collagen of which is unraveled by relaxin, with the result that the arches tend to fall and the foot can grow longer by a full shoe size during pregnancy [256].

As pregnancy proceeds, the abdominal muscles are stretched intensely so as to make room for the growing fetus. For this reason, one should do no *yogasana* work that calls for further stretching of these muscles (deep backbends, for example), and on the other hand, any pose that acts to tighten the abdominal muscles (*navasana*, for example) is also contraindicated, for one can ill afford to have the abdominal muscles contract prematurely.

In Lasater's most recent writing on the subject of *yogasana* and pregnancy [274], she expresses the opinion that though many students perform inversions routinely while pregnant without any apparent problems,

there is nonetheless a risk to the fetus involved in this, and that it is better to forgo all risks and just postpone inversions until after the birth. Risks include a breech presentation at delivery, and entanglement of the fetus in the placental cord, both brought about by the unnaturalness of the mother's inverted position.

The ability of a pregnant woman to balance will be changing rapidly as she adds 35–50 pounds of weight in a very asymmetric way. Standing on one leg for any length of time is especially to be avoided as this puts too much weight on the leg. On the other hand, during pregnancy, the body can be deficient in calcium having given so much to the baby, and this can lead to leg cramps, as can the low level of circulation in the legs (see *Respiratory and Cardiovascular Systems* below). In the latter case, wall-supported standing poses are recommended for avoiding such cramps.

Respiratory and Cardiovascular Systems

In response to the growing pressure that the fetus and uterus put on the ribs and diaphragm, the respiration rate increases, and at the same time, the soft tissues of the nose swell and make breathing difficult. At this point the pregnant yoga student needs to practice relaxing the breath, for this will be basic to all delivery techniques. As the size of the fetus increases, there will be more and more pressure put on the diaphragm, until in the final stage of pregnancy, breathing must involve the intercostal muscles much more, for the range of motion of the diaphragm is severely limited (Subsection 12.A, *Using the Diaphragm and Ribs to Breathe*, page 362).

The pressure of the baby on the femoral vein (Fig. 11.C-2) tends to trap blood in the legs and leads to swelling. If one chooses to do inversions at this time, the swelling is best relieved by inversions such as *sirs-*

asana, sarvangasana, or *viparita karani,* which also serve to reduce the constipation resulting from the pressure of the fetus on the intestines (however, see below). Blood that passes upward through the femoral veins empties eventually into the inferior vena cava, a large vein paralleling the spine and resting just anterior to it. There is danger during pregnancy that this important vein might be compressed by the weight of the fetus when the mother lies on her back for any length of time, especially after the fifth month. Because closing of the inferior vena cava takes so much blood out of circulation, the student may have a sense of light-headedness, dizziness or nausea as the amount of oxygen reaching the brain is inadequate. Even if no symptoms are evident, it is still a risk since the baby may be deprived of oxygen even though the mother feels no symptoms. Thus the necessary relaxing poses must be done on an inclined plane or while lying on the side body.

The Nervous and Digestive Systems

As the level of the hormone progesterone increases in the body of the pregnant student, the peristaltic action within the intestines (Subsection 18.A, page 447) decreases while the rising levels of relaxin lead to both constipation and indigestion. Furthermore, relaxin acts on the sphincter between the esophagus and the stomach to loosen its collagen fibers and so allows it to leak stomach acid into the esophagus, leading to massive heartburn.

The pressure of the growing fetus tends to press on the sciatic nerve as it passes out of the lumbo-sacral area, thereby generating pain in the buttocks and legs. This, however, can be relieved by the standard *yogasanas* that free the sciatic nerve from pressure by the piriformis muscle, Section 4.E, page 95. Carpal tunnel syndrome also can appear during pregnancy.

In terms of the autonomic nervous system, one wants to practice so as to relax the body during pregnancy, which is to say, work so as to shift the arousal away from the sympathetic side and toward the parasympathetic (Chapter 6, THE AUTONOMIC NERVOUS SYSTEM, page 133).

SECTION 19.C. MENOPAUSE

At about 40 to 50 years of age, nature begins to shut down the production of estrogen and progesterone by the ovaries, and menstruation becomes scanty and then stops. This change of hormonal activity, termed menopause, may require 2 to 5 years to run its course. Menopause is a natural stage in the life cycle of the female, and when viewed appropriately, it can show her much about who she is and who she is about to become. It certainly is not to be viewed as a disease or a medical crisis of any sort, though there are strong cultural influences directing how women might respond to this event.

The symptoms of menopause are many and varied, but most if not all of them relate to the relatively rapid changes of hormonal levels that characterize menopause. These symptoms include hot flashes (the most infamous symptom), mood swings, depression, night sweats, urinary problems, vaginal dryness, aching joints, reduced libido, and weight gain [269, 450].

When the amount of estrogen from the ovaries starts to decrease, the deficit can be made up by the production of this hormone by the adrenals and kidneys, if they have not been exhausted prematurely by stress [269]. Spinal twists and soft backbending can be used to stimulate the adrenals and kidneys at the time of menopause. During the period of low estrogen and progesterone, a more normal level of these compounds can be achieved by taking them from external sources, *i.e.,* hormone replacement therapy

(HRT). This medical approach decreases the risks of osteoporosis (Section 8.G, page 269) and heart disease, while increasing the risk slightly for breast cancer. If nothing is done to treat menopausal symptoms, a woman's body chemistry will slowly drift toward that of men, with disease patterns and frequencies much like those of older men [450].

Among the many symptoms that accompany the shift of hormonal activity in women at menopause, certain of these relate directly to *yogasana* practice in that they are either symptoms that impact on performance, and/or are antidotal for such symptoms. Several such effects that will especially interest the *yogasana* practitioner are listed below [450].

1) The major component of connective tissue (Subsection 9.A, page 273) is collagen, and estrogen receptors have been found on the fibroblasts that manufacture this structural material. As the estrogen concentration in the body drops after menopause, the quantity of collagen made by the fibroblasts decreases and so connective tissue becomes weaker, as do the bones and skin.

2) Declining levels of estrogen upset the balance between the bone-building cells (the osteoblasts) and the bone-destroying cells (the osteoclasts) in the body, in favor of the latter. The result is weak bones (wrist, vertebrae, and hip), subject to fracture more often than would occur otherwise. Strengthening of the bones during the premenopausal years through consistent *yogasana* practice will minimize the heightened risk of osteoporosis during and after menopause, Section 8.G, Osteoporosis, page 269.

3) With declining hormonal production, the muscular system loses strength, bulk, and stamina, and the joints may become stiff and painful. Again, *yogasana* practice can prevent or reverse these symptoms. Remember, at this point in life, that repair of muscle injuries will be slowed considerably,

so that one must not exceed one's capacity to work physically.

4) Hot flashes appear to be caused by the hormonal imbalance incurred when the ovaries are in the process of shutting down. This imbalance upsets the hypothalamus, which controls heart rate, sweating, and body temperature. When in this state, the heart rate increases, sweating may be profuse, and heat moves from the core of the body to the skin, where the temperature may increase by up to 7° F (hot flashes). These symptoms suggest a general activation of the sympathetic nervous system, Section 6.C, page 144, and that the yogic response for these symptoms would be strongly on the side of those *yogasanas* that are activating for the parasympathetic nervous system and therefore cooling.

Indeed, the cooling inversions such as *sarvangasana*, *niralamba sarvangasana*, and *viparita karani* are strongly recommended to moderate hot flashes [112, 269] as poses such as these lower heart rate, blood pressure, and promote vasodilation while reducing the hormones that cause retention of water and salt. Inversions stabilize the hormonal systems, and so are useful in all hormonal problems, menopausal or not.

5) Sweating is a mechanism whereby the body rids itself of heat through evaporation (Subsection 10.F, *The Sweat Glands*, page 307), however, the sweat glands do not seem to work as they normally did prior to menopause, for they now sweat profusely during hot flashes, yet there does not seem to be much of a cooling effect. Hot flashes at night are known as night sweats. In this case, sleep is very disturbed, with decreased REM durations, however, some measure of bodily rest nonetheless can be achieved through relaxing *yogasana* postures such as *savasana, etc.*

6) In the premenopausal female, the heart-healthy ratio of the waist-to-hip meas-

urement is less than 0.8. However, with the onset of menopause, the body's fat distribution will move toward that of men, the ratio in question will exceed 0.8, and the risk of cardiovascular problems will increase rapidly so as to approach that of men, unless one is involved in an active exercise program.

7) There are many sites on the surfaces of brain cells which are receptors for estrogen. When menopausal and beyond, the low levels of estrogen can negatively impact the ability to think, to perceive, to resist anxiety, and they can act to reduce the mental flexibility needed to accept new ideas. Low estrogen decreases the libido and raises the threshold for sexual arousal.

8) The brain's control of muscles, joints, and movement from within the cerebellum is very strongly dependent upon the levels of circulating estrogen in the body. When estrogen levels are low, tasks requiring fine control over these physical entities will be impaired. As nerve conduction slows with age, balance will be impaired, and memory also will wane.

With a life expectancy of 81 years, a woman can look forward to enjoying more than one-third of her life following menopause. Though the time of menopause is one of hormonal imbalance and emotional instability, once past menopause, a certain emotional/hormonal stability sets in that increases one's ability to focus on life's goals. It can be a time of peaceful introspection and accomplishment.

SECTION 19.D. SEXUAL FUNCTION

It is fascinating that the same hormones that function in the woman's body to signal the onset of puberty are also working in the man's body to the same end. In the young male as in the young female, at about age 12 to 14 there is a release of hormones from the hypothalamus to the pituitary gland, leading to the eventual production of the gonadotropins, FSH and LH. In the male body, the FSH promotes sperm production and maturation, whereas LH directs the production of testosterone and the secondary male characteristics: the male pattern of muscle and bone growth, enlargement of the sex organs, growth of coarse body hair, male pattern baldness, and an enlarged larynx [229, 473]. In the female's body, the generation of the gonadotropins leads to the appearance of breasts, pubic hair, a feminine voice and broader hips.

Testosterone in the male body increases the libido (sexual interest), and when it is present at only low levels, the libido too is depressed. There is no direct link between testosterone and the ability to have an erection [340a].

On reaching sexual maturity, sperm are manufactured in the testes, and stored there. Though the ovaries work best at body temperature (98.6º F, 37.0º C), this is too warm for the sperm in the testes, and so they are stored in the scrotal sac, outside the body where it is cooler. The testes prefer a temperature closer to 95º F, but in cold weather or when threatened by a blow, can be lifted reflexively more or less completely into the body for warmth or safety.

A large part of the mass of the penis consists of a spongy tissue carrying a large number of arteries, the smooth muscles of the artery walls being normally contracted due to sympathetic excitation. On sexual excitation, there is a shift to parasympathetic dominance which releases the muscle tone in the arterial walls of the penis, and it becomes engorged with blood. As with many situations of vasodilation, that in the penis leading to an erection involves the simple molecule nitric oxide. At the same time, the veins by which the arterial blood would exit the penis are compressed and so the blood is held in place in the erect penis. Exactly the same mechanism is at work in the female clitoris on excitation.

Circumstances that stimulate the sympathetic nervous system such as chronic stress, cold, fear, *etc.*, have a shrinking effect on the penis. In such cases, *yogasanas* performed to ease the level of stress also will have a beneficial effect on the man's virility. During the recurrent REM phases of sleep (Subsection 21.B, *The Sleep/Wake Cycle and Relaxation*, page 488), the sympathetic stress is turned off, and both men and women will experience periods of high sexual excitement 5–6 times per night.

As might have been expected, the hypothalamus plays a significant role in sexual arousal. In males, the preoptic area within the anterior portion of the hypothalamus, Fig. 6.B-1, is most critical for male sexual behavior. This nucleus is larger in males than in females, contains receptors for testosterone, and is excitatory for the parasympathetic nervous system. In females, Fig. 6.B-1, it is the ventromedial nucleus in the central portion of the hypothalamus that controls sexual behavior. This nucleus contains receptors for both estrogen and progesterone, and has neural connections to the periaqueductal gray area which in turn is connected to the spinal cord by way of the reticular formation. Damage to either the preoptic area in men or the ventromedial area in women will have profound effects on sexual behavior.

When there is physical stimulation of the penis, there is a reflexive action involving inhibitory interneurons that turns the sympathetic system off and stimulates the erection-generating centers between S3 and T12 in the lower spine [165]. Males in whom the spinal cord has been cut below the hypothalamus can still respond to genital manipulation with erection and ejaculation [120], however, they cannot be stimulated sexually by thinking sexual thoughts, as can men who have an intact connection between their hypothalamus and their penis.

At the moment of ejaculation, the autonomic dominance is said to shift from parasympathetic to sympathetic as striated muscles are energized to propel the sperm through the penis, however, the EEG at the moment of orgasm in both men and women is strongly right-hemisphere centered, as appropriate for parasympathetic release of tension [73]. As with *pranayama* and a sneeze, orgasm tends to open both nostrils.

Chapter 20

THE EMOTIONS

In this Section, three generally recognized and related mood disorders, depression, mania and anxiety, will be discussed along with the impact *yogasana* practice might have on them. That *yogasana* could be in any way prescriptive for these disorders is suggested by the fact that the symptoms for all three appear in part to involve the autonomic nervous system (Chapter 6, page 133), a system susceptible to control and change through *yogasana* practice. Because the emotions and the immune system are under the control of the autonomic nervous system, it is no surprise that the emotions have been shown repeatedly to have an impact on the immune system (Chapter 13, page 383). Similarly, it is understandable that mood and respiration have a reciprocally strong effect on one another [27], and that a particular mood can be strongly lateralized in the cerebrum. In regard the latter point, it is known that injection of sodium amital into the right carotid artery leads to a brief sense of elation, whereas injecting the same substance into the left carotid artery produces a momentary depression [225].

Of all the human senses, the olfactory system is unique in that its sensations are delivered directly to the amygdala, the emotional center within the brain, and to the hippocampus, a memory center within the brain. Thus the memory of past odors is strongly tied to emotional responses. Freud maintained that once we stood erect and lifted our noses away from the ground, our sense of smell began to degrade, leading to repression and mental illness.

It is one of the strong points of *yogasana* therapy that the *yogasanas* also are intimately tied to our emotions. Because unexpressed emotions, with their strong connection to the limbic system in the brain (Subsection 3.A, page 33), often are stored as muscular tension in the body (often in the shoulders, stomach, lower back, and jaw [345]), the release of muscular tension through *yogasana* frequently is accompanied by the release of emotional tension. The emotions that can lead to muscle tension include pleasure, pain, anger, rage, fear, sorrow, aggression, and sexual feelings.

Judging from the low rates of cure for emotional disorders such as depression, mania, and anxiety, and the variable responses to a particular drug, it appears that there are many varieties of each of these emotional disorders. Consequently, the effective *yogasana* routines might well be rather different for people suffering from what otherwise appear to be identical disorders. Nonetheless, there are certain broad areas in which *yogasana* can play a positive role. In almost every case, it seems true that the sooner an emotional disorder is treated, the more quickly it is overcome. Moreover, almost all of the drug therapies suffer from important side effects, which would be absent in a yogic course of treatment. Finally, *yogasana* practice can rebalance the autonomic nervous system, leading to a diminution of the symptoms of emotional disorder even if it does not cure it outright.

SECTION 20.A. DEPRESSION

Symptoms

Imagine the self-portrait of Vincent Van Gogh showing an old man with his head in his hands. This is a graphical depiction of the mental state of depression, and indeed, Van Gogh died by suicide. The depressed posture is one in which the body is bent forward at the waist, with the chest and the head bent forward, much like a beginner in *paschimottanasana*. The posture resembles as well the defensive postural reflex described in Subsection 7.D, *The Flexional Tonic Reflex*, page 214.

In addition to the postural, other physical symptoms of depression can include losses of appetite, energy, sexual desire, and memory, as well as excessive sadness, restlessness, retardation of thoughts and actions, constipation, decreased salivation and diurnal variation of the severity of symptoms [225, 333]. Five percent of the world's population suffers from major depressive illness [225], and in the United States, the rate of depression is twice as high among women than it is among men. Depression is the most common cause of headache [117], Subsection 3.B, *Headaches*, page 37. If the depression is not too deep, psychotherapy is about as effective as medication in curing the disorder, with placebos (Subsection 6.F, page 164) running not too far behind in effectiveness.

The mental/emotional aspects of the symptoms of depression are contained within Hamlet's words "How weary, stale, flat and unprofitable seem to me all the uses of this world." He spoke of symptoms that include a pervasive unpleasant mood, intense mental pain, inability to experience pleasure, generalized loss of interest in all things, difficulty in concentrating, indecisiveness, feelings of worthlessness and guilt, pessimistic thoughts and thoughts of dying and suicide [225, 333].

The broad category of depression has been divided into exogenous (reactive) and endogenous (physical) subclasses. In the former, there is an external precipitating event of great stress (loss of a loved one, loss of a job, *etc.*) in which the normal period of grief fails to come to an end, while in the latter, there is no external trigger. In both cases, there are strong genetic tendencies toward the illness. The general symptoms for exogenous and endogenous depression are listed in Table 20.A-1, but the dichotomy is not as sharp as implied by this Table.

The tidy picture painted up to this point is upset by the 15% of depressed patients who show symptoms opposite to those given in Table 20.A-1. In cases of atypical depression, patients show overeating and weight gain, extended sleeping periods and depression worse in the evening hours than in the morning! More will be said of this below.

Medicine Versus Depression

Many of the brain circuits use synapses involving serotonin, dopamine, and/or norepinephrine as neurotransmitters, and when there is a loss of activity in such circuits due to low neurotransmitter levels (see Section 5.D, The Neurotransmitters, page 128), the result often is depression. In contrast, the neurotransmitter acetylcholine is present in high concentrations in the brains of the depressed [153]. Because of the obvious link between the autonomic nervous system, the *yogasanas*, and norepinephrine (Section 6.C, The Sympathetic Nervous System, page 144), our discussion will focus on that part of depression involving norepinephrine. It is clear however, that low serotonin and dopamine levels also can be important factors in depression, and their involvement along with norepinephrine possibly explains

TABLE 20.A-1. COMPARISON OF THE CHARACTERISTICS OF EXOGENOUS AND ENDOGENOUS DEPRESSION [225]

Feature	Exogenous Depression	Endogenous Depression
Onset	Any age, but often below 40	Over 40
Recent stress	Yes	No
Familial depression	Absent	Present
Mood variation	Worse late in day	Worse in morning
Sleep pattern	Difficulty in falling asleep, but then stays asleep	Insomnia, middle of night or early morning; short REM phase
Appetite	May increase or decrease	None
Weight change	Little or no loss	Rapid loss; anorexia
Physical ailments	Fewer, less severe	Many, more severe
Mental activity	Mild slowing	Moderate to severe slowing
Attitudes	Self-pity, pessimism	Self-blame, remorse, guilt
Self-esteem	No loss	Complete loss
Interest	Mild/moderate loss	Pervasive loss in everything
Suicidal	Occasional	Common
Psychomotor level	Calm	Agitated
Mental pain	None	Considerable
Response to pleasure	Normal	None (anhedonia)

why there are so many different symptoms tied to this problem.

The route to the more common exogenous depression starts with the response of the body to stress; in this case, the hypothalamus releases CRF (corticotropin releasing factor) to the pituitary which in turn releases ACTH (adrenocorticotrophic hormone) into the blood stream, Fig. 15.B-1. On reaching the kidneys, the ACTH then acts on the adrenal cortex (see Section 6.C, The Sympathetic Nervous System, page 144), to eventually release among other things, the powerful chemical cortisol into the blood stream. Cortisol then promotes physiological changes to support the fight-or-flight response. The above can be called the hypothalamic-pituitary-adrenal (HPA) axis working under the prod of stress [333].

The cortisol produced by the HPA axis prompts the body to shut down all functions not related to self-protection. As cortisol delivers fuel to the muscles and heightens awareness, it also depresses the appetites for food and sex. Chronic excitation along the HPA axis is cause for depression. Indeed, in depressed patients, both the adrenals and the pituitary glands are enlarged, and cortisol is hyperexcreted, while the CRF levels in the cerebrospinal fluid also are high. It appears, then, that certain types of depression can be the result of a dysfunction along the HPA axis. Unusually high levels of cortisol also appear to mask the normal circadian rhythm of cortisol production (Section 21.B, page 474), and so lead to the desynchronization of other secondary oscillators in the body which otherwise are entrained with the cortisol rhythm.

Viewed in terms of the sympathetic-parasympathetic balance, the above explanation based upon high cortisol levels and low levels of the catecholamines would lead one to think that depression is a consequence of parasympathetic dominance, as can be seen by comparing Table 20.A-1 with Table 6.A-2.* It is to be noted however, that there is a negative feedback loop involving cortisol, Fig. 15.B-1, in which high levels of cortisol *inhibit* further release of ACTH from the pituitary, thus stabilizing high levels of cortisol in the blood as long as the stress continues.

At the same time that the cortisol level is being elevated via the adrenal cortex, the levels of epinephrine and norepinephrine in the brain are being depressed due to inactivity of the adrenal medulla, which otherwise floods the body with these hormones during times of stress by way of the sympathetic nervous system (Section 6.F, The Effects of Emotion and Attitudes on Stress, page 160). Because it is the symptoms of parasympathetic dominance that are most obvious in depression, any treatment that can raise the concentration of norepinephrine in the brain or increase its effectiveness is likely to have a positive influence on the course of treatment for depression.

In line with the "diagnosis" of depression as involving parasympathetic dominance [343], the standard medical treatment consists of giving drugs that either block the reuptake of norepinephrine from the brain's synapses or block the enzymes that otherwise clear norepinephrine from the synapses. In either case, the result is a higher, longer-lasting level of norepinephrine in the synapses of the brain, and a decrease in the symptoms of depression. Stimulation of the sympathetic branch of the autonomic nervous system [309, 360] leading to the release of the catecholamines also is effective. To the extent that depression is a response to a depleted level of norepinephrine in the brain, it is thought that an excess of norepinephrine in the brain leads to mania [333], Section 20.B, Mania and Bipolar Disorder, page 469.

Because the cortisol levels in some types of depression are chronically high whereas the catecholamine levels are depressed at

* There is evidence as well that some forms of depression relate to left-nostril dominance, whereas right-nostril dominance leads to hyperactivity/mania [120]. This is in accord with breathing through the left nostril promoting parasympathetic excitation in the right cerebral hemisphere, and breathing through the right nostril promoting sympathetic excitation in the left cerebral hemisphere (see Section 12.C, Nasal Laterality, page 374). Electroconvulsive therapy done only to the right cerebral hemisphere is extremely effective in curing depression while leaving the memory intact [153].

Brain-excitation studies [385] confirm the cerebrolateral nature of depression, for it is found that in depressed subjects there is a high level of alpha-wave activity in the left cerebral hemisphere (Section 3.E, Brainwaves and The Electroencephalogram, page 57) and a correspondingly low level on the right. Recall that alpha-wave activity is a signal for a deeply relaxed mental state, and that the left hemisphere is normally alert and charged with energy. This imbalance in alpha-wave activity is thought to arise from the breakdown of communication between the amygdala (the emotional center) in the brainstem and the relevant prefrontal cortices. The left prefrontal area that is so alpha-wave active in depressed patients is very inactive in subjects who are deeply in love. Interestingly, people who report high levels of happy feelings have larger and more active left prefrontal cortices than do the depressed [364]. Related evidence for the effects of brainwave activity on the occurrence of depression is given in Subsection 3.E, *Brainwave Frequencies and Mental Functioning*, page 60).

One wonders how the symptoms of atypical depression might be related to the 70% of left-handed people who have their dominant hemisphere for speech on the right side rather than on the left as do the 96% of right-handed people, Table 3.C-1. That is to say, perhaps those with atypical depression have atypical stimulation of the "wrong" hemisphere, and so show symptoms opposite to those expected.

the same time, it appears that the hormonal system under stress can be activated to produce cortisol, while at the same time the sympathetic nervous system is inactive and so produces an insufficiency of the catecholamines. This selective excitation of the adrenal cortex with respect to the adrenal medulla relates to our differing responses to situations that are seen as either a "threat" or a "challenge".

As for serotonin, it too seems out of balance in depressed people, and as with norepinephrine, drugs that maintain high levels of serotonin in the synapses can be effective in relieving depression. The neural paths that rely on norepinephrine and serotonin as neurotransmitters occur frequently in the limbic area. Therefore, deficiencies in these substances often lead to problems that have to do with emotions, appetite, or thought processing, all features of the limbic brain.

By involving the autonomic nervous system in depression, one implicitly involves the hypothalamus. Indeed, there is substantial evidence for the role that this organ plays in depression [225]. The early-morning rise of cortisol levels to abnormal levels in the depressed is known to originate with the release of CRF from the hypothalamus. In turn, the drugs that are effective in reducing the symptoms of depression work on the pathways in the locus ceruleus, a region in the brain which then activates the hypothalamus.

That the autonomic nervous system is tied to the problems of depression (and anxiety as well, Section 20.C, Anxiety, page 470) also is suggested by the observation that depressed people can fall asleep easily, but awaken at 4:00 to 5:00 AM with a depression headache and cannot return to sleep. Anxiety sufferers, on the other hand, have headaches in the evening and cannot fall asleep. These times of headache onset correspond in a striking way with the shifts of the autonomic nervous system from parasympathetic dominance to sympathetic dominance (between 4:00 to 6:00 AM, Fig. 21.B-3) and the reverse shift in the time period 5:00 to 8:00 PM, signaling a shift from sympathetic to parasympathetic dominance. Many symptoms of depression can be relieved for a short time by depriving oneself of sleep, for sleep is a very parasympathetic activity.

Once depressed, the depression exerts its effects on other systems of the body. Thus, severe depression correlates with a reduced functioning of the suppressor T cells of the immune system [346], and to death due to heart-related causes. If the depression is not too deep, then psychotherapy is about as effective as medication in curing the condition.

Yogasana Versus Depression

Given that both exogenous and endogenous depressions exhibit parasympathetic, right-hemispheric dominance, it is clear how certain *yogasanas* can work to dispel depression. Meyers [310], for example, has given a *yogasana* sequence designed especially for combating depression: it features many back-bending poses of long duration, both passive and active, along with vigorous handbalancing, and finally restful back-bending relaxations with the eyes open. Walden [474] presents a softer series of chest openings for relieving depression, but also encourages strong inhalations and a mental focus on the body in order to increase the prominence of the sympathetic nervous system [479]. Such chest-opening *yogasanas* are known to be energizing and warming, leading to increased circulation and heart rate, with the blood moving to the surface of the body to cool it [60], that is to say, stimulating to the sympathetic nervous system. As there is often an immunosuppression of the T cells (Chapter 13, THE IMMUNE SYSTEM, page 383) in cases of severe depression, it is no surprise that the *yogasanas* which are most effective in relieving depression are also the ones that act to revitalize the immune system.* If, however, a student showed signs of atypical depression, then the *yogasanas* would have to work the other end of the autonomic spectrum, stimulating the parasympathetic response.

A possible mechanism connecting backbending, EEG shifts, and depression is put forth in Subsection 3.E, *Brainwave Frequencies and Mental Functioning*, page 60. As depression involves an imbalance of the cerebral hemispheres, *yogasana* therapy for depression would be even more effective if the arousing postures could be done with a strong left-side accent (perhaps the above routine for depression, but with the left nostril blocked as done by Shannahoff-Khalsa and Beckett in dealing with obsessive-compulsive disorder [423]) in order to energize the right cerebral hemisphere and so decrease its alpha-wave activity. See Subsection 3.E, *Brainwave Frequencies and Mental Functioning*, page 60, for a possible way in which poses such as *urdhva dhanurasana* can help cure depression.

Not only will the backbending program work to banish that part of depression involving the autonomic nervous system, but in opening the chest, it may also reveal buried emotions and fears [242] which can leave the student feeling sad at first, but later relieved if the emotions are dealt with and then set aside. This obvious link between the physiological and the emotional works the other way as well, for there may well be hidden fears which keep us from opening the abdominal and solar plexus regions in backbends until those fears are confronted and rationalized (see Section 7.D, *Reflex Actions*, page 211). In such cases, attitude toward backbending may be critical [242].

In regard attitude and the *yogasanas*, note that if the performance of a *yogasana* is seen as a threat and so is laced with an attitude of fear, then excess cortisol will be released by the initial action of the hypothalamus, but release of the catecholamines will be repressed, whereas if the attitude is one of a welcome challenge, then only the catecholamines will be released and the high cortisol levels characteristic of depression do not appear.

Physiological studies on the effects of "hatha yoga" exercise have shown that they not only can combat depression temporarily, but are antidotes for anger, tension, sleeplessness, and fatigue [314, 364]. Psychologically, remember that "When we're feeling depressed, we long for genuine connections with others who accept us as we are, and we often can find that in yoga class" [479].

Colored Lights Versus Depression

There is general agreement that regular physical activity is associated with decreases in depression and anxiety for all ages and in both sexes [337], and this would include performing the *yogasanas*. It may be that the euphoria and sense of well-being that follow a *yogasana* practice are manifestations of the alpha waves that are known to be generated in the EEG pattern (see Subsection 3.E, *Brainwaves and The Electroencephalogram*, page 57) during moderate exercise, and which persist long after the exercise is finished. It is known that exercise increases norepinephrine and serotonin in the brain.

---

*There is also a very important time factor in the treatment of depression. Once the depressed attitudes become entrenched, even achieving the appropriate neurotransmitter balance will become an effective cure only a long time thereafter. The symptoms of depression are most easily combated in the early stages of their development [153].

Notice that the daily depressive low for those suffering from exogenous depression comes at the end of the day, just when cortisol levels are lowest (see Subsection 21.B, *Physiological Peaks and Valleys in the 24-Hour Period*, page 476). This suggests that if done with the proper attitude, backbending at this time of the day might have its largest positive effect (Subsection 21.B, *Yogasana and Chronotherapy*, page 486). To further stimulate the sympathetic system (see Subsection 16.D, *Color Therapy*, page 426), one could also introduce red-colored lights, as red is known to stimulate the sympathetic response. Similarly, the relaxed *yogasanas* recommended for the treatment of anxiety and mania would be even more effective if performed with blue lights.

Yet another aspect of depression is that experienced on a yearly basis. When the daylight hours are shorter and the sun is not so bright, the amount of ultraviolet light entering the eyes throughout the day is insufficient, and seasonal affective disorder (SAD) results. The SAD symptoms are much like those of depression. However, in this case, there are direct neural connections between the retina of the eyes and the suprachiasmatic nuclei within the hypothalamus, so that direct viewing of supplemental ultraviolet light is effective in lifting the depression (Subsection 16.D, *Color Therapy*, page 426).

SECTION 20.B. MANIA AND BIPOLAR DISORDER

Symptoms

If the catecholamine neurotransmitters in the brain are present in too high concentrations, then the mood symptoms are those of mania, and if the concentrations of the neurotransmitters change from too low to too high and back again, then a bipolar disorder is in full swing.

Approximately 25% of those showing major depression symptoms (Table 20.A-1) will also show periods of manic (euphoric) mood, with symptoms which are just opposite to those shown in the Table. In the manic phase, this alternating pattern of depression and mania (termed bipolar depression) is characterized by symptoms that may include elevated, expansive or irritable moods, grandiosity, hyperactivity, loquaciousness, increased sexual and physical energies, reckless involvements and little need for sleep [225]. The symptoms in the depression stage of bipolar disorder remain those for the unipolar case. It is generally thought that the manic phase of the bipolar disorder is the body/mind's attempt to keep from sliding into an irreversibly deep depression [47a].

One may swing between the extreme phases of the bipolar situation in a matter of weeks, or it may require years to go from one phase to the other [47a]. As one swings between these emotional extremes, the time at which the core temperature is maximum is 5:00 PM during the depressed phase of a bipolar disorder, but advances to 1:00 PM in the manic phase [321].

Treatment

In bipolar illness, the switch from depression to mania or the reverse can be almost instantaneous or long and drawn out. In the context of the discussion in Section 20.A, page 464, one imagines a rapid or slow shift of the autonomic system between sympathetic and parasympathetic dominance as the cause of the mood swings in bipolar depression. Indeed, the pharmacological treatment for mania is the use of powerful sedatives which inhibit sympathetic dominance.

Lithium is often used to treat mania, but it is not a cure and its mechanism of action is not understood. It is known, however, that lithium has the effect of lengthening the period of the X oscillator when it is free running so as to lengthen the period of the core temperature (see Section 21.B, Periodicity of Body Rhythms, page 474) [321]. That mania is more likely in the bright light of summer [389] may be due to the overstimulation of the hypothalamus by the retina. Were this the case, it would be a reversed SAD reaction (Subsection 16.D, *White-Light Starvation*, page 430).

In those cases where the root cause of mania is sympathetic dominance, the *yogasana* approach to dealing with bipolar disorder is to stress the relaxing and restorative poses, *i.e.*, just the opposite prescription given for depression. Consistency and regularity of one's day-to-day routines is a protective factor in combating bipolar disorder, and so could mean that a daily *yogasana* practice could be of help in overcoming this condition.

SECTION 20.C. ANXIETY

Symptoms

If a stress is a threat not to one's physical being, but instead to one's emotional being, to one's psyche, and at the same time one is afraid to act forcefully against the threat, then the result is anxiety. With anxiety, it is as if one suffers all of the physical symptoms associated with the fight-or-flight response of the sympathetic nervous system, but for a non-physical threat. Anxiety is ever-present in us all, but can reach pathological levels during panic attacks, phobia, obsessive-compulsive behaviors and post-traumatic stress disorder. In normal anxiety, there is a rapid cessation of anxiety symptoms once the stressful event is past, while the situation becomes more pathological if the person continues to hold on to the anxiety long after the event. Anxiety is always about the future [441].

Symptoms of anxiety include muscular trembling, sweating, rigid posture, heart palpitations, cold hands, muscle tension, heightened alertness, avoidance behavior, a feeling of dread, fatigue, and fear of losing one's balance [320]. Anxiety headaches appear at or close to bedtime, as the body swings from sympathetic dominance to parasympathetic dominance (Fig. 21.B-1). Just as depression is characterized by a parasympathetic dominance, anxiety is characterized by a sympathetic dominance which can be countered by taking sedating drugs such as tranquilizers. The characteristic symptoms of anxiety and depression are compared in Table 20.C-1. Note too that a severe case of anxiety is often accompanied by a secondary depression [311], and that anxiety, like depression, is immunosuppressive [346].

TABLE 20.C-1. SYMPTOMS THAT DIFFERENTIATE ANXIETY FROM DEPRESSION [311]

Anxiety	Depression
Hypervigilance	Psychomotor retardation
Severe tension and panic	Severe sadness and anhedonia
Perceived danger	Perceived loss
Doubt and uncertainty	Hopelessness; suicidal thoughts
Insecurity	Self-reproach
Phobic avoidance	Loss of libido

Anxiety and Yogasana

The gamma-motor efferent nervous system is under autonomic control and works to energize the muscles used for posture and balance. Because the gamma system is stimulated by anxiety, this disorder can lead to increased gamma discharge and a general tightening of the muscles [88]. On the other hand, *yogasanas* of the sort that can make us looser in a muscular sense, resulting in muscles of longer resting length (Subsection 7.B, *Resting Muscle Tone*, page 204) also can release feelings of anxiety.

From the yoga point of view, the anxious or panicked student is in need of those *yogasanas* which are relaxing and promote the parasympathetic response, while inhibiting the sympathetic (see [397], for example). A recent study of patients with anxiety has shown significant reduction in anxiety levels when meditating such that thoughts are centered on the body sensations of the moment, and not on external/environmental stimuli [314]. It is thought that, when in a state of relaxation, negative imagery is effectively blocked, thus preventing the right hemisphere from processing any anxiety-producing feelings [256]. Long-term relaxation will reduce anxiety.

Panic attacks are readily brought on by excess CO_2 in the blood, as when hyperventilating by making the inhalation long but the exhalation short. Perhaps improving ventilation through *pranayama* practice could be of help here in dealing with incipient panic attacks, when practiced in conjunction with relaxing and restorative *yogasanas* which promote parasympathetic dominance.

As with depression, those who exercise regularly acquire a demonstrable resistance to pathological anxiety [337]. Interestingly, though the same calming, anti-anxiety effect that is promoted by moderate exercise (*yogasana* for yoga students) also is promoted by meditative rest (*savasana* for yoga students), however, the benefits of exercise are longer lasting than those of meditative relaxation.

Other Disorders

As the emotion of anger is controlled by the hypothalamus, it is no surprise that passive *yogasanas* such as supported *halasana* are effective in defusing anger. As mentioned in Box 7.D-1, *Why Are Backbends Energizing?*, page 216, the emotion of fear can be overcome by the practice of backbending [242].

Obsessive-compulsive disorder (OCD) is thought to be a variety of anxiety disorder of a very recalcitrant type. Recent experiments show that OCD many times involves a lateralized cerebral deficit in the frontal or temporal lobes, and realizing the strong lateral effects of unilateral nostril breathing (Section 12.C, Nasal Laterality, page 374), Shannahoff-Khalsa and Beckett [423] have tested this method of treatment on several OCD patients. As the deficit is in the left cerebral hemisphere, gentle, seated exercises were performed while breathing through the right nostril, with the left nostril closed. Working in this way for one year led to significant reduction of OCD symptoms.

SECTION 20.D. EMOTION AND THE BREATH

The intimate connection between our emotional states and the qualities of the breath are obvious and unmistakable. For example, the holding of the breath in a moment of fear, or sobbing in happiness, *etc.* Fortunately, this bridge between the emotions and the breath can be crossed in both directions, so that the conscious use of the breath also can ease emotional pain [27, 441], as indicated in Table 20.D-1.

TABLE 20.D-1. EMOTIONAL DISTRESS AND THE BREATHING MODES THAT BRING RELIEF [441]

<u>Distress</u>	<u>Breathing Strategy</u>
Anger	As anger builds, divert thoughts to the flow of the breath through the nostrils.
Acute anxiety	Relaxed breath awareness often during the day, perhaps as often as hourly.
Sadness and depression	Breathe in an unbroken flow with breath deep and relaxed, avoiding pauses.
Physical pain	With deep breathing, mentally send the breath to join the pain, rather than fight the pain.

Chapter 21

TIME AND BODY RHYTHMS

SECTION 21.A. THE INNATE SENSE OF TIME

Within each of us, there are two types of clocks, each running at a regular pace, and each independently ticking off time subconsciously. Though many questions still remain, it is now known that one of these clocks rhythmically turns many of our biological processes on and off at characteristic times that stretch from fractions of a second to as long as a year. Often, these rhythms are independent of external input, and otherwise are only weakly dependent on external circumstances. Yet another internal clock within us senses elapsed time intervals, but is neither controlling of any biological process nor is it periodic in time. This Chapter explores the mechanisms by which these clocks operate, the effects of internal-clock time on various body/mind functions, and the relationship of body rhythms to *yogasana* practice.

Many cyclical functions in the body are clearly tuned to astronomical phenomena. Some have periods of a day, a month, or a year, corresponding to the earth's rotational period, the moon's rotational period and the time it takes the earth to circle the sun, respectively, while others are of the order of an hour or much less. For cyclic phenomena, the time elapsed between corresponding peaks is known as the period. For example, if the temperature varies rhythmically and is a maximum at 4:00 AM and again at 4:00 PM and a minimum at 10:00 AM and 10:00 PM, then the period for this rhythm is 12 hours.

In addition to the cyclic nature of our subconscious time sense, we also possess a noncyclical clock, again operating subconsciously, which is involved largely with elapsed time. This noncyclical clock is relevant as well, for as we practice *yogasana*, we become more fulfilled in the moment, and this has the effect of making us more patient in regard to the delayed fulfillment of other needs. With concentration on our practice, small things become less of a distraction, time seems to stretch out ahead of us in a more expansive way [21], and we develop a long-range view of life.

In contrast to periods of rhythmically-timed events, *e.g.*, temperature change, which do not change in any way as one ages, periods of elapsed time which are nonrhythmical, lengthen as we age. As described in earlier Sections, as we do our *yogasana* practice, our muscle response time lengthens, at least when we are younger. It is possible that this lengthening is related to the apparent slowing of the time sense in older students [17], caused by lower dopamine levels in the brain, for lower levels of dopamine can create a sense that time is passing more slowly than real-clock time. The stretching of real time is most obvious when the aged are busy; for example, subjects aged 60–65 who were asked to estimate the passage of 3 minutes while they worked at a clerical task required almost 5 minutes to do so [18].

473

SECTION 21.B. PERIODICITY OF BODY RHYTHMS

The cyclical appearance in time of a biological marker implies an oscillation in time of some controlling physiological function. One can imagine at least two ways in which such a physiological function could oscillate in time. First, a process would oscillate if it were triggered by some external factor which itself was oscillating in time, as for example, the sleep-wake-sleep cycle being triggered by the setting, rising, and setting of the sun with a 24-hour period. In fact, many of the body's rhythms have a 24-hour period, and are driven by this celestial oscillator.

For those phenomena that do not have 24-hour periods, another possibility is the following. Suppose that there are sensors in the body that signal when a certain body condition (blood acidity, for example) is too high, whereas other sensors signal when it is too low. On being triggered, each of the sensors promotes the opposite effect. That is to say, if the low-acidity sensor is activated, it triggers a process that sends the acidity up, whereas if the acidity is already too high, the high-acidity sensor will trigger a process that will send the acidity toward a lower value, Fig. 21.B-1. As shown in the Figure, with the setpoints of the two sensors placed somewhat apart, the acidity of the blood will rise to the upper setpoint level and then be sent to the lower level, which in turn will send it upward again to the upper setpoint. In this way, one sees that the acidity of the blood simply cycles up and down with a period between high-low-high points that depends upon where the acidity setpoints have been placed and how rapidly the system can move between them. This is the mechanism that has been advanced to explain the pulse of the cerebrospinal fluid in the central nervous system (Subsection 4.D, *Yoga and CSF Pulsations of the Medial Suture*, page 94), and would seem to be extendable to other body parameters such as temperature, heart rate, blood pressure, *etc.*, as long as they have high-low setpoints.

Ultradian Rhythms

Body functions that go from peak to valley and return to peak in 22 hours or less are termed "ultradian" [321]. Chief among these are the nasal rhythm in which the nostril used for breathing alternates sides left-to-right-to-left, *etc.*, within a period of about 4 hours (see Section 12.C, Nasal Laterality, page 374), while the cerebral hemispheric dominance also shifts with the same time period (see Section 3.D, Cerebral Hemispheric Laterality, page 49). REM excitation in sleep (Subsection 21.B, *The Sleep/Wake Cycle and Relaxation*, page 488), another ultradian process, has a period of 90 minutes, *i.e.*, it appears every 90 minutes during sleep. If the ultradian rhythms are to keep their peaks constant in time from one day to the next, then their periods must be submultiples of 24 hours, *i.e.*, 12, 8, 6, 4, 3, or 2 hours long. The phenomena of nasal alternation, cerebral hemispheric dominance, and REM excitation meet this expectation, and so have their peaks at the same times each day, all other factors such as bedtime being kept constant.

The periodic release of many hormones in the body shows an ultradian character with a period of somewhat less than 1 hour to somewhat more than 2 hours, and is thought to be related to other autonomic functions of the same periodicity which are governed by the hypothalamus [425]. As we go into puberty, intense spurts of hormones (estrogen for girls, testosterone for boys) are released into the bloodstream at approximately 90-minute intervals. The same internal clock may be driving both the release of insulin and sex hormones in teenagers, as each has a ninety-minute period.

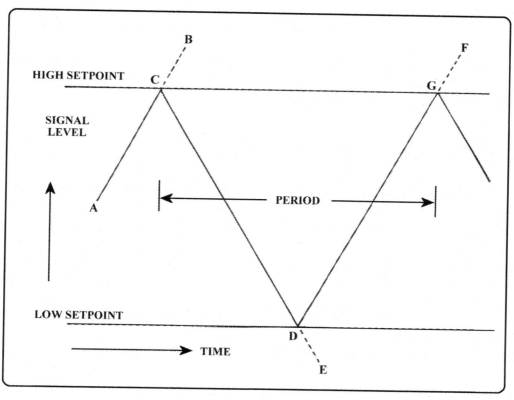

Fig. 21.B-1. Producing a signal oscillating in time using a pair of high-low setpoints. The signal level of some biological condition (temperature, for example) starts at **A** and rises in time toward **B**. However, a high-setpoint sensor is triggered at **C** and reverses the rise, sending the system toward **E** instead. As the system approaches **E**, a low-setpoint sensor is triggered at **D** and sends the system toward **F**. On its way to **F**, the system gets no further than **G**, where the high-setpoint sensor again intercepts it and sends it downward. The result of this action is a temperature that oscillates between the high and low setpoints with a period equal to the time interval between points **C** and **G**.

Of course, the breathing cycle (period *ca.* 10 seconds) and the heart beat (period *ca.* 1 second) are two of the body's key ultradian rhythms. A group of neurons having spontaneous rhythmic activity within the nucleus ambiguus of the medulla may be the respiratory pacemaker [195], whereas the resting heartbeat rate is generated within the heart itself by spontaneous polarization (Section 11.A, Structure and Function of the Heart, page 310), but is subject to strong input from both branches of the autonomic nervous system. Also to be mentioned in this category of ultradian rhythms are the less-obvious pulse of the cerebrospinal-fluid pressure, with a period of *ca.* 6–10 seconds (Subsection 4.D, *Yoga and CSF Pulsations of the Medial Suture*, page 94), and the period of gastrointestinal peristalsis, also about 10 seconds (Subsection 18.A, page 447).

It has been suggested [244] that the ultradian cycles with approximately 4-hour periods are vestiges of a very ancient biological system of activity and rest which has more or less faded in importance in modern man. As such, the effects of the 4-hour ultradian cycles can easily be masked by other, stronger influences, but they are still detectable by the alert student of *yogasana*. In any event, it appears that ultradian phenomena with periods much shorter than 24 hours are under the control of setpoint mechanisms of the sort described in Fig. 21.B-1.

The study of ultradian effects in the human body has been extended significantly by Shannahoff-Khalsa, *et al.* [424], who monitored a select group of subjects for the rhythmic variations of 21 different biological functions and found five broad periods within the time interval 40 minutes to 6 hours. Time variations across all variables revealed ultradian periods of 40–65, 70–100, 115–145, 170–215, and 220–340 minutes. All measurements were taken with subjects at rest in an inclined position. The levels of hormones ACTH, luteinizing hormone, epinephrine, norepinephrine and dopamine were measured separately in the blood of each arm, along with simultaneous measurements of the air flow through the left and through the right nostrils, cardiac output, heart rate, stroke volume, systolic pressure, diastolic pressure, and mean arterial pressure. While many of these correlated with the nasal flow, the strongest correlation across all of the variables was with the stroke volume of the heartbeat. Most interestingly, the catecholamines appear alternately in the blood of the left and right arms depending on the phase of the nasal cycle, implying that the hormonal action at the adrenals has a laterality that is tied in some way to the laterality of the nasal breath! All of these ultradian rhythms, autonomic, neuroendocrine, cardiovascular, immunological, and behavioral, appear to be under the control of the hypothalamus.

Circadian Rhythms; Physiological Peaks and Valleys in the 24-Hour Period

In spite of the tendency toward homeostasis (Subsection 6.A, page 133), life forms from algae to humans also function on a rhythmic basis, which is to say, they display functions that change in time rather than being static, and moreover, the changes are regular and occur at times that can easily be predicted. In those cases where the rhythmic process goes through a maximum, a minimum, and then returns to a maximum once in 24-hours, the rhythm is said to be circadian (*circa* = about, *dian* = *day*). Though the periods of such 24-hour circadian clocks are inborn, the times in the 24-hour cycle at which they reach maximum and minimum values are set by sleep patterns which in turn are strongly influenced by the light-dark illumination cycle of the rising and setting sun [153]. The details of the mechanism of circadian rhythms is now understood at the molecular level, as discussed briefly in Subsection 21.B, *The Mechanism of the Circadian Clock*, page 484.

Before going further into the specific details of periodic phenomena in the body, let us consider a few general characteristics of circadian rhythms. Many body processes show a maximum in their rate, or their concentration or their intensity once per day, and always at the same characteristic time of the day for each of the processes. Thus, for example, the core temperature of the body is maximal at 4:00 PM every day, the concentration of cortisol in the blood plasma is maximal every day at 9:00 AM, and the urinary excretion of K^+ is maximal every day at 2:00 PM. Minimum values of these functions are observed approximately 12 hours earlier (or later).

It is also known that many of the processes with apparent periods of 24 hours in fact show much longer periods when the subjects are shielded from external cues as to the length of the day, *i.e.*, they are kept in constant illumination and constant temperature, take their meals at random times, and have no social contact with the outside world through radio, TV, *etc.* In this state, called free running, many processes stretch out in time so as to have periods of up to 35 hours or so, whereas others stretch only somewhat to a period of 24.8 hours. All such free-running processes can be brought back into synchronization with the 24-hour clock by exposure to an external trigger having a definite 24-hour cycle such as sunrise-sunset, or a 24-hour drug regimen. This shift of the period from the free-running state to that of the 24-hour solar clock is called entrainment.

The fact that there are two (or more) clocks keeping time in the free-running human body at two (or more) different rates is apparent in the free-running circadian data of Fig. 21.B-2a. Once free-running, one sees clear peaks at 24.8 and 33.5 hours, and Moore-Ede, *et al.* [321], assign these to two desynchronized oscillators, X and Y, with free-running periods of 24.8 and 33.5 hours, respectively, Fig. 21.B-2b. It is known that oscillator X is the pacemaker for REM sleep, the core temperature, cortisol release, urinary volume, and K^+ excretion, and is thought to be located in the hypothalamus (possibly in the ventromedial hypothalamus). The Y oscillator is the pacemaker for slow-wave sleep, the rest-activity cycle, skin temperature, growth hormone, and Ca^{2+} excretion, and is located in the suprachiasmatic nucleus within the hypothalamus. Entrainment of the above processes by the light-dark cycle of the sun rising and setting results in a resetting of the periods of the free-running pacemakers to

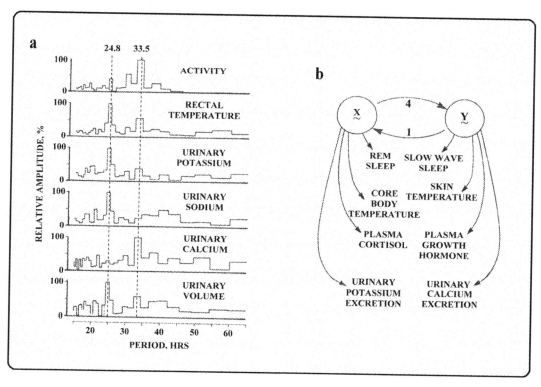

Fig. 21.B-2. (**a**) Spectral display of several biological rhythms in a free-running human subject. Two largely desynchronized rhythms are seen, with core temperature, urinary K^+, Na^+ and urinary volume largely following a 24.8 hour rhythm, whereas physical activity and urinary Ca^{2+} have a period of 33.5 hours. Each rhythm shows a small amount of the other. (**b**) The two rhythms are assigned to oscillator X (24.8 hours) and to oscillator Y (33.5 hours), with oscillator X controlling REM sleep and cortisol production in addition to the processes in (**a**) having the 24.8-hour period, and oscillator Y controlling slow-wave sleep, skin temperature and the production of growth hormone in addition to the processes in (**a**) having the 33.5-hour period. The admixture of X into Y is 4 times larger than the admixture of Y into X [321].

24.0 hours. Note too that there is mixed character to some of the processes in the Figure, with both periods appearing simultaneously.

For most biological processes, a rise in temperature of 10° C results in a doubling of the rate of the process. However, the pacemaker for the circadian rhythm apparently is temperature compensated, for the period of 24 hours is independent of body temperature [321], unless it is entrained to the 24-hour rotational cycle of the earth.

What physiological and psychological factors in the body then rise and fall over the span of a day, and when during the day are they maximal and when are they minimal? To answer these questions, all of these phys-

iological peaks and valleys that could be found in the literature are plotted as in Figs. 21.B-3, B-4, B-5, and B-6, along with their times of highest and lowest effect [178, 321]. In some cases, there is disagreement among authors by a few hours as to the times for maximum and minimum effects, but these have been averaged in the Figures. For ease of display, the 24-hour clock has been divided into quadrants, each covering a 6-hour time period. The data shown is that for individuals on a normal sleep schedule; abnormal sleep patterns or shifting time zones will rotate these patterns [178]. The times of maximum and minimum physiological effects are called circadian markers.

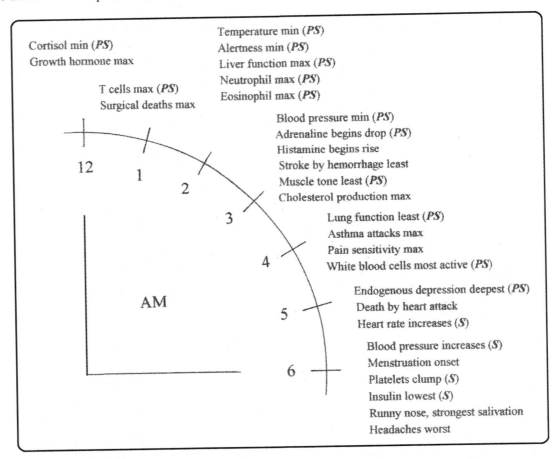

Fig. 21.B-3. The circadian shifts in bodily processes during the first six hours of the 24-hour day [178, 321, 387]. Changes that are induced by the dominance of the sympathetic nervous system are labeled (*S*), whereas those that are due to the dominance of the parasympathetic nervous system are labeled (*PS*). The maxima and minima are labeled "max" and "min", respectively.

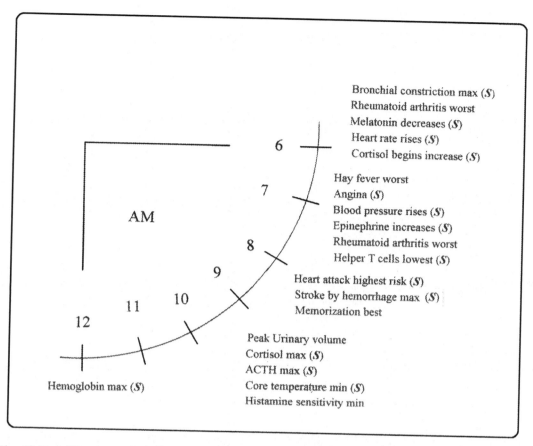

Fig. 21.B-4. The circadian shifts in bodily processes during the second six hours of the 24-hour day [178, 321, 387]. Changes that are induced by the dominance of the sympathetic nervous system are labeled (*S*), whereas those that are due to the dominance of the parasympathetic nervous system are labeled (*PS*). The maxima and minima are labeled "max" and "min", respectively.

In the hours between 12:00 midnight and 2:00 AM (Fig. 21.B-3), the body systems are essentially asleep and very little seems to be going on; digestion and cortisol levels in the blood are minimal, as are temperature, alertness, blood pressure, and muscle tone in this time interval, however release of the growth hormone is maximal at this time, as is metabolic activity of the cells lining the digestive tract.

A low cortisol level is a marker for low physical/mental activity. It is during this resting phase that the immune system (Chapter 13, page 383) strengthens itself, with maximum numbers of T cells, neutrophils and eosinophils in circulation, and maximum activity of the white blood cells

and lymphokines. Because asthma can be a symptom of an autoimmune response, the strong activity of the immune system in the hours around 3:00–4:00 AM leads to a preponderance of asthma attacks at this time (80% of breathing failures and 68% of asthma deaths occur between midnight and 8:00 AM [178]). On the other hand, the occurrence of stroke by hemorrhage in this time period is minimal as blood pressure is minimal and the epinephrine level starts to drop. Between midnight and 6:00 AM, liver action is at its peak, churning out cholesterol and glycogen. By comparison with the data of Table 6.A-2, each of the circadian markers in Figs. 20.B-3 to B-6 have been assigned an inferred connection to a branch

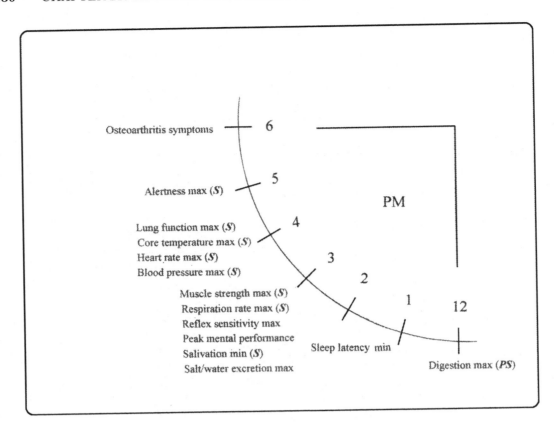

Osteoarthritis symptoms — 6

Alertness max (*S*) — 5

PM

Lung function max (*S*) — 4
Core temperature max (*S*)
Heart rate max (*S*) — 3
Blood pressure max (*S*)
                    2
Muscle strength max (*S*)
Respiration rate max (*S*)   1   12
Reflex sensitivity max
Peak mental performance
Salivation min (*S*)   Sleep latency min
Salt/water excretion max
                              Digestion max (*PS*)

Fig. 21.B-5. The circadian shifts in bodily processes during the third six hours of the 24-hour day [178, 321, 387]. Changes that are induced by the dominance of the sympathetic nervous system are labeled (*S*), whereas those that are due to the dominance of the parasympathetic nervous system are labeled (*PS*). The maxima and minima are labeled "max" and "min", respectively.

of the autonomic nervous system, either as sympathetic (*S*) or parasympathetic (*PS*). The general pattern of autonomic excitation would seem to be balanced between sympathetic and parasympathetic dominance at 12:00 midnight, but is moving toward clear parasympathetic dominance by 4:00 AM.

Between 5:00 AM and 6:00 AM, *i.e.*, at sunrise, the body-rhythms picture starts to change rapidly. One sees that death by heart attack following coronary arterial blockage or abnormal heart rhythms is three times as likely in the early morning hours between 6:00–9:00 AM. The incidence for stroke also peaks at 9:00 AM. At the same time, hormonal balances begin to shift and blood pressure and heart rate start to rise while platelets in the blood clump more easily and tend to form clots at this time. In the early morning hours, the nose is runny due to colds and nasal allergies, salivation is maximal [225], and rheumatoid-arthritis symptoms peak. Melatonin in the blood decreases with the rise of the sun, as does insulin, while the level of epinephrine increases. The hours between 6:00–9:00 AM mark the onset of strong sympathetic excitation of the autonomic nervous system, as one can see by comparing the circadian markers of Fig. 21.B-3 with the characteristics of Table 6.A-2.

In line with the excitation of the sympathetic branch of the autonomic nervous system in the early morning, the core body temperature as measured rectally has fallen to its lowest point by 9:00 AM as blood is

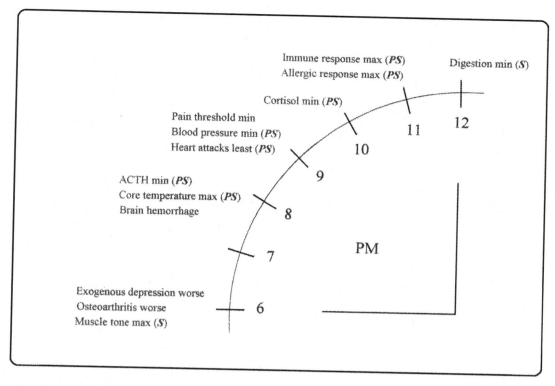

Fig. 21.B-6. The circadian shifts in bodily processes during the fourth six hours of the 24-hour day [178, 321, 387]. Changes that are induced by the dominance of the sympathetic nervous system are labeled (*S*), whereas those that are due to the dominance of the parasympathetic nervous system are labeled (*PS*). The maxima and minima are labeled "max" and "min", respectively.

moved from the visceral organs back into the muscles [225], while ACTH and cortisol levels (see Chapter 15, THE HORMONES, page 399) as well as urinary volume are at their peak values, readying the body for the day's battles.

The fever from a bacterial infection is highest from 5:00 AM to noon, whereas the fever from a viral infection is highest from 2:00–10:00 PM [387]. As regards the fever of bacterial infection, its time of maximum temperature does correspond to a low in immune-system response. Babies born in the morning hours are more likely to be healthy; babies born between 2:00–4:00 PM are more likely to have medical complications [387]. The level of hemoglobin in the blood is maximal at 12:00 PM, and the digestion is strongest at this time. It is also

to be noted that memorization is best in the period from 6:00–9:00 AM [387].

There seem to be no extreme values of body functions reached after 9:00 AM and before 3:00 PM, other than the power for digestion. Between 3:00 PM and 5:00 PM, the blood pressure maximizes, as do muscle strength, mental performance, lung function, and alertness [247]. Again, all of these responses are driven by sympathetic excitation. We assume that in the intervening hours between 10:00 AM and 2:00 PM when there are very few extremes of body function, the sympathetic and parasympathetic systems are closer to being in balance.

The steadily rising blood pressure peaks at 3:00 PM, along with peaks in muscular strength and mental performance [247]. The peak blood pressure may be 30% higher at 3:00 PM than it is at 3:00 AM. An hour later

(4:00 PM), lung function, core temperature, and heart rate (heart rate varies by up to 30 beats per minute in the span of 24 hours [387]) also reach their peak values. The ability to perform tasks which do not involve memory is greatest at the time that the core temperature reaches its maximum. Remember that at the temporal antipode (12 hours later), blood pressure was lowest at 3:00 AM as was the risk of stroke, and at that time, the epinephrine concentration in the body dropped and lung function decreased while at the same time histamine levels rose, further reducing lung function. It is clear from comparing the maxima of the physiological functions shown in Fig. 21.B-4 with the data of Table 6.A-2, that the sympathetic nervous system is in full swing between 3:00 PM and 5:00 PM, in strong contrast to the situation 12 hours earlier, *i.e.*, between 1:00 AM and 4:00 AM, when the autonomic dominance was parasympathetic.

One should not eat between 7:00 PM and 7:00 AM because "digestive fire" (*agni*, located in the solar plexus) is weakest at night (Fig. 21.B-5), is strongest when the sun is high in the sky (Fig. 21.B-4), and wanes as the sun sets [11].

Osteoarthritis symptoms peak at 6:00 PM, just 12 hours out of phase with the peak in rheumatoid arthritis symptoms (6:00 AM). It is clear that the rheumatoid arthritis symptoms appear when the autonomic balance switches from parasympathetic to sympathetic, whereas the osteoarthritis symptoms appear when the shift is the reverse. Similarly, mood variation is worse for endogenous depression at 5:00 AM and is worse for exogenous depression at 7:00 PM, Table 20.A-1. Notice that 5:00 AM marks the time of shift from parasympathetic to sympathetic dominance, while 7:00 PM marks the transition from sympathetic to parasympathetic dominance. Mood swings would be expected to be at their worst at these times of transition.

By 8:00–9:00 PM in the evening, the ACTH and cortisol levels are again minimal and core temperature peaks, the incidence of brain hemorrhage rises to its maximum and blood pressure falls. Oddly, the brain-hemorrhage rate is maximal at 8:00 PM, a time when the blood pressure begins to fall, and stroke is more common at 3:00 to 4:00 AM, the time at which the blood pressure is a minimum. Immune and allergic response are most severe at about 11:00 PM, but the death rate by heart attack is minimal at that time.

There is an interesting difference in the circadian markers of males and females in regard to enzyme activity: alcohol dehydrogenase works fastest to detoxify the body of ingested alcohol at 8:00 AM in men but is fastest in women at 3:00 AM [387]. Thus the tendencies of men and women toward inebriation vary differently depending upon the time of day.

Of course, the sleep cycle itself is based upon the circadian rhythm; however, within the sleep cycle there are several ultradian rhythms as well (see Subsection 21.B, *The Sleep/Wake Cycle and Relaxation*, page 488). In regard to circadian markers, we broadly can place sleep in the 8:00 PM to 5:00 AM domain, a time period already limited appropriately to parasympathetic action on the basis of other markers. Interestingly, the normal sleep cycle is thought to involve two intense periods, separated by a less intense period at about 12:00 midnight [46]. This accords nicely with the generalization that the time period 6 PM to 6 AM is home to two parasympathetic periods separated by a more balanced time at about 12:00 midnight [46].

When the times of various maximal and minimal body functions are plotted on a 24-hour cycle as in Figs. 21.B-3 through B-6, certain trends become clear as regards the natural times for parasympathetic *versus* sympathetic stimulation. Looking globally at the 24-hour clock, one sees that the sympathetic stimuli are strongest between 6:00 AM and 9:00 AM, are moderate from 10:00 AM to 2:00 PM, and then appear strongly again between 3:00–5:00 PM. This appears to be a baseline fight-or-flight sympathetic response in the body, independent of any specific threat or stress, but active during daylight hours, and least active around noontime. Although Cole [81] argues that mid-afternoon is a poor time for *yogasana* practice as students tend to fall asleep in *savasana* and otherwise seem to have no energy, this conflicts with the peaks of physical strength, alertness, and mental performance otherwise expected for the 3:00–5:00 PM time period, Fig. 21.B-4. The seeming conflict as to the amount of energy and awareness available to students in the 3:00–5:00 PM period may be age related, as this time period is more and more transformed from a time of strength and awareness into a time for rest as one ages.

In contrast to the times of sympathetic dominance, the parasympathetic responses cluster in the hours between 8:00–10:00 PM and between 2:00–4:00 AM, becoming moderate between 10:00 PM and 2:00 AM. It appears from Figs. 21.B-3 to B-6 that there are four periods of extreme autonomic stimulation, two sympathetic and two parasympathetic, each about 3 hours long, separated from one another by four periods of relative moderation, each about 3 hours long, in which it might be supposed that the autonomic system is more in balance. These daily shifts of autonomic dominance are natural body rhythms, driven subconsciously and entrained with the rising and setting of the sun. Because many of the maxima and their associated minima are separated by just 12 hours, they occur at the same time every day and so are in step with the rising and setting of the sun. It appears that in many other cases, the times of maximum and minimum effects are not separated by 12 hours, however. It is no accident that the pacemakers for circadian rhythm are located within the hypothalamus and that the autonomic processes so controlled are largely hypothalamic in nature.

Ayurvedic Rhythms

In Ayurvedic medicine [252], the hours of the day are divided into six periods, with rather close correspondences with the sympathetic/parasympathetic dominances uncovered in Figs. 21.B-3 to B-6. According to the Ayurvedic point of view, each of the three *doshas* (the active principles determining the biology, psychology, and pathology of the human body, mind, and con-

TABLE 21.B-1. COMPARISON OF THE AUTONOMIC AND AYURVEDIC TIME INTERVALS [252] DIVIDING THE 24-HOUR DAY.

Time	Autonomic Dominance	Active Dosha	Ayurvedic Characteristic
6:00 AM-10:00 AM	Sympathetic	Kapha	Energetic, fresh, a little heavy
10:00 AM-2:00 PM	Balanced	Pitta	Hungry, light, hot
2:00 PM-6:00 PM	Sympathetic	Vata	Active, light, supple
6:00 PM-8:00 PM	Balanced	Kapha	Cool, inert
8:00 PM-10:00 PM	Parasympathetic	Kapha	Cool, inert
10:00 PM-2:00 AM	Balanced	Pitta	Cool, energy low
2:00 AM-4:00 AM	Parasympathetic	Vata	Slow, dense, cold
4:00 AM-6:00 AM	Balanced	Vata	Dense, cloudy

sciousness [252]) is active in the time periods shown in Table 21.B-1. One sees that with a little manipulation, the Ayurvedic and autonomic time periods are amazingly close to one another over the 24-hour period, however, the correlation of autonomic dominance with the phases of the three *doshas* is not as obvious. For example, the 6:00–10:00 AM period is dominated by the sympathetic system and is *kapha* according to the *doshas*, yet in the 8:00–10:00 PM time slot, the dominant *dosha* is once again *kapha*, yet the autonomic dominance has become parasympathetic. In spite of this, the characteristics associated with the four quadrants of the day, Table 21.B-1, as assigned by Ayurveda are in general agreement with the circadian trends of sympathetic excitation during the day (energetic, light, hot) and parasympathetic at night (cool, inert, slow, dense).

According to Ayurveda, one should eat the first daily meal at 10:00 AM. With an average transit time of 18 hours for food to pass through the digestive system, excretion would then occur the following morning at 4:00 AM, this being an appropriate time since excretion would be driven by the parasympathetic action dominating at that time (Section 14.D, Body Wastes, page 396).

The yogic recommendation to commence *pranayama* at 4:00 AM and *yogasana* practice from 6:00–8:00 AM, is timed perfectly so that the former is done while in a state of parasympathetic relaxation while the latter takes advantage of the sympathetic energy flowing through the body at the later time. According to Fig. 21.B-4, the next best time for *yogasana* practice seemingly would be late afternoon (3:00–5:00 PM) when the sympathetic nervous system again asserts itself (Fig. 21.B-5), but not necessarily so for the older students.

Giving each phase of the nasal dominance a time period of four hours does fill the 24-hour span nicely, but it seems not to have any consistent effect on the 12-hour cycles of the other body functions. So, for example, the right nostril is open for breathing between 5:00–7:00 AM, which is consistent with a sympathetic arousal of the body during those hours, however, the same nostril also is active between 9:00–11:00 PM, a time when the observed dominance is parasympathetic. That little or no consistent effect is seen for the ultradian nasal cycle on the other circadian cycles is perhaps disappointing, but it is no surprise, for the circadian rhythms represent major physiological surges, whereas the effects of nasal laterality are far more subtle.

It is very interesting that the advice of modern medicine to be especially stress free in the early morning coincides with the yogi's traditional time for doing *pranayama*. However, since doctors [178] recommend that one do everything one can to reduce stress at this early morning time, as stress can precipitate a heart attack, the more strenuous *yogasana* practice perhaps should be left for the hours between 3:00–5:00 PM, when alertness, lung function, blood pressure, muscle strength, and mental performance are all at their maxima. If yogi's bodies are on the same schedules as those of the myriad subjects whose data led to the average times given in Figs. 21.B-3 to B-6, then those who practice *yogasana* at about 9:00 AM seem to be doing their most challenging work about 6 hours ahead of their peaks in physical and mental abilities. It would appear that the sympathetic dominance is stronger in the first half of the day (around 9:00 AM) than in the second (around 4:00 PM).

The Mechanism of the Circadian Clock

Some of the most obvious and important aspects of time in our physiological lives involve variations in bodily functions that occur once a day, *i.e.*, that are tied in some way to the rising and setting of the sun, but do not necessarily wax or wane at the times of rising and setting. Furthermore, though such circadian rhythms have 24-hour periods, they continue in their approximately 24-hour rhythm even when kept in total darkness for a week or more, showing that the circadian rhythm is innate rather than simply a momentary response to light and dark.

In humans, the seat of circadian control rests within the hypothalamus in a small cluster of cells known as the suprachiasmatic nucleus (SCN), Fig. 6.B-1. As one might guess from its name, the suprachiasmatic nucleus is located just above the optic chiasm. The cells within this nucleus have their own circadian rhythm, set in the womb before birth, and fully operational at the seventh month of gestation [387]. In the normal, uncontrolled situation, at sunrise, light penetrates the eyelids of the sleeping person and at the molecular level, stimulates a visual pigment in the retina which is different from the ones in the rods and cones responsible for normal vision [468], see Chapter 16, THE EYES AND VISION, page 411. This "wake up" signal travels from the retina to the SCN over dedicated neural channels within the optic-nerve bundle, but bypasses the cortex. On arrival at the SCN, the signal initiates the splitting of protein complexes within the cells of the nucleus, whereas when the sun sets, the protein complexes are reconstituted during the dark period and are ready then to split at the next burst of light [484]. The smooth changes of the concentrations of the associated and dissociated proteins within the SCN over the course of the day are coupled to hundreds of other aspects of our physiology and behavior, activating and deactivating them once every 24 hours [321]. It is this nucleus within the hypothalamus that is the pacemaker for the endocrine system,

turning it on and off in synchronicity with the light-dark pattern of ambient light perceived by the eyes.

As an example of the visual control of a circadian rhythm, consider that in the dark, the pineal gland releases melatonin, a hormone which promotes sleep, however, at the first light of dawn, the SCN is activated; it then indirectly signals the pineal to halt melatonin production, and so we become fully awake [92, 473]. Similarly, the oscillating protein concentrations in the SCN drive changes in the concentrations of vasopressin in the brain, with cyclical consequences in regard to rest and activity [55]. In the brain, vasopressin stimulates learning and memory; its concentration in the cerebrospinal fluid varies over a 24-hour cycle, and probably accounts for the circadian oscillation of our ability to learn and memorize throughout the day [389]. In animals, including man, loss of the SCN (a center rich in vasopressin) results in loss of the rhythms of corticosteroid release, feeding, drinking, and locomotor activity [225].

The chemistry of the visually-triggered, on-off process that controls circadian phenomena is an ancient one, and is innate within us, so that it actually functions with the same characteristic time periodicity (24 hours) even when there is no light to drive it [484]! Experiments with human subjects show that when the subjects are shielded from temperature changes and all visual cues as to light and dark, the circadian rhythms continue, but in some functions (sleep, for example) with periods more like 25–33 hours, whereas in other functions (rectal temperature in the same subjects, for example), with periods constant at 24.8 hours over many cycles [225]. In the case of sleep in constant darkness, the daily cycle in real time often tends to fall behind by about one hour per day, so that what was a ritual at 7:00 AM on every previous sunlit day will have shifted to 11:00 AM on going from

Monday to Friday with a 25-hour period in the dark. Ignoring the 24-hour clock on the week-ends and then trying to return to it on Monday is the cause of the "Monday-morning blues" during the work week.

At the present point in our evolution, the function of the external light and dark periods is to daily reset the time of the clock, but not to change its 24-hour character. That is to say, the core temperature of the body, for example, may rise and fall in a periodic way every 24 hours in all of us, but the times at which it will be maximal and minimal will depend upon our sleep habits, time zones, jet lag, *etc.* Through all this, the inherent frequencies of the circadian rhythms are independent of age [484], however the values of differences between maxima and minima decrease with age. That is, the differences between sympathetic and parasympathetic dominance fade with age.

Yogasana and Chronotherapy

It recently has been realized by doctors that *when* a medicine is taken often can be as important as *what* is in the medicine because taking a medicine at the "wrong" time of the day can decrease its efficiency while increasing unwanted side effects. To the extent that *yogasana* also is medicine, can it be that the *when* factor also can be important in addition to the *how* and *what* of our yoga practice? The element of *when* enters both yoga and medicine because the body actually is not homeostatic in the short term (Subsection 6.A, *Homeostasic Control; Feedback and Feedforward,* page 133), but, in fact, the productions of most of the physiologically important compounds in the body such as hormones, enzymes, neurotransmitters, *etc.*, rise and fall rhythmically over time. As these compounds are tightly coupled to physiological processes, their variations in time lead to process variations as well, *i.e.*, body rhythms.

The concept in Western medicine called "chronotherapy," in which the times at which drugs are administered are dictated by the peaks and valleys of the relevant circadian rhythms is both new and promising [58, 178, 205, 247, 362, 436]. Considerable evidence has been presented showing that the efficacy of certain drugs can be heightened considerably if their administration is synchronized with the normal circadian swings of body chemistry. For example, it is known that antihistamines, anaesthetics, analgesics, aspirin, and steroids work best when given at the appropriate times [82]. Consider, for example, the fact that the heart rate, blood pressure, and blood viscosity rise abruptly at 6:00 AM in most people as the autonomic nervous system goes strongly sympathetic at that time, Fig. 21.B-3. In response to this early-morning stress on the cardiovascular system, the incidence of heart attacks and angina discomfort is strongly peaked around this hour. Using chronotherapy in Western medicine, drugs are administered to hypertensive patients at a time such that the drugs will be most effective in relieving the sympathetic symptoms at the time of greatest cardiovascular risk, *i.e.*, 6:00 AM. A similar chronotherapeutic approach is now used to treat asthma, a condition with symptoms appearing strongly at about 4:00 AM, for which steroids are best inhaled between 3:00 and 5:30 PM [362]. In another application of the chronotherapy idea, it has been found that the toxicities of certain chemotherapeutic agents for healthy and cancerous cells vary with the time they are taken. Because normal cell processes run on a 24-hour cycle [387] whereas cancer cells run on a 20-hour cycle, the two cell types can have peak sensitivities to administered toxins at different times of the day; by injecting these drugs at the appropriate times, one can maximize the killing of cancer cells while minimizing the side effects on healthy cells, *i.e.*, the antitumor activity has been raised while the toxicity of the drug has been lowered.

Quite independently of Western medicine, yogic science has developed specific *yogasana* programs in response to student's health problems. At present, such yoga therapy is delivered without regard to where a student may be at any particular moment in his/her circadian cycles. Following the lead of Western medical science, one logically can ask, "Given a particular health condition and a prescribed *yogasana* routine as therapy, at what time of the day or night will the *yogasana* practice be most effective physiologically in regard to the condition?" To my knowledge, there is no work in the yoga community as yet on which to base an answer to the above question, however, one can make a guess.

If the risk of cardiovascular problems is greatest at 6:00 AM and is least at 6:00 PM, then it is most logical that the relaxing *yogasana* routine for such problems should be done just before 6:00 AM, or as close to it as possible, and that doing the same routine at 6:00 PM when cardiovascular risk is low would be of much less benefit. This timing runs counter to the usual recommendation of doing vigorous asana practice during the early morning hours and more restful work in the evening (see, for example [433]), however, from the chronotherapy point of view, such a schedule would be best for students who have no medical problems and least effective for students with cardiovascular complications. The suggestion that one perform the appropriate therapeutic *yogasana* work at the times of highest risk or discomfort assumes that the beneficial effects of the practice are immediate and not complicated by a chain of cause and effect which would otherwise delay the benefit.

A quick scan of the information on circadian markers in Figs. 21.B-3 to B-6, and the simple assumption that *yogasana* benefits are immediate, suggests the following times

as being the most appropriate for specific *yogasana* therapy practice:

depression: 5:00 PM
anxiety: 6:00 AM
asthma; bronchial constriction: 6:00 AM
cardiovascular problems/hypertension: 6:00 AM
rheumatoid arthritis: 6:00 AM
osteoarthritis: 6:00 PM
hot flashes in the evening: late evening

The "optimum times" quoted above are average times as appropriate to the average person; one must be careful in this that not everyone will fit into the "average" mold, and so one would profit from having a specific determination of just exactly when the circadian markers occur during the day. That is to say, the therapy should follow "body time" rather than "clock time", and one must be aware that students with central-nervous-system disturbances may have altered circadian rhythms, or even none at all. If a *yogasana* therapy routine does not seem to be effective when practiced at one time, then consider changing the time of practice.

This approach to the question of when is the best time to practice allows for individual variations in order to accommodate the fact that different students will have different but important circadian factors at work, possibly at different times. Considering that muscle strength, peak mental performance and peak lung function are found in the 3:00 to 4:00 PM time slot, Fig. 21.B-4, this would seem to be a good time for a vigorous *yogasana* practice for those younger students who are not "morning persons" and have no health problems.

Aged or not, if a pose is more difficult when performed on one side of the body than on the other, the human tendency is to spend less time on the more difficult side. Using a timer to balance the time spent on both sides would be wise. Moreover, one actually should spend even longer on the more difficult side in order to bring it up to the level of the easy side.

The Sleep/Wake Cycle and Relaxation

Little is known about why we need sleep, other than to say that apparently there are centers or neural networks in the brain that require a periodic rest from consciousness. It is known, however, that the transitions from wakefulness to sleep and from sleep to wakefulness are driven by centers in the brainstem, and that certain aspects of sleep actually show considerable mental activity. EEG studies (Subsection 3.E, page 57) confirm that there are close similarities of the brain states in certain of the sleep stages with those achieved in both relaxation and meditation [462].

Sleep is induced by the Raphe nuclei in the region of the lower pons and the medulla; the circuitry here uses serotonin as the neurotransmitter, and also sends inhibitory signals to the spinal cord to resist pain signals from moving upward into the consciousness. There is a possibility that the parasympathetic nervous system has a role in releasing into sleep, for excitations of the parasympathetic cranial nerves IX and X, involved with sucking/nursing and digestion after a large meal, respectively, do promote sleep, possibly by triggering the Raphe nuclei.

Once asleep, brain activity does not necessarily become quiet, but instead shifts in a cyclic way into other modes. There are five such modes or stages in the sleep/wake cycle that are recognized, each with its own characteristic EEG brainwave pattern, as shown in Fig. 3.E-1. On entering sleep, one moves from the awake stage with its attendant beta-wave EEG, and proceeds from there through sleep stages 1, 2, 3, and 4. Traversing these sleep stages once in sequential order and then returning in reverse order requires about 90 minutes, and

the cycle repeats itself five or six times during the night. Many hormonal cycles also have the 90-minute period.

The REM (rapid-eye-movement) phase of sleep (stage 1) is most paradoxical. Fig. 21.B-7 illustrates how several physiological variables are affected by the three sleep stages, awake, stage 2, and REM sleep. One sees that as the sleeper goes from awake to REM, the reticular formation becomes energized, but the neck muscles become slack and passive, as does the respiration. On the other hand, eye movement becomes excessive in the REM phase, seeming to follow the reticular activation. In the REM phase of sleep, the EEG is beta-like, *i.e.*, desynchronized and high frequency as appropriate for a level of high alertness. The heart rate and blood pressure are increased but irregular in the REM phase, respiration is rapid and uneven, and while all gastrointestinal movements cease as we go cold-blooded with little or no temperature regulation, penile and clitoral erections are common [225]. All but the last of these are characteristic of sympathetic nervous activity, whereas erection is a parasympathetic response, Table 6.A-2 and Section 19.D, Sexual Function, page 461, as are slack neck muscles and passive respiration.

The loss of muscle tone (atonia) in the REM phase arises because the actions of spinal motor neurons are inhibited. This atonia prevents us from acting out the active natures of our REM-sleep dreams; specific lesions in the brainstem can block this inhibition and so can lead to a very physical dreamlife.

Strangely, the rate of O_2 consumption in the brain during REM sleep is even larger than when one is involved in intense mental exercise, but otherwise does decrease in the order REM, stage 2, stage 3, stage 4 [50]. With all of these aspects taken together, it would appear that there is a paradoxical mixture of sympathetic and parasympathet-

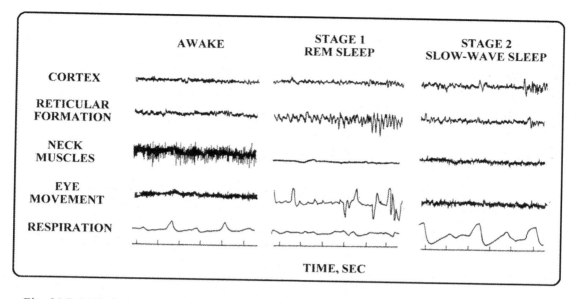

Fig. 21.B-7. Variation of several physiological features with changing levels of sleep. Note the extreme differences in most functions in the awake and REM phases.

ic symptoms present in the REM state. Dreams in the REM state are frequent, vivid and memorable.

The first REM period occurs about 90 minutes after first falling asleep, and then in each succeeding 90-minute period there is less of stages 3 and 4, and more of the stage-1 REM phase. REM sleep amounts to about 50% of the total sleep time in infants, 30% in children, and drops to 20% in those over 80 years old [230]. In an 8-hour sleep, one may have between three and five REM episodes, each lasting 5–30 minutes, and each longer lasting than the previous one. Normally, an adult spends about 15–25% of his/her sleep time in the REM state, however, in women who suffer from PMS, the REM sleep period is reduced to only about 5% of the total, and such sufferers will be irritable on awakening, even though they have had an 8-hour sleep.

Strictly speaking, REM sleep, with a period of only 90 minutes, is an ultradian rhythm, not circadian, but it is placed in the latter category since its repeating pattern occurs once per day. Note that there are several other physiological processes besides

REM sleep that have the 90-minute periodicity (Subsection 21.B, *Ultradian Rhythms*, page 474). The 90-minute period of the REM/ non-REM phenomenon in sleep is thought to be a phylogenetic remnant of an ancient rest-activity cycle in the human constitution [244], and is thought to assert itself during the waking hours as well (Section 12.C, Nasal Laterality, page 374). Though the purpose served by REM sleep is still being debated [225], it is clear that there are aspects of autonomic excitation involved.

Coleman [82] presents an interesting chart of circadian variations of physiological functions as they change through the sleep/wake cycle over two days, Fig. 21.B-8. It is no surprise that alertness drops as we sleep, and that we are most alert and awake when our temperature is the highest. Growth hormone, however, behaves oppositely, being almost zero during wakefulness, and maximizing during sleep-stage 3. Cortisol in the blood peaks in the early morning, as in Fig. 21.B-3.

It is known that certain chemicals produced in the brain during the waking hours act to induce sleep at night. Interestingly,

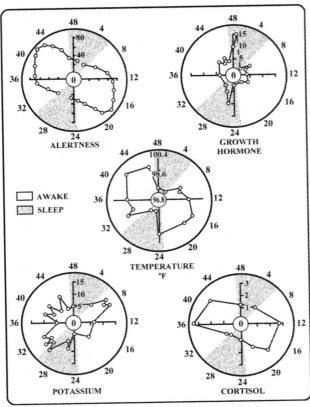

Fig. 21.B-8. Changes of various physiological functions according to the phases of the sleep/wake cycle. The figures surrounding the circles are the hours of the clock (6 being morning, 48 being midnight), the shaded parts are evenings, and the amplitude of the function is given as the length of the radius at any particular time during the 48-hour period.

many of these substances are active immunological agents in the human body. Furthermore, there would appear to be more going on than just repeatedly running through the sleep stages. Thus, there is substantial evidence that the most natural sleep cycle is broken into two equally long sleep phases separated by about 1 hour of wakefulness [46], the whole requiring 9–11 hours total. As discussed above, this expectation is born out by the pattern of circadian markers, Figs. 21.B-5 and B-6.

Adrenergic excitations in the reticular formation in the upper pons (Subsection 3.A, *The Spinal Cord and Brainstem*, page 29) are specifically arousing to the mind and

the body. When the body/mind is ready to come awake, a neural signal originates in the reticular formation and moves upward, through the thalamus to the cortex, bringing it awake first. Once awake, the cortex sends a descending signal to bring the muscles and reflexes into readiness by increasing the body's muscle tone.

It is most interesting to read that recent research strongly implicates the various sleep cycles in the learning and remembering of tasks such as the mechanics of *yogasana* performance [359]. As discussed further in Subsection 3.C, *Consolidation and Long-Term Memory*, page 45, the details of material newly learned during the day are transferred from the hippocampus to the cortex during periods of slow-wave sleep and then back again during REM phases. This conversation between the two brain areas while asleep results in the memory of the learned process being firmly implanted in the cortex while the hippocampus memory bank is cleared in order to receive the next day's input.

On relaxing in *savasana* after *yogasana* practice, one goes from the beta phase of wakefulness to an alpha brainwave state and thence to theta relaxation (sleep stages 3–4) [462]. Sleep stages 3–4 in turn are defined as having more than 50% theta waves, less than 50% alpha waves, and no beta waves present. In young adults, the latency period for attaining stage-2 relaxation (the time between feeling sleepy and actually entering sleep-stage 2) is about 10 minutes [79], possibly passing through a very brief REM period on the way. Consequently, one should allow at least this long with beginners in *savasana* in order to have some hope of achieving a restful state. Moreover, because norepinephrine released into the blood by *yogasanas* requires about 20 minutes to clear the bloodstream, a *savasana* of 10–20 minutes duration seems reasonable.

Inasmuch as research on circadian cycles shows that even when asleep, the penetration of the closed eyelids by dawn's early light is stimulating to the arousal response within the SCN (see above, *The Mechanism of the Circadian Clock*, page 484), it would seem prudent to use eyebags during *savasana*, unless the *yogasana* practice-room is in total darkness.

The sleep/wake cycle has a period of 24.0 hours because this particular body function is entrained with the rising and setting of the sun. If one flies across many time zones in the course of the day, then the sleep/wake cycle and the rising and setting of the sun become momentarily desynchronized, and one has jet lag until the entrainment can be re-established.

The quality of our sleep is more important than the quantity. While asleep, we cycle through 90-minute periods as shown in Fig. 3.E-1. In order to achieve a sense of rest and restoration, one needs to go through at least two full cycles of the sleep phases (3 hours) without any interruptions such as might occur during sleep apnea.* Sleep fragmented by apnea is devoid of the 90-minute cycles and so is far from restful. In contrast, relaxation following *yogasana* practice does not rely on any cyclic pattern of mental states, and so can be more restful than sleep itself. This is especially so if the sleep is only for an hour or so, since there is not sufficient time in this case to complete even one 90-minute cycle, whereas a 60-minute *savasana* can be most refreshing.

A circadian rhythm of sorts is observed in the flexibility of the body, for many experiments show that the range of motion for shoulder rotation and in *yogasanas* such as *uttanasana*, *paschimottanasana*, and *trikonasana* are least in the early morning and are then largest at 10:00–11:00 AM and again at 4:00–5:00 PM [5]. It would be most interesting to know if this were true as well for *yogasana* students, who are otherwise advised to practice in the early hours of the morning. Because of early-morning stiffness, there is a greater risk of injury when stretching in the morning (unless one warms up properly), and the range of motion will be larger later in the day.

Infradian Rhythms

Those bodily processes which require more than 24 hours to go through their cycle are termed "infradian." The most obvious is that of the menstrual cycle of women, where there are large upward swings of progesterone on a monthly basis (Subsection 19.A, *The Menstrual Cycle*, page 453). As with the circadian period, the monthly menstrual period is close to but not quite equal to the natural rhythm of the heavens, in this case the rotational period of the moon. It is said that the nasal cycle also has a monthly period [70]. The phenomenon of seasonal affective disorder (Subsection 16.D, *White-Light Starvation*, page 430) possibly is another infradian rhythm, in this case the period being one year.

*In sleep apnea, one cycles between deep sleep and no breathing, and light sleep with breathing restored. One remains unconscious of the nonbreathing episodes.

Chapter 22

AGING AND LONGEVITY

As yoga teachers, it is important that we understand those aspects of aging that are inevitable and those that are avoidable through yogic practices, for this will make our own lives more enjoyable as we age, and it also will allow us to work with and understand aging students in a more effective way. Though not all of our students necessarily will have heart problems, osteoporosis, hypertension, *etc.*, all of them sooner or later will become aged, as will we, and we must understand what that means in terms of abilities, attitudes, *etc*. Fortunately, it is here that yoga shines, for whereas so many other health/exercise regimes become less appropriate with age, that is not the case with *yogasana*. Moreover, we have many excellent personal examples of how *yogasana* benefits the aging and aged.

Actually, for those who survive to age 65, they are only slightly more likely to enjoy a robust old age than was possible 2000 years ago. Though our longevity has increased statistically over that time span, the aging seems to continue unabated regardless of whether we exercise or not. Exercise, diet, life-style changes, *etc.*, can prolong one's life, but not retard aging in any significant way. The positive effects of exercise fade away rapidly once we stop exercising [388].

As women age, they go through the menopausal stage of life, whereas men go through a less drastic shift called the climacteric. The consequences of menopause are described in Section 19.C, page 459, from the point of view of the *yogasana* practitioner and her physiology.

SECTION 22.A. SYMPTOMS AND STATISTICS

What to Expect

Problems of aging are becoming increasingly more important as the average age of the U.S. and of the world population increase. At the moment, the fastest growing segment of the U.S. population is the elderly, aged over 65, who will account for 21% of the population by the year 2030. Furthermore, today's babies can expect to live to age 75 on average, and if today's adult makes it to 65, he/she can expect another 16.7 years of longevity, though not necessarily of the highest quality, for reasons of compromised health. Among the elderly, heart disease takes more than 40%, cancer takes 20%, and 20% of those hardy enough to reach age 80 will suffer from Alzheimer's disease.

Appreciable aging begins in most people at 40–50 years, and is marked by several noticeable but not necessarily rapid changes [106]. Many lists have been compiled to document the symptoms of old age, and three of them will be considered here. Though the three parties involved in generating these lists have divergent professional interests, they are in almost total agreement as to the physical and mental/emotional effects of aging.

Nieman [337], an exercise physiologist, lists the effects of aging as including:

1. Loss of taste and smell

2. Periodontal bone loss; 50% of the U.S. population aged over 60 years has lost *all* teeth

3. Declining gastrointestinal function; less digestive juice, less absorption of nutrients, constipation

4. Loss of visual and auditory functions

5. Decrease in lean body weight, with increasing amount of body fat

6. Osteoporosis; bone weakness with diminished ability to repair fractures

7. Mental impairment; confusion, disorientation

8. Decreasing ability to metabolize drugs

9. Increase in chronic disease; diabetes, cancer, heart disease, high blood pressure, stroke, arthritis

10. Degradation of neuromuscular responses; reaction time, balance, strengths of muscles, tendons and ligaments all degraded

11. Urinary incontinence

12. Decreased size and function of liver and kidney

13. Decrease in heart and lung fitness; loss of 8–10% per decade of ability of heart and lungs to deliver oxygen (O_2) to muscles

To this we would add

14. Decrease in both physical and mental flexibility and range of motion

15. Lower levels of gonadal hormones.

Other aging criteria have been put forward by experts in the gerontology field. As George Burns noted: "You'll know when you're old when everything hurts and what doesn't hurt doesn't work; when you get winded playing chess; when you stop to tie your shoelaces and ask yourself, 'What else can I do while I'm down here?' and when everyone goes to your birthday party and stands around the cake just to get warm!"

An interesting but qualitative system-by-system description of "normal aging" in women has been presented recently by the Harvard Women's Health Watch [185]:

Skin: Loss of vital cells leads to skin which is thinner, less resilient, and less sensitive to temperature and pressure, but is more easily bruised or likely to bleed.

Brain: Perceptible loss of short-term memory in the 50's; general intelligence decreases in the 60's, and capacity for abstract thought lessens in the 70's.

Cardiovascular: Arteries become less elastic and accommodating as heart walls thicken. Contractile force falls off even if one is in good physical condition.

Respiratory: Lung function peaks in early 20's and then falls to about 75% by age 75 years.

Musculoskeleton: At menopause, demineralization rate within bones exceeds bone building as estrogen level starts to fall. Can lead to osteoporosis.

Digestive: Ages well, with little loss of function.

Reproductive: Most eggs are shed or reabsorbed and estrogen and progesterone production fall off at menopause, leading to hot flashes, *etc.*

Excretory: Small changes in urinary volume (increase) and timing (less during the day, more at night) with aging.

Immune: Thymus gradually degenerates and T cells decline in number and efficiency, leading to increased susceptibility to infection, but possible decrease in allergic reactions as well.

Endocrine: While many hormone levels fall, the endorphins increase to reduce sensitivity to pain. Thyroid and insulin outputs remain unchanged.

Sense Organs: These are most strongly hit by age. There are losses of sensitivity in hearing, seeing, tasting, and smelling.

Not all of the changes listed above are inevitable, and some in part actually are avoidable or reversible; for example, aboriginals not exposed to 20th-century noise often retain acute hearing into old age [473], and defective vision in old age still can be improved through yogic eye exercises [373]. Just how a number of these bodily functions change as one ages are graphed in Fig. 22.A-1 [337]. It is interesting to note how closely the symptoms of old age resemble those of weightlessness in space [482], physical inactivity [410], and bedrest [337].

Physical Aging

As we age, there is an unavoidable loss of muscle mass amounting to approximately 10% by age 50 years and 50% by age 80 years. This stands in contradistinction to the situation with heart muscle, which seems to enlarge with time rather than shrink. Not only do our skeletal muscles weaken with age, but there is a shift of the balance between slow-twitch (type-1) muscle fibers and fast-twitch fibers (types 2 and 3), Subsection 7.A, *Types of Muscle Fiber*, page 189, leading eventually to hybrid fibers of intermediate contraction velocity [6]. The

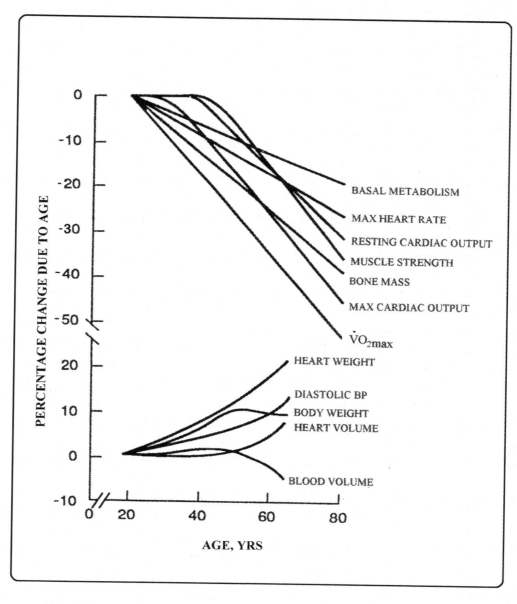

Fig. 22.A-1. Physiological changes in body function with increasing age as compared with the body at age 20.

intermediate-type fibers are not found in younger bodies.

Of the 14 physical and mental changes on aging listed above by Nieman, it is the thirteenth which is generally taken by gerontologists as the most direct *quantitative* measure of aging:

13. Decrease in heart and lung function; loss of 8–10% per decade of ability of the heart and lungs to deliver O_2 to muscles.

In particular, it is the quantity $\dot{V}O_{2max}$ that is readily measured and is of the greatest relevance according to Nieman.* $\dot{V}O_{2max}$ is a measure of the work capacity of the body, expressed as its ability to deliver O_2 to the muscles as they do their work. As discussed in Subsection 7.A, *Muscle Chemistry and Energy*, page 182, the ability of a muscle to do work over an extended time (beyond a few minutes) is dependent upon the delivery of oxygen to the mitochondria within the muscle cells; without sufficient oxygen in the blood, glucose cannot be oxidized, ATP is not produced and all muscular movement stops. Experiments on men and women show that $\dot{V}O_{2max}$ starts to decline by 8–10 % per decade after age 25. It is estimated that half of the decline in this quantity is due to lack of physical exercise, and half is innate and therefore unavoidable.

The avoidable half of the 8–10% decline in $\dot{V}O_{2max}$ seems to be more under our control. Experiments show that regular aerobic exercise can lead to the recovery of half of the decline in $\dot{V}O_{2max}$. This recovery holds up to age 75, at which point the decrease of $\dot{V}O_{2max}$ is independent of exercise. The largest single factor in forestalling the downward trends of aging is exercise, for this can increase lung capacity, build muscles and bone, and condition the heart and blood vessels.

This unavoidable decline in $\dot{V}O_{2max}$ is currently explained by two competing theories: 1) genetic errors accumulate and the body is unable to correct them, leading to inefficiency and disease, and 2) the body is inherently programmed so that cells divide only a fixed number of times and then regeneration slows or ceases, leading to disease and degeneration. At another level, natural selection in humans also plays a role in aging, as it selects against mutations that interfere with our reproductive years, but not against slow-acting mutations that only affect our later years [388].

In regard to these aging mechanisms, neurons (brain cells) and myocytes (heart cells) cease to divide at all after reaching maturity, and other cell types reproduce at slowly declining rates. As a result, the general effect of aging is a loss of cells and cell products such as enzymes, hormones, and collagen. Along with the decrease in hormonal levels, it also is thought [389] that the numbers of receptors for the hormones on the cell walls also decrease with age. Just as the hypothalamus gland initiates hormonal changes via the pituitary gland signaling puberty, it may also be that it changes the hormonal balance again as one goes into old age, signaling a physiological rollback [389].

Considered at the cellular level, aging is determined almost totally by cell loss and the concomitant loss of cell products. Of those cells that are replaced normally (and many are not), they are replaced at a slower rate as we age, and the products of cell function, hormones, enzymes, collagen, elastin,

---

* Note that the factor considered as prime by Nieman is not even mentioned specifically by the Harvard Women's Health Watch. This reflects the fact that $\dot{V}O_{2max}$ is the most quantifiable of the various factors but not necessarily the most important in terms of overall well being. With this caveat in mind, we focus on this quantity as being of special relevance to *yogasana* students and the athletically inclined.

and neurotransmitters, for example, are produced at slower and slower rates as well [185].

At the chemical level, much of the blame for aging can be placed at the feet of free radicals produced in the course of ATP production in the mitochondria. Free radicals are molecules with an odd number of electrons, meaning that not all of the molecular electrons can be involved in two-electron chemical bonds, and that the odd electron imparts a very high and nonspecific reactivity to the radical. When we are young, the ATP production is high and free-radical production is low, but as we age, the ratio shifts until the ATP supply becomes minimal and the free radicals become maximal in old age [478]. By virtue of their high reactivity, free radicals engage in many deleterious reactions, unless they are mopped up by antioxidants in the diet.

Yet another chemical factor in aging (thickening of the arteries, stiffening of the joints, feeble muscle action, failure of the organs, *etc.*) is due to the crosslinking of the amino acids in adjacent protein chains by glucose. Such crosslinks accumulate to eventually form hard, inflexible yellow-brown materials which closely resemble the products of the Maillard reaction in which meat is browned and hardened by roasting [307]. Free radicals also are involved in this reaction.

Physically, quantitative measures of the change in lumbar flexibility with increasing age have been summarized by Kapandji [228], Table 4.A-2. As can be seen in that Table, the maximum range of motion for lumbar extension and lateral bending is achieved in the teen years, and then falls to much less than half the maximum value in the years 65–77. This loss of spinal flexibility is important, for it will limit severely which physical activities can be enjoyed in the latter years. This loss of spinal flexibility with age is due to the fact that the inter-

vertebral discs dry out and shrink with age, encouraging the vertebrae to move toward one another and then to fuse. Regular practice of backbending, forward bending, *halasana,* spinal twists, and *sarvangasana* can work to slow if not stop this tendency.

The increase in the size of the heart as we age, Fig. 22.A-1, is at first sight perplexing, as the size of all other muscles is decreasing. This is explained as the result of the overwork performed by the aging heart in pushing blood through a vascular system that is more and more resistant to the flow of blood. On the other hand, the other striated muscles of the body become thinner and weaker as the nerves that innervate them die off through lack of use in old age.

Elderly persons (especially females) are predisposed to dizziness because of the aging process. Physiologic changes include a decline in proprioceptive (Section 7.C, Proprioception, page 208), visual (Subsection 16.A, *The Ocular-Vestibular Connection*, page 418), and vestibular reflexes (Section 17.B, The Vestibular Organs of Balance, page 437). The numbers of receptors and synapses in the visual and auditory channels are reduced as are the cerebral autoregulation and baroreceptor functions. All of the above lead to a diminished ability to regulate or compensate for the body's need for homeostasis [92].

Yet another aspect of aging which can impact on *yogasana* practice for the elderly is the question of foot pain. Such pain is a direct cause of falling in the elderly, and many times is the direct cause of physical inactivity as well. As we age, the feet lengthen and broaden, and the bottoms of the feet become thinner and less able to absorb the shock of footfall. The interference of foot problems with *yogasana* practice is especially a factor for aging women who have disfigured their feet through wearing fashionable but inappropriate shoes.

Longevity

For 99.9% of the time that human beings have populated the earth, the longevity has been no longer than 30–40 years. It is only relatively recently that this longevity figure has doubled, thanks to increasing awareness of sanitation, medical techniques, the cultivation of health habits, *etc*. The influence of health habits on mortality has been nicely set out by Breslow in [337] in terms of seven basic health habits:

1. Never smoke
2. Moderate alcohol consumption
3. Eat breakfast daily
4. No snacking
5. Get 7–8 hours sleep each night
6. Exercise regularly
7. Maintain ideal weight

Fig. 22.A-2 shows how ignoring these simple habits can become mortality factors. For both men and women, those who practice all 7 of the above have a 40% smaller death rate than those who practice only 4–5. These seven health habits are clearly compatible with the yoga lifestyle and are encouraged by it. On the other hand, if one practices only 0–3 of the health habits, the death rate increases by up to 60% over that for the median group.

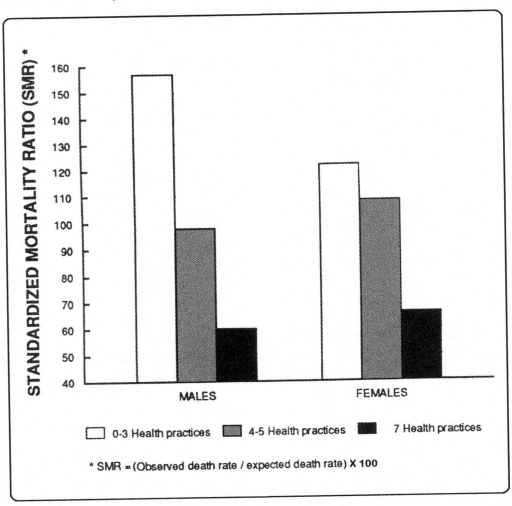

Fig. 22.A-2. The relation between the number of good health habits practiced by males and females and the standardized mortality ratio, defined as the ratio of the rate of deaths observed to the rate of deaths expected on average.

Note too that although a person with a 20 pack-per-year smoking history statistically will forfeit 3 years of life expectancy, there are other factors (stress, for example) affecting longevity other than direct health ones. For example, being a single male also will statistically reduce one's life span by 3 years, whereas being happily married adds two years [100].

Yoga, Sports, and Aging

Specific data is not available on the effects of aging on the *yogasana* student, however, there are some generalities for aging athletes that will apply across the board to all. Sports champions can use their speed to secure a competitive advantage in the age range 18–26 years, whereas champions in sports requiring coordination can extend their dominance for yet another decade beyond that. Power and endurance are strongest between years 30 and 40, with age being kinder to endurance performers than to power performers. Strength peaks at about 25 years but can plateau out to age 50, whence it then declines by 20% by age 65 and decreases continuously after that. Much of the strength loss is due to the loss of muscle mass and increased body fat. However, in these declining years, resistance training will slow strength loss as it helps to recruit motor units and promotes joint flexibility.

In summary, championship class athletes can expect to first lose their speed, then coordination, strength and endurance. It appears to be a different story for those practicing *yogasana* at noncompetitive levels, for Schatz [410] has published a list of how yoga practice can curtail or even reverse the aging process.

It is interesting and satisfying to compare her points in regard anti-aging and those of Nieman in regard aging, Table 22.A-1. Notice that for almost every item listed by Nieman as a negative change on aging, Schatz lists the positive effect *yogasana*

practice can have on that factor. This comparison illustrates in a very compelling manner how *yogasana* practice can work to combat the physical and mental decline usually associated with aging. Even more important, yoga done into "old age" can vastly improve the qualities of our lives and those of our students aside from the possibility of extending life, as it gives the practitioner a focus and commitment to a purpose greater than oneself [410].

It is interesting to see how the profile of leading medical problems and the leading causes of death change between the 19–39 year-old age group and the over-65 age group, Table 22.A-2. One sees there that the medical problems that newly appear once one reaches the older age group (osteoporosis, arthritis, hypertension, cardiovascular disease, and vision impairment) are all addressable through *yogasana* practice. A lifetime of sensible yoga practice will be a prophylactic against many of the items listed in Table 22.A-2, in agreement with the listings in Table 22.A-1.

SECTION 22.B. MENTAL AND EMOTIONAL EFFECTS OF AGING

Several of the physical factors that decline with aging would seem to have parallels in the mental/emotional sphere. In the latter case, most of the aging changes occur in the cerebral cortex [153] and as with the physical effects of aging, start at about age 40. Thus, the cortex of the 40–60 year old has 15–20% fewer cells than that of the 20 year old. By age 75 years, the cellular deficient is over 40%. With age, brain cells lose dendrites, are less responsive to neurotransmitters and have atrophied cell parts (Chapter 5, THE NERVES, page 107). With increasing age, dopamine-producing neurons decrease by 40% in certain parts of the brain and with falling dopamine levels, the

TABLE 22.A-1. COMPARISON OF THE EFFECTS OF
AGING [337] AND *YOGASANA* [410]

<u>Aging Effects</u> (Nieman)	<u>Yogasana</u> Effects (Schatz) [a]
1) Loss of taste and smell	1) Heightened senses of taste and smell
2) Periodontal bone loss	2) Can reduce TMJ syndrome
3) Declining GI function	3) Normalizes bowel function, improves digestion
4) Loss of visual and auditory sensitivity	4) Corrects refractive errors in vision, reduces visual headaches, sharpens hearing
5) Muscle loss/fat gain	5) Promotes muscle strength, endurance, and flexibility
6) Decrease of bone strength and density	6) Bone strength, bone density, and structural integrity of joints increase
7) Mental impairment	7) Increased ability to respond positively to stress. Increased mental acuity
8) Decreasing ability to metabolize drugs	8) Improved sensitivity to insulin; healthy metabolism of lipids and cholesterol
9) Increase in chronic disease	9) Increased immune function
10) Degradation of neuromuscular response	10) Increase of neuromuscular coordination
11) Urinary incontinence	11) Increase of neuromuscular control
12) Decreasing liver and kidney function	12) Increase in liver and kidney function
13) Decrease in heart and lung fitness	13) Increases in circulation and respiration efficiencies; increased tolerance to exercise
14) Loss of skeletal and mental flexibility and range	14) Striking increases in flexibility and range of motion
15) Increasing depression	15) Decreasing depression

----

[a] See also references [150, 373, 439, 465, 486].

sense of the passage of time slows. The locus ceruleus, an area of the brain rich in the norepinephrine needed for arousal, is smaller by 30% at age 70. By this age, the brain size is smaller by 11%, brain weight decreases and the open volume of the brain ventricles increases [153]. Blood flow to the brain and brain metabolism also decrease with age.

"Facts" such as these have led to the widely held belief that once mature, the number of brain cells decreases uniformly with age, with no replacement of old, dead cells possible. Imagine then the surprise when it was reported that in the human hippocampus, there is strong evidence for the creation of new neurons even in the elderly and that the renewal is spurred by exercise! [158]. It remains to be seen if such regeneration of neurons can occur in other areas of the brain. On the positive side, there are experiments that show that a reorganization of neural circuitry is possible as one ages which compensates for the declining numbers of neurons in the brain (Subsection 3.D, *Using Cerebral Hemispheric Laterality in Yoga*, page 55).

As with the physical side, mental response time increases with age. However, the general level of EEG activity (Section

TABLE 22.A-2. COMPARISON OF THE LEADING MEDICAL PROBLEMS AND THE LEADING CAUSES OF DEATH IN THE AGE GROUPS 19–35 YEARS AND OVER 65 YEARS [182]

Leading Medical Problems

19–39 Years	Over 65 Years
Nose, throat, upper respiratory infections	Nose, throat, upper respiratory conditions
Injuries	Osteoporosis and arthritis
Viral, bacterial, and parasitic infections	Hypertension
Acute urinary-tract infections	Urinary incontinence
Eating disorders	Cardiovascular disease
Violence, rape	Injuries
Substance abuse	Hearing and vision impairment

Leading Causes of Death

Motor vehicle accidents	Cardiovascular disease
Cardiovascular disease	Cerebrovascular disease
Homicide	Pneumonia and influenza
Coronary artery disease	Chronic obstructive pulmonary disease
AIDS	Colorectal cancer
Breast cancer	Breast cancer
Cerebrovascular disease	Lung cancer
Cervical cancer	Diabetes
Uterine cancer	Accidents

3.E, Brainwaves and The Electroencephalogram, page 57) does not decrease until one reaches age 80 or so. Perhaps this lengthening of response time is related to the apparent slowing of the time sense in the elderly [17], who sense that time is passing much more slowly than does real clock time, possibly due to lower dopamine levels. The stretching of apparent time is most obvious when the aged are busy.

Diet and/or exercise are generally held to be of no value in retarding the aging of the brain. This is understandable because almost all Western forms of exercise are repetitive and require no deliberate mental effort. In contrast, *yogasana* is rich in this mental component and so could be different in this regard.

The largest effect of aging on mental performance is loss of memory as mental resources decline. Most interesting, there is in a sense, a loss of mental flexibility with age, as one is less able to assimilate truly new ideas. "New knowledge" that simply builds upon already accepted ideas is easily incorporated by the aged, however, ideas that have no previous foundation are less and less acceptable with increasing age. Resistance to ideas that are too "new" for aged *yogasana* students can be a potent factor in retarding their progress (Section 3.C, Memory, Learning, and Teaching, page 42). The more closely "new ideas" in yoga are related to others already accepted, the more readily they too will be accepted.

Four factors have been put forward as key elements in maintaining mental competence into old age [187]: 1) maintain a high level of mental functioning through an activity that is intellectually engaging. Learn a new skill rather than watch TV and talk on the phone all day. 2) Maintain a high level of physical activity. 3) Maintain good lung function, and 4) Develop a feeling of "self-efficacy", so that one feels that he or she is in control of their life. In order to stay mentally bright, it is important to find mental and physical activities which are challenging, interesting, and enjoyable enough to keep one involved on a daily basis over a long period of time. It is difficult to think of anything better suited to these four goals than the daily practice of the *yogasanas*!

In regard aging, Nesse and Williams [335] point out that a gene can have multiple effects on the body, some good and some not so good, and that our present situation is a trade-off between longevity and quality of life. For example, the uric acid crystals which are responsible for the pain of gout are also strongly antioxidant and so possibly extend our life span. In the same vein, Nesse and Williams claim that strong immune defenses protect us from infection, but in the process they inflict low-level tissue damage. From this point of view, aging is seen not as a disease, but rather as a trade-off between life span and accumulating tissue damage that eventually works to our disadvantage.

Appendix I

YOGASANA ILLUSTRATIONS

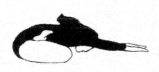

ADHO MUKHA
PADMASANA

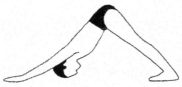

ADHO MUKHA
SVANASANA

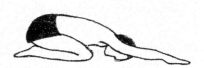

ADHO MUKHA
VIRASANA

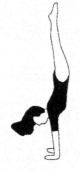

ADHO MUKHA
VRKSASANA

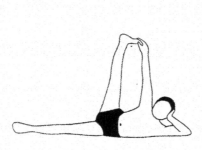

ANANTASANA

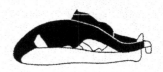

ARDHA BADDHA PADMA
PASCIMOTTANASANA

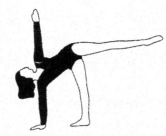

ARDHA CHANDRASANA

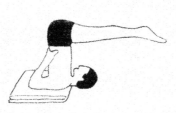

ARDHA HALASANA

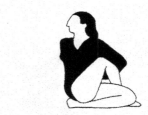

ARDHA MATSYENDRASANA I

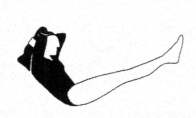

ARDHA NAVASANA

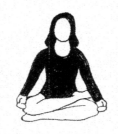

ARDHA PADMASANA

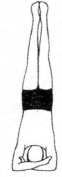

BADDHA HASTA SIRSASANA

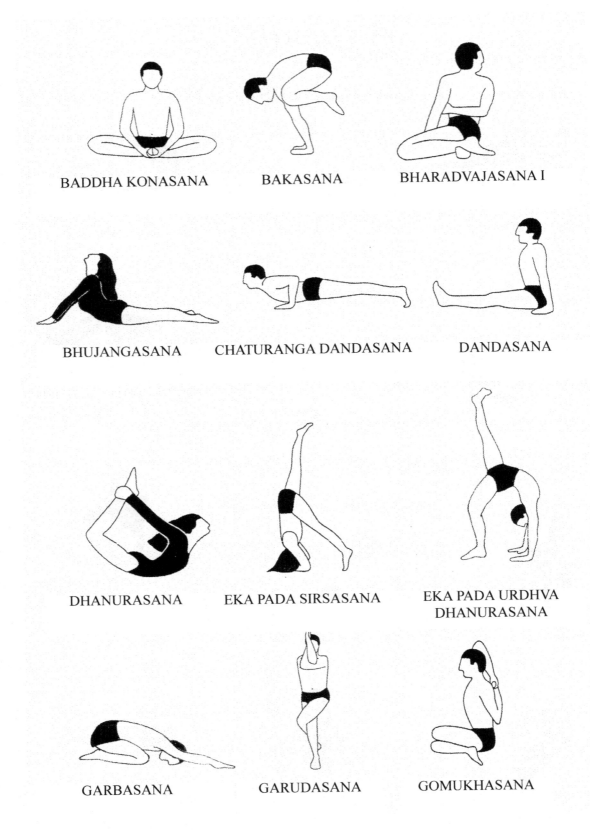

BADDHA KONASANA

BAKASANA

BHARADVAJASANA I

BHUJANGASANA

CHATURANGA DANDASANA

DANDASANA

DHANURASANA

EKA PADA SIRSASANA

EKA PADA URDHVA
DHANURASANA

GARBASANA

GARUDASANA

GOMUKHASANA

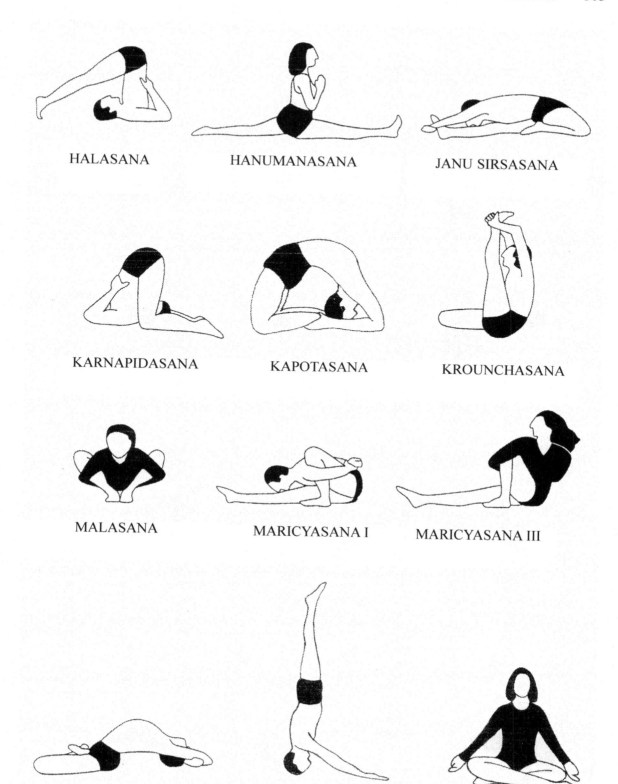

HALASANA

HANUMANASANA

JANU SIRSASANA

KARNAPIDASANA

KAPOTASANA

KROUNCHASANA

MALASANA

MARICYASANA I

MARICYASANA III

MATSYASANA

MUKTA HASTA SIRSASANA

MUKTASANA

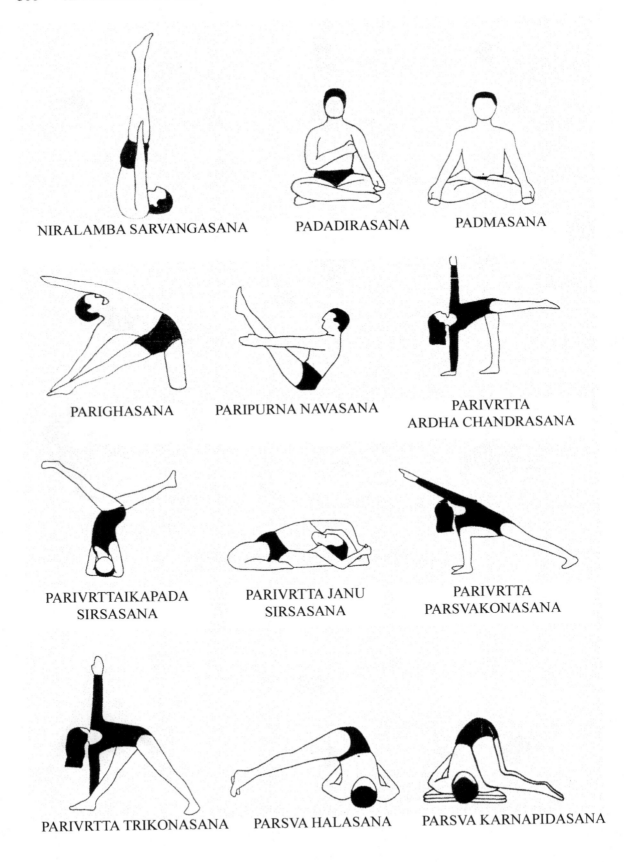

NIRALAMBA SARVANGASANA

PADADIRASANA

PADMASANA

PARIGHASANA

PARIPURNA NAVASANA

PARIVRTTA
ARDHA CHANDRASANA

PARIVRTTAIKAPADA
SIRSASANA

PARIVRTTA JANU
SIRSASANA

PARIVRTTA
PARSVAKONASANA

PARIVRTTA TRIKONASANA

PARSVA HALASANA

PARSVA KARNAPIDASANA

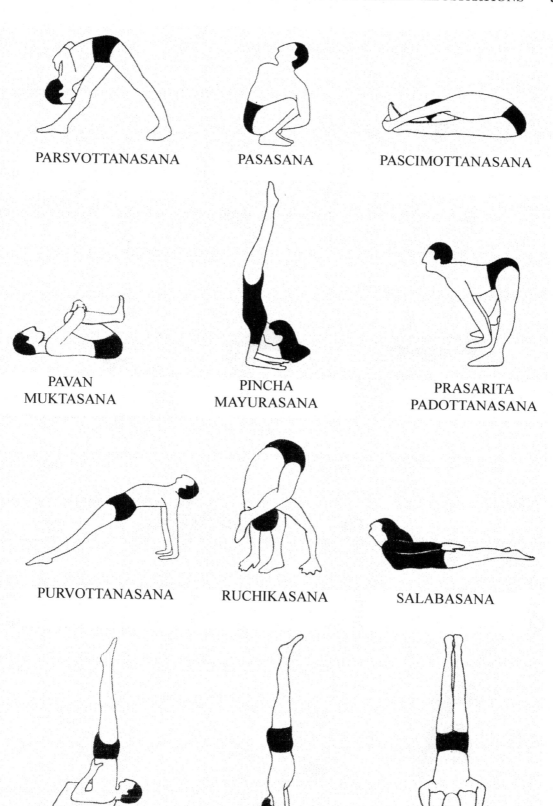

PARSVOTTANASANA

PASASANA

PASCIMOTTANASANA

PAVAN
MUKTASANA

PINCHA
MAYURASANA

PRASARITA
PADOTTANASANA

PURVOTTANASANA

RUCHIKASANA

SALABASANA

SALAMBA
SARVANGASANA

SALAMBA SIRSASANA I

SALAMBA SIRSASANA II

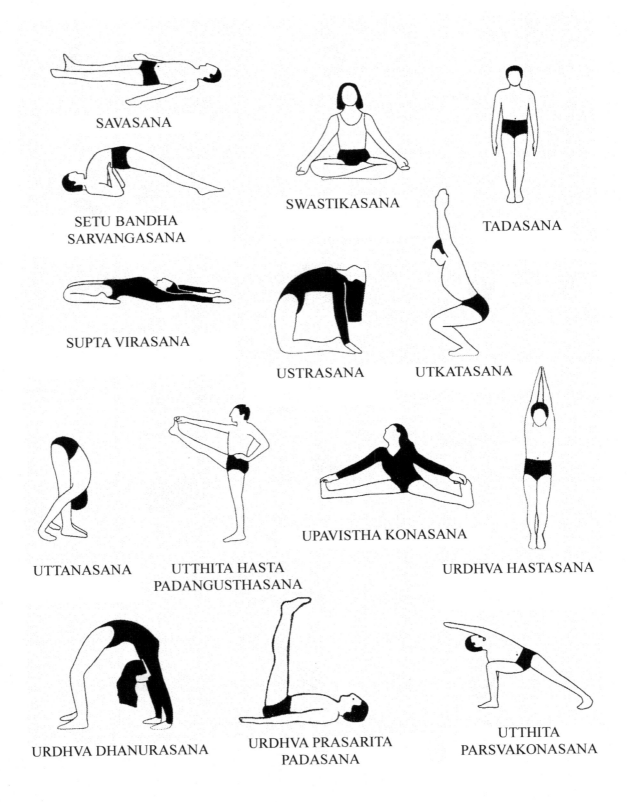

SAVASANA

SETU BANDHA
SARVANGASANA

SWASTIKASANA

TADASANA

SUPTA VIRASANA

USTRASANA

UTKATASANA

UTTANASANA

UTTHITA HASTA
PADANGUSTHASANA

UPAVISTHA KONASANA

URDHVA HASTASANA

URDHVA DHANURASANA

URDHVA PRASARITA
PADASANA

UTTHITA
PARSVAKONASANA

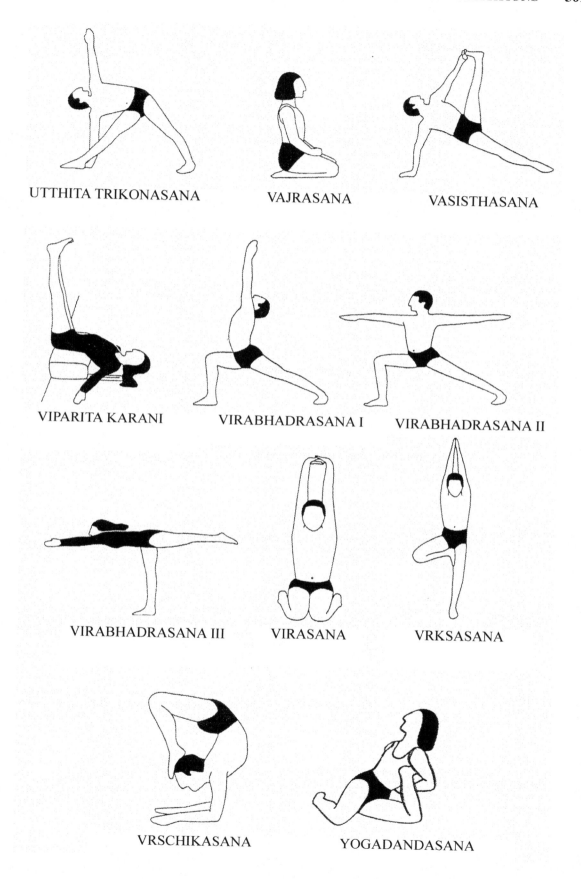

UTTHITA TRIKONASANA

VAJRASANA

VASISTHASANA

VIPARITA KARANI

VIRABHADRASANA I

VIRABHADRASANA II

VIRABHADRASANA III

VIRASANA

VRKSASANA

VRSCHIKASANA

YOGADANDASANA

Appendix II

INJURIES INCURRED BY IMPROPER YOGASANA PRACTICE

SECTION II.A. INTRODUCTION

Given that the practice of the *yogasanas* can have such a profoundly beneficial effect on a student's physiology, health, personality, philosophy, *etc.*, it is not surprising then that *yogasanas* performed improperly can lead to results that actually are harmful. That is to say, *yogasanas* are a powerful tool, and like a sharp razor, may do more harm than good in careless or unknowing hands.

"Improper" practice is taken to mean that the postures were done is such a way as to have led to an injury. Ignoring the many, many hearsay stories of injuries incurred in *yogasana* practice, there are nonetheless a significant number of scientific reports in the medical literature concerning such injuries, about which the *yogasana* teacher and practitioner should be aware. These medical reports of serious injury resulting from improper *yogasana* practice form the basis of this Appendix.

Unfortunately, the *yogasana* injury reports in question have been written by medical personnel who have no training in yoga, and though the reports are medically complete, they often seem to have omitted vital yogic information such as the style of yoga being practiced, the possible use of props, their teacher's instructions, which foot was placed on top of the other thigh, *etc*. Further, being unschooled in the art of *yogasana*,

these medical writers often conclude by condemning *yogasana* practice without understanding that there is a safe way to do these postures, but that the safe way requires an attentive student and a competent teacher. The situation is not unlike what it would be if a *yogasana* teacher were to pick up a scalpel and attempt surgery with little or no training, and then looking at the poor results, proclaim surgery to be nothing more than deceitful quackery and a sham!

The following Subsections touch briefly upon a few general situations which can lead to injury, as suggested by the specific case histories given in Section II.B, page 513.

Practicing Yogasanas from a Book, Without a Teacher

Because we so easily fool ourselves in regard our body and what it is doing at any moment, it generally is not a good idea to practice *yogasanas* using only a book (even a very good book), without input from a teacher (preferably a very good teacher). Those who do so either out of necessity or for philosophical reasons, at the very least run the risk of teaching the body the incorrect way to perform the asanas, and at the worst, risk injury. The student who has "learned yoga" from a book can be a big problem once he/she finds a competent teacher, for considerable erasing of the old technique often has to be done in order to implant the proper technique; indeed, old habits die hard.

Being Too Tired Can Lead to Injury

Even with proper technique, the tendency toward misalignment will intrude once one has been in the pose for a substantial time so that the mood has become more meditative and less concerned with mechanical technique. Related to this is the collapse that often occurs when the student is still in the pose, but receives the signal from the teacher to come out of the position. One notices, for example, that many more students lose their balance when coming out of *trikonasana* than when going into it, most likely for reasons of mental and physical fatigue. This premature relaxation of the body's alignment while still in a compromising position can lead to injury. Moreover, as Schatz [413] has pointed out, women who choose to practice demanding postures during their menstrual period may be working with diminished strength and energy, and so risk injury.

Being Too Ambitious Can Lead to Injury

It is natural that when a student is a quick learner, he or she becomes infatuated with *yogasana* practice and wants to try everything in the book as soon as possible. This ambitious attitude can place unwary students in deep water before they are ready for more demanding poses, and so sets the stage for an injury. My own experience in this is that the too-quick student will want to learn "how to stand on my head" and "how to do the lotus" positions, often before they understand how to do them safely. One must remind the student that *yogasana* practice is intended for a lifetime, and that all of the poses do not have to be mastered before age 21! Approaching these postures with cau-

tion is not only the safe way, but helps the students to control the tendency to go faster in all aspects of their lives.

Congenital Weaknesses

Even with an attentive student working with a competent teacher, there is still the possibility of injury due to an unsuspected congenital weakness in the student's body which is uncovered in a particular *yogasana*, even when done correctly. Thus, some students may be injured immediately on performing a particular *yogasana*, and others may do the same *yogasana* in the same way for a lifetime and not experience any problem. The difference here is that in the former case, the student was born with a congenital weakness that was exposed by the *yogasana*, whereas in the latter, the body was strong enough to tolerate the stress of the posture, at least for the short term. This inherent variability of susceptibility to injury must be kept in mind, and one must realize that even if everything in a pose is in alignment and is otherwise letter-perfect, a congenital weakness can still be present which sooner or later expresses itself as an injury. Further, what is proper for very experienced practitioners will not necessarily be appropriate for beginner and intermediate students, no matter how healthy they might be.

One can go too far in condemning *yogasana* practice on the basis of a few medically-certified injuries. Thus, Russell has pointed out [395] for example, the basilar-artery syndrome (see below) can be precipitated not only by incorrectly performing *yogasanas* such as *sarvangasana* or *bhujangasana*, but also in such innocent situations as tipping one's head back in the dentist's chair, during anaesthesia, having a shampoo at the hairdressers, picking fruit, painting a ceiling, driving a car, swimming the breast stroke, or presiding over a meeting [39, 479]. Certainly none of these are flagged by doctors or by the general public as being too dangerous to consider, and *yogasana* injuries should be given the same benefit of the doubt. Still, not to trivialize the risks in some of the *yogasanas*, students should work on these postures with a knowledgeable teacher, and avoid staying too long in static positions (see below).

Alter's book [5], *Science of Flexibility*, has an entire chapter on what he calls X-rated exercises, so called because of their risks; all of these X-rated positions are readily recognized as *yogasana* positions, or their variations. These include *triangamukhaikapada paschimottanasana* (risk to the knee of the bent leg), *supta virasana* (risk to the knees and spine), *malasana* (knees), *uttanasana* (lower back and knees), various backbends from *urdhva mukha svanasana* to *urdhva dhanurasana* (vertebral artery occlusion), gravity inversion (blood pressure), and *sarvangasana* and *halasana* (vascular and structural cervical problems). These concerns underline the need for working with an experienced teacher when a beginner first attempts these postures; there are no documented cases of injuries when these poses are practiced under the guidance of an experienced teacher.

SECTION II.B. SPECIFIC CASE HISTORIES

Neurological Damage

It is good and proper to encourage students to stay a little longer in the *yogasanas* than they are inclined to do otherwise. In most students, there is a rapid weakening of the nervous system as the pose is held, and an almost overpowering psychological need to come out of the pose. By keeping oneself in the pose just a little beyond the need to come out, one strengthens the neural circuits that drive the muscles holding the pose erect, and develops the will power necessary to progress in the practice. On the other hand, as the medical literature shows (below), one can stay far too long in the postures, to one's detriment. Ideally, one should work with effort, but not to the point of struggle, experiencing discomfort, but not pain. Done in this way, the poses will show strength and steadiness, and at the same time an ease and grace characteristic of the even, focused mind [111]. Resist the temptation to doze in postures which feel very comfortable.

In certain postures, one has bone pressing against bone, with muscles and nerves caught between, as with the shins in *padmasana* or the biceps/triceps pressing the femur in *maricyasana III*, whereas in yet others, there is a tourniquet effect and joints are closed so as to restrict the circulation of blood past the joint, as happens to the lower legs in *vajrasana*, for example. In such cases, the result is a slowing of the blood flow through the region in question with a consequent decrease in the oxygen being brought to the cells. This slow starvation of the nerves and muscles by compression is of little consequence when the *yogasana* is performed for a short time, but can become a serious factor when one feels comfortable in the position and so stays for an extended period. Nerve cells are especially sensitive to this "ischemia", for they do not tolerate a lack of oxygen (hypoxia) very well. As discussed below, staying in some poses for too long a time creates an ischemic condition resulting in temporary or even permanent injury to the associated afferent and efferent nerves, *i.e.*, a neuropathy.

In the case of an afferent nerve being injured by compression, the symptoms are a tingling sensation followed by a numbing loss of sensation. If, instead, it is the efferent nerve that is injured, then one has all degrees of loss of muscle control, deliberate and reflexive (Subsection 5.C, *Mechanical Effects on Nerves*, page 125).

In addition to ischemia, pressure on the nerves also may result in their demyelination, *i.e.*, a partial or total stripping of the fatty covering of the nerves that is so essential for their neural conductivity (Section 5.B, Nerve Conduction, page 114). Were this to happen, the nerve and the associated sensor or muscle is more or less incapacitated. Yet another possible consequence of external pressure on a nerve is the impediment to the vital flow of internal components within the axon, between the body of the neural cell and its axonal and dendritic tips.

Consider the case of a meditation student who is reported to have fallen asleep in full *padmasana* for more than three hours [301]. On the next day, the student felt a tingling from the hip to the upper knee on the right side, and after twenty-four hours, the tingling became numbness, with no sensations of pinprick, temperature or light touch in the area. Apparently the extended time in a position where the afferent sensory nerve on the right upper thigh was compressed by the opposite foot such that the nerve suffered ischemia was sufficient to deaden the response of the nerve for more than a month. Not only does the pressure of the ankle on the opposite upper thigh in *padmasana* compress the nerve directly and so interfere with its oxygenation, but it also contributes to a more general ischemia in that each foot and ankle rests upon the femoral artery of the opposite leg so as to attenuate the overall blood supply to the lower body.

In a somewhat similar case [471], another student of meditation spent two hours sitting with crossed legs, heels under thighs (presumably *muktasana* or a variation thereof); in this case the afferent sensory nerves were not damaged, however, the ankle-stretch reflex (foot drop) was affected, and was still inactive three weeks after the meditation due to the denervation of the muscles served by the peroneal and tibial components of the sciatic nerve (see below). Apparently, the weight of the body pressing down on the efferent nerves of the lower legs was sufficient to demyelinate the nerves locally, resulting in the loss of the relevant muscle responses [471].

Let us consider for a moment the structure and geography of the sciatic nerve. This nerve bundle is composed of five nerves, exiting the spine at vertebrae L4, L5, S1, S2, and S3 [170, 262], and travels diagonally left and right across the back of the pelvis, between the pelvic bones and the piriformis muscles deep within the buttocks.* Each of the bundles then travels down the back of its respective leg, and in the vicinity of the knee, branches into a smaller division that stays on the outer surface of the lower leg (the peroneal component), and a larger bundle that takes a route on the inside of the lower leg (the tibial component). Of the two branches, it is said that the tibial component is the more susceptible to injury by compression [452, 471]. A tributary of the sciatic nerve in the upper leg (the femoral cutaneous branch) innervates the inner, upper thigh [170].

In the case mentioned above of the student dozing in *padmasana*, the compressed nerve would appear to be the femoral cutaneous branch of the sciatic nerve, whereas for the student sitting in *muktasana*, the compression was below the knee, more likely where bone presses bone in the crossed-leg position, and most likely involved the

---

*Actually, the sciatic nerve penetrates the piriformis muscle in about 15% of the population, leading to sciatic discomfort that is severe but still treatable through *yogasana* practice.

tibial component of the sciatic nerve in the lower leg.

Yet another meditator commonly sat in *vajrasana* for up to six hours a day, "chanting for world peace" [64, 174]. The result was what is now called "yoga foot drop" in the medical literature, consisting of a loss of muscle strength in the ankles and toes such that the foot can not be flexed toward the knee. This outcome was attributed to peroneal neuropathy as a consequence of compression of the relevant efferent sciatic nerves.

Sciatic neuropathies can develop in many seemingly innocent situations. Thus, it is reported that loss of leg strength can occur when the sciatic nerve is compressed for hours on end as when lying in a coma, or when one is bed ridden and unable to move to a fresh position [447]. More bizarre are two independent cases of intense sciatic discomfort brought on by carrying a wallet stuffed with credit cards in the hip pocket of one's trousers [290]! In one of these credit-card cases, the patient earlier had been diagnosed as having a herniated disc, and had received chiropractic treatment for his problem.

The effects of compression leading to ischemia of an efferent nerve and paralysis of the relevant muscle are readily demonstrated in two situations familiar to *yogasana* students. First, being in *supta virasana* for many students brings on a temporary neuropathy of the nerves in the lower legs due to the heightened pressure at the backs of the folded knees, and to the restriction of blood flow below the knees. As a consequence of these effects, after 5 minutes in *supta virasana*, many students have momentary difficulty standing and walking. A similar momentary paralysis can occur in the arm by sitting cross legged with the arms in *gomukhasana*, and then carefully lying down on the back, thus pinning one arm between the floor and the back body

with its hand between the shoulder blades. The weight of the upper body pressing on the nerves of the upper arm for just a minute or two appears to be enough to paralyze the arm for a short time. For those who are susceptible to this type of compression-induced ischemia, it is frightening to think of what the results might be if they were to stay in positions such as these for an extended time.

Vascular Damage

The inner surfaces of the vascular system are tightly covered with endothelial cells which keep the platelets that circulate within the system from contact with any of the collagenous material in the outer layers; were there a rupture of the endothelial layer of the vascular system, the contact of the platelets with the collagen immediately initiates the formation of a blood clot at the site of injury. If the artery or vein is so compressed in a *yogasana* that the integrity of the endothelium is breeched, then platelets may gather at the exposed spot, forming a blood clot (a thrombosis). The thrombosis may grow to cut off circulation in the blood vessel in which it occurred, or may break loose to form an embolism that may then plug smaller vessels in other parts of the vascular tree. As the tendency to form blood clots is inherited [177], problems of this sort may show up as a congenital weakness in an otherwise strong *yogasana* student.

The *yogasana*-induced thrombosis/embolism scenarios are most often involved either with the blood vessels of the eyes (often in inverted poses), or with the vertebral arteries of the cervical spine (often with external pressure on the vertebrae or inappropriate turning of the head).

In traveling up the cervical spine, the vertebral arteries are threaded through openings in the bony transverse processes of vertebrae C6–C1, and then pass through the foramen magnum on their way to the back of the brain, Fig. 3.B-1. The blood supplies to the medulla oblongata, pons, mesencephalon and cerebellum are derived from the vertebral basilar-artery system [332]. Serious thromboses and/or occlusions in the brain can occur when the vertebral arteries are injured, as can happen when flexing the neck or turning the head.

There is a report in the literature [140] of an unfortunate student who performed *sirsasana* without adequate supervision, in her quest for "self-relaxation". In this, a young student is reported to have performed *sirsasana* without a teacher and with only two months home practice. After 5 minutes in the position, she felt a sharp pain in the neck, and two months after that, reported to her doctor that she had only partial feeling and weak muscle control on the right side of the body, and a declining level of consciousness. It was concluded that in doing *sirsasana*, she had injured the vertebral arteries in the neck, leading in time to a thrombosis in the basilar artery, which is fed by the vertebral arteries. In time, the thrombosis was set free in the vascular system, and the embolism so formed found its way into the left hemisphere of the brain where it interfered eventually with muscle action on the right side of the body.

In hindsight, one would guess that the student had placed her head on the floor too close to the hairline, and then went inverted without working the arms against the floor; this combination of errors would lead to a shearing action of the cervical vertebrae with respect to the vertebral arteries, Subsection 3.B, *Blood Flow through the Brain*, page 35. The student returned to near-normal after a year of therapy.

A similarly unfortunate outcome is reported for a yoga student again working without a teacher or proper instruction [175]. In this case, a young man performed an "inverted standing" (presumably *sarvangasana*) for 5 minutes every day for 18 months, without blankets under the shoulders, but with his shoulders and head pressed maximally against the bare floor. By the time the student went to the doctor, he was dizzy, was unable to walk, and had bruises over vertebrae C5, C6, and C7; after two months of therapy, he could walk again with a cane. His doctor reports a lesion in the medulla oblongata within the brainstem (Subsection 3.A, *The Spinal Cord and Brainstem*, page 29) as the causative factor, most likely induced by the intensity of the posture. The doctor concludes that "inverted standing" on the shoulders and head could be especially dangerous in the elderly, with their underlying vascular and arthritic problems.

Based on this unfortunate event, others have published blanket warnings against doing *halasana*, Fig. 11.F-2 [122, 337], without distinguishing between the harm that can come from performing the pose incorrectly, and the benefits that it gives when performed carefully, with proper preparation and attention to alignment and the lengthening of the spine. In response to these claims, Lasater has written eloquently, refuting their arguments in every detail [262]. In cases such as the above, the student was not being taught properly, if at all, and furthermore, were blankets used in the way prescribed for *sarvangasana* and *halasana* [216, 262], the chances for such unfortunate results would be considerably reduced.

Nagler [332] reports three cases of injury traced to active hyperextension (dorsiflexion) of the cervical spine. In the first, a young student in *adho mukha vrksasana* vigorously pulled his head back as he lost balance backward (overbalance, Appendix IV, BALANCING, page 525), inducing an obstruction of the vertebral artery; he was still in a wheelchair 18 months after the incident. A 55-year-old man performing what appears to have been *salabhasana* forcefully dorsiflexed the neck in the posture, and immediately found that he could not walk or lift his arms. Again, the diagnosis was an occlusion of the vertebral artery and the resulting ischemia. Lastly, a young "yoga enthusiast" while in *urdhva dhanurasana* with her head on the floor, was said to have suffered a cerebellar infarct due to the shutting off of the blood supply in the cervical area. Accidents of this sort are much more likely in those with a congenital disposition toward vertebral occlusion on dorsiflexion, however, one cannot know one's disposition in this regard until it is tested!

The vertebral artery is most subject to damage at the atlanto-axial joint between C1 and C2, the point of maximum movement when turning the head. Though no injuries are reported in this regard for *yogasana* students performing spinal twists, the medical literature is rife with reports of people who suffer seriously impeded blood flow to the brain and consequent neurological damage when they turned their heads abruptly, but in a seemingly benign manner [426].

Excessive effort in the *yogasanas* often reveals itself in the eyes. This is possibly due to a fragility of the veins in the eyes and to the fact that at the eyes, the hydrostatic pressure of the blood in inversions is not compensated by that of the cerebrospinal fluid, Section 11.F, Blood Pressure in Inverted *Yogasanas*, page 343.

A yoga teacher with many years experience was found to have a thrombosis (blood clot) in a vein serving one eye; it was concluded in her case that positions such as *sirsasana* in which the head is below the heart were a mitigating factor in the development of what was likely a congenital condition [74]. In a similar case, the connection between yoga and thrombosis about the eyes was thought to be much stronger. In this situation [296], the student had performed *sirsasana* for ten minutes, ten times daily for ten years, before noticing blue-purple nodules within the conjunctiva of the eyes. It was hypothesized that the thromboses were caused by the increased venous pressure in the eyes coupled with decreased venous outflow accompanying the inverted position, and were repaired surgically.

A student who daily performed *sirsasana* and *sarvangasana* for 15–20 minutes each, allowed his ophthalmologist to measure the intraocular pressures within his eyes as he performed a meditative seated pose, *urdhva dhanurasana*, *sarvangasana* and *sirsasana*, recording pressures of 18, 25, 28 and 32 mm Hg for these four positions [383]. All pressures returned immediately to the baseline pressure on returning to sitting. It was concluded that inverted poses such as these significantly increased intraocular pressure, and so should be discouraged in those with glaucoma or a tendency toward it.

Consider the case described by Fahmy and Fledelius [133], in which a woman who reported episodes of blurred vision following *yogasana* practice was found to have an elevated internal pressure in the fluid of the eyes (momentary glaucoma). Though this increased pressure did not appear after being in *sarvangasana* for one hour, it did appear following one hour in a face-down prone position. Normal pressure returned during the night. Investigation showed that the eyes in this particular case were formed in such a way so as to allow the lens and the iris to collapse upon one another in the face-down position (as in *salabhasana*), thereby pressurizing the internal fluid. This would be a case of a congenital defect in the structure of the eye, combined with an unfortunate choice of *yogasanas* for practice.

The types of eye problems discussed above can be brought about by any extreme effort in which one holds the breath and increases the internal abdominal pressure by tightening the abdominal muscles (the Valsalva maneuver). Beginners often resort to this action in an effort to amplify their strength, but this is clearly contraindicated for any but the most advanced *yogasana* practitioners. Perhaps it was this type of action that brought on the problem in the case cited above.

It is known that pressure on the inside of the upper arm acts to close the axillary vein and that this can lead to thrombosis [338]. Though there are no medical reports on this *vis-a-vis yogasana*, one easily imagines such a situation developing were a student to spend too long a time in either *maricyasana I* or *III*, for in both of these postures the axillary vein can be pressed tightly against the tibia.

It goes without saying that if one has a pre-existing vascular problem, such as varicose veins, one should not spend any length of time in poses that otherwise would further impede venous return from the area in question, *i.e.*, one should not do *padmasana*, for example, if one already has varicosities in the legs.

There is one tragic story in the literature of a young woman who died of a embolism said to be directly related to her practice of *pranayama* [91], however, it involved mouth-to-mouth breathing with another student, and the heavy use of marijuana.

Muscular Damage

Though the favorite topic of conversation among assembled yoga students is their latest muscle pull, spasm, or skeletal pain, I could find no record of such complaints having been taken to a doctor and then these finding their way into print. As discussed in Subsection 7.E, *Warming Up*, page 227, a proper warm up should precede any serious attempt at performing a *yogasana* that is challenging. This warm up will give the muscles a good stretch, lubricate the joints involved, and will start the flow of glucose from the liver. Only then is it safe to attempt the more difficult postures.

When doing any of the *yogasanas*, difficult or not, it is important that one does not try to stretch too quickly; if the student will allow himself to ease into the posture slowly, then there will be no tearing of the muscle fibers as they are stretched (Subsection 7.E, *When Stretching, Time Matters, and Time Is on Your Side*, page 224).

When done to excess, eccentric exercise can lead to rhabdomyolysis, a condition in which muscle tissue has been destroyed on a large scale, leading to the appearance of muscle-cell debris in the urine and a fatal blocking of the kidneys by myoglobin leaking from the damaged muscles [103].

Appendix III

BODY SYMMETRY

SECTION III.A. SYMMETRY, BEAUTY, AND HEALTH

It is clear that animals can be very selective in picking a mate. In this, one wonders just what criteria are used in rejecting one suitor and accepting another. For many animals, it appears that disease or weakness is reflected in a lack of left-right symmetry in the body. Indeed, experiments show that the criterion for selective mating in many animals is high left-right mirror symmetry, for high symmetry is synonymous with fertility, physical and mental health, optimal hormonal function and sexual prowess. Thus, by the simple assessment of lateral symmetry, animals can assure a strong, healthy mate, free of disease and weakness, and thereby increase the chances of having strong, healthy progeny [363, 473]. This criterion is known to be a factor in mate selection in insects, birds, many animals, and subconsciously in humans as well [14, 277, 363].

It is not unreasonable that humans as well tend to equate high skeletal symmetry with a strong and healthy mate who can supply strong and healthy progeny, whereas a lack of this left-right mirror symmetry implies physical collapse of some sort and less than perfect health. Among humans, symmetry also is a factor in beauty in all cultures and beauty in turn is very important again in choosing a mate. Tests of perceived facial beauty for both men and women consistently show that those who are thought to be "most beautiful" have the highest left-right facial symmetry [14, 363].

It must be mentioned that in spite of the superficial high symmetry of the body as seen from the outside, the inside of the body is quite asymmetrical. Due to packing difficulties, the left lung has two lobes but the right lung has three. Also the left and right bronchi are tilted a different angles so that if an object is inhaled into the lungs, it always will be found lodged in the right lung. The left side of the heart is larger and stronger than the right as it pushes blood through the entire body, whereas the right only pushes it through the lungs [3]. This aspect is discussed further in Section III.C, The Body's Inherent Lack of Symmetry, page 520. Note also that according to Ayurvedic thinking, the long-term lack of symmetry when breathing alternately through the nostrils (Section 12.C, Nasal Laterality, page 374) is a strong signal for incipient disease or an unhealthy condition [252].

Could this connection between geometry and health be related in some way to our striving for high left-right symmetry in the *yogasanas* when performed in the Iyengar way (*trikonasana*, for example), regardless of the overall inherent asymmetry of the pose? Quoting B.K.S. Iyengar, "Your whole being should be symmetrical. Yoga is symmetry. That is why yoga is a basic art" [210]. In fact, one of the basic principles of his style of *yogasana* teaching is the attempt to recover the high symmetry of *tadasana* even in the most asymmetric postures.

SECTION III.B. SYMMETRY AND YOGA

Continuing along this line of thinking, consider *tadasana* to be the standard of high symmetry, and thus indirectly, the standard of optimal strength and health. In going from *tadasana* to one of the less symmetric standing poses, *trikonasana* for example, is it not reasonable that we nonetheless perform the pose in such a way as to promote strength and health, *i.e.*, perform the pose with maximal symmetry? But how does one do an inherently asymmetric posture with maximal symmetry? The answer to this is to *perform these globally asymmetric poses in a way that the local symmetry is as high as it can be*, given the nature of the posture. Referring to *trikonasana*, we attempt to perform as many of the relevant *tadasana*-like actions as we can in *trikonasana*, trying to keep the local left-right mirror symmetry as high as possible and avoiding collapse in all parts of the body; see Box III.B-1 for a more detailed example of what is meant here.

Though not as obvious as handedness (Section III.D, page 523), our bodies have preferred sides for many other asymmetric motor tasks, such as which foot first steps onto the lowest step when climbing stairs, which eye opens first when slowly opening the eyes, which foot turns out more in *urdhva dhanurasana*, which index finger crosses over the other when interlacing the fingers, *etc.*

In addition to the unavoidable asymmetry imposed upon us by the placement of our organs (Section III.C, page 520), the preferential handedness in humans also affects our *yogasanas* in a purely mechanical way. For example, it is almost always more difficult for yoga students to place the right hand behind the back in *gomukhasana* than it is to place the left. This is due to habit, for right-handed people "live" in the forward-right quadrant of space, and so the backward-

right quadrant is foreign to them and thus a difficult place to visit. The same factor would come into play in *ardha baddha padma paschimottanasana*. Interestingly, the right-arm-behind-the-back problem for right handers doing *gomukhasana* does not appear as often for left handers when placing their left hands behind their backs, again showing that they are less committed to their handedness than are the right handers.

To the extent that our lack of left-right symmetry of the cerebral hemispheres may be a factor in the performance of the *yogasanas*, it is interesting to note that the proprioceptive sense of alignment is more accurate on the left side of the body.

In the general population, greater strength, coordination, balance and proprioceptive awareness are observed on the side of the dominant hand [5]. However, with the accent in yoga practice on working both the dominant and non-dominant sides, one would expect the lateral imbalances to be lessened (see Section 3.D, Cerebral Hemispheric Laterality, page 49).

SECTION III.C. THE BODY'S INHERENT LACK OF SYMMETRY

In the early stages of human embryonic development, the embryo is perfectly symmetric until the heart starts to form. From that point on, the asymmetries begin to accumulate. This is odd, for the human body as seen from the front appears to be highly symmetric across the medial plane dividing left from right. There are two equally-placed cerebral hemispheres, two eyes, two nostrils, two arms and two legs, *etc.*, and with only one mouth and one nose, even these are placed symmetrically on the medial plane. However, this symmetry is more apparent than real, since each of the pairs mentioned above has one partner of the pair which is functionally dominant, often in a

BOX III.B-1: PRESERVING THE SYMMETRY OF
TADASANA IN *TRIKONASANA*

Tadasana is as symmetric as one can get with respect to the left-right mirror plane of the body. Let us first list the symmetry elements present in *tadasana*:

1) Back body (back of head, scapula, buttocks, little fingers, calves and heels) in a vertical plane

2) Legs active and straight, with foot, ankle and knee of each leg in alignment

3) The axes of the spine (vertical) and of the pelvis (horizontal) are mutually perpendicular, whereas the axes of the shoulder girdle and of the pelvis are parallel

4) The distance from the right frontal pelvic bone to the lowest right rib is equal to that from the left frontal pelvic bone to the corresponding rib on the left

5) Normal spinal curvatures, with cervical vertebrae in line with those of the thoracic spine left to right

6) Lift the energy from the pit of the stomach into the chest, with scapula dropped away from the ears and tipped into the ribcage so as to open and lift it while lengthening the spine and spreading the collarbones

As compared with *tadasana* symmetry-wise, *trikonasana* has lost the left-right mirror symmetry totally, yet the proper action in *trikonasana* is such as to restore the local symmetry as outlined by the six points above, though of course one can not restore the global symmetry and still be in the pose. Consider the six points given above, but as applied to *trikonasana* to the right:

1) Rotate legs and ribs so that the back-body parts (back of head, scapula, buttocks, backs of the hands, calves and heels) as much as possible lie on a vertical plane

2) Legs active and straight, with the foot, ankle and knee of each leg in alignment

3) Tip the pelvis so that the axis of the pelvis remains perpendicular to the axis of the spine and parallel to the axis of the shoulders

4) Press the right sitting bone toward the left ankle and lift the right ribs away from the frontal pelvic bone on the right, so as to make the two sides of the upper body equally long

5) Maintain normal curvature in the spine, especially in the lumbar, and lift the head so as to keep the neck in line with the rest of the spine

6) Lift the energy from the pit of the stomach into the chest, with scapula dropped away from the ears and tipped into the ribcage so as to open and lift it while lengthening the spine and spreading the collarbones

When compared in this way, one sees immediately that at a certain low level, the work of *trikonasana* is largely that of trying to restore/preserve the local symmetry about certain key areas of the body while forfeiting the global symmetry. How many of the symmetry elements of *tadasana* can you find working in *parivrtta trikonasana*?

way that depends upon what the task is at the moment.

Looking within, Fig.18.A-1, asymmetry abounds. There are two lungs, but the left one is divided into three lobes whereas the right is divided into two. There is only one heart, but it is not placed symmetrically in the chest, nor is it itself right-left symmetric. The other internal organs are even more asymmetric: the liver, gallbladder, spleen, stomach, and colon are placed in the abdominal cavity on the basis of packing efficiency rather than symmetry. Furthermore, though the vagus nerve (cranial nerve X) branches to both the left and the right, the left branch reaches only to the upper stomach, whereas the right branch continues on to innervate almost all of the digestive organs, being far more extensive and important than the left branch [343].

One in every 25,000 babies is born with all of the internal organs transposed to the "wrong side" [33]. This seems not to be a serious threat to health and longevity, however, those born with two "right sides" rarely live past the first year, whereas those with two "left sides" have a normal life span.

Though the brain would seem to be left-right symmetric, the inner body's asymmetry penetrates into that region as well. As discussed in more detail in Section 3.D, Cerebral Hemispheric Laterality, page 49, the gross symmetry is deceptive, for the corresponding parts in the two hemispheres can have different sizes and the hemispheres themselves each have their special functions. Thus, in 95% of the population, the language functions are restricted to the left hemisphere, which is also dominant for manual motor skills in right-handed people. On the other hand, the right hemisphere is dominant for spatial ability, music and emotional behavior, Table 3.D-1.

That we think of each of the muscles as a distinct entity with a characteristic name is a useful approximation, but nonetheless it is still an approximation, for in truth the two most widely separated muscles are intimately connected by the web of fascia and connective tissue which surrounds all muscles down to the level of the sarcolemma; moreover this web incorporates the connective tissues that surround the bones and support the internal organs as well. Rolf [386] points out that if we could somehow extract all of the myofibrils from the body of a friend, leaving only the connective tissues, the result would still look recognizably like that person as we ordinarily know them.

Given then that the internal organs are left-right very asymmetrically placed within the body, and that they are held in place by webs of connective tissue which are themselves just a part of the larger web holding all of the body in its shape, it seems inescapable that the pull of these asymmetric organs on all the muscles of the body must in some small way make the muscle actions similarly asymmetric, as implied by Fig. 9.A-1. That is to say, *trikonasana* done to the left and to the right with sufficient inner awareness must feel different to some degree in spite of the efforts to make it otherwise. Similarly, even *tadasana*, the standard of high symmetry also must be asymmetric to some extent due to the basic asymmetry of the human-body plan. Nonetheless, we must work in the direction of perfect left-right symmetry even though it is unattainable.

This line of thinking brings us to an odd impasse: when doing the asymmetric *yogasanas*, one must work to retain as much local symmetry as possible, yet even in the most symmetric pose, *tadasana*, one should sense a great local asymmetry, for that is the nature of our inner construction. See also Box IV.E-2, *Physical Crossover Requires Neural Crossover*, page 543, for an example of how the body's neural crossover can impact on our sense of left-right balance.

SECTION III.D. HANDEDNESS

That 97% of humans show a left-hemisphere dominance [230] accounts for the fact that 90% of the population is right-handed, thanks to decussation of the efferent nerves in the spinal cord (Section 4.B, The Spinal Cord, page 83). As shown in Table 3.D-2, the dominant hemisphere for speech is the left one for not only right-handed people, but for many of the left-handed as well as the ambidextrous, however, this tendency is much stronger in the right-handed than in the others. In general, left-handed people are more symmetrical than are the right-handers, which is to say, they are less committed to their handedness.

If one defines the cerebral hemisphere that controls verbal expression as the dominant hemisphere, then 96–99% of right-handed people have a dominant left hemisphere. More specifically, the dominant center resides in the left frontal lobe. For people who are left handed, 60–70% also have a dominant left hemisphere; in those cases where the cerebral dominance is on the right side, the center in question is the right frontal lobe [225]. People with a strong excitation in the right prefrontal cortex tend to be more nervous and pessimistic, whereas, when the left prefrontal cortex is strongly excited preferentially, the patients show depression.

The parietal lobe of the dominant hemisphere plays a significant role in calculation, writing and the reading of words. As the temporal lobes of the brain are closely associated with hearing, injury to the temporal lobe on the dominant side leads to an inability to understand spoken words [340]. Cerebral laterality also seems to have its effect on sexual orientation, for the proportion of left-handed lesbians is double that of left-handed women in the general population, and the more left-handed you are, the larger is the corpus callosum, that nerve bundle which serves as the communications highway between the right and left cerebral hemispheres [325].

Appendix IV

BALANCING

SECTION IV.A. INTRODUCTION

Because mechanical balancing is more or less a part of virtually every *yogasana*, it is of special importance to the *yogasana* student. In any posture, if one falls before the *yogasana* is brought to completion, then fully one-third or more of the going-into-the-pose/remaining-in-the-pose/coming-out-of-the-pose, three-part cycle has been lost. Maintaining balance can be especially difficult when the posture requires (a) being inverted on the head, as in *sirsasana*, (b) balancing on the hands, either inverted as in *adho mukha vrksasana* or nominally upright as in *bakasana*, (c) standing on one leg, as in *vrksasana*, (d) moving from one balanced position to another, as when going from *ardha chandrasana* to *virabhadrasana III*, (e) balancing on the ischium (sitting) bones of the pelvis, as in *navasana*, and (f) rotating in a balanced position such that the left and right sides of the upper body are reversed with respect to the lower parts, as in *parivrtta trikonasana*. Of course, there are poses which combine aspects of the points listed here, as for example, *vasisthasana*, an inclined balancing pose involving support on one arm and one leg. Additionally, to lose one's balance is to fall, and because the fear of falling is a natural one, strong and ever-present, it can inhibit our attempts at being totally in the posture. Fortunately, the balancing senses can be sharpened by practice.

All inanimate systems when left to themselves move naturally and spontaneously to the state of lowest energy; in the case of an object in the earth's gravitational field, the state of lowest energy is reached when the centers of the object and the earth are as close to one another as possible, for they experience a mutual gravitational force which is attractive in inverse proportion to the square of the distance between them (Appendix V, GRAVITY, page 553). Translated into the practical world of the *yogasana* student, this means that in every pose, the student is pulled by gravity toward the center of the earth and onto the floor! Our work in *yogasana* practice is to resist the effects of this natural attraction of our body for the floor in all of the postures, except for *savasana*.

Even in a *yogasana* in which balance is not a factor, as with *adho mukha svanasana*, for example, the effect of gravity nonetheless is to pull the body down onto the floor; it is the work of the arms and legs that keeps the pelvis lifted up and back, resisting gravity with no thought given to maintaining balance. However, in a balancing pose such as *adho mukha vrksasana*, the effect of gravity becomes doubly disadvantageous, for it requires that the body be kept in balance in spite of gravity, and at the same time, that it be extended upward, again in spite of gravity. However, as will be discussed below, the act of yogic extension against gravity actually serves to make the balancing easier in almost all cases.

There are four distinct sensory systems in one's body which are relevant to the act of balancing in the *yogasanas*: (1) The positions and rates of motion of the various body parts with respect to one another are sensed by the proprioceptors in the muscles (see Section 7.C, Proprioception, page 208) and joints (see Section 8.E, The Joints, page 260) and a map of the body in space is constructed by the brain from this information. (2) Deep-pressure sensors in the skin (see Section 10.B, page 290) detect the pattern of pressure within the skin as it presses the floor. This shifting pattern of pressure is readily translated into a sense of balancing or falling. (3) Two types of sensors deep in the inner ears monitor the relative static positions of the head with respect to the downward pull of gravity as well as the rotational motion of the head (see Section 17.B, The Vestibular Organs of Balance, page 437), and (4) the eyes can sense the relative orientation of the line between their centers with respect to the horizon. All four of these sensor modes working more or less simultaneously keep the body in mechanical balance during *yogasana* practice. Of the various balancing systems, the proprioceptive is the most rapidly responding, with the visual and vestibular apparatus significantly slower [225]. Moreover, the relative importance of the different balancing sensors may differ from one person to the next and from one *yogasana* to the next. As we age, the first balancing mechanism to fail is that of the vestibular apparatus.

SECTION IV.B. MECHANICAL ASPECTS OF BALANCING

Balancing a Rigid Block

Let us first consider what is mechanically involved in balancing a solid, inanimate object. The rule is simple: an object will rest on the floor without falling over if the line between its center of gravity (Appendix V, GRAVITY, page 553) and the center of the earth passes through the surface common to the object and to the floor. If the line of centers does not pass through this surface, called the base of the object, then the object will tumble until a surface does come onto the floor for which the line of centers does fall within the base. Looking at the object in Fig. IV.B-1, it is seen that configurations a, b and c are stable (balanced) because in these cases, the lines of center pass through the respective bases, A, B and C. However, the same object when placed in configuration d does not have its line of centers within the area of surface D, and so will fall so as to place surface B on the floor. Should there be two or more points of contact on the floor as with object 1 in Fig. IV.B-2, then the effective area for balancing includes the stippled area between the points in contact with the floor.

If the line of centers lies within the base, but very close to one edge, as for object 2 in Fig. IV.B-2, then a very small tipping toward the left or the right will be enough to pull the line of centers outside the base and so topple the object. Object 3, Fig. IV.B-2, similarly will fall for the same reason if given a small push to the left.

The simple exposition given above applies not only to blocks of wood, but to yoga students (especially the very stiff) in any *yogasana* supported on the floor without props.

In order to balance with any surface of the body (hands, feet, pelvis, *etc.*) in contact with the floor, the line between the center of gravity of the body and the center of the earth must lie within the effective area of that surface of the body.

For a person of normal weight and proportions standing with the arms relaxed (*tadasana*), the center of gravity of the body is just below the navel and about half way back toward the lumbar spine. That person

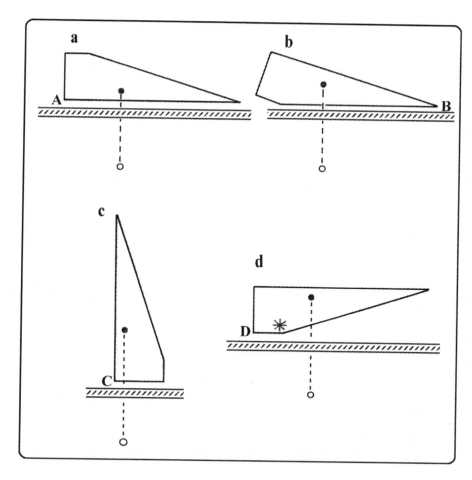

Fig. IV.B-1. A chisel-shaped block of wood in four orientations (**a**, **b**, **c**, **d**) having four bounding surfaces, **A**, **B**, **C**, and **D** placed with each of the faces sequentially on the table; the dashed lines represent the lines between the centers of gravity of the earth (o- -) and the block (•- -).

will stand balanced as long as the line between this point within the body and the center of the earth falls within the area delineated by the placement of the feet. However, it is not necessarily the case that the center of gravity of the body lies within the body. In *urdhva dhanurasana*, for example, the center of gravity rises more toward the solar plexus because the arms are lifted overhead, and is positioned in the empty space behind the dorsal spine because the spine is lifted well above the line connecting the heels and the wrists; the area of the base is that delineated by the placement of the hands and feet on the floor.

Though it is possible to recover from a slight loss of balance using the great strength of the supporting limb or its part in contact with the floor, the student will find this tiring, and from there will come to see that the use of strength to maintain balance is secondary to remaining constantly aware of the balanced position and not letting the body move too far into the falling position.

Intelligent Balancing of a Block

Actually, the unstable block in configuration D (Fig. IV.B-1d) does not simply "fall" to the right, but more precisely, in falling, it rotates about the point marked * in a clockwise way as viewed by the reader. When the line of centers falls outside the area of the base as in configuration D, a rotational force

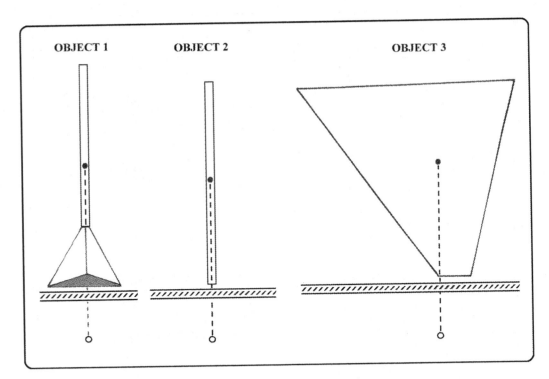

Fig. IV.B-2. Object 1 has a base area (stippled) defined by its widely separated triangular feet, with the dashed line between its center of gravity (•- -) and the center of the earth (o- -) well within the effective area of the base; for this reason, object 1 will be very stable. Objects 2 and 3, each with its line of centers just barely within the area of its base will be much more unstable with respect to small oscillations which can carry this line outside the area of the base.

called "torque" is developed. Torque unopposed leads to rotation and falling. One way to keep such a block from falling on the floor is to lean it against the wall instead, *i.e.*, have it fall onto the wall instead of onto the floor (Section IV.D, Other Aids to Balancing in the *Yogasanas*, page 533).

If, however, the block were articulated, *i.e.*, had a joint, and also contained moveable parts and motors to move them, a torque sensor, and a computer, then it would be possible for this intelligent block to balance without leaning on the wall. To do this, it must sense the clockwise "falling" torque, and with the aid of the computer and motors, move the block's mechanical parts in a way so as to generate a counterclockwise torque which would counterbalance the original imbalance. This is a more realistic model of balancing in the body, with

the movable parts being the limbs, the motors being the muscles, the sensors being the four balancing modes discussed in Section IV.A, page 525, and the computer being the central nervous system. Most importantly, the counterclockwise torque which preserves the balance often cannot be generated internally, but comes instead from pressing an appropriate part of the body against the floor at the appropriate time.

Consider now a half-human model of balancing using countertorque, consisting of a broomstick balanced vertically on the extended index finger, eyes, a computer, and a moveable hand. In this combination, there is a joint, in effect, where the broomstick rests on the finger. As the broomstick rotates clockwise in falling in the gravitational field, the eyes sense the resultant change of position due to the unbalanced torque, and with the aid of the computer and the muscles of the wrist, the hand supporting the broomstick is swung in a counterclockwise way so as to generate a countertorque and so preserve the balance. However, if the countertorque is too large, it brings the broomstick past vertical and starts a falling/rotation in the counterclockwise sense. In response to this, the eye again alerts the computer, and the hand then is sent in a clockwise arc so that the broomstick rotates counterclockwise.

In this metronomic *pas de deux*, it is as if there are two swinging pendula (the broomstick and the hand), the motions of which are synchronized to keep the net torque on the vertical broomstick averaged to zero over time. The motions of the two pendula are essentially out of phase, *i.e.*, when the wrist swings to the left, it sends the broomstick to the right, and *vice versa*.

Balancing in the *yogasanas* amounts to having a continuous sense of the falling torques, and the continuous development of countertorques within the body that bring it back into balance, *i.e.*, that keeps the line of centers within the base of the posture. In speaking of conscious action, William James describes it as "the marksman ends by thinking only of the exact position of the goal, the singer only of the perfect sound, the balancer only of the point of the pole whose oscillations he must counteract" [131].

SECTION IV.C. BALANCING THE BODY

The balancing of a block on a table is a static process, however, the balancing of the body in *yogasana* is a dynamic process. Interestingly, it is the extreme flexibility of the body as compared with a block of wood that makes balancing the body so much more difficult, and at the same time, it is the extreme flexibility of the body/mind that

allows one to maintain the balance of the body! The description given in the previous Section for balancing a broomstick on the end of the finger holds the essence of what must be done to balance the body in the *yogasanas*. In order to balance, one must keep certain parts of the body as immobile as a broomstick while at the same time, one must maintain a mobile joint close to the floor, which joint is given 100% of the responsibility for keeping the whole structure in balance. It does this by sensing the falling torque and generating a countertorque.

On Becoming a Broomstick

Because Object 2 in Fig. IV.B-2 essentially is a broomstick, it is mechanically stable as long as there are no external or internal disturbances, however, even a slight tipping to the side will take the line of centers beyond the minuscule base, initiating a fall. With the broomstick balanced on the end of the finger, this poses no problem, as long as the eye and the joint formed at the point of contact of the hand with the broomstick, work together so as to maintain balance.

Now imagine that Object 2 has been cut horizontally into 10 pieces and that a thin elastic band has been placed between each pair of adjacent slices. As will be seen below, this is a more realistic model of a student attempting to balance, for example, in a standing pose. In this case, the broomstick has become eleven individual but strongly interacting pendula by the introduction of ten joints along its length, with each pendulum representing the motion about a particular collapsed but all-too-mobile joint in the student's body.

In theory, the eye-hand combination of the supporting arm could move in a complicated way such as to keep all the relative torques of the eleven individual pendula sufficiently compensated so as to maintain balance, at least for a short time. However, all too quickly the complexity of keeping the torques of eleven independent pendula in balance becomes overwhelming, with the result that the center of gravity of the broomstick soon falls outside the base of its support and irreversible falling begins. How much easier and more sensible it is to replace the elastic bands with stout metal sleeves, making the broomstick integral again, with only the one joint between finger and broomstick responsible for balancing!

Correspondingly, the best plan for balancing in a standing pose, for example, is to focus all of the attention on the ankle joint, and keep all of the other joints immobile. In all upright standing poses, it is the proprioceptive feedback from the ankles (the primary joint for balancing in this type of posture) and from the Pacinian corpuscles in the soles of the feet that are crucial for the control and maintenance of the balance [225]; the involvement of the other joints (secondary joints) unnecessarily complicates the picture if they too are allowed to oscillate.

How then does one inhibit motion about the secondary joints when balancing on the foot so as to localize the balancing action in the foot? The extraneous motion about joints other than the ankle can be minimized by energetically opening each of these joints in the body maximally, making each of the joints taut (Iyengar says "poker stiff"), and the body monolithic. The stabilization of the secondary joints follows naturally from the yogic extension of the body normally performed in the pose when bringing it into alignment and extension. Nothing more is needed than to realize that the extra effort on extension of the secondary joints also serves the sense of balance, and that placing this then on second attention after stabilizing the secondary joints, one then gives undivided attention to the action of the ankle joint working the floor. With practice, one then works to minimize the amplitudes of the oscillations in the ankle so as to make the balance-conserving motions imperceptibly small.

Generating a Countertorque

Given that one has learned how to transform the body into a broomstick for the purposes of balancing, how then does one achieve the second necessary action for balance, the generation of a torque counter to that of falling? The answer to this is best illustrated by the exercise described in Box IV.C-1.

When the body in standing position is momentarily tipped off balance as in the *uttanasana* described in Box IV.C-1, it has been shown [225] that the first reaction is for the balls of the feet to be pressed into the floor by contraction of the gastrocnemius (calf) muscles, in order to generate a countertorque. This is then followed by further countertorques generated by contraction of the hamstrings and paraspinal muscles. These successive reflex actions are set in motion by the simultaneous activation of the four receptor modes mentioned above, *i.e.*, cutaneous, vestibular, proprioceptive, and ocular. The sequence of actions in this balancing is that the muscle closest to the base is activated first, while those more distant are activated at later times.

Conscious action in regard to balancing requires time to receive the off-balance signal, evaluate it, compute a new course of action, transmit the action plan and finally execute it. When time is too short for this, the body takes the reflex route to quick action, bypassing the higher brain centers (see Section 7.D, Reflex Actions, page 211). Postural response time is shortest when the imbalance is sensed proprioceptively by the muscle spindles (70–100 milliseconds), while response times are perhaps twice as long when the off-balance signal is vestibular or ocular [225]. If there is no need for

BOX IV.C-1: HOW TO USE THE FLOOR WHEN BALANCING

In order to discover the counter-rotating force so useful in balancing, stand with your feet 18 inches from the wall, lean your seat onto the wall and fold into *uttanasana*. Using your hands, gently push off the wall so as to be in classical *uttanasana*, legs vertical, weight distributed evenly on the balls of the feet and on the heels. Now tip your weight forward and see how pressing the base of the toes (especially those of the big toes, Box IV.E-1, *You Have More Sensitivity in Your Big Toe than You Ever Imagined*, page 539) into the floor tips one backward and so brings one back into balance. That is to say, by pressing the base of the toes into the floor, Fig. IV.C-1a, you generate a torque counter to that appropriate to falling forward, and so come back to the upright position, provided the countertorque is of the proper size and comes at the proper time. This clearly shows how one works the floor in order to generate a countertorque that maintains balance.

In contrast, now allow the weight to fall backward when in free-standing *uttanasana*; because there are no toes at the back of the foot to press onto the floor, a countertorque can not be generated at the ankle, and one ends up falling backward onto the wall. The simple lesson illustrated by the above applies to any standing pose, on one leg or two, regardless of the position of the upper body: keep the weight slightly forward toward the toes in order to avoid falling backward over the heels. Falling too far forward is avoided by pressing the base of the toes gently into the floor, so that the forward lean does not become excessive. Falling backward is to be avoided because one cannot generate a countertorque in this case, and falling is certain. It is because Nature has placed the ankle over the heel and far from the toes, that a countertorque can be generated by leaning forward, but not backward. The awareness of the action of the toes, foot and ankle on the floor in this exercise should be uppermost in the minds of the students as they practice balancing in the standing *yogasanas*.

When on the feet as in *tadasana* (or on the hands as in *adho mukha svanasana*), the toes (or fingers) rest on the floor, stretching forward from the ankles (wrists). Neither the toes nor the fingertips try to grip the floor in these poses. However, when one comes to balance on one foot (or the hands), it is then advantageous to move the weight somewhat forward onto the toes (or fingertips) in order to generate the necessary countertorque for balancing.

The student will readily appreciate the advantage of having a base of large area when balancing by comparing the increasing difficulty of balancing after tipping into *uttanasana* first with the feet hip-width apart, then with the feet successively together, with one foot in *ardha padmasana*, and finally when standing on just the toes of one foot. Similarly, compare the ease of balance in *sarvangasana* with that in *niralamba sarvangasana*, a posture with a much smaller base. When balancing on the hands or other parts of the anatomy, the same principles of "broomstick and countertorque" to keep the line of centers within the base still must be enforced.

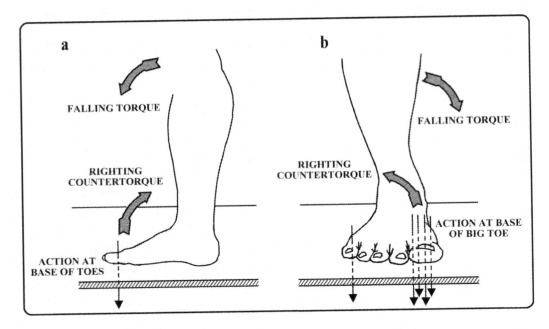

Fig. IV.C-1 (**a**). As one falls forward in *uttanasana*, the base of the toes are pressed into the floor so as to generate a countertorque opposing that generated by falling forward. (**b**) Schematic of the right leg and foot as they stand on the floor in *vrksasana*. If the leg/torso falls clockwise (upper arrow), then the reflexive action is for the big-toe side of the foot to press the floor, generating a counterclockwise but balancing torque (lower arrow).

haste, then the conscious mind can intercede in the decision making, though the elapsed time for action will be longer.

The broomstick-countertorque approach to balancing on one foot assumes that one can raise and lower the inner arch of the foot (arch 1-3 in Fig. 8.D-4). If this arch has fallen and can not be activated, then the broomstick-countertorque technique will not work to maintain the balance in the standing poses.

There is a unique aspect of the balancing reflex that should be encouraging to the *yogasana* student. Whereas the patellar knee-jerk reflex (see Section 7.D, Reflex Actions, page 211), for example, remains always the same, the balancing reflex becomes both quicker and more refined with practice. That is to say, one eventually can balance on one's hands by practicing, for the balance reflex can maintain balance for a longer and longer time with less and less

effort through practice [225]. This is possible because our bodies are capable not only of *responsive feedback* (a reaction to an imbalance already in motion), but also to *responsive feedforward*, a process in which the imbalance is anticipated and adjustments made in preparation for it. So, for example, in the case of falling forward in *sirsasana I*, the reflexive action in the elbows may be too strong at first, and the body then starts to fall backward. With practice, one can reflexively anticipate the over-reaction and both moderate the first response and at the same time be prepared to counter it with the second by anticipating it. In this way, practice sharpens the balancing ability and makes progress possible.

In discussing the mechanism of balancing in the body, note must be made of the cerebellum and the basal ganglia of the brain (see Subsection 3.A, *The Limbic System*, page 33), for these two centers are intimately involved in the act of balancing. The proprioceptive sensors (Section 7.C, Proprioception, page 208) relay their information in a constant stream to the hemispheres of the cerebellum, where this detailed information is transformed into a total-body map indicating where the various muscles and limbs of the body are located, which are moving, how fast they are moving, and in which directions. At the same time, signals from the vestibular apparatus in the inner ears (Section 17.B, The Vestibular Organs of Balance, page 437) also converge upon the cerebellum, indicating the position of the head in the gravitational field and its angular motion, if any. Ocular information is also of great importance here, but the information does not go to the cerebellum, but directly to the occipital lobe instead, from which it spreads to many other areas of the brain. With the proprioceptive, visual, deep pressure, and vestibular information in hand, the cerebellum and basal ganglia then work together to devise a muscular strategy so that balance is maintained with smooth but corrective movements. If the movement in question involves a conscious act of balance, then the plan devised by the cerebellum and basal ganglia is sent upward to the motor cortex of the cerebrum, and from there, downward to the relevant muscles. If, on the other hand, the balancing is more postural or reflexive, then the cerebellar plan does not involve the cortex, but instead is loaded directly into the medulla for transmission downward to the muscles.

Because the afferent signals from the vestibular apparatus go to the brainstem and the returning efferent nerves activate the muscles in the head and upper back, it is an interesting question then as to whether such upper-body sensors are of any value when balancing on the feet. Indeed, the brainstem nuclei involved in vestibular balancing do have tracts to the cerebellum (Subsection 17.B, *Innervation of the Vestibular Tract*,

page 440), but from this point, there are efferent nerves to muscles in the foot and ankle which can control the balance when standing.

SECTION IV.D. OTHER AIDS TO BALANCING IN THE *YOGASANAS*

There are several things one can do in aid of balancing in the *yogasanas*, in expectation of eventually using the "broomstick and countertorque" model in the middle of the room. In order to balance in *yogasanas*, the student must be sensitive to changes in one or more of the receptor modes, whether the body is upright, inclined, horizontal, or inverted, and must be able to activate the proper response. Until that higher level of performance is reached, there are several aids to balancing that can be instituted when the student's balancing organs are not yet up to the demands of the posture. These aids to balancing are discussed here, as adjuncts to the discussion in Section IV.C, Balancing the Body, page 529. Note, however, that the information/advice given in this Subsection will aid balancing for the beginning student, but as mentioned below, it tends to promote a habit that eventually must be broken if one is to progress in *yogasana* study.

Vision and Balance

As more than one-third of the neurons in the brain are involved in some way in the visual process, it is no surprise that the eyes might be involved in balancing. Students can readily test for themselves the truth of this statement by performing the simple exercise described in Box IV.D-1, *Using Your Eyes to Balance*, page 534, in which the head is immobile and the eyes lock onto an immobile object in the far field, all in aid of balancing.

BOX IV.D-1: USING YOUR EYES TO BALANCE

More so than one might think, we use our eyes to sense the horizon in order to adjust our verticality. As any seasick person can tell you, our sense of balance is dependent in part upon the eye's view of the horizon and the steadiness of this view. The general truth of this statement for the student of *yogasana* is easily shown. Come into *vrksasana* as you normally do, and then close your eyes and see how much more challenging the balancing has become. The key factor here in using the eyes to balance is the presence in the eye of receptive fields (Subsection 16.A, *Vision and Neuroanatomy of the Eye*, page 415), many of which are sensitive to the angular alignment of straight lines in the visual field. As one starts to fall, the changing angle of the horizon as sensed by the eyes serves to initiate corrective actions to preserve balance.

Because the eyes are so important to balancing, one concludes that there must be an optimum way of using them to stabilize a standing pose. Indeed, the eyes can be used to the best advantage when balancing in the following way. Having first come into the position, pick a stationary object on the far wall and keep it attentively in the center of your field of view. As long as the object does not move and as long as you keep it centered in the visual field, the signals from the eye's receptive fields will not change, and this will serve to keep you balanced. Of course, staring at a blank wall having no feature onto which the eyes can focus will be disorienting, and you are sure to fall, the closer you are to such a wall. This will also be the case if you have other students in your field of view who are wobbly and/or falling! Only with intense mental concentration can the balance be kept if the visual field is either unmarked or is in motion. That the balance is not affected in *vrksasana* by closing only one eye shows that the visual effect on balancing does not involve stereoptical vision.

Simple testing of the visual anchor in different balancing *yogasanas* shows that the eyes can aid balance in both upright and inverted positions, but that in the latter, they are less useful the closer the eyes are to the floor. That is to say, they are of great value when balancing in *adho mukha vrksasana* and in *vasisthasana*, but they are of no value when balancing in *anantasana*, *sirsasana* or *sarvangasana*. Moreover, yoga experience shows that in standing balances with the eyes open, the visual support of balance is greatest when the eyes look down, is less so when looking straight ahead, and is least when the head is turned to look upward. The truth of this statement is easily tested by doing *vrksasana* with each of the three head positions. These differences probably involve both using different parts of the vestibular apparatus when balancing in the different head positions, and also the fact that we are more habituated to looking downward (walking, *etc.*), than we are to looking upward, and so the visual-balancing mechanism is more effective in the head-down position. Whether looking up at the ceiling, across the room, or down at the floor, having a point of visual focus will be mechanically stabilizing in the standing poses.

The other side of the visual-fixation coin is that one can become habituated to this mode of balancing, always using the same objects on which to focus. When this becomes the case, trying to balance in a different environment can be very destabilizing. Moreover, using the eyes in this way promotes a certain tension in the visual system (Section 16.B, Stress, Vision, and Yoga, page 419) which can be counterproductive in the long term.

In situations in which one is moving while balancing, as when going from *virabhadrasana I* into *virabhadrasana III*, for example, locking the eyes onto a fixed point is impractical. In this case, imagine a black line painted on the floor and running through the forward foot. Keep this imaginary "runway" well lit and centered in your visual field as you lean forward, lifting the back leg for take off, and lowering it to land. As you become more adept at balancing in the *yogasanas*, the less you will need to rely on the eyes to hold you up.

An oculomotor reflex comes into play when one starts in *ardha chandrasana* and then slowly turns into *parivrtta ardha chandrasana*, keeping the arms outstretched throughout. The balancing difficulty arises in the transition between the postures where neither hand is on the floor. In cases such as this, pick a point on the floor on which to focus the gaze. As the head and body turn, the vestibular-oculomotor reflex (Section 16.A, Structure and Function of the Eyes, page 411) automatically will turn the eyes at the same rate but in the opposite direction as the head so as to keep the focal object centered in the field of view even though the head is in motion. This action will not cover the full 180° range of motion of the head, but can be done in a few angular increments, advancing the point of visual fixation with each increment. Putting a coin on the floor as a visual marker can be of great help in such balances.

It is known that muscular actions in response to visual cues are slowest in dim light and fastest in bright light [190, 196]. This means that balancing in *yogasanas* will be easiest with bright illumination because the responsivity is quicker, and conversely, will be more difficult in very dim light. It is conceivable that poor vision could interfere with using the eyes to advantage in balancing. Try *vrksasana* with and without your glasses to see if this is the case.

Using the Wall as Support in Balancing Yogasanas

When learning to balance in the *yogasanas*, use of the wall can be both a great teacher and an impediment to growth, in more ways than one. Being just another prop, the wall can help the beginner in many ways approach a difficult position, but in doing so, the student runs the risk of becoming married to the prop, unable to function without it. Once we are comfortable working against the wall, we must take the next step of cutting the umbilical cord connecting us to the wall, and work then to take our place in the larger world without props. The same philosophy applies to using the eyes to balance (Subsection IV.D, *Vision and Balance*, page 533); they are useful props, but the intent of our practice eventually is to cut ourselves free of these aids.

With the above caveat in the minds of the students and their teachers, the students can then use the wall to great advantage in the following ways:

(A) Use the wall to steady the pose so that the student can feel more comfortable in the position, without fear of falling. *Ardha chandrasana* is a good example of a pose that beginners will struggle with in the middle of the room, but take special delight in doing with the support of a wall at their back and a block under the hand.

(B) Once supported by the wall, the student then can devote full attention to the extension and alignment of the pose without worrying about falling. In this case, the wall is not only a support for balance, but is a reference plane onto which one works to place key points of the back body, *i.e.*, the back of the head, the shoulder blades, the backs of the hands, the buttocks, and the heel of the up leg. Again, *ardha chandrasana* performed with support of the wall is a good example of working on extension and alignment while postponing the issue of balance.

(C) When using the wall for support, the student should work sufficiently close to it that the wall can be reached without distorting the body's alignment in the process. For example, if the feet and supporting hand are placed 12 inches from the wall in *ardha chandrasana*, and the student then uses the wall for balance by placing the back of the hand of the upward arm on the wall, then the two arms will not necessarily be in the ideal alignment that otherwise is enforced when the pose is set up closer to the wall in the beginning.

(D) In standing poses such as *vrksasana*, *hasta padangusthasana*, and *parivrtta trikonasana*, *etc.*, where balance is a major factor, and in seated poses such as *paripurna navasana*, have the students lean slightly backward (or forward or sideward) onto the wall for support and alignment, then shift their weight slightly off the wall to attempt a free-standing balance.

Making Your Own Wall for Balancing

For those students with less than perfect balance who nonetheless are ready to wean themselves away from the wall and work in the middle of the room, the internally-generated wall can be of great value. Consider the balancing pose, *salamba sarvangasana*. According to Iyengar [209], *salamba* means supported or propped up, as the bent arms support the torso. In a sense then, one has created an "internal wall" with the arms in *salamba sarvangasana*, against which one can lean the rest of the body for support.

Though other postures are not identified by the word "*salamba*", they too can use the internal prop for balancing support. By way of example, consider the balancing pose *anantasana*. With one arm supporting the head and the other connected to the toe of the extended up leg, the balance on the side of the body can be precarious if all of the body parts are appropriately in-line. However, if the ankle of the down leg is flexed so that the toes point toward the knee, then the little toe is off the line of the body on the floor, and tipping the body forward onto the little toe provides an internal wall onto which one can lean forward as effectively as when one leans backward on a masonry wall. Practice *anantasana* with the toes of the down leg pointed first away from the knee and then toward the knee all the while keeping the body weight rolled slightly forward, in order to see the advantage of the latter position in regard to balance. Note also that once the weight is allowed to roll backward in *anantasana*, it makes no difference what the toes are doing: the battle is lost and one rolls out of the pose and onto one's back.

The balancing situation is exactly the same in *ardha chandrasana* as in *anantasana* in that if the fingers of the arm touching the ground are placed in line with the foot on the ground, the effective base of the pose is much smaller than if one places the fingers instead to the little-toe side of the standing foot and then leans back on the arm. That is to say, placing the fingers off the line of the foot in *ardha chandrasana* provides an internal wall onto which one can lean so as to stabilize the balance of the pose. With balancing practice, the fingers can be brought more and more onto the line of the standing foot, just as with practice one can move from *salamba sarvangasana* to *niralamba sarvangasana*.

Many other balancing *yogasanas* such as *parivrtta trikonasana*, *parivrtta ardha chandrasana, pincha myurasana, sarvang-asana, etc.*, are performed by constructing such an internal wall and then leaning against it. In fact, this is what we do each time we press the floor in order to generate a countertorque. The generation of a countertorque in aid of balancing is described in more detail for *vrksasana* in Subsection IV.E, *Localizing the Balancing Action in Vrksasana*, page 538.

Redistributing the Mass in the Aid of Balance

Visualize the circus acrobat balancing on the high wire, carrying her long pole held crosswise to the wire. Though this pole does not in any way increase the area of the performer's base (sole of the foot on the wire), it does aid greatly in stabilizing the left-right balance. In the standing *yogasanas*, you too can be helped by this balancing-pole action if the synchronization of falling-body torque and foot countertorque cannot be realized. Rather than working to extend the arms upward as in many standing poses, extend them outward to the sides instead, and feel the stability that comes from this redistribution of mass which more easily generates a useful (if not totally correct) counterbalancing torque. Students having trouble balancing in *vrksasana* or *virabhadrasana III*, for example, profit from redistributing their mass by placing their arms to the sides so as to form balancing poles in these postures.

A moment's reflection on the basic theorem of balance, Subsection IV.B, *Balancing a Rigid Block*, page 526, convinces one that any change of an asana which redistributes its weight so as to lower its center of gravity will make it more stable with respect to tipping over. Just as with sports cars, if the center of gravity is low, then the *angular*

displacement that is allowed before the body (or the car) falls is much larger than when the center of gravity is higher. Thus, from the center-of-gravity point of view, balancing in *vrksasana* is more difficult with the arms extended overhead (as in *urdhva hastasana*) than with the arms at the sides of the body, because in the former, the center of gravity is raised and so a smaller angle of body tilt will suffice to cause a fall. However, there is a compensating feature of the arms-over-head position that make it the preferred manner of performing this *yogasana, i.e.,* it promotes a tautness in the secondary joints that eradicates unnecessary wobble (Subsection IV.C, *On Becoming a Broomstick*, page 529). Arguing in the same vein, *malasana* performed by standing on one foot (the other extended parallel to the floor) is more stable than *hasta padangusthasana* because its center of gravity is much lower. Thus it is seen that the more extended position which we always seek in our practice is not necessarily the most stable one mechanically.

One often can see multi-jointed pendula in the circus, stabilized using several of the balancing principles given in this Chapter, as discussed in Box IV.D-2, *The Human Balancing Tower*, page 538.

All of the general points described in the discussion above in regard to foot balancing will apply generally as well to the inverted *yogasanas*, Section IV.F, page 544. In order to illustrate the basic facts of balance, the balancing aspects of several specific *yogasanas* (standing balances, hand balances, and a few others) which are well known to all who practice this discipline, are discussed below. In this, we will integrate the information in the previous Sections (IV.B, Mechanical Aspects of Balancing, page 526, 16.A, Structure and Function of the

---

BOX IV.D-2. THE HUMAN BALANCING TOWER

The human-tower circus stunt begins with acrobat 2 standing on the shoulders of acrobat 1. Acrobat 3 then climbs up to stand on the shoulders of acrobat 2, making a three-high tower. Should the lights go out at this point, the tower will fall immediately, for keeping this thing in the air requires many visual cues, especially because there are so many flexible joints in the construction. If the circus is a good one, they will then attempt to stand acrobat 4 on the top of the three-high, making a four-high tower. Because the weight on the shoulders of acrobat 1 is becoming appreciable, acrobat 4 will be a young child, who is often flung to the top of the tower. Balancing such a tower is a mighty feat, even with the lights on, as there is independent movement at the "joints" of the tower formed by the feet of acrobat 1 on the floor, by the feet of acrobat 2 on the shoulders of acrobat 1, and so on up the tower. Balance can be maintained for only a few seconds before the tower falls (always forward), and acrobat 4 is caught by bystanders. The balancing of an equally long and heavy pole is trivial compared to the problems of balancing four pendula moving independently, as when stacking four acrobats.

Much more stable constructions can be built of acrobats if several of them are positioned close to one another in a bottom layer. The acrobats of the second layer then place their feet on one shoulder each of the adjacent acrobats in the first layer, and the tower is built layer by layer. This approach illustrates how interlacing acrobats can minimize the allowed motions of the whole by lowering the center of gravity, and especially how broadening the base will make the structure much more stable. We try to do both when balancing in the *yogasanas*.

Eyes, page 411, and 17.B, The Vestibular Organs of Balance, page 437).

SECTION IV.E. BALANCING IN THE STANDING *YOGASANAS*

Localizing the Balancing Action in Vrksasana

With the feet placed properly in *vrksasana*, the pose resembles the broomstick labeled "Object 2" in Fig. IV.B-2, and like Object 2, is easily tipped out of balance. To balance on the right leg in *vrksasana*, start first in *tadasana*. With both feet still on the floor, first imperceptibly shift the weight from the left leg onto the right leg. If you try lifting the left leg without first shifting, you

will fall immediately. Better then to slowly move the weight off the leg to be lifted and transfer it onto the standing leg; in general, it is most effective to try and achieve a balanced position as you are entering the pose rather than trying to find it in the confusion of being in the pose while off balance.

As one brings weight onto the standing leg, select a stationary object across the room as a visual anchor, and keep its image centered in your field of view. With practice, you will be able to release your visual hold on the anchor and allow your gaze to become broad and soft. Extending the fingertips to the ceiling will then serve to open all of the secondary joints fully, keeping them taut and immobile.

Consider next that the posture starts to fall. As shown schematically in Fig. IV.C-1b, if the right leg tends to fall counterclockwise, then pressure applied by the big-toe side of the right foot to the floor will generate a clockwise torque within the foot-ankle-leg; the foot and ankle in *vrksasana* play the roles of the hand and wrist in the broomstick balance. This action in *vrksasana* essentially is one in which the foot pendulum creates a countertorque to balance the falling torque. Balance is restored and maintained by pressing first one side of the foot to the floor and then the other so as to always (in time and space) counterbalance (countertorque) with the foot and ankle, the falling imbalance (torque) of the upper body. Because the big toe is so much stronger than the little toe, one can stay up

in *vrksasana* longer if the weight on the standing foot is deliberately kept slightly on the big-toe side. See Box IV.E-1, below, for a further discussion of the big toe.

With the arms over head in *vrksasana*, the upward lift of the body in the course of opening the joints leads to the sensation of hanging by your fingertips from the ceiling rather than standing with your foot on the floor. While balancing in *vrksasana*, the mind focuses totally on the *countertorquing* motions of the ankle joint, but ignores the other joints of the body because they are extended and thus immobilized.

Having reduced the act of balancing in *vrksasana* to localizing the action in the foot

---

BOX IV.E-1: YOU HAVE MORE SENSITIVITY IN YOUR BIG TOE THAN YOU EVER IMAGINED

In Fig. 10.C-1, there is a plot of the measured mean separation between surface pressure receptors in various parts of the body. The larger this mean separation is, the fewer the number of sensors in this area and the lower the resolution of the touch, *i.e.*, the coarser the sense of touch. In accord with the very large areas of the cerebral cortex devoted to the areas of the lips, tongue, fingers, and thumbs (Figs. 2.A-4 and 7.A-6), these areas have the finest resolution for touch. It is the exacting command over the movements in these areas that make speech and toolmaking possible for human beings. Notice however, that the resolution in the palm of the hand is no higher than that of the big toe (hallux), and that the resolution of the touch sensors of the big toe is finer than those of the sole of the foot, the calf, thigh, belly, back, forehead, shoulder, upper arm, or forearm!

What can it possibly mean that the big toe would have such a high resolution for pressure on its underside? I interpret this as showing that in our evolution to bipedalism, we have developed extraordinary strength and sensitivity in the area of the big toe in order to balance on two feet, using the pressure sensors in and around the big toe as the prime sensors. From the point of view of the *yogasana* student, this interpretation should seem logical in hindsight, for in the *yogasanas*, we often depend strongly on the actions of the big toe against the floor to maintain both alignment and balance.

In making this argument, I have used the fact that the distribution of light-pressure sensors appropriate to Fig. 10.C-1 which are active in sensing the weight distribution on the big toe when standing is mirrored by that of the deep-pressure sensors used in sensing any falling torque. The idea proposed here receives support from the sensory cortex, which shows about as much cortical area devoted to foot and toe sensors as to hand and finger sensors [225]. When balancing in *vrksasana*, trust your big toe and keep the body's primary intelligence in the toes, foot and ankle of the balancing leg.

and ankle of the standing leg, we now consider how the ankle keeps the body balanced in the pose. With the cervical vertebrae in line with those below it, the balanced position in *vrksasana* is aided by the sensing of the vertical position by the utricles of the inner ears, by the appropriate receptive fields in the retinas of the eyes, by the proprioceptive sensors throughout the body, and especially by the pressure-sensitive Pacinian receptors on the bottom of the foot. Should these sense an imbalance, the off-balance condition is reported both upward to the higher centers of the brain and downward to the muscles of the body in reflex arcs that automatically right the body. Note however, that because of the flexibility of the cervical spine, the head may be truly balanced according to the vestibular organs, while the rest of the body is not. Thus, verticality of the entire body along the length of its axis must involve the participation of proprioceptors other than the vestibular organs if the head, torso and legs are to be in the proper aligned relationship [477]. If, while in *vrksasana*, one turns the head in small circles at a modest speed, all balance will be lost as the confusing signals from the vestibular apparatus swamp those from the Pacinian and joint-capsule sensors in the sole of the foot. Keep the head still and let the sensors in the foot and the visual cues control the balance.

If *vrksasana* is wobbly, stability can be gained by broadening and lengthening the standing foot, and by spreading the arms laterally. For students seeking more challenge, coming up on the toes of the foot of the straight leg in *vrksasana* makes the base yet smaller and hence the pose even more difficult to keep balanced.

Though the body is left-right symmetric while we stand in *urdhva hastasana*, this is no longer the case in *vrksasana*, for if we balance on the left leg, the lumbar spine tends to move to the right, the thorax to the left and the cervical spine to the right again [228]. However, these lateral curvatures are very much reduced if the body is extended upward as recommended for better balancing, for this acts to straighten the spine. When standing on one leg as in *vrksasana*, the pelvis on the unsupported side tends to drop from lack of support, but the gluteus medius muscle (Fig. 7.A-2) on the unsupported side then contracts to hold the pelvis in balance.

Often with the beginner, the falling is so rapid that one has no time in which to organize a muscular rebuttal before one is irrevocably out of the pose. In this case, placing the pose against the wall will prove to be of value, for it removes the time element while still allowing the student to practice coming back into balance once he/she is ready to lean away from the wall (Subsection IV.D, *Using The Wall as Support in Balancing Yogasanas*, page 535).

In the case of the muscles, too rapid a stretching of the muscle spindles leads to a reflexive contraction of the stretched muscle (Section 7.B, Muscle Sensors; The Mechanoreceptors, page 198). Just as happens with the spindles in the muscles, if the head is moved impulsively (as when rotating it in a circular motion in the discussion above), there is a strong torque within the semicircular-canal sensors, prompting an immediate reflexive righting action to occur which often is destabilizing in the long run. However, if we move the head slowly from head down to head up in *vrksasana*, for example, then vestibular response is slow, smooth and under conscious control, just as for slow, conscious stretching of the muscle, and there is no reflexive countermotion.

It is said that the "elderly" are unable to balance while standing on one leg [153]. Thus, the average balancing time on the dominant leg has been reported to vary with age in the following way (time in seconds): age 40–49 (15.5–7.2), age 50–59 (8.7–3.7), age 60–69 (4.5–2.5) and age 70-79 (2.6–1.5) [180]. This rapid falling off of the balancing time (about 50% every decade) is thought to be the result of incidental damage to the afferent sciatic nerve running from the leg to the base of the spine, the longest in the body, for it is considered unlikely that such a long single neuron could remain intact and functioning over a lifetime. That "elderly" yoga students daily are able to do *vrksasana* for minutes rather than seconds shows that this idea is in error.

Once a sprained ankle is in its healing mode and can bear weight without pain, circulation into and out of the sprained area can be very healing. This circulation is promoted by balancing on the affected ankle in *vrksasana*, for early mobilization of the ankle speeds recovery and lessens the pain of injury.

Balancing in the Other Standing Yogasanas

Considerable attention as been given to the balancing aspect of *vrksasana*, the prototype balancing posture in the standing poses. With these points now out in the open, much less need be said about the other standing poses, for the balancing points are essentially the same.

In both *anantasana* and *vasisthasana*, the balancing problem is front-to-back, whereas the ocular support, being generally from left-to-right, would be of reduced value in these postures. Balancing will be easier in *vasisthasana* than in *anantasana* because of the high torque that can be generated by the hand on the floor in the former pose and because with the hand on the floor, the countertorque can be either clockwise or counterclockwise. The hand on the floor for

vasisthasana should be as broad as possible to allow one to generate the maximum countertorque and to provide the largest base for balancing.

Consider the student bending to the right, coming into *trikonasana*. Because the feet are widely separated in *trikonasana*, there is no problem with wobbling or falling in the left-right direction, while front-to-back there is no less stability than in feet-together *tadasana**. Leaning to the right in *trikonasana* will activate that semicircular canal having its axis parallel to that of the rotational axis (pubis to coccyx). According to the physiologists, this action will not stimulate the vestibular-ocularmotor reflex (see above) since this reflex involves only the canal in each ear having its axis parallel to the body's long axis, however, the utricle in each inner ear does sense the deviation of the head from verticality. Nonetheless, if you go into *trikonasana* with your eyes closed, you will tend somewhat more to fall forward-backward, showing again the utility of consciously using the eyes for balancing in *trikonasana* as you did in *vrksasana*. Note too that the student needs static balance when balancing in *trikonasana*, but dynamic balance when going in both directions between *tadasana* and *trikonasana*. To the extent that the vestibular apparatus of the inner ears is involved in moving in and out of *trikonasana*, congestion and stuffiness in this area can upset one's balance. If *trikonasana*-to-the-right is further embellished by turning the head so as to look at the upraised left hand, then the vestibular-ocularmotor reflex would come into play as the rotation of the head is about the proper internal body axis.

*As pointed out to me by Carol Wipf, beginning students actually are more stable in *trikonasana* when they are bent at the waist, with the chest far forward of the triangle of the legs and the seat pushed backward. This can be understood as a front-to-back balance enhanced by the mass redistribution (Subsection IV.D, page 537) in the front-to-back direction resulting from pressing the chest forward and the seat backward.

Balancing signals from the left vestibular and ocular organs are processed in the right cerebral hemisphere, which in turn activates muscles on the left side of the body. Similar decussations (lateral crossings) occur for signals originating on the right side. If, as we lean to the right for *trikonasana*, we instead place the left hand down and rotate the spine so as to look backward (*parivrtta trikonasana*), the eyes still could be of great use in balancing. However, note that on leaning to the right, we are accustomed to having the right ear and the right eye closer to the ground than are those organs on the left, whereas in *parivrtta trikonasana*, it is the left ear and the left eye that are closer to the ground, even though the tilt is to the right! Furthermore, with respect to the face, the directions of "front" and "back" also have been reversed in *parivrtta trikonasana*. This means that the inputs from the left and right vestibular sensors, from the left and right eyes, and possibly from the right and left edges of the soles of the feet must be mentally reversed left-to-right at some point in the neural arc if the balance is to be maintained. This mental adjustment can be slow to develop at first, and so *parivrtta trikonasana* is often much more wobbly than *trikonasana* itself.

Pulling the inner thighs toward one another in *parivrtta trikonasana* stabilizes the legs and pelvis in this pose, and so makes balancing easier by removing any possible oscillation in this area and returning full control to the feet and ankles. However, the pressing of the inner thighs in *parivrtta trikonasana* is an action, not a movement (Chapter 7, THE SKELETAL MUSCLES, page 167), and so the thighs actually do not press on one another, as this would collapse the groins. See Box IV.E-2 for further discussion of the effects of physical crossover on balancing.

The general rules elaborated above for *vrksasana* would apply to balancing in *virabhadrasana III*. Start in *urdhva hastasana*, with all of the secondary joints extended and stabilized, and keeping the balance in the consciousness, pivot slowly (front-to-back) over the standing leg. The joints of the body other than the standing ankle are fully opened and thus too taut to wobble, and the gaze is focused on a line on the floor, real or imagined, which runs from the sole of the foot to the forward wall. Like landing lights on a airport runway, this line will guide you and hold you steady if you keep it centered in your field of view as you slowly and with intense consciousness move in and out of *virabhadrasana III*, all the while working the ankle of the standing foot against the floor to generate the countertorque needed to balance. Additional stability of balance in *virabhadrasana III* comes from keeping the palms facing one another while rotating the biceps of the upper arms outward [161] so as to keep the upper body taut.

The balancing pole-effect is already working for you in *virabhadrasana III* as the torso and the up leg are stretched forward and backward, respectively, to aid balance along this line. In order to gain the same advantage along the left-right line in *virabhadrasana III*, one can extend the arms sideways rather than forward. In this position, you are now fully the airplane landing and taking off from the runway on the floor.

As one moves from the vertical to the horizontal head position coming into *virabhadrasana III*, the saccules will become active as the balancing organs in the face-down position. Of course, the proprioceptors will be active in all body orientations and especially the pressure-sensitive receptors on the sole of the foot of the supporting leg also contribute to the balance, as do the eyes and joint capsules. As in *vrksasana*, balance in *virabhadrasana III* is more readily accomplished if the weight on the stand-

BOX IV.E-2. PHYSICAL CROSSOVER REQUIRES NEURAL CROSSOVER

Perform the following simple *yogasana* work to see the unbalancing effect of taking a part of the body normally on the right and placing it on the left. In this crossed-over orientation, maintaining balance requires that the balancing reflex signals received by the higher centers in the "wrong" side of the brain transfer the signals to the corresponding part of the "correct" side of the brain, and correspondingly re-route the efferent signals to the muscles to the opposite side of the body. One might guess that this left-to-right transfer of neural signals is achieved via the corpus callosum, a large bundle of nerves connecting the left and right hemispheres of the brain. However, there is specific evidence that neither the hands nor the feet are associated via the corpus callosum, and so a more indirect mechanism must be at work. Transfer of neural signals via the corpus callosum is said to be aided by walking for a short time with opposite arms and legs swinging together [357].

A) Assume the table position on hands and knees, with the hands under the shoulders and separated by shoulder width, and the knees set under the hips and placed hip-width apart. Now straighten the right leg and hold it parallel to the floor. Balancing in this position is trivial because of the large area of the base formed by the two hands and the knee (and foot) of the bent leg. Repeat, lifting the left leg instead.

B) Assume the table position, but with the knees together and the hands as close to one another as possible, adjacent fingers of each hand touching one another and thumbs touching. Perform the right-leg lift again, noting how much more difficult the left-to-right balancing is with the area of the base so much smaller. Notice as well how the inner and outer edges of the hands sense the imbalance and so work against the floor in order to generate the appropriate countertorques for maintaining balance. As closing the eyes in this pose does not change the balance, visual cues are unimportant here.

C) Set up as in B above, hands touching, but now cross the right arm over the left so that it is the little fingers that touch rather than the thumbs. With the right leg lifted, the balancing action of the hands on the floor now must be deliberately reversed left-to-right in the brain in order to keep from falling. Note the increasing levels of concentration necessary to keep from falling as one goes from A to B to C. If the student is unable to maintain balance in the crossed-over position, try the opposite-arm-leg walk for a few minutes and then test again in the crossover table position C.

D) Similar crossover balancing problems arise in *parivrtta trikonasana* and when doing *adho mukha svanasana* with arms crossed and one leg lifted. Practicing these and similar poses in the crossover positions will promote a keener sense of balance overall, and is excellent exercise for reconnecting the mind to the body. See also Subsection 3.D, *Brain Laterality Can Lead to Body Laterality and Vice Versa*, page 56, for further discussion of the topic of neural crossover.

ing foot is kept somewhat to the big-toe side and the arches of the foot are kept broad.

Other aids to balancing are available to the student practicing balancing in the upright position. See, for example, Box IV.F-1, *Resistive Balancing*, page 545, Subsection IV.F, *Balancing in the Inverted Yogasanas*, page 544, and Section IV.G, General Points on Keeping Your Balance, page 551.

SECTION IV.F. BALANCING IN THE INVERTED *YOGASANAS*

Aids to Balancing in the Inverted Yogasanas

The neural confusion that is inherent when balancing in the left-to-right crossover position as discussed above is likely to be compounded when the student is top-to-bottom inverted. Expect beginning students to be totally disoriented and out of touch with their muscle control when they are inverted for the first time. Though many of the points made in the discussion of upright balancing on the feet (Sections IV.C, page 529, and IV.D, page 533) apply as well to inverted balancing on the hands and on the head, there are several useful points not mentioned in the earlier Section as they apply most readily to the inverted positions.

Balancing in *adho mukha vrksasana* (full arm balance) is best learned by first using the wall for support. The ideal body alignment in this pose is that of *urdhva hastasana*, however, if the student places the hands 12 inches or more from the wall and then uses the wall to hold the heels steady, then the body is necessarily in a banana shape, *i.e.*, belly forward and lumbar collapsed. Because this posture has the heels too far overhead, encouraging compression in the lumbar spine, it is called overbalancing, whereas underbalancing refers to the heels being too far in front of the face, en-

couraging bending at the hips when inverted. As beginners become more accomplished in this *yogasana*, they should be encouraged to move the hands ever closer to the wall in order to bring the arms, spine, and ribs into *urdhva hastasana* alignment (however, see below).

Once proper alignment and extension are achieved at the wall, the student next should be encouraged to work away from the wall in order to develop independence. With this latter point in mind, in the inverted poses, set the balancing point on the floor at a distance from the wall equal to the heel-to-shin length of the legs. If the student then overbalances from here, bending one leg will bring the toes to the wall without bending the rest of the body out of position.

Depending upon the student's aptitude, inverted balancing postures should be performed either close to the wall, a shin's length removed from the wall, or very far from the wall. Do not let students practice the balance at a distance of, say, three feet from the wall, for if they start to fall backward from there, the wall is too far away to support their balance, and they otherwise will fall heavily into the wall and possibly be injured.

Fear of falling backward is a strong emotion for students in inverted postures [416], and may lead to a permanent relationship with the wall. In order to overcome this, it is useful to set students in the center of the room, away from the wall, and practice deliberately falling backward from inverted positions. Use helpers to lower the performing student's body onto the heels and back as they slowly fall with a helper's support into the unknown. Once this fear of falling backward is conquered, then the student can practice the balance unassisted in the center of the room.

Assuming that the students are using the one-legged kick to come into *adho mukha vrksasana* in the middle of the room, it is

BOX IV.F-1: RESISTIVE BALANCING

For practice in resistive balancing, first hold the student in the balanced position, and then slowly push him/her out of balance, either to underbalance (feet too far forward) or overbalance (feet too far backward), but maintain the support in the unbalanced position. The holding in the unbalanced position is minimal; for inverted *yogasanas*, usually just placing the tips of the thumb and index finger of one hand on the upper thighs (front or back) is enough. From the position of supported imbalance, the student then works as in Fig. IV.F-1 to generate a countertorque which overcomes the imbalance and brings the position back to stability. By working with support while in the off-balance position, the student has the time to sort out the proprioceptive and vestibular signals and try various righting strategies. Over time, this results in the training of the various neuromuscular groups necessary for activating the complex balancing patterns. The technique of resistive balancing can be used as well in standing poses such as *ardha chandrasana, parivrtta trikonasana, etc.*

Using the support given in resistive balancing also can be very useful in implanting in the student's mind the consequences of letting a balance become too far underbalanced. For example, support a student in *adho mukha vrksasana* in the overbalanced position, Fig. IV.F-2a, and the student will be able to work the hands against the floor to recover the balance point. However, if the same student is supported in the underbalanced position, Fig. IV.F-2b, he/she will quickly discover that recovery is not possible while keeping the arms straight, and so learns to avoid that situation in the future.

Once the resistive-balancing exercise is finished, have the student return to the beginning position (feet on the floor) slowly, with as little help as possible. This latter is a resistive strengthening exercise involving eccentric isotonic work (Subsection 7.A, *Types of Muscle Contraction*, page 187), and will quickly build the strength needed to go up into the inverted *yogasana* without jumping or kicking, as does increasing the duration of the inverted poses.

wise to coach them into pulling the armpits forward as they go up (that is, in the direction appropriate to *adho mukha svanasana*), as the opposite action at the shoulders is apt to drop the student onto his head or back following the kick.

Imagine our beginning student trying unsuccessfully to balance away from the wall in *sirsasana I*. For many such students, the proper muscle actions for balancing in *sirsasana I* seem not to be accessible when inverted, or the falling is so rapid that they cannot be brought into play quickly enough to save the pose. One way around these problems for some is to practice the technique of resistive balancing [106], described in Box IV.F-1.

Performing the Inverted Yogasanas

There are many excellent articles describing why students should be doing *adho mukha vrksasana*, and how to get into the inverted position [134, 209, 261, 415, 433], however, there is precious little on how to stay there without leaning against the wall. Similar expositions are readily available for wall-supported *sirsasana* [209, 263, 433] and *pincha mayurasana* [209, 433]. At this

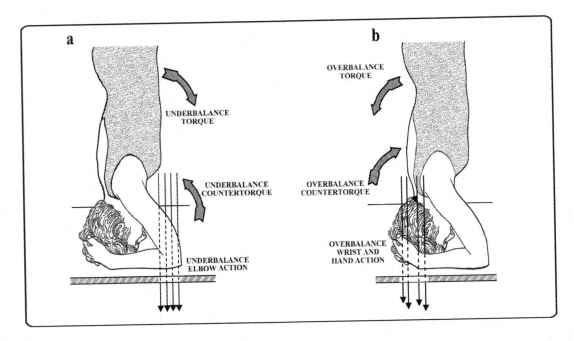

Fig. IV.F-1. (**a**) Schematic representation of the forearm and wrist in *sirsasana*, with the torso underbalanced and rotating clockwise. In this case, the counterbalancing torque is generated by pressing the elbows into the floor. (**b**) If the torso is overbalanced so that it would fall in a counter-clockwise sense, then application of the wrists to the floor will generate the necessary counter torque and so restore balance.

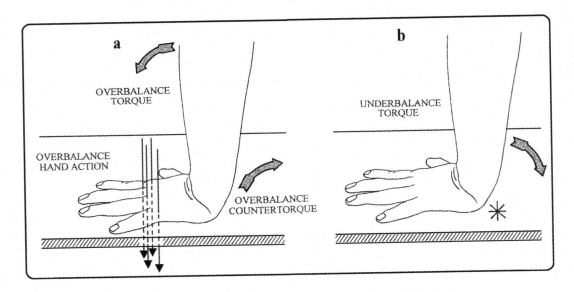

Fig. IV.F-2. (**a**) Schematic representation of the forearm, wrist and hand in *adho mukha vrksasana*, with the torso overbalanced and rotating counterclockwise. Selective pressure at the fingers and base of the knuckles generates a counterbalancing torque to restore alignment. (**b**) When the pose is underbalanced (torso rotating clockwise), there is no way to press the wrist in order to generate a coutertorque, and the torso falls, rotating around the point marked *.

point, we discuss how to stay up, once in these inverted postures.

Begin *adho mukha vrksasana* at the wall, and following the previous Subsections:

a) work with the hands at least shoulder width apart and with maximum length and width of each hand so as to maximize the area of the base of the pose

b) use nothing soft under the hands

c) with the eyes open, fix the gaze on a point on the floor just forward of the finger-tips [134], tilting the head so as to lift the chin away from the sternum; gazing at a coin placed forward of the fingertips can be very stabilizing

d) begin the asana in full *adho-mukha-svanasana* extension and alignment, step one of the feet half way toward the hands, and then kick the body into the inverted position, retaining the hand and shoulder actions of *adho mukha svanasana*. In Box 7.A-4, *The Hands Help Wag The Shoulder Blades in Adho Mukha Svanasana*, page 196, a chain reaction of sorts is described in which the specific action beginning at the bases of the thumbs and index fingers on the floor in *adho mukha svanasana* results in specific movements of the collar bones, ribcage, and shoulder blades. The action of the thumb and index finger in *adho mukha vrksasana* is parallel to that of the same appendages in *adho mukha svanasana*. Progress from the one-legged kick to jumping up (or pressing up) with both legs together.

e) kick gently and with deliberation into the final position so that the momentum of the kick does not lead to excessive overbal-ance, and to allow the vestibular-organ signals to change smoothly as you come into the inverted position. You will want to kick into a position of approximate balance, and then use the feedforward reflex (Subsection 6.A, *Homeostatic Control; Feedback and Feedforward*, page 133) to pull the body in a controlled way into the final posi-

tion. If you do not learn how to kick into the inverted position without either overbalancing or underbalancing, you will never learn how to get into the pose in the middle of the room

f) in the inverted pose, keep all of the secondary joints open and taut as the body is extended upward from above the wrists to the heels. In *vrksasana*, this is done by stretching the arms up and pulling the ribcage away from the pelvis. In *adho mukha vrksasana*, this is done by lifting the heels and bases of the big toes toward the ceiling so as to pull the pelvis away from the ribcage. Give full attention to the actions of the hands and wrists on the floor

g) once in the position, do not move the head as this will only create extraneous noise within the vestibular organs, which already have enough to do without this added burden. The outward look of full-arm balance is very much like that of *urdhva hast-asana*, with the exception that in the former the head is decidedly thrown back more than is proper for the latter [209]. This head-back position, in fact, is absolutely neces-sary for all hand-balancing *yogasanas* which in general are very difficult with the head turned down, chin to sternum. Note that this head position for inversions is op-posite to that recommended for erect posi-tions (see Section IV.E, Balancing in the Standing *Yogasanas*, page 538), even with the eyes open

h) slowly bring the buttocks off the wall, yet keep the weight somewhat heavy on the fingertips. Just as the leg is stronger than the arm, so are the foot and ankle stronger than the hand and wrist. This means that one can afford to lean far forward in *vrksasana* and the strength of the ankle can supply enough countertorque to keep the body from falling further, whereas the wrist and hand, being much weaker, will tolerate only a much smaller overbalance in full-arm balance before being overcome

i) with the body off the wall yet leaning slightly backward, heels lightly on the wall, press the fingers of the hands against the floor so that the body is torqued slightly in the falling-forward direction. It is this compensation of the overbalancing action of falling backward with the counterbalancing action of the fingers on the floor that keeps the pose stable mechanically. This torque is stronger yet if the fingers are bent so that only the tips and lowest knuckles of the fingers press the floor, in addition to the palms, of course. On the other hand, if the falling torque is clockwise (underbalancing) as shown in Figure IV.F-2b, there is little or no countertorque that can be generated because the bones of the wrist are at the very heel of the hand, and the balance is lost by rotating about the spot marked *. That is to say, if you want to stay balanced with the arms straight in this pose (and in *bakasana*), you must actually stay a little overbalanced,

with the weight of the body always heavier on the fingers and base of the knuckles than on the heels of the hands

j) as a variation, start with the hands well away from the wall, and in the inverted position, extend one leg forward while the other is extended backward (as in beginning *parivrttaikapada sirsasana*), so as to gain a balancing-pole advantage in the front-to-back direction. Once in this position, gently tip the back leg off the wall, but remain slightly overbalanced; do not swing the legs excessively, but work more from the wrists.

The yogic full-arm balance, Fig. IV.F-3a, is very different from that often seen in the circus. For circus performers, the principal concern is keeping balance rather than gaining yogic extension. To that end, the circus full-arm balance is often done with an extreme backbend in the lumbar region, with the abdomen and chest very forward of the arms and the heels far behind the head,

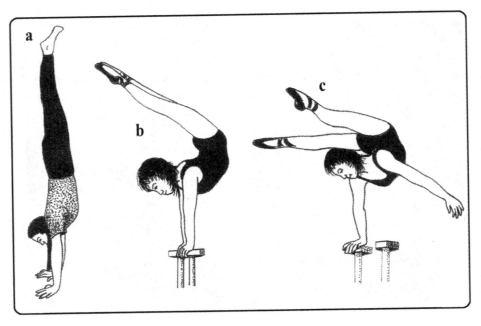

Fig. IV.F-3. The two styles of *adho mukha vrksasana*. (**a**) The yogic position, with maximal spinal lengthening and verticality (Theresa Rowland), and (**b**) the circus posture, with extreme spinal extension so as to gain the balancing-pole advantage in the front-to-back direction. (**c**) In the one-arm hand balance, circus style, the legs also separate left-to-right so that the performer now has both front-to-back and left-to-right balancing-pole advantages. Notice that the body is positioned so that the center of gravity is progressively lower on going from **a** to **b** to **c**, thereby increasing the stability of the posture.

Fig. IV.-3b. This posture works for them because the trunk of the body itself serves as a front-to-back balancing pole, rather like the situation with beginners in *trikonasana* (Section IV.E, Balancing in the Standing *Yogasanas*, page 538), and the extreme spinal extension (backbending) lowers the center of gravity. When the equilibrist shifts to balance on one arm, Fig. IV.F-3c, the legs are then separated left to right, thus acting as an additional balancing pole for imbalance in that direction. Needless to say, the "banana" or "circus handstand" is a totally inappropriate posture for yoga work for beginners or intermediate students, and any tendency in this direction is to be discouraged [134, 261] (however, see *vrscikasana* [209]).

Much of what has been outlined above for balancing in *adho mukha vrksasana* can be carried over *in toto* for balancing in poses such as *bakasana* and *pincha mayurasana*. In these poses, lean so as to develop a slight overbalance torque and then compensate this with a countertorque generated by pressing the fingers or parts of the forearms (Appendix V, GRAVITY, page 553) against the floor appropriately. If, in any of these *yogasanas*, the pose becomes underbalanced, then there is no way to regain balance (unless one can bend the arms), and one must start over, remembering to keep the weight somewhat heavy in the overbalanced direction. In all of these poses, coming down slowly with control will help build the shoulder, chest and back strengths needed for performing the poses without the support of the wall.

In the context of what has been said above in regard to balancing in inversions, *sirsasana I* is especially interesting from several points of view. First, unlike *adho mukha vrksasana*, balancing in *sirsasana I* is much easier: its base area is larger, the center of gravity is lower, there are fewer joints above the floor which can go into

motion, and the placement of the hands on the floor (Fig. IV.F-1) allows both clockwise and counterclockwise compensating torques to be applied for balance. This last point does not apply to those variations of *sirsasana* in which both the hands and elbows are forward of the head, Appendix I, page 503. In these cases, one must stay slightly underbalanced in order to not overbalance and roll backward.

In preparation for going up in *sirsasana I*, take *adho mukha virasana*, with the weight of the head pressing the brow onto the floor for several minutes. Pressure at this point in the head promotes the vagal heart-slowing response (see Section 11.F, Blood Pressure in Inverted *Yogasanas*, page 343) and so lowers the blood pressure before inverting. This could be useful for all inversions where increased blood pressure upon inversion is a problem.

Lasater [263] points out that in *sirsasana*, beginners tend to go up into the inverted position using the strength of their arms, and then balance with their legs, whereas one should do the reverse. As Farhi says with respect to balancing in *adho mukha vrksasana*, one should instead keep a neutral position of the legs with respect to the pelvis [134], *i.e.*, do not swing the legs back and forth in order to maintain balance. I agree with this totally, and feel the same reasoning applies in the other inverted balances.

In *sirsasana*, if one extends the body straight up to take all of the looseness out of the joints (the body is taut), then the balancing action is in the hand and wrist, as it should be. If the body is loose instead, then balancing action reverts to points far above the point of contact with the floor, and complex body oscillation ensues. Not only is the balance impaired by this upper-body motion, but maintaining the motion is very energy draining. Finally, only in *sirsasana I* and *savasana* are we unable to see any part of the body; all of the alignment then must be via the proprioceptive system of the body [264].

Most interestingly, the very strong positive-feedback effect that one gets from the eyes in the other inverted postures is not a factor at all in *sirsasana I!* Not only is *sirsasana I* stable with the eyes closed (try it), but it is even more so than *tadasana* with the eyes open. Why is this so?

To answer this question, note first that *sirsasana I* can be more stable than *tadasana* both because the area of the base is larger and because the center of gravity of the body in *sirsasana I* is much more over the center of the base, whereas in *tadasana*, the center of gravity is more toward the heels and so is less tolerant of any backward motion. As for closing the eyes having no impact on balancing in *sirsasana I*, this is at first quite a surprise since it is very important in *vrksasana* and *adho mukha vrksasana*, for example. Notice however, that the contribution of the eyes to balancing comes from their sense of the visual field shifting as the head moves. But in *sirsasana I*, the head is pinned to the floor and because it does not move, the eyes are of no value in determining the balancing response! As regards the semicircular canals (see Section 17.B, The Vestibular Organs of Balance, page 437), they too are unresponsive in *sirsasana I* since they only respond to accelerating rotations of the head. Similarly, the utricle and saccule of the inner ear could help balance the body if the head position reflected the body position, however, with the head firmly on the floor, these organs will give constant signals independent of the body position*. Hence, balancing in *sirsasana I* is largely a matter of proprioceptive sensing and adjustment, with significant input from the pressure sensors in the lower arms.

In *sarvangasana*, do not look at the ceiling, as this is an eyes-up position and thus would serve to activate the intellect in a pose that does not require it. Similarly, do not look at the solar plexus, as this tends to pull the eyes in toward the nose, thus creating tension. Looking at the knees in *sarvangasana* is a good neutral position for the eyes in this pose. Regarding body position, keep the weight slightly overbalanced in *sarvangasana*, so that the weight is somewhat shifted off the neck and more toward the elbows. Inasmuch as one can see only oneself in *sarvangasana*, it is an ideal pose for self-examination [255]. In contrast, in the counterpose, *sirsasana I*, one can see everything except one's self.

As described more clearly in Section 4.A, The Spinal Column, page 63, each of the cervical vertebrae has a bony arch, through which the spinal cord passes. Each of the arches is itself in contact with the arches above and below, through facet joints. Because the bones of the arches are set at 45° with respect to the line of the vertical spine, only a gliding motion of one cervical vertebra with respect to the next is relatively stress free. This allowed motion is either forward and upward as when one tips the head in flexion (chin to chest as in *jalandhara bandha*), or the opposite which is backward and down, as when placing the head in extension (head back). It is also safe to tip the head to the right and downward as well, as this slides the joints on the right forward and upward while those on the left go backward and down. Trying to turn one's neck to look to the side while in *sarvangasana* or *halasana* is strongly not advised as these motions risk fracturing the bones of the facet joints (Section 4.A, The Spinal Column, page 63) when they are loaded as they are in these positions [271], or interfer-

---

*Actually, the mat of sensor cells in the utricle lies in a horizontal plane with the gelatinous mass above it when standing upright. When inverted, it is possible that the gelatinous mass pulls away from the sensor hairs and thus the hairs are not bent in response to an imbalance.

ing with the arterial blood flow through the vertebral arteries (Subsection 3.B, *Blood Flow through the Brain*, page 35). On the other hand, in *parsva halasana* and in *parsva karnapidasana* the cervical spine retains its *jalandhara-bandha* orientation while the remainder of the spine is rotated. Similarly, rotations while in variations of *sirsasana I* are to be done with the cervical spine as in *tadasana*, with all of the twisting to be done in the thoracic and lumbar regions where the loading is not so great and where there is more freedom of movement because the vertebrae are not pinned to the floor by the weight of the body.

Elderly students, especially women, are predisposed to dizziness as a consequence of the aging process, as aging implies a physiologic decline in proprioceptive, visual and vestibular reflexes, all of which serve normally to keep us in balance. The performance of older yoga students who have practiced *yogasanas* for a long time suggests that this decline in the balancing senses does not necessarily have to occur or can be slowed significantly by *yogasana* work. Balancing questions aside, one must use care and good judgement when bringing new students into the inverted positions, especially the elderly, as discussed in Appendix II, INJURIES INCURRED DURING IMPROPER *YOGASANA* PRACTICE, page 511.

SECTION IV.G. GENERAL POINTS ON KEEPING YOUR BALANCE

Many of the specific points raised in the Sections above can be generalized so as to apply to any and all balancing positions in yoga, whether upright or inverted, inclined or horizontal. These generalities regarding the balancing aspects of the *yogasanas* are gathered together in this place.

(1) It is very difficult to balance on one or more appendages when said appendages are barely strong enough to hold up the pose. Any work that strengthens these appendages in general will correspondingly make the balancing easier.

(2) Make the area of the base of the pose large so that the line between the center of gravity of the student and the center of the earth is well within the area of the base. This does not mean that practicing *adho mukha vrksasana* with the hands as far apart as possible will help the balancing, because the balancing problem in this *yogasana* is forward-backward, and separating the hands only aids in the left-right direction. On the other hand, putting the hand on the floor in *ardha chandrasana* so that it is behind the standing foot rather than in line with it does aid the balance tremendously. Spread the hand so that the span of the knuckles is maximal; spread the foot so that the span of the base of the toes is maximal.

(3) Enlarge the area of the base so as to avoid wobble. Balance means not only not falling over, but a steadiness in the position which signals complete control of the body.

(4) The closer the center of gravity of the student is to the floor, the easier is the balance, in part because the time available for response is longer if the student starts to fall.

(5) The surface supporting the pose must be solid and unyielding. Try balancing in *vrksasana* while standing on a soft foam block or on a multiply-folded sticky mat to see how important it is that the support be firm.

(6) Keep all of the joints of the body (except the lowest) fully extended to avoid unnecessary wobble at these joints. Assuming that the balancing is being done on the floor, use the joints that rest on or close to the floor to do the balancing, keeping all others fully open but immobile. The big toe will be very important in standing poses, both for reasons of strength and balance.

(7) When balancing on the hands (feet), let the weight of the body fall lightly on the

fingers (toes), and with the body's secondary joints fully extended, work the floor with the fingers (toes) so as to generate a compensating countertorque to the falling-body torque.

(8) Appendages held out to the side or front-to-back will stabilize balance in the plane of the appendages. This is the balancing-pole effect often used in the circus, and by small children walking on top of narrow walls.

(9) Once in the pose, keep the head still. When the head moves, the motion sensors in the inner ear will activate reflex arcs that may conflict with the balancing efforts of the joints on the floor.

(10) When balancing on the feet, keep the head in the neutral position so that the cervical vertebrae are in alignment with the remainder of the spine. This will not necessarily be true when in the inverted *yogasanas* where the head-up, chin-away-from-the-chest position is more appropriate.

(11) Keep the eyes open when balancing; fix the gaze on an immobile object in the far visual field and keep the object centered in the visual field. In those cases where balance is involved in moving into the *yogasana*, imagine a line painted on the floor; keeping the line centered in the visual field while moving is very stabilizing. Avoid trying to balance when the visual background is in motion, and avoid having to look at a blank wall having no distinguishable features. Balancing in the open with no walls for visual support can be an added burden [161]. Try wearing glasses in order to see if poor vision could be a factor in balancing.

(12) Balancing will be easier if the same background is present as when the *yogasana* was first learned. Face the same wall each time so that the same visual anchors are present during the practice. Once these visual tricks are mastered, then work to disengage from the anchors, so that the pose can be done facing in any direction, in any room or open space. At this point, the eyes can be kept with the gaze broad and defocused so as to relax the muscles of the eyes.

(13) Move slowly and with awareness into the final position of balance, starting in a balanced position and adjusting the balance as you go, so that there is a minimum of readjusting to be done once in the pose. Moving slowly also promotes the mental steadiness that is required for physical steadiness. Your steadiness in a balance at a particular moment will reflect your emotional stability at that time; do not be surprised if a balance that was easy on one day appears difficult on the next.

(14) One comes most smoothly into the balanced position by leaning the pose first on a wall and then gently moving the weight off the wall so as to balance freely.

(15) When kicking into an inverted position, do not try to kick into exact balance, but instead, either overkick or underkick slightly, and using the feedforward reflex (Subsection 6.A, *Homeostatic Control; Feedback and Feedforward*, page 133), catch the pose and then either push or pull it into position in a controlled way.

(16) Practice; the balancing reflexes are refined by practice, practice, practice.

One final point should be made with respect to the safety of the teacher when teaching inversions. The time will come when some of your students will have to be hoisted into the inverted positions because they do not kick hard enough to reach the wall on their own and/or need shoulder support from behind. In this situation, your face will be in the direct line of fire of their heels unless your students understand *when* they are to kick, and you then turn your head away from the action at the appropriate moment. If you neglect to turn away, sooner or later you will get kicked in the face [261].

Appendix V

GRAVITY

SECTION V.A. EXERTING PRESSURE ON THE FLOOR

You Have No Choice

Gravity affects us as *yogasana* students in several important ways. First, let us look at the inviolable Law of Universal Gravitation first deduced by Sir Isaac Newton. Given two objects of mass m_1 and m_2 separated by a center-to-center distance of d, the gravitational force F attracting each of the objects to the other is given by Newton as

$$F = G\, m_1\, m_2\, /d^2$$

where G is a fixed number called the gravitational constant. When we do yoga on the floor at the surface of the earth, then F is our weight, m_1 is our mass, m_2 is the mass of the earth and d is the earth's radius. As F is the force with which the soles of our feet press onto the floor in *tadasana*, and G, m_2 and d are fixed quantities, the only way we can change the force with which our feet press into the floor (our weight) is to change our mass m_1, *i.e.*, eat a cheesecake, slim down, or hold a sandbag.

Note that there is no room in the above equation for personal choice or will power. Contrary to what is said by many teachers in *yogasana* classes, you cannot simply:

a) "Press your feet into the floor," as in *tadasana*. If you could press your feet into the floor on command, then you could change your weight as measured on the bathroom scale at will, instantaneously. Your feet press into the floor in *tadasana* whether you want them to or not, and how hard they press into the floor cannot be changed as long as you stay in *tadasana* and do not change your weight.

b) "Come up by pressing your feet into the floor" in *trikonasana*. Actually, your feet unavoidably are pressing into the floor as you start the pose, remain pressing while you are in the pose and press the floor as you come out of the pose; this pressure of your feet on the floor does not change unless your weight changes. The only way to press your weight more into the floor on coming up from *trikonasana* is to start eating more and exercising less.

c) "Press your forearms into the floor" in *pincha mayurasana*. Just as when standing with your weight on your feet, your weight on the floor in *pincha mayurasana* will not respond to your teacher's advice to press the floor harder or heavier in this posture, because Newton's Law got there first.

One has the illusion that the weight can be pressed into the floor because we are generally not aware of the pressure on the soles of the feet resulting from the Earth's gravitational pull on our mass. However, when the teacher says, "Press the feet," we become quickly aware of the pressure and so think that the teacher's instruction immediately made the pressure increase. Actually, the pressure has stayed constant, but the awareness of the pressure increased when the teacher gave her command.

Though you cannot change the weight that presses your feet onto the floor in *tadasana*, what you can change is the *distribution* of your weight among the various body

553

parts touching the floor. That is to say, in *tadasana*, you can be heavier on your heels by being lighter on the balls of your feet, and you can move the weight from the inner edges of the feet to the outer edges, *etc*. You can press your feet more strongly into the floor in *adho mukha svanasana* by shifting your weight away from your hands and toward your feet. When coming up from *trikonasana*, one shifts the weight between the left and right feet, and also between different parts of each foot, but "pressing the feet into the floor" has no meaning. And though you simply cannot "Press your forearms into the floor" in *pincha mayurasana*, you can lift your upper arms away from your forearms to achieve the same end, or you can be heavier on the hands and lighter on the elbows, *etc*.

Actually, there is a yogic way of pressing your feet into the floor in *tadasana*: if in this pose, you will press your arms upward against the ceiling with a force of Q pounds, then the weight on the soles of your feet will increase by Q pounds. If you are standing on your partner's thighs while doing this, he will feel the extra push. However, if while standing you reach vigorously into the air above you, you do not lessen the weight with which your feet press onto the ground. Strangely, you can increase the pressure of your feet on the floor (slightly) when in *tadasana* by coming into *malasana*, as explained in the following Section.

SECTION V.B. THE CENTER OF GRAVITY

When standing in *tadasana*, the different body parts are at different distances d from the center of the earth and so each body part is pulled with a slightly different force, *i.e.*, has a different weight. The single force (weight) that you register on the bathroom scale when in *tadasana*, is equivalent to what you would exert if all of your mass were concentrated at one particular point in space, a point called the center of gravity. In the human body when in *tadasana*, the center of gravity is a few inches below the belly button and half way back along the line from front to back.

Mechanically, your body acts/reacts as if all of its mass were at the center of gravity; the center of gravity is the single point about which the body rotates freely and the point at which the body can be supported from below or above and remain balanced in any orientation without rotating. Once in *tadasana*, the center of gravity rises when we raise our arms into *urdhva hastasana*, whereas when we crouch in *malasana*, the center of gravity is closer to the center of the earth. Theoretically, we weigh more when our center of gravity is lowered (d is smaller and F is correspondingly larger) and less when our center of gravity is raised (d is larger and F is correspondingly smaller), but these changes are microscopic.

Often what is sought by "pressing the feet into the floor" is a lengthening of the distance between two points in the body, one of which is constrained to the floor. The lengthening does not press the hands, feet, or forearms more into the floor, but does lift the center of gravity. Thus to be more accurate, we should be saying things such as, "lift your center of gravity by lengthening the distance between your feet and your pelvis." The work involved in doing the *yogasanas* is largely the work of lifting the center of gravity of the body away from the center of gravity of the earth, and correspondingly, the body is most relaxed when its center of gravity is closest to the center of the earth, *i.e.*, in *savasana*.

The concept of the center of gravity is most useful to *yogasana* students in another context. In order to avoid falling in balancing poses, the line between the center of the earth (its center of gravity) and the center of gravity of the body must pass through the area of the base of the body in contact with the earth (Subsection IV.B, *Balancing a Rigid Block*, page 526). One can remain balanced in a pose only as long as the line between the centers of gravity of the body and the earth falls within the area of the base of the pose.

SECTION V.C. GRAVITATIONAL EFFECTS ON *YOGASANAS*

For the yoga student, the physiological effects of gravity are threefold:

1) The gravitational force that keeps us fixed to the earth also works to pull us flat onto the floor, however, thanks to the rigidity of our bony skeleton, we remain more or less upright. The endless work of the asanas to "lift up" is done in response to this downward pull. Actually, we work against the downward pull of gravity when we work to raise our center of gravity. This lifting is highest and most sustainable when the bones of the body are positioned so as to bear the most weight (gravitational stress) and the muscles are used only to keep the bones in alignment (*tadasana*, for example). Of course, nonaligned positions are also possible (*utkatasana*, for example), but here a larger part of the gravitational stress falls on the muscles, and so the pose cannot be held as long. Bones fatigue in the course of years, muscles in the course of minutes. Nonetheless, both bones and muscles are strengthened by resisting the pull of gravity, and both wither in a gravity-free environment or in an environment where there is gravity but no effort to resist its pull.

In zero gravity, muscles atrophy, and in some muscles, the slow-twitch fibers so necessary for muscle strength are converted instead into fast twitch muscles which are quick acting but not as long lasting. As the bones demineralize and become brittle, the demineralizing bone raises serum levels of Ca^{2+} to dangerous levels. The immune system seems also to be adversely affected by weightlessness, as is sleep quality and motor coordination. All of the above observations parallel many of the body changes observed in the aging process and in prolonged bedrest. Clearly a regular *yogasana* practice works against all of the negative effects of too little gravitational pull on the body, by keeping us out of the sick bed and by giving us opportunities for actively responding to gravity's pull.

2) Though the skeleton can support the flesh against the pull of gravity, it is not as effective in shielding the body fluids from this downward pull. Thus these fluids tend to pool in that part of the body closest to the floor, *i.e.*, when standing, in the legs, when sleeping, on the side of the body closer to the mattress. In regard *yogasanas* performed in the supine position, there is a more efficient filling of the right atrium when horizontal, and in consequence of this, the volume receptors in the atrium report a high value to the hypothalamus, which in turn decreases the heart rate as compared to the situation where the posture is performed in a standing position. However, even in the standing position, there are indirect ways of using the bones and muscles to elevate fluid as well (see Subsection 11.C, *Venous Flow Against Gravity*, page 332, and Section 11.G, The Lymphatic System, page 352), and these keep the fluid distribution more or less uniform.

Weightlessness has a strong negative effect on body fluids. First, without gravity, fluids move more to the head when standing and so cause stuffiness and congestion. The senses of taste and smell degrade, and in zero gravity, each leg loses about one liter of fluid, with overall plasma volume decreasing by 20%. Once plasma volume decreases, red blood cell production shuts down and anemia sets in.

3) The gravitational pull of the body toward the earth's center gives us a proprioceptive handle on our orientation in space (see Appendix IV, BALANCING, page 525), so valuable for balancing. Note however, that the body's sensors can not distinguish between the gravitational force and any other external force that is unavoidably present when the body is in accelerating or decelerating motion, other than the gravitational force is always toward the center of the earth and the other external forces can be in any direction.

In this regard, we continuously monitor subconsciously where our limbs are in space by integrating visual cues with information from our vestibular system (Section 17.B, The Vestibular Organs of Balance, page 437), from proprioceptors on bones, muscles and joints (Section 7.C, *Proprioception*, page 208), and from mechanoreceptors on our skin (Subsection 10.B, *Deep Pressure*, page 290). Of these balance sensors, all but the visual cues depend partly or completely on our body's response to gravity.

The effects of weightlessness on the human body are of interest to us not only because they point out several important factors here on earth that we have come to ignore due their constancy, but also because the effects of weightlessness seem to mimic closely those of old age, (Chapter 22, AGING AND LONGEVITY, page 493) [482]. Space travelers are off balance when they return to earth's gravitational field and mental deterioration sets in: they suffer from motion sickness, vomiting, headache, poor concentration, and loss of appetite.

Certain of the *yogasanas* are relatively unaffected by the pull of gravity, as for example, *supta padangusthasana*, whereas others are strongly affected, *chaturanga dandasana*, for example. With respect to the latter, in the presence of gravity, lowering from the plank position to *chaturanga dandasana* involves an eccentric isotonic extension of the triceps, whereas the same motion in the absence of gravity would involve a concentric isotonic contraction of the biceps (Subsection 7.A, *Types of Muscle Contraction*, page 187). To experience what *yogasana* practice would be like in the zero gravity of outer space, try the poses while submerged in your swimming pool.

GLOSSARY

Many but not all of the technical terms used in this Handbook are adequately defined in the text and can be found using the Index. In case the Index is of no help, is inadequate, or is too slow, then this Glossary can be used for succinct definitions. The definitions given in the Glossary are not the widest possible, but are suited to the level of technical discussion used in this Handbook.

ABDUCTORS – muscles that lift the limbs away from the center line of the body

ACETYLCHOLINE – one of several neurotransmitters released into the neuromuscular synaptic gap in the course of nerve conduction.

ACTIN – one of the two protein strands in skeletal muscle (the other is myosin) responsible for its contraction

ACTION POTENTIAL – the voltage that propels the neural signal down the axon and toward the waiting synapse. This voltage is generated by the selective motions of various ions through channels in the cell membrane

ADAPTATION – the loss of a receptor's sensitivity over a period of time as a result of continuous stimulation

ADDUCTORS – muscles that pull the limbs toward the center line of the body

ADENOSINE DIPHOSPHATE (ADP) – the chemical product formed from the energy-producing reaction of ATP with water

ADENOSINE TRIPHOSPHATE (ATP) – the key biological chemical used to produce energy in the body

ADRENAL GLAND – an endocrine gland resting on top of the kidney, and composed of the cortex (secreting corticosteroids such as cortisol) and the medulla (secreting epinephrine and norepinephrine)

ADRENERGIC – said of synapses in the body that involve the catecholamines as neurotransmitters

ADRENOCORTICOTROPHIC HORMONE (ACTH) – a pituitary hormone that stimulates the adrenal cortex to release cortisol. Production of ACTH is initiated by hormonal release of corticotropin releasing factor (CRF) from the hypothalamus

AEROBIC OXIDATION – pertaining to oxidation processes within the body that require oxygen pulled from the air

AFFERENT FIBER – a nerve fiber which conducts impulses from a sensory receptor to the central nervous system, or from lower to higher levels in the sensory projection systems within the central nervous system

AGONIST – one half of a pair of muscles each of which moves a body part in a direction opposite to that moved by the other; *see* ANTAGONIST

ALDOSTERONE – a hormone released by the adrenal cortex which promotes water retention

ALLERGEN – a substance that produces an allergic reaction; the response to an allergen is called an allergy

ALPHA BRAINWAVES – electrical voltage waves sensed in the scalp at a rate of 8–13 Hz, indicating relaxed wakefulness, early stages of meditation and sleep, and receptivity to ESP; a creative state of mind

ALPHA-MOTOR NEURON – an efferent neuron originating in the ventral horn of the spinal cord and terminating on a muscle fiber

ALPHA RECEPTORS – generally responsive to norepinephrine, causing a constriction of the smooth muscles in the organs of the gastrointestinal tract

ALVEOLI – the smallest branches of the bronchial tree, being the sites at which gas exchange of oxygen and carbon dioxide between blood and breath take place

AMENHORREIC – lacking in menstrual periods

AMINO ACID – a molecule bearing both an amino group ($-NH_2$) and a carboxylic acid group ($-COOH$). Amino acids combine chemically to form proteins

AMPHETAMINES – stimulants to the central nervous system, increasing blood pressure

ANALGESIA – the loss of sensitivity to pain without loss of consciousness or the other sensory qualities

ANALGESIC – a drug that relieves pain

ANAEROBIC OXIDATION – pertaining to oxidation processes within the body that obtain their oxygen from sources other than the air

ANDROGEN – a male hormone responsible for the development of male characteristics

ANEURYSM – a swelling in the wall of a blood vessel

ANGIOTENSIN – a neuropeptide promoting drinking of water

ANGSTROM – a unit of length measurement on the atomic scale, equal to one hundred millionth (10^{-8}) centimeter; the diameter of the hydrogen atom is 1.2 Angstroms

ANOXIA – the condition in which tissue is deprived of oxygen

ANTAGONIST – a muscle which produces a result opposite to that produced by the contraction of its agonist muscle, *i.e.*, if the biceps is considered to be the agonist, then its antagonist is the triceps

ANTERIOR – the front part of the body

ANTERIOR HYPOTHALAMUS – that forward part of the hypothalamus, controlling the excitation of the parasympathetic nervous system

ANTIBODY – a protein, also called an immunoglobulin, which binds to the surface antigen of a particular infectious organism and kills it.

ANTIDEPRESSANT – a drug or *yogasana* that is mood elevating

ANTIDIURETIC HORMONE – *see* OXYTOCIN

ANTIGEN – a foreign protein that triggers the formation of antibodies by the immune system.

AORTA – the large artery leaving the left ventricle of the heart and supplying oxygenated blood to the entire body

APOCRINE GLANDS – located mainly in the armpits and surrounding the genitals, release a smelly fluid when the body is under emotional or physical stress

APONEUROSIS – a broad band of tendon, connected to several bones

APOPTOSIS – process by which cells kill themselves

AQUEOUS HUMOUR – the fluid filling the space between the cornea and the lens of the eye

ARTERIOLES – small arteries positioned between the larger arterial branches and the capillaries, controlling the rate of flow of blood from the heart and hence the blood pressure

ARTICULAR PROCESSES – the protruding wings on each side of the vertebral bodies, each of which is used in forming a vertebral facet joint

ARTICULATION – the formation of a joint by bringing two bones together

ATLANTO-OCCIPITAL JOINT – the cervical joint between the atlas of the skull and C1 of the vertebral column

ATLAS – the first cervical vertebra

ATRIUM/ATRIA – the right and left upper chambers of the heart, which collect blood from the body and the lungs, and then pump it to their respective ventricles

AUTOIMMUNE – pertaining to the attack of the body's immune system on one of its own cell types

AUTONOMIC GANGLIA – nerve plexi serving the autonomic nervous system

AUTONOMIC NERVOUS SYSTEM – referring to that part of the nervous system that operates without conscious control, as with the nerves that innervate the internal organs, the smooth muscles, and the glands

AUTOREGULATING – organs that are self regulating

AVASCULAR – tissue such as cartilage that lacks blood vessels

AV NODE – the point in the ventricles of the heart that triggers ventricular contraction

AXON – the part of a nerve cell that conducts the neural signal away from the cell body, and forms a synapse to a neighboring cell, be it neuron, muscle, or gland

BALLISTIC STRETCHING – a very rapid stretching limited by the protective response of the muscle spindles which promote muscle contraction; the opposite of *yogasana* stretching

BARORECEPTOR – a sensor within the body which is sensitive to pressure, transducing it into a neural signal

BASILAR ARTERY – an artery at the base of the brain, connecting the carotid and vertebral arteries

B CELLS – lymphocytes that are produced in the bone marrow, and that produce antibodies; they are responsible for antibody memory

BETA BLOCKER – a medication that decreases the heart's activity and prevents blood vessels from dilating (among other effects) by binding to the beta receptors and preventing their stimulation by epinephrine and norepinephrine

BETA BRAINWAVES – asynchronous brainwaves in the 13–30 Hz range, signaling a state of arousal and energy

BETA RECEPTORS – found in the heart and respond to epinephrine, the effect being to increase the heart rate, the strength of contraction, and to dilate the vascular system of the skeletal and cardiac muscles

BIFURCATING – the branching of a single vessel into two

BIPOLAR DISORDER – a psychosis in which periods of depression alternate with periods of mania

BIOELECTROCHEMISTRY – processes in the body simultaneously involving elements of biology, electricity and chemistry; said of the process of neural conduction

BIOFEEDBACK – a technique in which instruments detect the level of body function and display this to the conscious awareness of the subject who then responds physiologically/mentally so as to change or maintain the level

BIOGENIC AMINES – organic compounds within the body bearing the amino group $-NH_2$ as with the catecholamines

BIORHYTHMS – the regular variation in time of the body's basic functions, with repeat periods that stretch from seconds to years

BONE SPURS – sharp, bony projections that grow to eventually press painfully upon nerves

BLOOD/BRAIN BARRIER – a membrane surrounding the brain which allows only small molecules such as glucose to pass from the blood into the brain

BOW LEGS – legs in which the knees fall outside of the straight line between the hip and the ankle

BRAIN – that part of the central nervous system above the spinal cord and within the cranium

BRAINSTEM – that part of the brain between the cortex and the spinal cord, including the medulla oblongata, the pons, and the midbrain, but excluding the cerebrum and cerebellum

BRAINWAVES – electrical signals on the scalp detected with an electroencephalograph, indicating the state of cortical activity

BREATHING CENTERS – those neurological nuclei within the brainstem controlling the mechanics of inhalation and exhalation of the breath

BRONCHIOLE – a small airway in the respiratory system; a subdivision of the bronchial tree lying in size between the bronchi and the alveoli

BURSA – a small fluid-filled sac serving as lubrication between bone and muscle

CANCELLOUS BONE – porous bone of light weight but high strength, also called trabecular bone

CAPILLARY – a short blood vessel of very thin walls, standing between the arterial and venous systems, allowing the passage of nutrients and waste products between the fluids inside and outside the capillary wall

CARDIAC MUSCLE – the contractive muscle within the heart

CARDIAC OUTPUT, $\dot{Q}$ – the rate at which blood is pumped through the heart, milliliters/minute

CARDIOPULMONARY SYSTEM – pertaining to the heart and lungs

CARDIOVASCULAR SYSTEM – pertaining to the heart and associated arteries and veins

CAROTID ARTERIES – arteries within the neck that carry blood to the forward part of the brain

CAROTID SINUS – an expanded portion of the carotid artery containing the baroreceptor sensor which measures the blood pressure at that point and then sends the message to the central nervous system

CARBON DIOXIDE, CO_2 – a product of the reaction of sugar (fuel) and oxygen (oxidant), carried by the blood to the lungs and expelled on exhalation

CARTILAGE – a form of collagenous tissue, avascular, dense and weight-bearing, as found in the larynx, trachea, nose and joints

CATECHOLAMINES – the neurotransmitters epinephrine, norepinephrine and dopamine

CELESTIAL OSCILLATORS – the sun as it rises and falls daily; the moon as it waxes and wanes monthly

CENTER OF GRAVITY – that point inside or outside of the body, about which the body would rotate were it unsupported. In *tadasana*, the center of gravity is just below the navel and half way back from the front body

CENTRAL NERVOUS SYSTEM, CNS – the brain and spinal cord lying within the skull and the spinal column, respectively

CENTRAL-PATTERN GENERATOR – a neural plexis in the spine capable of driving a repeating muscular pattern such as walking when triggered by higher centers

CEREBELLUM – the coordination center within the brain for posture and equilibrium, situated above the pons and medulla

CEREBRAL CORTEX – the convoluted outer layer of the gray matter covering the cerebral hemispheres

CEREBROSPINAL FLUID – a fluid resembling blood plasma in which the brain and spinal cord float

CEREBRUM – the posterior part of the brain lying above the thalamus and basal ganglia

CERVICAL – pertaining to the neck, for example, the cervical vertebrae

CHAKRAS – the points along the center line of the body which are the common intersections of the *sushumna*, the *ida*, and the *pingala nadis*; several *chakras* correspond to nerve plexi

CHELATION – the binding of metallic ions to organic molecules having a claw shape

CHOLINERGIC – said of synapses in the body that involve acetylcholine as the neurotransmitter

CHRONOTHERAPY – a therapeutic program in which consideration is given to the time at which the therapy is applied in order to increase its effectiveness

CHYME – the partially digested semisolid that passes from the stomach into the small intestine

CILIARY MUSCLES – controlling muscles that alter the shape of the lens of the eye and so adjust its ability to focus

CIRCADIAN MARKER – the point in time during the day when a particular biologic process is either at a maximum or a minimum

CIRCADIAN RHYTHM – a rhythmic process within the body that maximizes and minimizes once per day, always at the same time each day, *i.e.*, it has a 24-hour period

CLAUDICATION – a cramping muscle pain, caused by an inadequate blood flow

COCCYGEAL – pertaining to the four fused vertebrae at the base of the spine

COCHLEA – the spiral organ within the inner ear that transduces sound waves into auditory nerve signals

CO-CONTRACTION – the simultaneous contraction of the two components of an agonist/antagonist muscle pair

COLLAGEN – a fibrous protein from which many body parts, from soft tissue to bones, are constructed; it is a principal component of connective tissue

COLOR THERAPY – the exposure of the eyes to various colors as a therapeutic mode for nonvisual problems

COMMISSURAL FIBERS – tracts of nerve fibers that connect opposite sides of the brain or spinal cord

COMPRESSIVE STRESS – the mechanical stress imposed on an object when its ends are pressed toward one another

CONCENTRIC ISOTONIC ACTION – the contraction of a muscle as it works isotonically to move a load

CONDYLES – the enlarged rounded ends of bones

CONES – the light-sensitive elements in the retina of the eyes, used for daylight vision, with sensitivity to red, green or blue light

CONROTATORY – a spinal twist in which the ribcage and the pelvis rotate in the same sense

CONSOLIDATION – the process whereby memories are moved from fleeting short-term memory to permanent long-term memory

CONTRALATERAL – said of two structures on the opposite sides of the body

CORE TEMPERATURE – the temperature of the interior of the body, usually measured rectally

CORNEA – the transparent outer coating of the eye

CORPUS CALLOSUM – a thick bundle of nerve fibers connecting the left and right cerebral cortices of the brain to one another

CORTEX – the outer covering of an organ, such as the cortex of the brain or the cortex of the adrenal glands. In the brain, the cortex is the site of consciousness and the initiator of deliberate action

CORTICAL BONE – the dense form of bone

CORTISOL – a hormone released by the adrenal cortex when the body is under stress, as when the sympathetic nervous system is activated

CRANIAL NERVES – a set of twelve nerves exiting the skull at the base of the brain, serving the region of the head and neck without passing through the spinal column

CROSS BRIDGE – the molecular fragment between the actin and myosin filaments of the muscle fiber which is responsible for their relative motion when the muscle contracts

CROSS-BRIDGE HEADS – molecular knobs at the ends of the crossbridges, responsible for the attachment and detachment of the myosin crossbridges to the actin chains within muscle

CROSSLINK – a short molecular bridge joining two longer molecular polymer chains

DECUSSATION – a crossing of a nerve from one side of the body to the other

DEFIBRILLATOR – an electrical device used to shock the heart's four chambers into beating rhythmically at appropriate rates

DELTA BRAINWAVES – synchronous electrical waves in the brain of very low frequency (1–4 Hz), appearing during sleep

DEMYELINATION – the stripping of the myelin sheath from around a myelinated nerve fiber, as in multiple sclerosis

DENDRITE – part of the nerve-cell body that receives messages from other nerve cells and transmits them toward the cell body

DEPHOSPHORYLATION – a chemical process in which a phosphate group, PO_4, is split from a larger molecule

DEPOLARIZED – the condition of a neuron that has received an electrical signal from a nearby neuron and as a result, has a potential of –65 millivolts or less, as compared with –70 millivolts when in the resting state

DERMATOME – the area of skin innervated by a single sensory root of the spinal cord

DETRAINING – to stop a physical training program

DIAPHRAGM – a thin, domed muscle spanning the bottom of the ribcage, the contraction of which helps fill the lungs with air

DIAPHYSIS – the shaft of a long bone such as the femur, bounded on the ends by the epiphyses

DIASTOLE – the phase of the cardiac cycle during which the atria fill with blood while the ventricles rest

DIFFUSION – the motion of molecules from a region of high concentration to one of low concentration

DISC PROLAPSE – *see* HERNIATION

DISLOCATION – the movement of a bone from its normal position

DISROTATORY – a spinal twist in which the ribcage and the pelvis are rotated in opposite senses

DISSOCIATION – an abnormal mental state in which it is felt that one is leaving the body

DISTAL – the furthest point from a given point

DORSAL – toward the back of the spine (posterior) in four-footed animals

DORSIFLEXION – the bending onto itself of the back body, as for example, the bending backward of the head at the neck

DOWAGER'S HUMP – *see* KYPHOSIS

ECCENTRIC ISOTONIC ACTION – the elongation of a muscle as it works isotonically to move a load

ECCRINE GLAND – a gland that releases its secretions into a duct; a sweat gland used for cooling the body

EDEMA – a swelling of the body tissue with excess fluid

EFFECTOR ORGAN – the target site for an efferent neuron

EFFERENT FIBER – nerve fiber that carries impulses away from the central nervous system to muscles, or from higher to lower centers in the central nervous system

ELASTIC – the mechanical behavior or property of a stressed material to return to its original dimensions when the stress is relieved

ELECTROCARDIOGRAM – a graph of the heart's electrical activity in time

ELECTROENCEPHALOGRAM (EEG) – a recording of the electrical activity of the cortex, usually through electrodes placed on the scalp

EMBOLISM – matter such as a blood clot (thrombus) that travels in the vascular system to eventually occlude (block) an artery; if within the brain, an embolism can cause a stroke

ENDOCRINE GLANDS – ductless organs which secrete hormones directly into the blood

ENDOGENOUS – originating or produced internally

ENDORPHINS – natural, morphine-like substances produced in the body

ENDOSTEUM – the inner lining of a hollow bone

ENDOTHELIUM – the cells forming the capillary wall, allowing the transfer of gases and nutrients across the wall

END PLATE – the plate-like ending of an efferent axon, forming the neuromuscular synaptic junction to a muscle fiber

ENTERIC NERVOUS SYSTEM – the totally independent nervous system within the gut

ENTRAINMENT – said of biorhythms that are synchronized with the 24-hour period of the rising and setting sun

ENZYME – a chemical which accelerates a chemical reaction without itself being consumed

EPIDERMIS – the outer layer of the three layers of the skin, consisting largely of dead cells

EPIPHYSES – the knobs on the ends of the long bones, separated by the bone shaft

EPITHELIUM – the innermost lining of hollow tubes in the body such as blood vessels, *etc.*

ERECTILE TISSUE – tissue that becomes engorged with blood when stimulated to do so

ERECTOR SPINAE – muscles paralleling the spine, used to keep the spine erect and in alignment

ESTROGEN – sex hormones responsible for maturation of the female genitalia

EXOGENOUS – originating or produced externally

EXTENSION – movement of the bones tending to open the joints; to extend a part of the body; backbending is a front-body extension

EXTRACELLULAR FLUID – any fluid which is not contained within the cells, but lies outside of them

EXTRAFUSAL MUSCLE FIBER – muscle fiber that is not part of the muscle spindle

FASCICULUS – a bundle of muscle fibers, usually with a common function

FAST-TWITCH MUSCLE FIBERS – muscles that are able to contract rapidly and with great force, but only for a short time, also known as Type-3 fibers

FEEDBACK – the return of sensory information to its source, resulting in a change of activity of the source

FIBRILS – small bundles of fibrous molecules

FIBROCARTILAGE – dense connective tissue found between the vertebrae and in joint capsules and related ligaments

FIGHT-OR-FLIGHT SYNDROME – the active response of the sympathetic nervous system to a perceived threat

FLEXION – movement of the bones tending to close the joints

FLEXOR – a muscle that bends the body by closing one or more joint angles

FORAMEN/FORAMINA – an opening between two larger vessels in the body

FORCED UNILATERAL BREATHING – breathing through one nostril only due to the forceful closing of the other by mechanical means

FOVEA – the spot on the retina having the highest resolution, and having only the color-sensitive cones as receptors

FREE NERVE ENDINGS – sensors found in the skin which are sensitive to tissue damage; they function as pain receptors when connected to nociceptive neurons

FRONTAL LOBE – the most forward lobe of each of the cerebral hemispheres

GAMMA-MOTOR NEURON – a motor neuron with cell body in the ventral horn of the spine and terminating at the intrafusal fibers of the muscle spindle; intimately involved with the tension in and stretching of the skeletal muscles

GANGLION – an aggregate of nerve-cell bodies, usually outside the central nervous system

GAP JUNCTION – a variety of fast-acting synapse, not using a neurotransmitter, but transmitting ionic current directly across the synaptic junction, as in the heart

GASTROINTESTINAL TRACT – the digestive tract from the mouth to the anus

GLAND – an organ specialized for secretion, usually of a hormone or of body waste

GLIA – cells within the nervous system which support the nerves mechanically and perform many housekeeping chores in the vicinity

GLUCAGON – a liver enzyme that promotes the conversion of glycogen to glucose

GLUCOSE – a simple sugar used by the body as a source of fuel for oxidation by oxygen, *etc.*

GLYCOGEN – a polymer of glucose

GOLGI TENDON ORGAN – a stretch-sensitive receptor in the muscle tendon

GRAY MATTER – slowly conducting, unmyelinated nerves in the nervous system

GROWTH HORMONE – a stimulant for the growth of the body prior to sexual maturation

HABITUATION – the process in which the response to an innocuous stimulus decreases the more it is experienced

HALLUX – referring to the big toe

HEAT-LOSS CENTERS – nuclei in the anterior hypothalamus that promote cooling of the body

HEMATOCRIT – the percentage of red blood cells in whole blood

HEMORRHAGE – heavy bleeding from a damaged blood vessel

HERNIATION – a rupture of the annulus of an intervertebral disc, allowing the nucleus pulposus to leak out; also known as disc prolapse

HERTZ – a measure of frequency, *i.e.*, the number of times an event occurs in a second. An EEG wave that rises and falls 23 times in a second has a frequency of 23 Hertz (Hz). 1 Hz = 1 cycle per second (cps)

HIP JOINT – the ball-and-socket joint formed by the juncture of the head of the femur and the acetabulum of the pelvis

HISTAMINE – a chemical released when tissue is injured; responsible for the pain sensation when its presence is sensed by the free nerve endings

HOMEOSTASIS – refers to the many processes through which the body maintains a state of internal equilibrium as reflected in, for instance, temperature, heart rate, blood pressure and the chemistry of tissues and body fluids

HORMONE – a chemical substance liberated by an endocrine gland, which then circulates throughout the body activating other organs

HYDROLYSIS – a chemical reaction involving the splitting of H_2O into H and OH radicals and the reactions of these radicals with a second, different molecule

HYDROXYAPATITE – the hard, mineral component of bone and teeth, containing calcium and phosphate

HYPERFLEXIBILITY – the ability to stretch into positions that are so far beyond proper alignment that they risk damage to the ligaments

HYPERPOLARIZED – a condition of a nerve fiber wherein its potential is above –65 millivolts and so is inhibited from conducting a neural current

HYPERTENSION – persistently high blood pressure, systolic and diastolic, usually taken as a reading above 140/90, systolic/diastolic

HYPERTROPHY – increasing in size, as of an exercised muscle

HYPERVENTILATION – breathing at a rate of more than 14 per minute, with the exhalation shorter than the inhalation

HYPOTENSION – persistently low blood pressure, usually taken as below 100/60, systolic/diastolic

HYPOTHALAMUS – a part of the diencephalon, beneath the thalamus; an important brain center for the autonomic nervous system

HYPOXIA – a state in which there is a deficiency of oxygen

IATROGENIC – pain or other medical problems arising as a result of medical treatment

IDA – the *nadi* originatig at the right side of the coccyx and terminating at the left nostril after crossing the *sushumna* several times

IDIOPATHIC – of unknown cause, seemingly appearing spontaneously as with an illness

IMMUNE SYSTEM – the system with which the body identifies foreign proteins and destroys them

IMMUNOTRANSMITTER – a molecule allowing communication between different parts of the immune system

INCUS – one of three bones of the middle ear, the "anvil"

INFARCT – a portion of tissue which is occluded by an embolism and is dying from this cause

INFERIOR VENA CAVA – the major vein returning blood to the heart from the legs and trunk

INHIBITION – a neural blockage of the response to a stimulus

INNERVATION – nerves serving tissue or organs; not all tissues or organs are innervated

INSULIN – an important hormone that converts glucose into glycogen and facilitates the transfer of glucose through the cell membrane

INTERNEURON – a type of neuron that always acts to hyperpolarize its synaptic neighbor, thereby halting neural conduction

INTEROSSEUS TISSUE – nonmuscular tissue binding two bones together

INTERVERTEBRAL DISCS – soft pads of tissue separating neighboring vertebrae

INTRAOCULAR – within the eyeball

ION – an electrically charged atom or molecule, called a "cation" if the charge is positive or "anion" if the charge is negative

ION CHANNEL – a pore within a membrane that allows certain ions to pass through it

IPSILATERAL – said of two structures on the same side of the body

IRIS – muscles surrounding the pupil of the eye, controlling its size

ISCHEMIA – a condition in which an area of the body is underserved by the vascular system, as in muscles rarely used, flesh under external pressure, *etc.*

ISOKINETIC – the action of a muscle against a resistive load, moving it at a constant velocity

ISOMERIZATION – a change of molecular geometry while retaining the molecular constitution. Ethyl alcohol and dimethyl ether have the same chemical formula, C_2H_6O, but different spatial geometries, and so are geometric isomers

ISOMETRIC – a static muscle contraction in which tension is generated in the muscle but there is no change in muscle length

ISOTONIC – the action of a muscle in moving a load having a constant resistance

KINESTHESIA – the sense of the positions of the body's parts and their rates of movement using muscle-tendon-joint sensors

KNOCK KNEES – legs in which the knees fall to the inside of the lines joining the hips to the ankles

KYPHOSIS – a condition of the spine in which the thoracic vertebrae are excessively rounded backward

LACRIMAL – referring to tears and the tear ducts

LACTATE ION/LACTIC ACID – chemicals produced by the muscles through their oxidation of glycogen

LATERAL – outward; to the side; opposite to medial

LATERAL FLEXION – bending to the side, as in *trikonasana*

LEFT BRAIN – the left cerebral hemisphere, responsible for excitation of the sympathetic nervous system

LIGAMENT – connective tissue that joins two bones to form a joint

LIMBIC SYSTEM – a group of nuclei within the brain responsible for emotions, *etc.*

LIPID BILAYER – the outer cell membrane formed by a double layer of end-to-end phospholipid molecules

LOAD/LOADING – the stress imposed on an object, as for example, the weight of the body stressing the bones of the legs when standing

LONG-TERM MEMORY – memory that is stable for a very long time, formed by consolidation of events stored first in short-term memory

LORDOSIS – a condition of the spine in which the lumbar vertebrae are excessively pressed forward

LOWER HINGE – the hip joints, as opposed to the upper hinge formed by the sacroiliac joints and the lumbar spine

LUMBAR – that part of the back body and sides, being between the lowest ribs and the top of the pelvis

LUMBAGO – lower-back pain, often attributed to a herniated intervertebral disc in the lumbar region

LUMEN – the empty spaces within the organs of the digestive tract

LYMPHOCYTE – a cell of the immune system having but one nucleus and residing mostly in the lymph; lymphocytes produce antibodies, fight tumors and respond to viral infections

LYMPHOKINE – an immunotransmitter in the immune system

MACROPHAGE – a large cell residing in tissue which attacks invading cells recognized as other than self

MALLEUS – the "hammer", one of the three bones of the middle ear

MANIA – periods of unusually elevated mood, interest and engagement, in contrast to depression

MASSETERS – the muscles connecting the lower jaw to the skull, used in mastication (chewing)

MASTER GLAND – the pituitary gland

MECHANORECEPTOR – a sensor within or upon the body which is sensitive to mechanical pressure

MEDIAL – referring to the inner aspect of the body, closer to the center line; the opposite of lateral

MEDULLA – the central part of an organ, surrounded by the cortex

MEISSNER'S CORPUSCLE – an encapsulated organ of the skin, sensitive to touch

MELATONIN – a hormone produced by the pineal gland, involved with the light/dark and sleep cycles

MEMBRANE – a thin structure composed mainly of lipid molecules surrounding each cell of the body

MEMBRANE POTENTIAL – the voltage appearing across a membrane due to the differing numbers of charged particles (ions) on its two sides

MENINGES – the three-layer covering of the brain and the spinal cord

METABOLISM – the sum of all energy-changing chemical processes that take place in an organism

METALLOPROTEIN – a protein containing one or more metal atoms in it as well; hemoglobin, containing four iron atoms per molecule, is a metalloprotein

MICROGLIAL – one of the prevalent cell types in the brain, used largely for housekeeping rather than signaling

MICRON – a metric unit of length, equal to one millionth of a meter, *i.e.*, 0.00004 inches, or one thousandth of a millimeter

MIDBRAIN – the brainstem between the pons and the thalamus

MIDDLE EAR – the chamber between the eardrum and the inner ear, containing the three bones, the malleus, the incus, and the stapes

MILLIMETER, MM – one thousandth part of a meter; 1 mm = 0.04 inches

MINERALIZATION – the process whereby soft organic tissue is reinforced by crystals of the mineral hydroxyapatite, turning the tissue to bone

MITOCHONDRION – an organelle within cells responsible for the generation of ATP for the cell's energy needs

MONOCYTES – cells that clean up debris after neutrophils do their work on invading bacteria

MOTIVATIONAL SYSTEM – a function within the limbic system that dictates the level of effort to be applied toward performing a certain task

MOTOR CORTEX – that part of the cortex containing the neural machinery that stimulates the skeletal muscles

MOTOR END PLATE – that part of an efferent neuron which synapses to a muscle fiber and energizes it

MOTOR UNIT – a motor nerve, its branches, and the assembly of contractive muscle fibers connected to it

MUSCLE MEMORY – the subconscious memory of how to use the muscles to perform a learned task, for example, how to work the legs in *dandasana*; also called reflexive memory

MUSCLE SPINDLE – a receptor structure within a muscle giving feedback information for adjusting and controlling the extent and speed of muscle elongation

MUSCULOSKELETAL – pertaining to the muscles and the skeleton

MYALGIA – pain in a muscle

MYOFIBRIL – a subunit of the muscle fiber

MYOGLOBIN – the oxygen-carrying metalloprotein serving slow-twitch muscle fibers

MYELIN – the fatty material surrounding certain nerves, making them rapid conductors of nerve impulses; myelin consists of a wrapping of Schwann cells

MYOFASCIA – the connective tissue surrounding muscles and binding the muscle fibers to one another

MYOSIN – one of the two proteins within muscle fibers responsible for its contractile properties

MYOTACTIC STRETCH REFLEX – the reflexive recoil of the body from a situation in which certain muscles are being overstretched or are in pain

NEGATIVE FEEDBACK – a biological process in which an effect is produced, but which effect acts to retard further production of the effect

NEURAL – relating to the nervous system

NEURAL CROSSOVER – the neural shift from left to right that accompanies the physical shift which occurs when a part of the right side of the body is placed on the left, and *vice versa*

NEURALGIA – a sharp pain usually associated with a pathology within the nerve itself

NEUROENDOCRINE – the chemical-electrical interaction between elements of the neural and hormonal subsystems

NEUROGENESIS – the formation and growth of nerves to replace those that have died

NEUROMUSCULAR JUNCTION – the synapse between the axon of a stimulating efferent neuron and the receptor site on the muscle fiber to be energized

NEURON – a nerve cell consisting of a bulbous cell body, trees of signal-detecting dendrites and a long axon extending from the cell body and carrying neural signals to other cells

NEUROPATHY – a malfunction or affliction of the nerve

NEUROPEPTIDE – a short peptide capable of acting as a neurotransmitter

NEUROTRANSMITTER – a molecule that carries neural information across the synaptic gap, from one neuron to the next

NEUTROPHIL – a white blood cell that forms the first line of defense against foreign substances, bacteria, *etc.*

NOCICEPTOR – a receptor especially sensitive to noxious stimuli, *i.e.*, those capable of producing tissue damage; the afferent neurons that carry pain signals to the brain

NOISE – random fluctuations of current/voltage within the neural circuitry, present even when there is no significant signal from the receptors

NONSTEROIDAL ANTIINFLAMMATORY DRUGS (NSAIDS) – aspirin-like agents (ibuprofen and indomethacin) which reduce swelling and reduce pain

NORADRENALINE – *see* NOREPINEPHRINE

NOREPINEPHRINE – a neurotransmitter hormone released by the adrenal medulla into the blood, acting in the sympathetic nervous system and in the brain

NUCLEUS PULPOSUS – the soft central component of the intervertebral disc

O_2 – the oxygen molecule

OCCIPITAL – at the back of the head

OCCIPUT – the base of the skull at the rear

OCCLUSION – a mobile clot in the blood stream, lodged in a too-small blood vessel; also a shrinking of the diameter of a vessel by outside pressure

OCULAR-VAGAL REFLEX – *see* VAGAL HEART-SLOWING REFLEX

ONTOGENY – a history of the development of an individual

OPTIC CHIASM – the point within the skull where the optic nerves from the inner (nasal) retinas cross left to right

OPTIC DISC – on the retina, the point of exit of the optic nerve, this being a blind spot with no visual receptors

ORGANELLES – the discrete organs within a cell such as the mitochondria, the nucleus, *etc.*

OTOLITH – a small stone of calcium carbonate within the balance sensors of the inner ear

OVERBALANCE – to fall backward when in an inverted balance posture

OXIDATION – the chemical reaction of a fuel such as glucose with oxygen to yield the energy necessary to sustain biological processes

OXIDATIVE PHOSPHORYLATION – the oxidation process whereby ADP is converted into ATP

OXYTOCIN – a hormone released by the posterior pituitary, which acts to contract smooth muscle, as in the uterus during childbirth

PAIN – a protective mechanism signaling the brain that there is something wrong in the body that requires attention

PALMAR CONDUCTANCE or RESISTANCE – the electrical conductance or resistance of the skin of the palm due to stress-induced sweating

PALPATE – to touch from outside the body

PALPITATIONS – usually of the heart; regular or irregular rapid beating of the heart

PARACRINE – cells that secrete hormones locally for use by adjacent cells only

PARALLEL PROCESSING – the ability to perform different mental tasks simultaneously, as in the right cerebral hemisphere

PARASYMPATHETIC NERVOUS SYSTEM – a major branch of the autonomic nervous system, responsible for the 'relaxation" response following the activation of the sympathetic nervous system; it stimulates vegetative functions using the cranial and sacral nerves

PATHOGEN – a virus, bacterium or parasite that invades the body and produces disease

PERIOSTEUM – the outer covering of bone, interwoven with the attached tendons and ligaments

PERIPHERAL NERVES – those bundles of nerve fibers that connect sensory or motor organs to the central nervous system; the cranial and spinal nerves and the peripheral ganglia lying outside the central nervous system

PERISTALSIS – a progressive muscular movement down the gastrointestinal tract, designed to move its contents in the mouth-to-anus direction

PERMEABILITY – the ability of a membrane to allow certain chemicals to pass through it

PHASIC REFLEX – an instantaneous and short-lived muscular response to a stimulus, as when stepping on a sharp object in bare feet

PHOSPHOLIPID – a highly polar molecule based upon a glycerol backbone, fatty sidechains and a charged phosphate group; cell membranes are formed by a double layer of phospholipid molecules

PHYLOGENY – a history of the development of a species

PIEZOELECTRIC EFFECT – appears when certain materials are stressed and develop a very intense electric field on their surfaces; bone is piezoelectric material

PILOMOTOR RESPONSE – the lifting of a hair by excitation of smooth muscles at its base

PHYSICAL CROSSOVER – to displace a body part from the right-hand side of the body to the left and *vice versa*, as in *pari-vrtta trikonasana*, for example

PINGALA – the *nadi* originating at the left side of the coccyx and terminating at the right nostril after crossing the *sushumna* several times

PITUITARY – the master gland, located just below the hypothalamus, that directs many other hormonal processes, the forward portion of which is itself under the neural control of the hypothalamus; also known as the hypophysis

PHOSPHORYLATION – a chemical reaction in which a phosphate group, PO_4, is joined to another chemical group, often a protein

PLACEBO – a Latin word meaning "I will please"; often an inert pill or solution of salt or sugar given in place of an analgesic agent

PLASMA – the fluid portion of blood when freed of suspended cells

PLATELET – a disc-like cellular component of blood that is responsible for clot formation at the site of vascular damage

POLYMER – a very large organic molecule formed by the joining together of many smaller molecules either all of the same kind, or of related types. Example, collagen is a polymer of the amino acids glycine and proline and cellulose is a polymer of glucose molecules

POLYMODAL – said of nerve endings that are sensitive to more than one type of stimulus, *i.e.*, temperature, pressure, pain, *etc.*

POSTERIOR HYPOTHALAMUS – the rear part of the hypothalamus, controlling the excitation of the sympathetic nervous system

POSITIVE FEEDBACK – a biological process in which a compound is formed and its formation promotes further production

POSTGANGLIONIC NEURON – a part of the autonomic nervous system, originating in the outlying ganglia and terminating at effector organs

POSTURAL MUSCLES – those muscles having an ongoing muscle tone of a relatively low level, but which hold the body in an upright posture for long periods of time

PROLAPSE – to fall out of place, as of an organ, *etc.*

PROPHYLAXIS – steps taken to prevent a disease or harmful condition

PROPRIOCEPTION – a subconscious sense of where the various body parts are in space, and in what direction and how fast they are moving; the sensors reside in the muscles, tendons, joints, and the vestibular organs

PROTEIN – large networks of amino acids joined to one another

PREGANGLIONIC NEURON – a part of the autonomic nervous system originating in the central nervous system and terminating in an outlying ganglion

PROGESTERONE – a hormone produced by the ovaries, and significant in both menstruation and pregnancy

PROSTAGLANDINS – cellular compounds that are released when cells are injured, causing swelling and inflammation

POWER STROKE – that phase in the cardiac cycle where the left ventricle contracts in order to pump oxygenated blood through the aorta

PULMONARY CIRCULATION – the movement of blood from the heart to the lungs and the return of the blood to the heart

PYROGEN – a substance in the body which promotes a high fever

RADIATING PAIN – pain sensations which move away from the spine toward the extremities with time

RATE OF CHANGE OF LENGTH – how rapidly a muscle's length is changing on being stretched or contracted

REBOUND HEADACHE – the headache which may follow once a particular treatment modality for headache is withheld

RECEPTOR – a cell specialized for sensitivity to a particular physiologic variable

RECEPTIVE FIELD – a group of sensor cells in the retina which work together to detect a particular geometric or kinetic aspect within the visual field, such as a horizontal straight line, or a slanted line moving from left to right, *etc.*

RECRUITMENT – the employment of specific motor units, depending upon the task to be performed

REFRACTORY PERIOD – the brief period during a neural impulse during which no second impulse is possible

RELAXATION – not contracted, a state of restful alertness; the aspect of alertness differentiates relaxation from sleep

REFLEX – the simple, innate response of a system to a particular stimulus

REFLEX ARC – the direct link between the receptor and the effector organ via the central nervous system

REM SLEEP – a phase of sleep characterized by rapid eye movement, dreaming, muscular paralysis and a desynchronized EEG. Occurs about every 90 minutes during a night's sleep

RENIN – an enzyme released by the kidney in times of low blood volume, which acts ultimately to restrict urination

RESPIRATORY SINUS ARHYTHMIA (RSA) – the difference between the heart rate when inhaling and exhaling

RESTING MUSCLE TONE – the degree of muscle contraction (tonus) when in a restful state

RETICULAR ACTIVATING SYSTEM – *see* RETICULAR FORMATION

RETICULAR FORMATION – the center in the brainstem from the lower medulla to the diencephalon, involved with arousal, alertness, and modulation of neural traffic ascending and descending the central nervous system

RETINA – the light-sensitive cells and the associated neural networks at the back of the eyeball

RIGHT BRAIN – the right cerebral hemisphere, promoting excitation of the parasympathetic nervous system

RIGHT VAGUS NERVE – the right branch of the vagus nerve (cranial nerve X), extending from the hypothalamus to the lower regions of the digestive system

RODS – the light receptor cells in the retina functioning only in dim light, and without color sensitivity

SACCULE – a vestibular receptor in the inner ear, for sensing lateral head tilt

SACRAL – referring to the fused vertebrae (the sacrum) at the base of the spine

SACROILIAC JOINT – the joint at the base of the spine joining the sacrum of the spine and the ilium of the pelvis

SARCOLEMMA – the connective-tissue sheath surrounding a bundle of myofibrils within a muscle

SARCOMERE – the bundle of interleaved myosin and actin myofibrils between adjacent Z lines in a myofibril. When the muscle contracts, the actin fibers are pulled along the myosin fibers and the Z lines move toward one another

SCAPULA – a shoulder blade

SCHWANN CELL – a fatty cell which is wrapped about an axon, thereby myelinating it and significantly increasing its conduction velocity

SCIATICA – discomfort in the buttocks and legs arising from impingement on the sciatic nerve

SCOLIOSIS – a deviation of the spine in the lateral direction

SEMICIRCULAR CANAL – one of three perpendicular semicircular organs within the inner ear sensing the rate, sense, and axial direction of head rotation

SENSITIZATION – an increasing sensitivity to pleasurable sensations with time

SENSORIMOTOR INTEGRATION – the interaction of the sensory and motor systems of the body to accomplish a specific task

SEROTONIN – a pituitary hormone and neurotransmitter found throughout the body, implicated in depression, and having other functions in the body as well

SETPOINTS – the upper and lower limits of a physiological variable (temperature, pH, *etc.*) between which a regulatory mechanism operates; the body adjusts automatically so as to keep the variable at a value between the setpoints

SHORT-TERM MEMORY – the storage area for briefly storing memories before they are either erased or moved to long-term memory

SINUS NODE, SN – heart muscle fibers within the atria of the heart, triggering their contraction

SKELETAL MUSCLE – striated muscles used to open and close joints

SKIN TENSION – the tension detected by sensors in the skin due to tension in the muscles underlying the skin

SLOW-TWITCH FIBERS – type-1 muscle fibers that contract relatively slowly, but which are capable of contraction for a long time

SLOW-WAVE SLEEP – stages of deep sleep in which the EEG displays synchronous waves of low frequency

SMOOTH MUSCLES – not striated muscles, usually under autonomic control as those within the intestines, blood vessels, *etc.*

SOMATIC – referring to the muscles of the body

SPASM – an involuntary muscle contraction

SPHINCTER – a ring of smooth muscle that opens or closes an orifice of the body

SPINAL APPENDAGES – primarily the skull and pelvis, but indirectly the arms and legs as well

SPINAL FLEXION – forward bending

SPINAL ROOT – a spinal nerve bundle consisting of afferent fibers from the dorsal spine and efferent fibers from the ventral spine

SPINAL STENOSIS – a narrowing of the spinal canal, possibly placing pressure on the spinal cord

SPINOUS PROCESS – the posterior aspect of each of the spinal vertebrae, forming the chain of bumps that can be felt as the spinal column from the outside

SPONTANEOUS POLARIZATION – the spontaneous development of an action potential in a muscle cell leading to contraction without any initial stimulation by an efferent nerve, as with cardiac muscle

SPRAIN – a sudden or violent twist or wrench of a joint which injures the ligaments at that joint

STAPES – one of the bones of the middle ear, shaped somewhat like a stirrup

STEM CELLS – the basic cells that give rise to each of the types of tissue, such as brain, lung, muscle, *etc.*

STERNAL NOTCH – the depression at the point where the clavicles meet the manubrium in the front upper thorax

STRAIN – a muscle or its tendon injured or weakened by maximal extension, most often by overuse, misuse or excessive pressure. Also, the fractional change in length of a substance following an applied stress

STRESS – mechanical or emotional pressure applied to the body/mind

STRESS FRACTURE – a microfracture of bone that grows into a full-blown fracture due to on-going applied stress

STRESSOR – an emotional or physical factor that leads to emotional or physical stress in the body

STROKE VOLUME – the volume of blood pumped by one cycle of the heart beat

SUBCORTICAL – referring to centers in the brain at a level lower than that of the cortex, *i.e.*, the thalamus, for example

SUBLUXATION – a momentary decrease in the normal area of contact between bones in a synovial joint

SUPERIOR VENA CAVA – the large vein draining blood from the head, arms and chest into the right atrium of the heart

SUPRACHIASMATIC NUCLEUS – a nucleus within the brain resting just above the optic chiasm, and responsible for many of the body's circadian rhythms

SUPRASPINAL – involving brain centers higher than those in the spinal cord, and more likely to add a conscious component to the spinal reflex mode

SYMPATHETIC NERVOUS SYSTEM – a major branch of the autonomic nervous system, responsible for the "fight-or-flight" response to a threatening situation

SYNAPSE – the very narrow space between the ends of adjacent neurons, this being the relay junction between them

SYNCHRONICITY – brainwaves of a particular frequency in the EEG that reach their peak voltages at the same time in different areas of the scalp

SYNERGIST MUSCLE – a muscle that participates in a muscular action, but only in a supporting role

SYSTOLE – the period of the heart action during which the ventricles contract and blood pressure rises

T CELLS – as part of the immune system, T cells identify foreign cells in the body and attack and destroy them

TEMPORAL ANTIPOD – the halfway point in a biorhythm cycle, which is the time of minimum activity of the function

TENSILE STRESS – the mechanical stress imposed on an object when the ends are pulled away from one another, as when stretching a muscle, bone, or nerve

TESTOSTERONE – the most important sexual hormone (androgen) found in men

THERMOREGULATION – the process whereby an organ or body controls its temperature over a narrow range

THORACIC – pertaining to the chest

THROMBUS – a blood clot formed within a blood vessel

TONIC REFLEX – a muscular reflex of low intensity and long duration, as with the resting muscle tone

TRACT – a bundle of nerves all beginning and ending at common points

TRACTION – putting a bone or muscle under tensile stress in order to lengthen, immobilize or align it

TRANSDUCTION – the conversion of a sensory stimulus (light, pressure, *etc.*) into an electrical signal in the associated afferent neuron

TRIGLYCERIDE – a compound formed by the union of one molecule of glycerol with three molecules of a fatty acid

TRIPARTITE BRAIN – the division of the brain into the forebrain, the midbrain and the hindbrain, the latter being the oldest and most primitive part

TUMOR – a benign or malignant abnormal tissue growth

ULTRADIAN – biorhythms with periods shorter than 24 hours, as for example, the heart beat

UNDERBALANCE – to fall forward when in an inverted balance posture

UNILATERAL BREATHING – breathing through one nostril only for a prolonged time, either naturally or forced by mechanical closure of the opposite nostril

UNIPOLAR DEPRESSION – periods of depression that do not alternate with periods of mania

UPPER HINGE – bending of the body in the area of the sacroiliac joint and the lumbar vertebrae, as distinct from bending at the lower hinge

UTRICLE – a vestibular organ for sensing forward/backward tilt of the head

$\dot{V}O_2$ – the rate of consumption of oxygen while working at a constant rate

$\dot{V}O_{2max}$ – the maximum rate of oxygen consumption while working at the maximum rate

VAGAL – referring to the vagus nerve (cranial nerve X), and responsible for much of the parasympathetic control of the heart, stomach, and intestines

VAGAL HEART-SLOWING REFLEX – the reflexive slowing of the heart rate when the orbits of the eyes are pressed

VALSALVA MANEUVER – squeezing the abdominal muscles while holding the breath, allowing one to generate momentary strength in the thorax

VARICOSITY – a swelling of a vessel or organ

VASCULAR HEADACHE – a headache brought on by tension in the smooth muscles of the vascular system in the brain

VASOCONSTRICTORS – the nerves or substances that cause blood vessels to narrow, causing a slowing of the blood flow

VASODILATORS – nerves or substances that cause blood vessels to widen, causing an accelerated blood flow

VENTRAL – referring to the front side of the body

VENTRICLES – the lower chambers of the heart that pump blood through the arteries of the body; also empty spaces within the brain, filled with cerebrospinal fluid

VENTRICULAR NODE (VN) – the point within the ventricles of the heart at which ventricular excitation and contraction originate

VENULE – a small vein, lying in size between the capillaries and the veins

VERTEBRAE – the 23 or so block-like bones that form the spinal column, found in the cervical, thoracic, lumbar, sacral and coccygeal regions

VERTEBRAL ARTERIES – arteries that are threaded through foramina in the cervical vertebrae and serve the rear portion of the brain

VERTEBRAL WEDGING – having wedge-shaped vertebrae and/or discs, leading to an excessive curvature of the spine

VERTIGO – dizziness and nausea caused by head motions that confuse the vestibular apparatus

VESICLE – a small vessel filled with a particular compound or mixture which can release its contents into the body fluids by rupturing the vessel's walls; prominent in neural transmission across the synaptic cleft

VESTIBULAR APPARATUS – organs within the inner ear, responsible for many aspects of balance and equilibrium, sensing the orientation in the gravitational field and rates of angular motion

VISCERA – the internal organs of the abdomen

VISCOELASTIC – a solid such as muscle, showing both viscous and elastic mechanical properties; when stressed briefly it appears to be elastic, but when stressed for an extended time, it appears to be viscous

VISCOUS – a very thick fluid or solid which moves only slowly when stressed mechanically and does not return to its original shape when the stress is removed

VISUAL CROSSOVER – the crossing over of a branch of the optic nerve of an eye on one side of the head to the cerebral hemisphere on the other side, the crossing occurring at the optic chiasm

VITREOUS HUMOUR – the viscous fluid filling the chamber between the lens and retina of the eye

WATER BALANCE – control of the salt concentrations in the body by intake and voiding of water

WHITE MATTER – the rapidly conducting nerves of the nervous system which are myelinated, *i.e.*, covered by Schwann cells

Z LINES – the two zones at the ends of a sarcomere that are pulled toward one another when the muscle fiber contracts

REFERENCES

[1] B. S. Aaronson, "Color Perception and Affect," *Am. J. Clin. Hypn.* **14**, 38 (1971).

[2] I. Abraham, "Prolotherapy for Chronic Headache," *Headache* **37**, 256 (1997).

[3] C. Ainsworth, "Left, Right and Wrong," *New Scient.*, Jun 17, 2000, p. 40.

[4] R. McN. Alexander, *Bones: The Unity of Form and Function*, MacMillan, NY, 1994.

[5] M. J. Alter, *Science of Flexibility*, 2nd Ed., Human Kinetics, Champaign, IL, 1996.

[6] J. L. Andersen, P. Schjerling, and B. Saltin, "Muscles, Genes and Athletic Performance," *Sci. Am.,* Sep 2000, p. 48.

[7] S. Anderson, "The Supple Spine," *Yoga Intern.*, Jul/Aug 1994, p. 14.

[8] S. Anderson, "A Play of Opposites," *Yoga Intern.*, Jun/Jul 2000, p. 17.

[9] C. Angus, "Don't Let Osteoarthritis Get the Best of You," *Yoga Intern.*, Feb/Mar 1998.

[10] Anon., "The 1998 Nobel Prizes in Science," *Sci. Am.*, Jan 1999, p. 16.

[11] Anon., "Making Waves," *Discover*, Oct 1998, p. 24.

[12] Anon., *Sci. Am.*, Jun 1999, p. 10.

[13] Anon., "Pricking for Endorphins," *Sci. Am.*, Aug 1999.

[14] Anon., "Birds Do It, Bees Do It," *The Economist*, US Ed., Aug 30, 1997, p. 59.

[15] Anon., "Healthy Serenades," *New Scient.*, Feb 5, 2000, p. 25.

[16] Anon., "Exercise May Toughen Immune System," *Yoga J.*, May/Jun 1990, p. 14.

[17] Anon., "Housecalls," *Health*, Jul/Aug 1998, p.128.

[18] Anon., "Why Does Time Seem to Speed Up as I Get Older?" *Health*, Jul/Aug 1998, p. 128.

[19] Anon., "The Rhythm of Mind," *Discover*, Jan 2000, p. 24.

[20] Anon., "Neural Ties That Bind Perception..." *Sci. News* **155**, 122 (1999).

[21] S. Atmarupananda, "What Can We Expect from a Life of Vedanta?" *Yoga Intern.*, Jun/Jul 1999, p. 24.

[22] K. Baier, "What Is an Asana?" *Yoga Rahasya* **2**, 89 (1995).

[23] B. Balasubramanian and M. S. Pansare, "Effect of Yoga on Aerobic and Anerobic Power of Muscles," *Ind. J. Physiol. Pharmacol.* **35**, 28 (1991).

[24] R. Ballentine, "Clinical Significance of the Nasal Cycle," *Res. Bull. Him. Intern. Inst.* **2**, 9 (1980).

[25] R. Ballentine, "Breathing: The Chest Cavity, Part I," *Res. Bull. Him. Intern. Inst.* **2**, 8 (1980).

[26] R. M. Ballentine, Jr., "Nasal Functioning," *Res. Bull. Him. Intern. Inst.* Winter, 1980, p. 11.

[27] C. Bass and W. Gardner, "Emotional Influences on Breathing and Breathlessness," *J. Psychosom. Res.* **29**, 599 (1985).

[28] W. H. Bates, *The Bates Method for Better Eyesight Without Glasses*, Holt, Rinehart and Winston, NY, 1968.

[29] T. Baumgart, "Brain Rejuvenation," *Yoga J.*, Nov/Dec 1998, p. 20.

[30] T. Beardsley, "Truth or Consequences," *Sci. Am.*, Oct 1999, p. 21.

[31] K. Behanan, *Yoga, A Scientific Evaluation*, Dover, NY, 1937.

[31a] M. Bekoff, "Beastly Passions," *New Scient.*, Apr 29, 2000, p. 32.

[32] T. Belay, "Stress Express," *New Scient.*, May 27, 2000, p. 21.

[33] J. C. I. Belmonte, "How the Body Tells Left from Right," *Sci. Am.*, Jun 1999, p. 46.

[34] B. E. Benjamin, *Listen to Your Pain*, Penguin, NY, 1984.

[35] D. Bennett, "Don't Tickle My Funny Bone," *Muscles and Fitness*, May 1998, p. 212.

[36] H. Benson, *The Relaxation Response*, Morrow, NY, 1976.

[37] T. K. Bera, M. M. Gore, and J. P. Oak, "Recovery from Stress in Two Different Postures and in Savasana—A Yogic Relaxation Posture," *Indian J. Physiol. Pharmacol.* **42**, 473 (1998).

[38] M. Berg and M. Basta Boubion, "Zapping Postexercise Pain," *Muscle and Fitness*, May 2000, p. 106.

[39] G. B. Beringer and G. S. Golden, "Beauty Parlor Stroke: When a Beautician Becomes a Physician," *J. Am. Med. Assoc.* **270**, 1198 (1993).

[39a] M. J. Berridge, "The Molecular Basis of Communication within the Cell," *Sci. Am.*, Oct 1985, p. 142.

[40] O. P. Bhatnagar, A. K. Ganguly, and V. Anantharaman, "Influence of Yoga Training on Thermoregulation," *Ind. J. Med. Res.* **67**, 844 (1978).

[41] R. B. Blackwelder, *Alternative Medicine*, Monograph, Edition 219, Home Study Self-Assessment Program. Kansas City, MO, *Amer. Acad. Fam. Phys.*, Aug 1997.

[42] E. B. Blanchard and L. D. Young, "Self-Control of Cardiac Functioning: A Promise As Yet Unfulfilled," *Psychol. Bull.* **79**, 145 (1973).

[43] D. Bodanis, *The Body Book*, Little Brown, Boston, MA, 1984.

[44] S. Bonnick, *The Osteoporosis Handbook*, Taylor, Dallas, TX, 1994.

[45] C. Bowe, "Body Briefing: The Endocrine Glands," *Lear's Mag.*, Jan/Feb 1989, p. 69.

[46] B. Bower, "Slumber's Unexpected Landscape," *Sci. News* **156**, 205 (1999).

[47] B. Bower, "Schizophrenia May Involve Bad Timing," *Sci. News* **156**, 309 (1999).

[47a] B. Bower, "Pushing the Mood Swings," *Sci. News* **157**, 232 (2000).

[48] A. J. Bowman, R. H. Clayton, A. Murray, J. W. Reed, M. M. Subhan and G. A. Ford, "Effects of Aerobic Exercise Training and Yoga on the Baroreflex in Healthy Elderly Persons," *Eur. J. Clin. Invest.* **27**, 443 (1997).

[49] G. Brainard, V. Pratap, C. Reed, B. Levitt, and J. Hanifin, "Plasma Cortisol Reduction in Healthy Volunteers Following a Single Session of Yoga Practice," *Yoga Res. Soc. Newslet.*, Philadelphia, PA., Apr/Sep 1997, p. 1.

[50] D. R. Brebbia and K. Z. Altshuler, "Oxygen Consumption Rate and Electro-encephalographic Stage of Sleep," *Science* **150**, 1621 (1965).

[51] W. F. Brechue and M, D. Beekley, "What Does the Body/Muscle Remember?" *Women's Health Digest* **2**, 221 (1996).

[52] G. Broden, A. Dolk, C. Frostell, B. Nilsson, and B Holmstrom, "Voluntary Relaxation of the External Anal Sphincter," *Dis. Colon Rectum* **32**, 376 (1989).

[53] B. B. Brown, *New Mind, New Body*, Harper and Row, NY, 1974.

[54] B. Calais-Germain, *Anatomy of Movement*, Eastland Press, Seattle, WA, 1993.

[55] M. Caldwell, "Mind Over Time," *Discover*, Jul 1999, p. 52.

[56] D. Campbell, "The Mozart Effect and More," *New Visions*, Sep 1998, p. 6.

[57] N. R. Carlson, *Physiology of Behavior*, 3rd Ed., Allyn and Bacon, Boston, MA, 1986.

[58] B. L. Carter, "Optimizing Delivery Systems to Tailor Pharmacotherapy to Cardiovascular Circadian Events," *Am. J. Health Syst. Pharm.* **55**, S17 (1998).

[59] R. Carter, "Tune In, Turn Off," *New Scient.*, Oct 1999, p. 30.

[60] C. Cavanaugh, "Urdhva Mukha Svanasana," *Yoga J.*, May/Jun 1991, p. 34.

[61] E. Chaney, *The Eyes Have It*, S. Weiser, York Beach, ME, 1987.

[62] C. S. Chen, M. Mrksich, S. Huang, G. M. Whitesides and D. E. Ingber, "Geometric Control of Cell Life and Death," *Science* **276**, 1425 (1997).

[63] I. S. Chohan, H. S. Nayar, P. Thomas and N. S. Geetha, "Influence of Yoga on Blood Coagulation," *Thromb. Haemostas.* **51**, 196 (1984).

[64] J. Chusid, "Yoga Foot Drop," *J. Am. Med. Assoc.* **217**, 827 (1971).

[65] J. Clarke, "Resting Breath Pattern," *Res. Bull. Him. Intern. Inst.* **3**, 15 (1981).

[66] J. Clarke, "The Nasal Cycle, Part II," *Res. Bull. Him. Intern. Inst.* **2**, 3 (1980).

[67] J. Clarke, "Respiration, Heart Rate, and the Autonomic Nervous System," *Res. Bull. Him. Intern. Inst.* **3**, 4 (1981).

[68] J. Clarke, "Slowing Down: The Practice of 2-to-1 Breathing," *Yoga Intern.*, Nov/Dec 1994, p. 56.

[69] J. Clarke, "Asana and Aerobics," *Yoga Intern.*, Jan/Feb 1994, p. 31.

[70] J. Clarke, "The Nasal Cycle. Ancient and Modern Studies of Body-Mind Balancing," *Yoga Intern.* Reprint Series, 1995, p. 13.

[71] J. Clayton, "Caught Napping," *New Scient.*, Feb 26, 2000, p. 43.

[71a] B. Clennel, "A Woman's Yoga Practice," *Iyengar Yoga Assoc. Greater New York Newslett.*, Summer/Fall, 1999, p. 7.

[72] A. Coghlan, "Beg, Steal or Borrow," *New Scient.*, May 20, 2000, p. 17.

[73] H. D. Cohen, R. C. Rosen, and L. Goldstein, "Electroencephalographic Laterality Changes During Human Sexual Orgasm," *Archiv. Sex. Behav.* **5**, 189 (1976).

[74] J. Cohen, D. H. Char, and D. Norman, "Bilateral Orbital Varices Associated with Habitual Bending," *Arch. Ophthalom.* **113**, 1360 (1995).

[75] P. Cohen, "Forget Me Not," *New Scient.*, Jul 1, 2000, p. 12.

[76] K. H. Coker, "Meditation and Prostate Cancer: Integrating a Mind/Body Intervention with Traditional Therapies," *Seminars on Urologic Oncology* **17**, 111 (1999).

[77] R. Cole, "Physiology of Yoga" in *Newsletter, B. K. S. Iyengar Yoga Institute of Southern Africa,* Dec 1988, p. 26.

[78] R. Cole, "Science Studies Yoga," as reported by A. Cushman in, *Yoga J.*, Jul/Aug 1994, p. 43.

[79] R. J. Cole, "Postural Baroreflex Stimuli May Affect EEG Arousal and Sleep in Humans," *J. Appl. Physiol.* **67**, 2369 (1989).

[80] R. Cole, "Relaxation Physiology and Practice," unpublished notes, 1994.

[81] R. Cole, personal communication, 1999–2000.

[82] R. M. Coleman, *Wide Awake at 3:00 A. M. By Choice or by Chance?* Freeman, NY, 1986.

[83] C. Collins, "Yoga: Intuition, Preventative Medicine, and Treatment," *J. Obstet. Gyn. Neonatal Nursing* **27**, 563 (1998).

[84] B. Cook, "Controlling Diabetes," *Yoga Intern.*, Feb/Mar 1998, p. 51.

[85] R. Coontz, "The Planet That Hums," *New Scient.*, Sep 1999, p. 30.

[86] R. S. Cooper, C. N. Rotimi, and R. Ward, "The Puzzle of Hypertension in African-Americans," *Sci. Am.*, Feb 1999, p. 56.

[86a] P. Copeland, "Yoga and the Endocrine System," *Yoga J.*, Jul/Aug 1975, p. 9

[87] P. Copeland, "Pranayama and Physiology," *Yoga J.*, Nov/Dec 1975, p. 9.

[88] P. Copeland, "Yoga, Mind and Muscle," *Yoga J.*, Mar/Apr, 1976, p. 27.

[89] P. Copeland, "Yoga, the Heart and the Breath," *Yoga J.*, May 1975, p. 6.

[90] S. Coren, *The Left-Hander Syndrome,* Free Press, NY, 1992.

[90a] W. L. Cornelius and K Craft-Hamm, "Proprioceptive Neuromuscular Facilitation Flexibility Techniques: Acute Effects on Arterial Blood Pressure," *Physician Sports Med.* **16**, 152 (1988).

[91] G. E. Corrigan, "Fatal Air Embolism after Yoga Breathing Exercises," *J. Am. Med. Assoc.* **210**, 1923 (1969).

[92] M. V. Corrigan, C. V. Tyler, Jr., *Common Problems in Elderly Persons*, Monograph Ed. No. 223, Home Study Self-Assessment Program, Am. Acad. Fam. Physicians, Kansas City, MO., Dec 1997.

[93] J. Couch, "How to Teach Yoga in Industry," *Yoga J.*, Jul/Aug 1981, p. 27.

[94] J. Couch, "In Defense of Stretching," *Yoga J.*, Jul/Aug 1983, p. 11.

[95] D. Coulter, "Self-Preservation," *Yoga Intern.*, Nov/Dec 1994, p. 67.

[96] D. Coulter, "Moving Gracefully: The Role of the Knee-Jerk Reflex," *Yoga Intern.*, Jul/Aug 1994, p. 55.

[97] D. Coulter, "For Clarity of Mind; the Diaphragmatic Breath," *Yoga Intern.* Reprint Series, 1999, p. 9.

[98] J. E. Councilman, *The Science of Swimming*, Prentice Hall, Englewood Cliffs, NJ, 1968.

[99] G. Couzens, "PMS Workout," *Self*, Oct 1991, p. 150.

[100] G. Cowley, "How to Live to 100," *Newsweek*, Jun 30, 1997, p. 54.

[101] A. McQ. Crawford, "Hormones Demystified," *Yoga J.*, May/Jun 1997, p. 34.

[102] E. Criswell, *How Yoga Works: An Introduction to Somatic Yoga*, Freeperson Press, Novato, CA, 1987.

[103] T. Dajer, "Deadly Knee Bends," *Discover*, May 1999, p. 38.

[104] A. S. Dalal and T. X. Barber, "Yoga, Yogic Feats, and Hypnosis in the Light of

Empirical Research," *Am. J. Clin. Hypn.* **11**, 155 (1969).

[105] A. R. Damasio, "How the Brain Creates the Mind," *Sci. Am.*, Dec 1999, p. 112.

[106] R. C. Darling, "Physiology of Exercise and Fatigue," in, *Therapeutic Exercise*, S. Licht, Ed., Waverly Press, Baltimore, MD, 1958, p. 21.

[107] J. P. Das, "Yoga and Hypnosis," *Intern. J. Clin. Hypn.* **11**, 31 (1963).

[108] K. K. Datey, S. N. Deshmukh, C. P. Dalvi, and S. L. Vinekar, "Shavasan: A Yogic Exercise in the Management of Hypertension," *Angiology* **20**, 395 (1969).

[109] H. Davson, *A Textbook of General Physiology*, Little, Brown, Boston, MA, 1959.

[110] D. C. Dennett, *Consciousness Explained*, Little, Brown, Boston, MA, 1991.

[111] T. K. V. Desikachar, *The Heart of Yoga*, Inner Traditions Intern., Rochester, VT, 1995.

[112] J.-M. Derrick, "A Routine for Menopause," *Iyengar Yoga Assoc. Greater N.Y. Newslet.*, Summer/Fall, 1999, p. 4.

[113] G. Devereux, "Hatha Yoga and the Five Energies of Nature," *Yoga Intern.*, Aug/Sep 1999, p. 30.

[114] R. A. Deyo, "Low Back Pain," *Sci. Am.*, Aug 1998, p. 48.

[115] J. Diamond, "Dining with the Snakes," *Discover* **15**, 48 (1994).

[116] M. C. Diamond, A. B. Scheibel and L. M. Elson, "*The Human Brain Coloring Book*," Harper Perennial, NY, 1985.

[117] S. Diamond, *Hope For Your Headache Problem*, Second Ed., Intern. Univ. Press, Madison, CT, 1988.

[118] S. Diamond, *The Hormone Headache*, Macmillan, NY, 1995.

[119] L. J. DiCarlo, P. B. Sparling, B. T. Hinson, T. K. Snow, and L. B. Rosskopf, "Cardiovascular, Metabolic, and Perceptual Responses to Hatha Yoga Standing Poses," *Med. Exerc. Nutr. Health* **4**, 107 (1995).

[120] S. Dimond, *Introducing Neuropsychology*, C. S. Thomas, Springfield, IL, 1978.

[121] J. E. Dodes and M. J. Schissel, "Letter to The Editor," *Discover*, Oct 1999, p. 16.

[122] R. H. Dominguez and R. Cajda, *Total Body Training*, Scribner's, NY, 1982.

[123] R. Donelson, G. Silva and K. Murphy, "Centralization Phenomenon: Its Usefulness in Evaluating and Treating Referred Pain," *Spine* **15**, 211 (1990).

[124] P. G. Donohue, "Ear-Muscle Contraction Renders Clicking Noise," *Star Ledger*, Oct 2, 1998, p. 70.

[125] J. Douillard, *Body, Mind and Sport*, Harmony, NY, 1994.

[126] C. P. Dunavan, "Blindsided by Tetanus," *Discover*, Jan 2000, p. 39.

[127] S. Dunn, "How Yoga Saved My Life," *Yoga J.*, August, 2000, p. 78.

[128] R. Eccles, "The Central Rhythm of the Nasal Cycle," *Acta Otolaryngol.* **86**, 464 (1978).

[129] D. L. Eckberg, F. M. Abboud, and A. L. Mark, "Modulation of Carotid Baroreflex Responsiveness in Man: Effects of Posture and Propranolol," *J. Appl. Physiol.* **41**, 383 (1976).

[130] M. Eliade, *Yoga, Immortality and Freedom*, Princeton Univ. Press, Princeton, NJ, 1969.

[131] E. V. Evarts, "Brain Mechanisms of Movement," *Sci. Am.*, Sep 1979, p. 164.

[132] W. J. Faber and M. Walker, *Pain, Pain, Go Away*, Ishi Press, Mountain View, CA, 1990.

[133] J. A. Fahmy and H. Fledelius, "Yoga-Induced Attacks of Acute Glaucoma," *Acta Ophthalom.* **51**, 80 (1973).

[134] D. Farhi, "Asana: Handstand," *Yoga J.*, Jan/Feb 1993, p. 35.

[135] D. Farhi, "Holding Your Breath," *Yoga J.*, Mar/April, 1996, p. 75.

[136] D. Farhi, "Padmasana," *Yoga J.*, Nov/Dec 1999, p. 84.

[137] D. Farhi, "Karnapidasana: Pain in the Ear Pose," *Yoga J.*, Nov/Dec 1993, p. 40.

[138] A. Feinstein, *Training the Body to Cure Itself*, Rodale, Emmaus, PA, 1992.

[139] L. Fitzgerald and R. Monro, "Follow-up Survey on Yoga and Diabetes," *Yoga Biomed. Bull.* **1**, 61 (1986).

[140] K. Y. Fong, R. T. Cheung, Y. L. Yu, C. W. Tai and C. M. Chang, "Basilar Artery Occlusion Following Yoga Exercise: A Case Report," *J. Clin. Neurosci.* **30**, 104 (1993).

[141] S. Francina, "The Fountain of Youth," *Yoga J.*, May/Jun 1997, p. 87.

[142] C. C. Francis, *Introduction to Human Anatomy*, 4th Ed., C. V. Mosby, St. Louis, MO, 1964.

[143] D. Frawley, "Yoga and Sound," *Unity in Yoga News*, **2**, Winter, 1990, p.1.

[144] D. Frawley, "Mantra and the Energetics of Sound," *Clarion Call* **3**, 35 (1990).

[145] D. Frawley, "The Chakras and Modern Science," *Yoga Intern.*, Sep/Oct 1993, p. 5.

[146] J. Funderburk, *Science Studies Yoga*, Himalayan Press, Honesdale, PA, 1977.

[147] E. Funk and J. Clarke, "The Nasal Cycle. Observations over Prolonged Periods of Time," *Res. Bull. Him. Intern. Inst.*, Winter, 1980, p. 1.

[148] E. Funk, "Biorhythms and the Breath: The Nasal Cycle," *Res. Bull. Him. Intern. Inst.*, Winter, 1980, p. 5.

[149] M. R. Gach, *Accu-Yoga*, Japan Public., Tokyo, 1981.

[150] C. Gallup, "A Yoga for the Eyes," *Yoga J.*, Nov/Dec 1986, p. 19.

[151] J. Gardner, *Color and Crystals, A Journey Through the Chakras*, The Crossing Press, Freedom, CA, 1988.

[151a] M. S. Garfinkel, A. Singhal, W. A. Katz, D. A. Allen, R. Reshetar and H. R. Schumaker, Jr., "Yoga Intervention for Carpal Tunnel Syndrome: A Randomized Trial," *J. Am. Med. Assoc.* **280**, 1601 (1998).

[152] J. Gavin, "Understanding Psycho-anatomy," *IDEA Health and Fitness Source*, May 2000, p. 61.

[153] M. S. Gazzaniga, *Mind Matters: How Mind and Brain Interact to Create Our Conscious Lives*, Houghton-Mifflin, Boston, MA, 1988.

[154] R. M. Gerard, *Differential Effects of Colored Lights on Psychophysiological Functions*, Ph. D. Dissertation, Univ. California, Los Angeles, 1958.

[155] M. D. Gershon, *The Second Brain*, HarperCollins, NY, 1998.

[156] N. Geschwind and W. Levitsky, "The Human Brain: Left-Right Asymmetries in the Temporal Speech Region," *Science* **161**, 186 (1968).

[157] N. Geschwind, "Specializations of the Human Brain," *Sci. Am.*, Sep 1979, p. 180.

[158] W. W. Gibbs, "Dogma Overturned," *Sci. Am.*, Nov 1998, p. 19.

[159] P. R. Gillespie, "Beyond Relaxation," *Yoga J.*, Jul/Aug 1988, p. 37.

[160] S. Gillespie, "Taking Yoga to Heart," *Yoga Intern.*, Mar/April, 1995, p. 19.

[161] G. Giubilaro, personal communication.

[162] J. Glausiusz, "Brain, Heal Thyself," *Women's Health Digest* **2**, 224 (1996).

[163] W. H. Glazier, "The Task of Medicine," *Sci. Am.* **228**, 13 (1973).

[164] D. Goleman, "Too Much Rest Prolongs Muscle Pain," *The New York Times*, May 19, 1988.

[165] I. Goldstein, "Male Sexual Circuitry," *Sci. Am.*, Aug 2000, p. 70.

[166] J. Goodrich, "Freeing the Inner Eye" *East West*, Apr 1990, p. 54.

[167] K. S. Gopal, V. Anantharaman, S. D. Nisith, and O. P. Batnagar, "The Effect of Yogasanas on Muscular Tone and Cardio-Respiratory Adjustments," *Indian J. Med. Sci.* **28**, 438 (1974).

[168] K. S. Gopal and S. Lakshmanam, "Some Observations on Hatha Yoga: The Bandhas," *Indian J. Med. Sci.* **26**, 564 (1972).

[169] M. Grady, "Tempering the Mettle: The Practice of Bellows Breathing," *Yoga Intern.*, Jan/Feb 1994, p. 56.

[170] H. Gray, *Anatomy, Descriptive and Surgical*, Running Press, Philadelphia, PA, 1974.

[171] R. L. Gregory, *Eye and Brain*, Princeton Univ. Press, 5th Ed., Princeton, NJ, 1997.

[172] S. Grillner, "Neural Networks for Vertebrate Locomotion," *Sci. Am.*, Jan 1996, p. 64.

[173] T. Gura, "Roots of Immunity," *New Scient.*, Feb 19, 2000, p. 24.

[174] E. Haga, "Yoga," *J. Am. Med. Assoc.* **218**, 98 (1971).

[175] S. H. Hanus, T. D. Homer, and D. H. Harter, "Vertebral Artery Occlusion Complicating Yoga Exercises," *Arch. Neurol.* **34**, 574 (1977).

[176] W. Harman, "Science and Yoga, Friends at Last?" *Yoga Intern.*, Jul/Aug 1991, p. 21.

[177] *Harvard Medical School Family Health Guide*, A. L. Komaroff, Ed., Simon and Schuster, NY, 1999.

[178] *Harvard Women's Health Watch*, "Chronotherapy," Vol. III, April, 1996, p. 2.

[179] *Harvard's Women's Health Watch*, "High Blood Pressure," Vol. III, Jul 1996, p. 2.

[180] *Harvard Women's Health Watch*, "Exercise," Vol. III, January, 1996, p. 5.

[181] *Harvard Women's Health Watch*, "Excess Hair," Vol. V, Sep 1997, p. 4.

[182] *Harvard Women's Health Watch*, "Prevention," Vol. IV, 1997, p. 2.

[183] *Harvard Women's Health Watch*, "Sciatica," Vol. V, Sep 1997, p. 2.

[184] *Harvard Women's Health Watch*, "By the Way Doctor," Vol. V, Sep 1997, p. 8.

[185] *Harvard Women's Health Watch*, "What Is Normal Aging?" Vol. IV, Jun 1997, p. 3.

[186] *Harvard Women's Health Letter*, "A Special Report on Headache," Revised, Harvard Med. School, Health Pub. Grp., Boston, MA, 1999.

[187] *Harvard Women's Health Watch*, "Aging, Memory and the Brain," Vol. VII, No. 11, Jul 2000, p. 1.

[188] J. Harvey, "Patterns of Response to Stressful Tasks; the Biofeedback Stress Profile," *Res. Bul. Him. Intern. Inst.* **2**, 4 (1980).

[189] E. Haseltine, "Your Better Half. How to Tell Which Side of Your Brain Is Controlling Your Life," *Discover*, Jun 1999, p. 112.

[190] E. Haseltine, "Slow Pain Coming'" *Discover*, Aug 1999, p. 88.

[191] E. Haseltine, "Gre-t Exp-ct-ti-ns:- What You See Is Rarely What You Get," *Discover*, Sep 1999, p. 107.

[192] E. Haseltine, "How Your Brain Sees You," *Discover*, Sep 2000, p. 104.

[193] I. Haslock, R. Monro, R. Nagarathna, H. R. Nagendra and N. V. Raghuram, "Measuring the Effects of Yoga in Rheumatoid Arthritis," *Brit. J. Rheum.* **33**, 788 (1994).

[194] J. Hedstrom, "A Note on Eye Movements and Relaxation," *J. Behav. Ther. and Exp. Psychiat.* **22**, 37 (1991).

[195] L. Heimer, *The Human Brain and Spinal Cord*, 2nd. Ed., Springer-Verlag, NY, 1995.

[196] L. Helmuth, "Slow Motion Sets in When the Lights Dim," *Sci. News* **155**, 228 (1999).

[197] L. Helmuth, "Neural Teamwork May Compensate for Aging," *Sci. News* **155**, 247 (1999).

[198] B. Hendrick, "Love: Research Says It's Symmetry, Not Chemistry," *Dallas Morning News*, Oct 14, 1997, p. 4C.

[199] E. R. Hilgard, "Illusion That the Eye-Roll Sign Is Related to Hypnotizability," *Arch. Gen. Psychiatry* **39**, 963 (1982).

[200] P. Hirsch, personal communication, 1985.

[201] J. Hoenig, "Medical Research on Yoga," *Confin. Psychiatr.* **11**, 69 (1968).

[202] K. Hoffman and J. Clarke, "A Comparative Study of the Cardiac Response to Bhastrika," *Res. Bul. Him. Intern. Inst.* **4**, 7 (1982).

[203] K. Hoffman, "Moving with the Current: Observations on Nostril Dominance," *Yoga Intern.*, Sep/Oct 1993, p. 10.

[204] K. Hoffman, "Nostril Dominance: Experiencing Subtle Energy," *Yoga Intern.* Reprint Series, 1995, p. 10.

[205] W. J. Hrushesky, "Cancer Chronotherapy: Is There a Right Time in the Day to Treat?" *J. Infus. Chemother.* **5**, 38 (1995).

[206] D. H. Hubel and T. N. Weisel, "Brain Mechanisms of Vision," *Sci. Am.*, Sep 1979, p. 150.

[207] D. H. Hubel, *Eye, Brain, and Vision*, Sci. Am. Lib., New York, NY, 1995.

[208] A. Hymes and P. Nuernberger, "Breathing Patterns Found in Heart Attack Patients," *Res. Bul. Him. Intern. Inst.* **2**, 10 (1980).

[209] B. K. S. Iyengar, *Light on Yoga*, Schocken, NY, 1966.

[210] B. K. S. Iyengar, in *Iyengar, His Life and Work*, M. Manos, Ed., Timeless Books, Porthill, ID, 1987.

[211] B. K. S. Iyengar, *The Tree of Yoga*, Fine Line Books, Oxford, Eng., 1988.

[212] B. K. S. Iyengar, "Chakras, Bandhas and Kriyas," *Iyengar Yoga Inst. Rev.* **9**, 1 (1989).

[213] B. K. S. Iyengar, *Body the Shrine, Yoga Thy Light*, B. I. Taraporewala, Ed. and Pub., 1978.

[214] B. K. S. Iyengar, *The Art of Yoga*, HarperCollins, New Delhi, 1993.

[215] B. K. S. Iyengar, *Light on Pranayama*, Crossroad Pub. Co., NY, 1999.

[215a] B. K. S. Iyengar, *Yoga The Path to Holistic Health*, Dorling Kindersley, London, 2001.

[216] G. S. Iyengar, *Yoga, A Gem for Women*, Timeless Books, Palo Alto, CA, 1990.

[217] G. S. Iyengar, "Effect of Inverted Yoga Postures on Menstruation and Pregnancy," *Yoga Rahasya* **4**, 29 (1997).

[218] S. A Jella and D. S. Shannahoff-Khaksa, "The Effects of Unilateral Forced Nostril

Breathing on Cognitive Performance," *Int. J. Neurosci.* **73**, 61 (1993).

[219] S. Johnsen, "Transparent Animals," *Sci. Am.*, Feb 2000, p. 81.

[220] B. E. Johnson, *Adult Rheumatic Disease*, Monograph, Edition 216, Home Study Self-Assessment Program, Kansas City, MO, *Am. Acad. Fam. Phys.*, Jul 1997.

[221] N. Jones, "Soothing the Inflamed Brain," *Sci. Am.*, Jun 2000, p. 24.

[222] D. Juhan, *Job's Body: A Handbook for Bodywork*, Station Hill Press, Barrytown, NY, 1987.

[223] T. Kamei, Y. Toriumi, H. Kimura, S. Ohno, H. Kumano and K. Kimura, "Decrease in Serum Cortisol During Yoga Exercise Is Correlated with Alpha Wave Activation," *Percept. Mot. Skills*, **90**, 1027 (2000).

[224] E. Kandel, "Small Systems of Neurons," *Sci. Am.*, Sep 1979, p. 67.

[225] E. R. Kandel, J. H. Schwartz and T. M. Jessell, *Principles of Neural Science*, Third Ed., Appleton and Lange, Norwalk, CT, 1991.

[226] I. A. Kapandji, *The Physiology of the Joints, Vol. I, Upper Limb*, Churchill Livingstone, Edinburgh, 1982.

[227] I. A. Kapandji, *The Physiology of the Joints, Vol. II, Lower Limb*, Fifth Ed., Churchill Livingstone, Edinburgh, 1987.

[228] I. A. Kapandji, *The Physiology of the Joints. The Trunk and the Vertebral Column. Vol. III*, Second Ed., Churchill, Livingstone, Edinburgh, 1974.

[229] W. Kapit and L. M. Elson, *The Anatomy Coloring Book*, HarperCollins, NY, 1977.

[230] W. Kapit, R. I. Macey and E. Meisami, *The Physiology Coloring Book*, Addison Wesley, Menlo Park, CA, 1987.

[231] S. V. Karandicar, *Yoga Therapy in Spinal Disorders*, Private Publication, Pune, India.

[232] M. L. Kathotia, *Color Therapy for Common Diseases*, Hind Pocket Books, Delhi, India, 1996.

[233] D. Keller, "Reconcilable Differences," *Yoga J.*, Nov/Dec 1999, p. 104.

[234] S. Keen, "Fear in the Belly," *Yoga J.*, May/Jun 1999, p. 58.

[235] D. C. Kerrigan, M. K. Todd and P. O. Riley, "Knee Osteoarthritis and High-Heeled Shoes," *The Lancet* **351**, 1399 (1998).

[236] C. Kilham, "Nada Yoga: Sound Current Meditation," *Yoga J.*, Sep/Oct 1981, p. 47.

[237] A. Kilmurray, "Studying with Dona Holleman," *Inst. Yoga Teacher Education* **3**, 1 (1982).

[238] A. Kilmurray, "Gravity, Newton's Third Law and Asana," Am. Yoga Newslet. **1**, 5 (1983).

[239] A. Kilmurray, "The Safe Practice of Inversions," *Yoga J.*, Nov/Dec 1983, p. 24.

[240] A. Kilmurray, "Understanding Twists," *Yoga J.*, Sep/Oct 1984, p. 31.

[241] A. Kilmurray, "Sarvangasana," *Yoga J.*, Sep/Oct 1990, p. 33.

[242] A. Kilmurray, "Urdhva Dhanurasana," *Yoga J.*, Nov/Dec 1990, p. 30.

[243] D. Kimura, "The Asymmetry of the Human Brain," *Sci. Am.* **228**, 70 (1973).

[244] R. Klein and R. Armitage, "Rhythms in Human Performance: 1½ Hour Oscillations in Cognitive Style," *Science* **204**, 1326 (1979).

[245] J. Koch-Weser, "Sympathetic Activity in Essential Hypertension," *New Eng. J. Med.* **288**, 627 (1973).

[246] L. K. Kothari and O. P. Gupta, "The Yogic Claim of Voluntary Control over the Heart Beat: An Unusual Demonstration," *Am. Heart J.* **86**, 282 (1973).

[247] M. Kraft and R. J. Martin, "Chronobiology and Chronotherapy in Medicine," *Dis Mon* **41**, 501 (1995).

[248] G. Krishna, "*The Awakening of Kundalini*," Dutton, NY, 1975.

[249] P. Kumar, *Yoga Intern.*, Sep/Oct 1993, p. 34.

[250] G. Kurian, N. K. Sharma, and K. Santhakumari, "Left Arm Dominance in Active Arm Positioning," *Percept. Mot. Skills* **68**, 1312 (1989).

[251] T. Kurz, "*Stretching Scientifically*," Stadion, Island Pond, VT, 1994.

[252] V. Lad, *Ayurveda, The Science of Self-Healing*, Lotus Light, Wilmot, WI, 1984.

[253] L. Lamberg, "Dawn's Early Light to Twilight's Last Gleaming," *J. Am. Med. Assoc.* **280**, 1556 (1998).

[254] H. E. Landsberg, *Weather and Health*, Doubleday, Garden City, NY, 1969.

[255] J. Lasater, "Eka Pada Sarvangasana," *Yoga J.*, Sep/Oct 1981, p. 48.

[256] J. Lasater, "Yoga and the Pregnant Woman," *Inst. Yoga Teacher Education Rev.* **2**, 7 (1981).

[257] J. Lasater, "Understanding the Neck," *Inst. Yoga Teacher Education* **1**, 1 (1981).

[258] J. Lasater, "Sarvangasana," *Yoga J.*, Jan/Feb 1982, p. 49.

[259] J. Lasater, "Muscle Tension and Breech Presentation," *Inst. Yoga Teacher Education Rev.* **3**, 15 (1982).

[260] J. Lasater, "Posture and its Effects," *Inst. Yoga Teacher Education Rev.* **3**, 7 (1982).

[261] J. Lasater, "Asana: Handstand," *Yoga J.*, Jul/Aug 1983, p. 7.

[262] J. Lasater, "The Plough: Good or Bad?" *Yoga J.*, Jan/Feb 1983, p. 7.

[263] J. Lasater, "Headstand, Part Two," *Yoga J.*, Sep/Oct 1984, p. 13.

[264] J. Lasater, "Salamba Sirsasana," *Yoga J.*, Jul/Aug 1984, p. 15.

[265] J. Lasater, "Incorporating Backbends into Your Practice," *Yoga J.*, Nov/Dec 1986, p. 41.

[266] J. Lasater, "Touching: The Essence of Non-Verbal Communication," *Inst. Yoga Teacher Education Rev.*, Summer, 1989, p. 16.

[267] J. Lasater, "Healthy Backbends," *Yoga J.*, May/Jun 1991, p. 14.

[268] J. H. Lasater, "Yoga for the Overly Flexible," *Yoga J.*, Jan/Feb 1993, p. 6.

[269] J. Lasater, *Relax and Renew*, Rodmell Press, Berkeley, CA, 1995.

[270] J. Lasater, "Stability Revisited: Realigning the Sacrum in Asana," *Yoga Intern.*, Apr/May 1999, p. 43.

[271] J. Lasater, "Saving Your Neck: the Cervical Spine in Yoga Poses," *Yoga Intern.*, Oct/Nov 1999, p. 47.

[272] J. Lasater, "Heading Off Headaches," *Yoga Intern.*, Aug/Sep 1999, p. 51.

[273] J. Lasater, "Breathing Lessons," *Yoga J.*, May/Jun 1999, p. 104.

[274] J. Lasater, "Inversions?" *Yoga Intern.*, Jun/Jul 2000, p. 10.

[275] J. Lasater, "Building Strength," *Yoga Intern.*, Dec/Jan 2000, p. 56.

[276] J. Lee, "Metabolic Powerhouse," *New Scient.* Life Sci., No. 135, Nov 11, 2000, p. 1.

[277] B. Lemley, "Isn't She Lovely," *Discover*, Feb 2000, p. 42.

[278] V. Lepicovska, C. Dostalek, and M. Kovarova, "Hathayogic Exercise Jalandharabandha in its Effect on Cardiovascular Response to Apnoea," *Act. Nerv. Super. (Praha)*, **32**, 99 (1990).

[279] E. Leskowitz, "The Third Eye: A Psycho-endocrine Model of Hypnotizability," *Am. J. Clin. Hypn.* **30**, 209 (1988).

[280] E. Leskowitz, "Seasonal Affective Disorder and the Yoga Paradigm: A Reconsideration of the Role of the Pineal Gland," *Med. Hypoth.* **33**, 155 (1990).

[281] J. Liberman, *Light: Medicine of the Future*, Bear and Co., Santa Fe, NM, 1991.

[282] D. B. Lindsley and W. H. Sassaman, "Autonomic Activity and Brain Potentials Associated with 'Voluntary' Control of the Pilomotors," *J. Neurophysiol.* **1**, 342 (1938).

[283] B. Lipinski, "Biological Significance of Piezoelectricity in Relation to Acupuncture, Hatha Yoga, Osteopathic Medicine and Action of Air Ions," *Med. Hypotheses* **3**, 9 (1977).

[284] E. Lipson, "Yoga Works!" *Yoga J.*, Winter, 1999, p. 6.

[285] N. K. Logothetis, "Vision: A Window on Consciousness," *Sci. Am.*, Nov 1999, p. 69.

[286] J. W. Long, *The Essential Guide to Prescription Drugs*, Harper and Row, NY, 1980.

[287] I. Lorch, "Total Vision," *East West*, April, 1990, p. 49.

[288] E. G. Lufkin and M. Zilkoski, *Diagnosis and Management of Osteoporosis*, Am. Family Physician, Monograph No. 1, 1996.

[289] F. M. Luskin, K. A. Newell, M. Griffith, F. F. Marvasti, M. Hill, K. R. Pelletier, and W. L. Haskell, "A Review of Mind/Body Therapies in the Treatment of Musculoskeletal Disorders with Implications for the Elderly," *Altern. Therap.* **6**, 46 (2000).

[290] E. G. Lutz, "Credit-Card Wallet Sciatica," *J. Am. Med. Assoc.* **240**, 738 (1978).

[291] R. I. Macey, *Human Physiology*, Prentice-Hall, Englewood Cliffs, NJ, 1968.

[292] L. Mackinnon, *Advances in Exercise Immunology*, Human Kinetics, Champaign, IL, 1999.

[293] J. MacMullen, "Yoga and the Menstrual Cycle," *Yoga J.*, Jan/Feb 1990, p. 65.

[294] A. Malathi and V. G. Parulkar, "Effect of Yogasanas on the Visual and Auditory Reaction Time," *Indian J. Physiol. Pharmacol.* **33**, 110 (1989).

[295] J. Marchant, "Reading Your Mind," *New Scient.*, Aug 12, 2000, p. 20.

[296] C. E. Margo, J. Rowda and J. Barletta, "Bilateral Conjunctival Varix Thromboses Associated with Habitual Headstanding," *Am. J. Ophthalom.* **113**, 726 (1992).

[297] E. N. Marieb, *Human Anatomy and Physiology*, Benjamin/Cummings, NY, 1992.

[298] P. Marks, "Blast from the Past," *New Scient.*, Feb 19, 2000, p. 11.

[299] G. G. Matthews, *Cellular Physiology of Nerve and Muscle*, 3rd Ed., Blackwell, Oxford, England, 1998.

[300] R. Matthews, "Death by Crucifixion," *New Scient.*, Jan 23, 2000.

[301] T. G. Mattio, T. Nishida, and M. M. Minieka, "Lotus Neuropathy: Report of a Case," *Neurology* **42**, 1636 (1992).

[302] J. McCrone, "Rebels with a Cause," *New Scient.*, Jan 22, 2000, p. 22.

[303] J. W. McDonald, "Repairing the Damaged Spinal Cord," *Sci. Am.*, Sep 1999, p. 65.

[304] J. McDougal, in B. Baptiste and K. F. Mendola, "Rx for Runner's Cramps," *Yoga J.*, Mar/Apr 1999, p. 36.

[305] R. H. Mehta, "Our Digestive System," *Yoga Rahasya* **2**, 157 (1995).

[306] S. Mehta, M. Mehta and S. Mehta, *Yoga the Iyengar Way*, A. A. Knopf, NY, 1997.

[307] L. Melton, "AGE Breakers," *Sci. Am.*, Jul 2000, p. 16.

[308] R. Melzack and P. D. Wall, *The Challenge of Pain*, Basic Books, NY, 1983.

[309] *"The Merck Manual of Diagnosis and Treatment*," Merck, Sharp and Dohme Research Laboratories, 1966.

[310] B. Meyers, "Sequence for Depression," IYA of Greater New York Newsletter, Spring 1994, p. 15.

[311] P. J. Michels, *Anxiety*, American Academy of Family Physicians, Monograph No. 212, Home Study Self-Assessment Program, Jan 1997.

[312] E. B. Miller, "Yoga for Scoliosis," *Yoga J.*, May/Jun 1990, p. 66.

[313] J. Miller, *The Body in Question*, Random House, NY, 1978.

[314] J. J. Miller, K. Fletcher and J. Kabat-Zinn, "Three Year Follow-Up and Clinical Implications of a Mindfulness Meditation-Based Stress Reduction Inter-vention in the Treatment of Anxiety Disorders," *Gen. Hosp. Psychiatry* **17**, 192 (1995).

[315] R. C. Miller, "The Psychophysiology of Respiration: Eastern and Western Perspectives," *J. Intern. Assoc. Yoga Therapists*, Vol. 2, No. 1, 1991.

[316] R. C. Miller, "The Therapeutic Application of Yoga on Sciatica—A Case Study," *J. Intern. Assoc. Yoga Therapists* **3**, 2 (1992).

[317] R. Monro, R. Nagarathna and H. R. Nagendra, "Yoga Therapy: The Eyes Have It," *Yoga Intern.*, Apr 1998, p. 45.

[318] R. Monro and L. Fitzgerald, "A Scientific Look at Yoga and Diabetes," *Yoga Biomed. Bull.* **1**, 71 (1986).

[319] W. Montagna, *"Comparative Anatomy*, John Wiley, NY, 1959.

[320] A. Montagu, *Touching. The Human Significance of the Skin*, 3rd Ed., Harper and Row, NY, 1986.

[321] M. C. Moore-Ede, F. M. Sulzman, and C. A. Fuller, *The Clocks That Time Us*, Harvard Press, Cambridge, MA, 1982.

[321a] K. Morris, "Meditating in Yogic Science," *The Lancet* **351**, 1038 (1998).

[322] S. N. Motiwala and R. H. Mehta, "Treating Chronic Ailments with Yoga. Acidity," *Yoga Rahasya* **2**, 28 (1995).

[323] S. N. Motiwala and R. H. Mehta, "Treating Chronic Ailments with Yoga II (Cervical Spondylosis)," *Yoga Rahasya*, **3**, 29 (1996).

[324] S. N. Motiwala and R. H. Mehta, "Treating Ailments with Yoga IV (Chronic Fatigue Syndrome)," *Yoga Rahasya*, **4**, 32 (1997).

[325] A. Motluk, "Dicing with Albert," *New Scient.*, Mar 18, 2000, p. 43.

[326] A. Motluk, "No, No, this Way: Why Men and Women Argue over Which Route to Take," *New Scient.*, Mar 25, 2000, p. 13.

[327] A. Motluk and A. Raine, "Not Guilty," *New Scient.*, May 13, 2000, p. 42.

[328] A. Motluk, "Fingered," *New Scient.*, Jun 24, 2000, p. 32.

[329] D. Moyer, "Sarvangasana," *Yoga J.*, Sep/Oct 1987, p. 30.

[330] R. Nagarathna and H. R. Nagendra, "Yoga for Bronchial Asthma: A Controlled Study," *Brit. Med. J.* **291**, 172 (1985).

[331] R. Nagarathna, H. R. Nagendra and R.

Monro, *Yoga for Common Ailments*, Gaia Books, London, 1990.

[332] W. Nagler, "Vertebral Artery Obstruction by Hyperextension of the Neck: Report of Three Cases," *Arch. Phys. Med. Rehabil.* **54**, 237 (1973).

[333] C. B. Nemeroff, "The Neurobiology of Depression," *Sci. Am.*, Jun 1998, p. 42.

[334] K. Nespor, "Psychosomatics of Back Pain and the Use of Yoga," *Intern. J. Psychosom.* **36**, 72 (1989).

[335] R. M. Nesse and G. C. Williams, "Evolution and the Origins of Disease," *Sci. Am.*, Nov 1998, p. 86.

[336] J. Netting, "Wink of an Eye," *Sci. Am.*, May 1999, p. 26.

[337] D. C. Nieman, *Fitness and Sports Medicine*, Bull Publishing, Palo Alto, CA, 1990.

[338] R. A. Norman, M. E. Norman and R. Holtz, "Stress Thrombosis," *Osteopath. Med. News*, Apr 1990, p. 26.

[339] K. V. Noveen, R. Nagarathna, H. R. Nagendra and S. Telles, "Yoga Breathing through a Particular Nostril Increases Spatial Memory Scores without Lateralizing Effects," *Psychol. Rep.* **81**, 555 (1997).

[340] A. D. Novitt-Moreno, *How the Brain Works*, Ziff-Davis Press, Emeryville, CA, 1955.

[340a] R. Nowak, "Life in the Old Dog," *New Scient.*, Jul 22, 2000, p. 36.

[341] P. Nuernberger, "Effects of Breath Training on Personality Test Scores," *Res. Bull. Him. Intern. Inst.* **3**, 9 (1981).

[342] P. Nuernberger, "Stress: A New Perspective," *Res. Bull. Him. Intern. Inst.* **3**, 7 (1981).

[343] P. Nuernberger, *Freedom from Stress*, Himalayan Intern. Inst., Honesdale, PA, 1981.

[344] P. Nuernberger, "Stress: A New Perspective," in *The Quiet Mind*, J. Harvey, Ed., Himalayan Press, Honesdale, PA, 1988.

[345] A. Olsen and C. McHose, *Body Stories*, Station Hill Press, Barrytown, NY, 1991.

[346] R. E. Ornstein, *The Psychology of Consciousness*, Harcourt Brace, Jovanovitch, NY, 1977.

[347] J. Ott, "Responses of Psychological and Physiological Functions to Environmental Light. Part I," *J. Learning Disabil.* **1**, 18 (1968).

[348] S. Overeem, G. J. Lammers and J. G. van Dijk, "Weak with Laughter," *The Lancet* **354**, 838 (1999).

[349] J. Pacheco, "Red Light, Green Light. Somatics and Yoga," *Yoga Intern.*, Feb/Mar 1999, p. 17.

[350] A. Palkhivala, personal communication, 1999.

[351] Parker Chiropractic Research Foundation, *Chart of Effects of Spinal Misalignment*, 1975.

[352] C. Patel and M. Marmot, "Can General Practitioners Use Training in Relaxation and Management of Stress to Reduce Mild Hypertension?" *Brit. Med. J.* **296**, 21 (1988).

[353] R. Patel, "The Yoga Sutras and Asana Practice," *Inst. Yoga Teacher Education* **1**, 8 (1981).

[354] E. Patterson, personal communication, 1999.

[355] W. G. Penfield and T. B. Rasmussen, *The Cerebral Cortex of Man: A Clinical Study of Localization of Function*, Macmillan, NY, 1950.

[356] S. Perkowitz, "Feeling Is Believing," *New Scient.*, Sep 1999, p. 34.

[357] C. B. Pert, *Molecules of Emotion*, Touchstone, NY, 1997.

[358] J. Peterson, "Ten Reasons Why Warming Up Is Important," *Health and Fitness J.*, Jan/Feb 1999, p. 52.

[359] H. Phillip, "Perchance to Learn," *New Scient.*, Sep 25, 1999, p. 26.

[360] *Physicians Desk Reference*, 51st Ed., 1997.

[360a] T. G. Pickering, "Why is Hypertension More Common in African Americans?" *J. Clin. Hypertens.* **3**, 50 (2001).

[361] M. Pierce, "Breathing for Modern Life," *Yoga J.*, Sep/Oct 1998, p. 104.

[362] D. J. Pincus, T. R. Humiston, and R. J. Martin, "Further Studies on the Chronotherapy of Asthma with Inhaled Steroids: The Effect of Dosage Timing on Drug Efficacy," *J. Allergy Clin. Immunol.* **100**, 771 (1997).

[363] S. Pinker, *How the Mind Works*, Morton, NY, 1997.

[364] A. Pirisi, "Yogis Score High on Happiness," *Yoga J.*, May/Jun 2000, p. 33.

[365] D. W. Plocher, "The Auditory Response to Inverted Posture," *Arch. Otolaryngol.* **111**, 135 (1985).

[366] M. Pohl, A. Rosler, I. Sunkeler, H.-J. Braune, W. H. Oertel, and S. Lautenbacher, "Insertion Pain in Needle Electromyography Can Be Reduced by Simultaneous Finger Slapping," *Neurology* **54**, 1201 (2000).

[367] A. A. Pollack and E. H. Wood, "Venous Pressure in the Saphenous Vein at the Ankle in Man During Exercise and Changes in Posture," *J. Appl. Physiol.* **1**, 649 (1949).

[368] D. J. Ponte, G. J. Jensen and B. E. Kent, "A Preliminary Report on the Use of the McKenzie Protocol versus Williams' Protocol in the Treatment of Low-Back Pain," *J. Orthopedic Sports Phys. Ther.* **6**, 130 (1984).

[369] Prakasha, "Science and Yoga," *Ascent*, Summer, 2000, p. 16.

[370] M. Radnot, "Effects of Testicular Extirpation upon Intraocular Pressure," *Annals NY Acad. Sci.* **117**, 614 (1964).

[371] J. Raloff, "Medicinal EMF's," *Sci. News* **156**, 316 (1999).

[372] S. Rama, R. Ballentine and S. Ajaya, *Yoga and Psychotherapy*, Himalayan Institute, Honesdale, PA, 1976.

[373] S. Rama, *Joints and Glands Exercises*, Himalayan Institute, Honesdale, PA, 1977.

[374] S. Rama, R. Ballentine and A. Hymes, *Science of Breath*, Himalayan Intern. Inst., Honesdale, PA, 1979.

[375] S. Rama, "The Science of Prana: Basic Breathing Exercises," *Res. Bull. Him. Intern. Inst.* **2**, 1 (1980).

[376] S. Rama, "Pranayama," *Res. Bull. Him. Intern. Inst.* **3**, 1 (1981).

[377] B. Ramamurthi, "Yoga: An Explanation and Probable Neurophysiology," *J. Indian Med. Assoc.* **48**, 167 (1967).

[378] K. Raman, "Migraine and Yoga," *Yoga Rahasya* **3**, 57 (1996).

[379] K. Raman, *A Matter of Health*, Eastwood Books, Madras, India, 1998.

[380] S. Rao, "Yoga and Autohypnotism," *Brit. J. Med. Hypnot.* **17**, 38 (1965).

[381] S. Rao, "Metabolic Cost of Headstand Posture," *J. Appl. Physiol.* **17**, 117 (1962).

[382] R. Restak and D. Mahoney, *The Longevity Strategy: How to Live to 100 Using the Brain-Body Connection*, Wiley, NY, 1999.

[383] R. Rice and R. C. Allen, "Yoga in Glaucoma," *Am. J. Ophthamol.* **100**, 738 (1985).

[384] C. Rist, "The Pain in the Brain," *Discover*, Mar 2000, p. 57.

[385] J. Robbins, "Wired for Sadness," *Discover*, April, 2000, p. 77.

[386] I. P. Rolf, *Rolfing*, Healing Arts Press, Rochester, VT, 1977.

[387] K. J. Rose, *The Body in Time*, Wiley, NY, 1988.

[388] M. R. Rose, "Can Human Aging Be Postponed?" *Sci. Am.*, Dec 1999, p. 106.

[389] E. L. Rossi, *The Psychobiology of Mind-Body Healing*, Norton, NY, 1986.

[390] B. Rothenberg and O. Rothenberg, *Touch Training for Strength*, Human Kinetics, Champaign, IL, 1995.

[391] F. P. Ruiz, "What Science Can Teach Us About Flexibility," *Yoga J.*, Mar/April, 2000, p. 92.

[392] F. P. Ruiz, "Bodhi Building," *Yoga J.*, Jul/Aug 2000, p. 84.

[393] F. P. Ruiz, "Insight for Sore Eyes," *Yoga J.*, Sep/Oct 2000, p. 74.

[394] E. Ruoslahti, "Stretching Is Good for a Cell," *Science* **276**, 1345 (1997).

[395] W. R. Russell, "Yoga and the Vertebral Arteries," *Brit. Med. J.*, Mar 11, 1972, p. 685.

[396] A. Rychner, "Getting Out from Under. Asana for Relieving PMS," *Yoga Intern.*, Mar/Apr 1995, p. 57.

[397] E. Sander, "Menopause: The Yoga Way," *Yoga J.*, Jan/Feb 1996, p. 61.

[398] L. Sarasohn, "Honoring the Belly," *Yoga J.*, Jul/Aug 1993, p. 76.

[399] S. Saraswati, *The Effects of Yoga on Hypertension*, Second Ed., G. K. Kejriwal, Bihar, India, 1984.

[400] S. Saraswati, *Health Benefits of Inverted Asanas*, Second Ed., G. K. Kejriwal, Bihar, India, 1992.

[401] S. Saraswati, *Health Benefits of Backward Bending Asanas*, Second Ed., G. K. Kejriwal, Bihar, India, 1992.

[402] J. E. Sarno, *Healing Back Pain; the Mind-Body Connection*, Warner Books, NY, 1991.

[403] J. E. Sarno, "How to Say No to Back Pain," *Bottom Line/Personal*, Jun 15, 1991, p. 13.

[404] S. Satyananda Saraswati, *Health Benefits of Forward Bending Asanas*, Bihar School of Yoga, Bihar, India 1992.

[405] A. G. Schauss, "Tranquilizing Effect of Color Reduces Aggressive Behavior and Potential Violence," *J. Orthomol. Psychiat.* **8**, 218 (1979).

[406] M. P. Schatz, "Inversions and Menstruation," *Yoga J.*, Nov/Dec 1983, p. 30.

[406a] M. Schatz, "Stress and Relaxation: Hypertension and Yoga," *Iyengar Teacher Ed. Rev.*, 1984, p.7.

[407] M. Schatz, "Yoga, Circulation and Imagery," *Yoga J.*, Jan/Feb 1987, p. 54.

[408] M. P. Schatz, "Yoga, the Mind and Immunity," *Yoga J.*, Jul/Aug 1987, p. 42.

[409] M. P. Schatz, "You Can Have Healthy Bones," *Yoga J.*, Mar/Apr 1988, p. 43.

[410] M. P. Schatz, "Yoga and Aging," *Yoga J.*, May/Jun 1990, p. 58.

[411] M. P. Schatz, *Back Care Basics*, Rodmell Press, Berkeley, CA, 1992.

[412] M. P. Schatz, "In a Slump? Unrounding Your Lower Back," *Yoga Intern.*, Oct/Nov 1998, p. 55.

[413] M. P. Schatz, "A Woman's Balance: Inversions and Menstruation," *http://www.iyengar.ch/Deutsch/text_menstruation.htm*, Aug 24, 2000.

[414] V. Schneider, "The Healing Power of Color," *Yoga J.*, Jan/Feb 1987, p. 7.

[414a] G. H. Schueller, "Thrill or Chill," *New Scient.*, April 29, 2000, p. 20.

[415] J. Schumacher, "Preparing for Arm Balances," *Yoga J.*, Jul/Aug 1989, p. 69.

[416] J. Schumacher, "Preparing for Inversions," *Yoga J.*, Jul/Aug 1990, p. 68.

[417] C. Seibert, "The Chakras and Modern Science," *Yoga Intern.*, Sep/Oct 1993, p. 5.

[418] W. Selvamurthy, V. S. Ray, K. S. Hegde, and R. P. Sharma, "Physiological Responses to Cold (10° C) in Men after Six Months Practice of Yoga Exercise," *Intern. J. Biometrology* **32**, 188 (1988).

[418a] W. Selvamurthy, K. Sridharan, U. S. Ray, R. S. Tiwari, K. S. Hegde, U. Rahhakrishna and K. C. Sinha, "A New Physiological Approach to Control of Essential Hypertension," *Indian J. Physiol. Pharmacol.* **42**, 205 (1998).

[419] H. Selye, *The Stress of Life*, McGraw Hill, NY, 1956.

[420] E. Serber, "Yoga Cures for Headaches," *Yoga Intern.*, Jan/Feb 1999, p. 42.

[421] S. Shankardevananda Saraswati, *The Practice of Yoga for the Digestive System*, Bihar School of Yoga, Bihar, India, 1987.

[422] D. S. Shannahoff-Khalsa and B. Kennedy, "The Effects of Unilateral Forced Breathing on the Heart," *Int. J. Neurosci.* **73**, 47 (1993).

[423] D. S. Shannahoff-Khalsa and L. R. Beckett, "Clinical Case Report: Efficacy of Yogic Techniques in the Treatment of Obsessive Compulsive Disorder," *Intern. J. Neurosci.* **85**, 1 (1996).

[424] D. S. Shannahoff-Khalsa, B. Kennedy, F. E. Yates, and M. G. Ziegler, "Ultradian Rhythms of Autonomic, Cardiovascular, and Neuroendocrine Systems Are Related in Humans," *Am. J. Physiol.* **270**, R873 (1996).

[425] D. S. Shannahoff-Khalsa, B. Kennedy, F. E. Yates and M. G. Ziegler, "Low-Frequency Ultradian Insulin Rhythms Are Coupled to Cardiovascular, Autonomic, and Neuroendocrine Rhythms, *Am. J. Physiol.* **272**, R962 (1997).

[426] D. G. Sherman, R. G. Hart, and J. D. Easton, "Abrupt Change in Head Position and Cerebral Infarction," *Stroke* **12**, 2 (1981).

[427] T. Shipley, "Rod-Cone Duplexity and Autonomic Action of Light," *Vision Res.* **4**, 155 (1964).

[428] Shyam Sundar Goswami, *Hatha-Yoga*, L. N. Fowler, London, 1959.

[429] K. W. Sieg and S. P. Adams, *Illustrated Essentials of Musculoskeletal Anatomy*, Mega Books, Gainsville, FL, 1985.

[430] S. Simpson, "Pain, Pain, Go Away," *Sci. News* **155**, 108 (2000).

[431] V. Singh, A. Wisniewski, J. Britton and A. Tattersfield, "Effect of Yoga Breathing Exercises (Pranayama) on Airway Reactivity in Subjects with Asthma," *The Lancet* **335**, 1381 (1990).

[432] N. E. Sjoman, *The Yoga Tradition of the Mysore Palace*, Abhinav Press, New Delhi, 1996.

[433] B. Smith, *Yoga for a New Age*, Prentice-Hall, Englewood Cliffs, NJ, 1982.

[434] C. U. M. Smith, *The Brain: Towards an Understanding*, Capricorn, NY, 1972.

[435] R. Smith, "The Timing of Birth," *Sci. Am.*, Mar 1999, p. 68.

[436] M. H. Smolensky and F. Portaluppi, "Chronopharmacology and Chronotherapy of Cardiovascular Medications: Relevance to Prevention and Treatment of Coronary Heart Disease," *Am. Heart J.* **137**, S14 (1999).

[437] P. J. Snyder, "Effects of Age on Testicular Function and Consequences of Testosterone Treatment," *J. Clin. Endocrinol. Metab.* **86**, 2369 (2001).

[438] S. H. Snyder, "The Molecular Basis of Communication Between Cells," *Sci. Am.*, Oct 1985, p. 132.

[439] R. Sovik, "Keep Your Nose Clean," *Yoga Intern.*, Feb/Mar 1998, p. 61.

[440] R. Sovik, "Energy Rising. How to Establish Sushumna," *Yoga Intern.*, Feb/Mar 1999, p. 57.

[441] R. Sovik, "Breathing Through Emotions," *Yoga Intern.*, Feb/Mar 2000, p. 61.

[442] L. Sparrowe, "Menstrual Essentials," *Yoga J.*, Sep/Oct 1999, p. 74.

[443] M. Stefanick, "Effects of Inverted Poses on Cardiovascular Physiology," *Inst. Yoga Teacher Education Rev.* **3**, 1 (1983).

[444] D. Stein, *The Women's Book of Healing*, Llewellyn, St. Paul, MN, 1996.

[445] K. Stephan and G. Iyengar, "A Visit with Geeta Iyengar," *Newsletter of IYA, GNY and MA*, Spring/Summer, 1990, p. 1.

[446] K. A. Stevens and J. M. Parrish, "Neck Posture and Feeding Habits of Two Jurassic Sauropod Dinosaurs," *Science* **284**, 798 (1999).

[447] J. D. Stewart, E. Angus and D. Gendron, "Sciatic Neuropathies," *Brit. Med. J.* **287**, 1108 (1983).

[448] M. T. Stiles, "Know Your Knees," *Yoga Intern.* Reprint Series, "Yoga Therapy for Knees and Shoulders," 1998, p. 3.

[449] M. T. Stiles, "Wings of the Heart: Working with the Shoulders," *Yoga Intern.* Reprint Series, "Yoga Therapy for Knees and Shoulders," 1998, p.12.

[450] M. Stoppard, *Menopause*, Dorling Kindersley, London, 1994.

[451] N. Suda, "Earth's Background Free Oscillations," *Science*. **279**, 2089 (1998).

[452] S. Sunderland, "The Relative Susceptibility to Injury of the Medial and Lateral Popliteal Divisions of the Sciatic Nerve," *Brit. J. Surg.* **41**, 300 (1953).

[453] R. E. Svoboda, *Aghora II: Kundalini*, Brotherhood of Life, Albuquerque, NM, 1993.

[454] Swami Veda Bharati, "What Is the Opposite Sex? *Yoga Intern.*, Sep/Oct 1993, p. 7.

[455] L. W. Swanson, "The Hypothalamus" *in Handbook of Chemical Neuroanatomy, Integrated Systems of the CNS*, A. Bjorkland, T. Hokfelt, and L. W. Swanson, Eds., Elsevier, Amsterdam, 1987.

[456] M. Talbot, "The Placebo Prescription," *NY Times Mag.*, Jan 9, 2000, p. 34.

[457] C. Taylor, "Death by Crucifixion," *New Scient.*, Jan 23, 2000.

[458] S. Telles, R. Nagarathna, and H. R. Nagendra, "Breathing through a Particular Nostril Can Alter Metabolism and Autonomic Activities," *Indian J. Physiol. Pharmacol.* **38**, 133 (1994).

[459] S. Telles, R. Nagarathna and H. R. Nagendra, "Physiological Measures of Right Nostril Breathing," *J. Altern. Complement. Med.* **2**, 479 (1996).

[460] R. Ornstein and C. Swencionis, eds., *The Healing Brain*, Guilford Press, NY, 1990.

[461] J. Thomas and M. G. Mawhinney, *Synopsis of Endocrine Pharmacology*, University Park, Baltimore, MD, 1973.

[462] P. R. Tigunait, "Psychology of Consciousness," *Res. Bul. Him. Intern. Inst.* 3, 1 (1981).

[463] R. Tigunait, "Mind Games; How We Make Ourselves Sick," *Yoga Intern.*, Jun/Jul 2000, p. 25.

[464] C. Tomlinson, "20/20 Vision Quest," *Yoga J.*, Mar/April, 1999, p. 120.

[465] Dr. B. Trachtenberg, personal communication, 1998.

[466] J. Travis, "Boning Up," *Sci. News* **157**, 41 (2000).

[467] J. Travis, "Mom's Eggs Execute Dad's Mitochondria," *Sci. News* **157**, 5 (2000).

[468] J. Travis, "Protein May Help the Eyes Tell Time," *Sci. News* **157**, 120 (2000).

[469] J. E. Upledger, *Cranial Sacral Therapy I Study Guide*, UI Pub., 1991.

[470] A. Vescovi, R. Galli, U. Borello, A Gritti, M. G. Minasi and C. Bjornson, "Skeletal Myogenic Potential of Human and Mouse Neural Cells," *Nature Neurosci.*, Oct 3, 2000, p. 986.

[471] C. M. Vogel, R. Albin, and J. W. Albers, "Lotus Footdrop: Sciatic Neuropathy in the Thigh," *Neurology* **41**, 605 (1991).

[472] S. Vogel, *Cat's Paws and Catapults*, Norton, NY, 1998.

[473] A. von Hippel, *Human Evolutionary Biology*, Stone Age Press, Anchorage, AK, 1994.

[474] P. Walden, "Asanas to Relieve Depression," *Yoga J.*, Nov/Dec 1999, p. 45.

[475] M. Walker, "Pressure Gets to You," *New Scient.*, Aug 1999, p. 16.

[476] J. Watkins, *Structure and Function of the Musculoskeletal System*, Human Kinetics, Champaign, IL, 1999.

[477] A. Weil, "Activity and Rest," *Yoga Intern.*, Oct 1998, p. 49.

[478] R. Weindruch, "Caloric Restrictions and Aging," *Sci. Am.*, Jan 1996, p. 46.

[479] A. Weintraub, "The Natural Prozac," *Yoga J.*, Nov/Dec 1999, p. 40.

[480] M. I. Weintraub, "Beauty Parlor Stroke Syndrome," *J. Am. Med. Assoc.* **269**, 2085 (1993).

[481] M. A. Wenger, B. K. Bagchi and B. K. Anand, "Experiments in India on 'Voluntary' Control of the Heart and Pulse," *Circulation* **24**, 1319 (1961).

[482] R. J. White, "Weightlessness and the Human Body," *Sci. Am.*, Sep 1998, p. 57.

[482a] R. Yee, personal communication, 2000.

[482b] *Yoga Calendar*, Yoga Journal, Berkeley, CA, 1993.

[483] Y. Yoshikawa, "Everybody Up Side Down," *Yoga J.*, Sep/Oct 2000, p. 94.

[484] M. W. Young, "The Tick-Tock of the Biological Clock," *Sci. Am.*, Mar 2000, p. 64.

[485] C. Zimmer, "Circus Science," *Discover* **19**, 56 (1996).

[486] C. Zimmer, "Into the Night," *Discover* **19**, 10 (1998).

INDEX

A

Abdomen, and the flexional reflex, *215;* psychoanatomy of, *163;* tension in, *215*

Abdominal aorta, *327*

Abdominal breathing, *370, 371;* action of the diaphragm in, *363, 364, 370;* and emotions, *374;* and *langhana*, *374;* and peristalsis, *371;* and RSA, *368;* and the tidal volume, *366;* and *viparita karani*, *370;* and visceral massage, *370, 371;* see also **Diaphragmatic breathing**

Abdominal contraction, and the central tendon, *363;* control of, *366;* and its cross inhibition with the diaphragm, *364;* and the diaphragmatic breath, *371;* and exhalation, *363;* and inhalation, *363;* when sneezing, *373;* and spinal curvature, *361;* and thoracic breathing, *372*

Abdominal muscles, Caesarian section and stretching of, *457*

Abducens nerve, see **Cranial nerve VI**

Accommodation, *413;* and yogic eye exercises, *419*

Acetabulum, as a joint, *97, 247, 249, 250, 260;* location of, *97, 237, 247*

Acetate ion, *116*

Acetylcholine, *115–117, 122, 128–130, 144–146, 400;* in bronchi, *359;* effect on the brain, *128;* excitatory action of, *123, 129;* in the heart, *315, 317;* and immunity, *386;* inhibitory action of, *123, 129;* in muscle action, *178;* and muscle fiber type, *189;* receptors for, *174*

Achilles tendon, reflex arc in, *213;* rupture of, *264*

Acoustic nerve, see **Cranial nerve VIII**

Acquired immunity, *383;* and lymphocytes, *384*

Acromion, *250;* and the glenoid fossa, *254, 258*

Actin, *172, 180;* overlap with myosin, *181, 185, 190, 194;* structure of, *178, 179, 190*

Action potential, *114, 117–119, 121, 123, 128;* and adaptation, *286;* in muscles, *173–175, 190*

Acupuncture meridians, *105*

Adaptation, *285–287;* in Meissner's corpuscles, *290;* in Merkel receptors, *291;* in muscle spindles, *202, 203;* of neurons, *116;* in Pacinian corpuscles, *290;* rapid, *286, 418;* in Ruffini corpuscles, *208;* slow, *286*

Adenosine diphosphate (ADP), in muscles, *182, 183*

Adenosine triphosphate (ATP), and cross bridges, *182, 183;* in dead muscles, *184;* as energy source, *116;* and exercise, *321, 496;* and free radicals, *497;* and hemoglobin, *369;* in muscles, *182–184, 191;* and stomach acidity, *445*

Adho mukha padmasana, and constipation, *398*

Adho mukha svanasana, *69, 152, 195, 230, 241;* and the carrying angle, *259;* and the epidermis, *283;* and exhalation, *364;* and gravity, *525;* head supported, *39, 220;* and neural crossover, *543;* and pelvic motion, *100;* and pressure on the floor, *554;* and rotation of the femur, *249;* and redistributing the mass, *554;* and humerus, *250, 547;* and the scapulae, *196, 258, 259*

Adho mukha virasana, and blood pressure, *349;* head supported, *39;* and the heart, *321;* and the ocular-vagal heart-slowing reflex, *549*

Adho mukha vrksasana, *42, 127, 191, 196, 349;* and balancing, *525, 534, 544–548;* and filament overlap, *186;* and the glenoid fossa, *255, 256;* and gravity, *525;* and resistive balancing, *545;* and skeletal alignment, *186, 241, 258, 259;* torque and countertorque in, *546;* and the vertebral arteries, *516;* and vision, *534;* yogic balance *versus* circus balance in, *548*

Adipose tissue, *279*

Adrenal cortex, aldosterone and salt regulation in, *405;* and androgens, *405;* and corticosteroids, *405;* and cortisol, *403, 405, 406;* and estrogen, *403, 405;* and the glenoid fossa, *255;* and glucose, *405, 406;* neural and hormonal stimulation of, *406;* and sex steroids, *405;* and stress, *156*

Adrenalcorticoids, see **Catecholamines**

Adrenal glands, *1, 405, 407;* and the ANS, *139;* and the hypothalamus, *399–403;* location of, *402;* relation to *chakras, 103;* and thoracic misalignment, *80*

Adrenal medulla, *128, 405;* and the ANS, *139, 145;* and the catecholamines, *403, 405, 406;* and endorphins, *147;* release of its hormones, *136;* and threat *versus* challenge, *466–468*

Adrenergic synapses, *407*

Adrenocorticotropic hormone (ACTH), and adrenal cortex, *403;* and anterior pituitary, *404;* and the ANS, *139, 143, 148;* and circadian rhythms, *479, 481, 482;* and cortisol, *404;* and immunity, *385;* and memory, *47;* mode of action of, *385;* ultradian release of, *476*

Aerobic oxidation, *184;* and *surya namaskar, 184*

Afferent neurons, *18, 84, 86, 172, 173;* compression of, *513;* in muscles, *175;* types of, *120*

Aging, *493–502;* and allergies, *494;* and Alzheimer's disease, *493;* and arthritis, *494;* and comparison to bedrest, *495;* and body fat, *494;* and bones, *244;* and brain plasticity, *113, 500;* and brain size, *500;* and cancer, *493, 494;* and cardiovascular conditioning, *494, 495, 500;* and cell division, *496;* and the cerebral cortex, *499;* and circadian rhythms, *486;* and collagen, *414, 496, 497;* and crosslinking of connective tissue, *279;* and dehydration of ground substance, *279;* and depression, *500;* and diabetes, *494;* and digestion, *494;* and dopamine, *500, 501;* effects of, *494–502;* and the EEG, *500, 501;* and exercise, *496;* and flexibility, *494;* and free radicals, *497;* and hearing, *437, 494, 495;* and the heart, *322, 493–497;* and homeostasis, *341;* and hot flashes, *494;* and hypertension, *337, 494;* and immunity, *390, 391, 500;* and intervertebral discs, *497;* and kidneys, *500;* and lateral bending, *497;* and the liver, *500;* and the locus ceruleus, *500;* and lumbar vertebrae, *82, 84, 93, 497;* and the lungs, *494–496;* and memory, *494, 501, 502;* and menopause, *494;* and mental alertness, *494;* and muscle-fiber type, *192, 495, 496;* and muscle strength, *192, 494, 495;* and neurogenesis, *500;* and norepinephrine, *500;* and osteoporosis, *494, 495;* and periodontal bone loss, *494;* and proprioception, *497;* and range of motion, *494;* and respiration, *494, 495;* and the sciatic nerve, *540;* and the sense of smell, *494;* and the sense of taste, *494;* and the sense of time, *473, 500, 501;* and the skin, *494;* and length of spine,

89, 90; and spinal mobility, *497;* and stroke, *494;* and T cells, *494;* and testosterone, *409;* and urinary incontinence, *494;* and $\dot{V}O_{2max}$, *496;* and vestibular balance, *497, 526;* and vision, *494;* and *vrksasana, 540;* and weightlessness, *556;* and *yogasana* practice, *496, 497, 499, 501;* see also **Brain Aging**

Agonist/antagonist pairs, *10, 189, 193–196;* and Golgi tendon organ, *206;* effect of interneurons on, *124*

AIDS virus, and lung infection, *388;* and T lymphocytes, *385–388;* and *yogasana* practice, *390*

Air, turbulence in the breath, *374*

Airways, diameters of, *359;* filtering by nose, *375;* and turbulence in, *374*

***Ajna chakra**, 103;* location of, *104*

Alcohol, dehydrogenase in males and females, *482;* and longevity, *498;* and osteoporosis, *270;* and effect on reticular formation, *33*

Aldosterone, and adrenal cortex, *403, 405;* and angiotensin II, *150, 335, 407;* and the ANS, *139, 149;* and salt regulation, *404;* as steroidal hormone, *401;* times of max/min concentration, *402*

Alertness, and the ANS, *147, 150;* and cortisol, *149;* time of minimum, *478–480;* and sleep/wake cycle, *489, 490*

Allergic reactions, *384, 387, 388;* and aging, *494;* and allergens, *383;* and B lymphocytes, *384;* and circadian rhythms, *481, 482;* and histamine, *388;* and the hypothalamus, *388;* and the spine, *79*

Alpha-motor neurons, *172–174;* dorsal-root locations of, *305;* in motor units, *113;* and nerves, *200–202;* effect of pressure on, *221;* and reflexes, *212, 222;* and the vestibular organs, *440*

Alpha receptors, and the arteries, *138;* and epinephrine, *129;* and the heart, *137;* and norepinephrine, *129, 407*

Alpha waves, and the ANS, *57, 59, 60, 138, 140, 150;* and color viewing, *427;* in depression, *50, 51, 466;* in the EEG, *32, 33, 59, 60, 138;* and the prefrontal cortex, *50, 153;* in psychosis, *61;* and relaxation, *44, 166;* and *savasana, 421, 490;* during sleep, *490;* and TV, *33;* and *yogasana* practice, *337, 468*

Alveoli, function of, *323, 358, 362, 364;* location of, *311;* stretch receptors in, *203;* structure of, *357, 358;* surface tension of, *374*

Alzheimer's disease, *40, 389;* and aging, *493*

Amacrine cells, *416*

Ambition, and *yogasana* injuries, *512*

Amenorrhea, *455;* and estrogen, *455;* and over-training, *455*

Amino acids, and the blood-brain barrier, *325;* in collagen, *273*

Amphetamines, and reticular formation arousal, *33, 130, 150*

Amygdala, and the emotions, *463;* function of, *34, 43;* and the hypothalamus, *143;* location of, *34;* and the sense of smell, *463*

Anaerobic oxidation, *183;* of glucose, *183, 191;* in type-3 muscle fibers, *191*

Anaesthesia, *33;* and the joints, *198, 264, 265;* and Na⁺ channels, *130;* and soft music, *437*

Anahata chakra, *75, 102, 103, 309;* location of, *104;* and immunity, *387;* and *nada* sound, *436;* and the thymus, *405*

Analgesia, *38, 302, 303*

Anantasana, *247;* balancing in, *541;* vision and balance in, *534;* and the internal wall, *536*

Androgens, and the adrenal cortex, *403, 405;* and the testes, *409;* and testosterone, *409*

Anemia, *324, 369;* and zero gravity, *555*

Anger, *155, 463;* and the breath, *472;* and *halasana*, *226, 471;* and the hypothalamus, *142, 471;* and muscle tension, *463*

Angina, and circadian rhythms, *479*

Angiotensin II, and aldosterone, *335, 407;* in brain and kidneys, *130;* and renin, *150;* as a vasoconstrictor, *335, 338*

Angiotensinogen, and renin, *335, 338*

Ankle, balancing on, *537–542;* blood circulation in *vrksasana*, *540;* motion of, *252, 253*

Annulus fibrosus, *87*

Anoxia, *435*

Antagonist muscles, *185;* see also **Agonist /Antagonist Pairs**

Anterior hypothalamus, *138;* and control of the ANS, *14;* function of, *144, 203;* location of, *141*

Anterior pituitary, *400;* and ACTH, *404;* and gonadotropin RF, *404;* and growth hormone, *404;* and prolactin, *404;* and thyroid SH, *404*

Anterior thalamic nuclei, location of, *34*

Antibodies, and antigens, *384;* and immunoglobulins, *384*

Anticholinergic drugs, and motion sickness, *440*

Antidiuretic hormone (ADH), see **Vasopressin**

Antigens and antibodies, *384;* and B lymphocytes, *384*

Antioxidants, *502*

Anus, *16;* and coccygeal misalignment, *80;* location of, *443;* pressure in and *uddiyana bandha*, *447;* sphincters of, *397*

Anxiety, *463, 470, 471;* and the anterior hypothalamus, *203;* and the apocrine glands, *395;* and blue lights, *469;* and the breath, *472;* and cancer, *387;* and chronotherapy, *487; versus* depression, *470;* and headache, *38, 481;* and immunity, *471;* and inversions, *349;* and menopause, *461;* and muscle tone, *471;* and the placebo effect, *164, 165;* and relaxation, *471;* and stressors, *154–156;* symptoms of, *470;* and thoracic breathing, *372;* and type-A PMS, *454;* and *yogasana* practice, *471*

Aorta, *329;* blood flow through, *329, 331;* blood pressure in, *310, 311, 314, 329;* function of, *312, 314, 325, 326;* and inversions, *346;* location of, *310, 311, 360, 443;* oxygen sensors in, *367;* stress-strain curve for, *278*

Aortic arch, and baroreceptors, *339, 340;* blood pressure and inversions, *345;* and EEG shifts, *341;* location of, *310, 339*

Apana **energy**, and menstruation, *455*

Aponeuroses, *235, 262*

Apoptosis, of nerves and muscles, *112, 128*

Appendicular skeleton, *236, 247–260;* and arms, *254–260;* and feet, *252–254;* and legs, *247–253, 255;* see also **Arms**, **Forearms**, **Feet**, **Legs**, etc.

Appendix, location of, *443*

Aqueous humour, location of, *414*

Arachidonic acid, and pain, *126*

Arachnoid layer, *93*

Arch of the foot, collapse of, *280;* and pregnancy, *458*

Ardha baddha padma paschimottanasana, *127;* and muscle compression, *221, 222*

Ardha chandrasana, *11, 33;* and balancing, *418, 525, 535, 536;* and resistive balancing, *545;* and rotation of the femur, *249;* against the wall, *536;* and the internal wall, *536*

Ardha halasana, and type-H PMS, *455*

Ardha matsyendrasana I, *91*

Ardha navasana, *220;* and breathing, *365*

Ardha padmasana, *266, 531*

Arms, psychoanatomy of, *163;* rotation of, *78, 79, 256–259;* structure of, *254–256;* and thoracic misalignment, *80;* see also **Forearm** and **Glenoid fossa**

Arousal, and amphetamines, *33, 130, 150;* see also **Reticular formation**

Arteries, *311, 329;* blood of, *313;* blood flow through, *329, 331;* blood pressure in, *329;* and the catecholamines, *406;* collapse of, *185;* diameter of, *327;* and elastin, *275, 494;* function of, *325;* and headaches, *334;* musculature of, *326–328;* pulmonary, *310, 326;* vasoconstriction and the ANS, *139;* vasodilation and the ANS, *139;* wall structure of, *328, 330, 331*

Arterioles, *311, 312, 329;* and blood flow, *327–329, 331, 340, 341;* blood pressure in, *329;* dilation by epinephrine, *129;* function of, *325–327;* muscle tone of, *312, 331, 346;* and pressure drop in, *330, 331*

Arthritis, *5, 6;* and aging, *494;* and joint lubrication, *265, 267, 271;* and obesity, *271;* and thoracic misalignment, *80;* and the weather, *267*

Asana, *6, 9*

Ascending colon, location of, *443*

Ascending information, *16, 32, 85, 86*

Ashtanga yoga, *9*

Aspartate ion, as a neurotransmitter, *129*

Aspirin, *5;* and menstrual pain, *456;* and the prostaglandins, *296, 456*

Asthma, *359;* and allergens, *359;* and the ANS, *166;* and chronotherapy, *486, 487;* and cigarettes, *359;* and circadian rhythms, *478, 479;* and the diaphragmatic breath, *372;* and exhalation, *359;* and the immune system, *387;* and over-training, *359;* placebo treatment of, *164;* and *pranayama*, *359;* and thoracic misalignment, *80;* precipitated by *yogasana* practice, *372*

Astrological signs, and the placebo effect, *164*

Asymmetry, in the brain, *49–57, 522;* of the breath, *519;* of the colon, *522;* and connective tissue, *522;* of cranial nerve X, *522;* in embryos, *522;* and poor health, *519;* of proprioception, *520;* of the viscera, *522*

Atherosclerotic plaque, *331;* and hypertension, *338;* and *savasana*, *338*

Atlanto-axial joint, and spinal twists, *517;* and the vertebral arteries, *517*

Atlanto-occipital joint, *67, 74*

Atonia, in REM sleep, *488*

Atrial baroreceptor, function of, *342;* in inversions, *345*

Atrial volume receptor, and diastolic blood pressure, *341;* in supine postures, *555;* and urination following inversion, *351, 396, 397*

Atrium, function of, *312, 313, 318;* location of, *310*

Atroventricular (AV) node, and the heart beat, *309, 315–317;* and Purkinje cells, *316*

Atypical depression, *464;* and handedness, *466;* and SAD, *431*

Attitudes; *468;* and gamma-motor neurons, *202, 214;* and immunity, *386;* negative/positive, *152;* and rheumatoid arthritis, *388;* and stress, *160*

Audition, see **Hearing**

Auditory cortex, *18, 19, 28;* location of, *27*

Auditory memory, and eye motion, *425*

Authority-patient relationship, *166*

Autism, and oxytocin, *404;* and excess testosterone, *410*

Autoimmune reaction, *387, 388;* and rheumatoid arthritis, *388;* and stress, *155*

Autonomic nervous system (ANS), *5, 11, 13–15, 17, 133–166, 317, 386, 387;* balancing of, *159, 160;* and beta waves, *60;* and bipolar disorder, *469;* and bones, *246;* branches of, *136, 137, 144–153;* and the breath, *139;* and the CNS, *442;* and cerebral laterality, *138, 422;* and cigarette smoke, *147;* and the clitoris, *461;* and the colon, *145;* and colored lights, *426–430;* conscious control of, *135, 156–158, 161, 317;* and cortisol, *139, 148, 149, 386;* and CRF, *139, 148, 153;* and defecation, *150, 397;* and depression, *467, 468;* and digestive secretions, *448;* dominance of and circadian rhythms, *480, 482;* and the EEG, *138;* and the emotions, *160–166;* and the endocrine glands, *400;* and endorphins, *139;* and the eyes, *138, 145, 150, 151;* and fatty acids, *139, 147;* and feedback, *134;* and finger temperature, *158;* and the gastrointestinal organs, *138;* and glucagon, *139, 147;* and glucose, *138, 139, 147;* and glycogen, *138, 139;* and habituation, *138;* and the heart, *137, 145, 147, 150, 364;* and homeostasis, *150;* and hunger, *442;* and the hypothalamus, *135;* and insulin, *139, 150;* and intraocular pressure, *138;* and lactic acid, *139;* and lie detectors, *60, 159, 293;* and the liver, *145, 153;* and the lungs, *145;* and the lymph nodes, *386;* and lymphocytes, *386;* and the motor unit, *145;* and mucus, *139, 393, 394;* and muscles, *139;* and nutrients, *13;* and osteoblasts, *246;* and osteoclasts, *246;* and piloerection, *140, 148, 150;* response to color, *422;* and salivation, *139, 145, 150;* and serotonin, *137;* and tears, *139, 150, 393;* and type-A PMS, *454;* and ultradian rhythm, *476;* and vasoconstriction, *138;* and vasodilation, *138;* and visual stress, *420;* and *yogasana* practice, *156–158, 463*

Axial skeleton, *235*

Axilla, and nasal laterality, *139, 159, 377, 379;* and *padadirasana*, *379;* and sweat glands, *395*

Axon, *108, 121, 122;* plate of, *109;* effect of pressure on, *125;* transport in, *128*

Ayurveda, and breathing, *355;* and color therapy, *426;* and the *doshas*, *483, 484;* and the fear center, *216;* hourly rhythms of, *483, 484*

B

Back, density of skin receptors on, *288*

Backbending, benefits of, *83, 84;* and depression, *467;* and epinephrine, *216–218;* and fear, *215–218, 471;* and the flexional reflex, *215;* and immunity, *389;* and inhalation, *356;* and the kidneys, *216;* and the lumbar spine, *75, 93, 497;* and menopause, *459, 460;* and norepinephrine, *217;* and rotation of the femurs, *250;* and sexual stimulation, *216;* supported, *218, 389;* see also **Spinal extension**

Bacteria, *13, 155, 325, 383;* and balance, *447;* in colon, *446;* and infection, *481;* and killer T cells, *385;* and lymphocytes, *384, 386;* and saliva, *393, 394;* in the small intestine, *447;* and tears, *395;* and vitamins, *446*

Baddha konasana, *78;* conscious action in, *223;* and menstrual cramps, *231;* and rotation of femurs, *249, 262, 266*

Bakasana, *98, 177;* balancing in, *525, 548, 549*

Balancing, *20, 525, 552;* and the basal ganglia, *532, 533;* using the big toe, *538, 539;* as a broomstick, *528, 538, 539;* and the center of gravity, *554, 555;* and the corpus callosum, *543;* and the eyes, *45, 411;* general points on, *551, 552;* and center of gravity, *526;* and gravity, *525, 556;* and head position, *534;* and inverted poses, *542–552;* and the light level, *422, 535;* and mechanoreceptors, *556;* and *navasana*, *525;* and Newton's Law, *553;* and neural crossover, *543;* and the Pacinian corpuscles, *526, 530, 539, 540;* and proprioception, *556;* and receptive fields, *417, 539;* and redistributing the mass, *536, 537;* of rigid blocks, *526–529;* in standing poses, *537–542;* and strength, *527;* and torque/countertorque, *528–530;* in *uttanasana*, *530;* and the vestibular-ocular motor reflex, *418, 535;* and vestibular organs, *33, 67, 438–440, 526, 533, 556;* and vision, *526, 533–535, 542*

Balancing-pole effect, see **Redistributing the mass**

Balasana, and type-A PMS, *454*

Baroreceptors, *198, 338–341;* in carotid arteries, *37;* and cranial nerve X, *339;* and *halasana*, *347, 348;* and the heart, *340, 341;* and hypertension, *335;* and inclined/inverted postures, *341, 348;* and interneurons, *340;* and laughter, *341, 351;* and the medulla, *339, 340;* and reflex arcs, *340, 341;* lack of sensitivity of, *337, 338*

Bhakti yoga, *9*

Ballistic stretching, *226*

Basal ganglia, *18;* and balance, *533;* connections to other centers, *173, 222, 533;* function of, *34, 35, 177*

Basilar-artery syndrome, and *bhujangasana*, *512,* and *sarvangasana*, *512*

Basilar membrane, *433*

Bastrika, *382*

Beauty, *13;* and health, *519;* in man, *519;* and symmetry, *519*

Bedrest, and relation to aging, *495;* effect on bones, *241;* and osteoporosis, *270*

Beta receptors, and the arteries, *137;* and the bronchioles, *406;* and the catecholamines, *129, 406;* and the heart, *137, 406;* and the pancreas, *407, 408*

Beta waves, and the ANS, *60;* arousal and, *50;* and colored lights, *430;* in depression, *50, 51;* in the EEG, *32, 59–61, 138, 140;* in psychosis, *61;* relation to cerebral hemispheres, *140;* during sleep and relaxation, *33, 44, 488*

Bharadvajasana I, *78*

Bhujangasana, *69;* and the basilar-artery syndrome, *512*

Bicarbonate ion (HCO₃⁻), in blood, *367*

Biceps brachii, *191;* and its antagonist, *193;* and forearm rotation, *257;* inhibition of by triceps, *196;* and isometric contraction, *187;* location of, *168, 197;* muscle attachments to, *171;* reflex arcs in, *212;* action on scapulae, *196;* and speed of contraction, *172*

Biceps femoris, location of, *169;* and patellar knee-jerk reflex, *212, 213;* and reciprocal inhibition of, *195*

Big toe, use in balancing, *539;* pressure receptors in, *539;* use in *vrksasana*, *539;* see also **Hallux**

Bile, and the gallbladder, *401, 448*

Bioelectrochemistry, *108*

Biofeedback, *114, 144*

Biorhythms, and headache, *39;* and hormones, *142, 403;* and pregnancy, *457;* see also **Circadian rhythms**, **Infradian rhythms**, and **Ultradian rhythms**

Bipolar cell, function of, *112;* structure of, *109, 110;* in vision, *132, 416*

Bipolar disorder, *469, 470;* and blue light, *469;* and the catecholamines, *469;* and core temperature, *469;* and lithium, *469;* relation to mania, *469;* and SAD, *470;* and *yogasana* practice, *470*

Black Americans, and hypertension, *338*

Bladder, and the ANS, *147, 212;* and cranial nerve X, *151;* dermatome for, *306*

Blinking, *20, 413;* and the ANS, *138, 413;* and dirty corneas, *414;* and forced unilateral breathing, *379;* and stress, *413;* and the superior tarsal muscle, *413;* and tears, *395;* and *yogasana* practice, *413*

Blood, acidity of, *246, 373, 367;* and bones, *235;* function of, *322, 323;* hemorrhage, *352;* and hormones, *323;* and hyperventilation, *372, 373;* and the immune system, *323;* and nutrients, *323, 406;* plasma, *323;* viscosity and chronotherapy, *486*

Blood-brain barrier, and glucose, *325;* and immunity, *388, 389;* and white blood cells, *325*

Blood-air mixing, *358*

Blood clotting, and the ANS, *147, 148;* and blood flow, *162, 243*

Blood flow, *330–332;* and the ANS, *136, 147;* through brain, *79;* and clotting, *162, 243;* and headaches, *162;* healing effects of, *162;* and immunity, *162, 384;* and inversions, *349;* through the lungs, *358;* and muscle contraction, *332;* and pressure drop, *331;* rates of, *323;* rerouting of, *177, 178, 323;* resistance to, *331;* shift of supply, *320;* and turbulence, *332;* types, *323, 324;* through the vertebral arteries, *330;* and vascular diameters, *334;* and vasopressin, *47;* velocity *versus* area, *329–331;* and warming up, *227;* in *yoganidrasana, 161, 162;* see also **Circulation** and **Heart**

Blood pressure, *11, 20;* and the ANS, *137, 147, 148, 150;* and the baroreceptor reflex, *340;* and breathing, *364;* and chemoreceptors for, *342;* and chronotherapy, *486;* and circadian rhythms, *478–482;* diastolic, *311, 312, 315, 322;* gender differences and, *160;* and green color, *427;* and homeostasis, *338, 341;* and inversions, *342, 349–351;* and peripheral resistance, *340;* in REM sleep, *488;* and renin, *335;* and stressors, *153, 155;* systolic, *311, 312, 315;* unilateral breathing, *54;* and vasopressin, *404;* in venules, *329;* and *yogasana* practice, *337*

Blood sensors, atrial fractional volume, *341;* stroke volume, *342*

Blood vessels, *1;* in the spine, *81, 88*

Blue-color viewing, and anxiety, *469;* effects of viewing, *427;* and emotions, *429, 469;* and

mania, *469;* and muscle strength, *429;* and norepinephrine, *469*

B lymphocytes, and allergies, *384;* and antigens, *384;* and bone marrow, *384;* and lymph nodes, *384;* response to bacteria, *384;* and rheumatoid arthritis, *388;* and the spleen, *384*

Body clock, *134, 421, 422, 473–491;* and the endocrine system, *422*

Body fat, and aging, *494, 499;* and longevity, *498;* and menstruation, *454*

Body intelligence, and B.K.S. Iyengar, *130*

Body maps, in the brain, *209, 210;* in the eye, *176;* in the foot, *176;* in the hand, *176;* see also ***Homunculi***

Bones, *1, 235–272;* of the appendicular skeleton, *236;* of the axial skeleton, *236;* and blood, *235, 246;* cranial, *96;* and estrogen/progesterone balance, *408;* facial, *96;* fibers in, *273;* flat, *235, 237;* and growth hormone, *236, 244;* and B lymphocytes, *384;* and ligaments, *235;* long, *235, 236, 240;* oligomenorrhea and loss of, *455;* and platelets, *238;* and testosterone, *408*

Bone chemistry, and blood acidity, *246;* and Ca^{2+}, *235, 242, 243;* and cartilage, *235;* and collagen, *236, 241, 242;* and detoxification, *242, 243;* and hydrochloric acid, *242;* and hydroxyapatite, *235, 236, 240–242;* and lead, *243;* and phosphorus, *235;* and zero gravity, *555*

Bone density, *241, 242;* and estrogen/progesterone balance, *408, 409;* and osteoporosis, *241, 269, 272;* and *yogasana* practice, *241*

Bone marrow, *22, 238, 239;* and leucocytes, *383;* and red blood cells, *369*

Bone remodeling, *64, 236, 244–246;* and repair, *236, 244*

Bone strength, and aging, *494;* and bedrest, *242;* and hydroxyapatite, *246;* and mechanics, *240, 241;* and muscle tone, *240;* and *yogasana* practice, *241, 500*

Bone structure, *241, 269;* cancellous, *63, 236, 239, 240, 269;* and collagen, *236, 241, 242;* and connective tissue, *238;* cortical, *236, 239, 240, 269;* and the epiphyseal line, *236, 238, 239, 251, 260,* innervation of, *238–240;* and ligaments, *235;* vascularization of, *238–240*

Bottom brain, *24*

Bottom hinge, *249*

Bow legs, *100, 247, 248*

Brachialis, location of, *168, 197;* action on scapulae, *196;* inhibition by triceps, *196*

Brachioradialis, location of, *168;* use of, *197*

Braille, *289*

Brain, *14, 16, 18, 20;* and the ANS, *138;* asymmetry of, *49–57, 522;* and blood flow, *35–37, 84;* and cerebrospinal fluid, *93;* and higher centers, *87, 125, 195;* interactions amongst centers, *173;* and cell connections, *21;* cell death in, *21, 22;* development and maturation, *40;* gender differences, *41;* gray matter, *93, 107;* immune system of, *388, 389;* inhibition in, *29;* hemorrhage and circadian rhythm in, *481, 482;* and hypertension, *40;* movement on breathing, *364;* movement in *savasana, 364;* myelination of, *39;* neurogenesis in, *40;* and noncentralization of function, *24, 25, 29;* and nutrients, *93;* overheating of, *375;* oxygenation of, *84;* pain in, *37;* plasticity of, *21, 42, 43, 46, 113, 500;* relation to retina, *418;* reptilian, *133;* ventricles of, *93;* weight and size, *21, 35, 40, 500;* and white matter, *107*

Brain aging, cells of, *496;* and exercise, *501,* and diet, *501,* and size, *500;* and *yogasana* practice, *501*

Brainstem, *14–18, 20, 22, 25, 30;* connections to other centers, *173, 202;* and salivation, *393*

Brainwave frequencies, and mental functions, *60, 61;* and learning/memory, *60, 61*

***Brahmarandra**, 101*

Breast cancer, and excess estrogen, *410;* and hormone replacement, *460;* and melatonin, *404*

Breasts, and estrogen/progesterone balance, *408;* hormones and development, *408*

Breath, and the endorphins, *303;* and depression, *472;* illness and odor of, *365;* and pain, *472*

Breathing, *1, 20, 30;* in *ardha navasana, 366;* and the ANS, *139;* control centers for, *365;* and emotions, *63, 374, 471, 472;* and gas exchange, *372, 373;* and the heart rate, *364, 379;* and interneurons, *365;* and *maricyasana III, 366;* and old age, *373;* and personality, *162;* and posture, *373;* and relaxation, *202;* and rib motion, *363;* and symmetry, *519;* and ultradian rhythm, *475, 476;* and venous blood flow, *367;* see also **Abdominal breathing, Diaphragmatic breathing, Thoracic breathing,** and **Respiratory system**

Breathing rate, pacemaker for, *365*

Breech presentation, and muscle tension, *457;* and *yogasana* practice, *457*

***Brmhana**, 355, 356;* and *pranayama, 382;* properties of, *356;* and the sympathetic NS, *374;* and the thoracic breath, *374*

Brodmann areas, *28, 29*

Bronchi, *144;* and circadian rhythms, *479;* contraction and the parasympathetic NS, *359, 479;* diameters of, *359;* dilation and the sympathetic NS, *359;* location of, *311, 356, 357;* mucus and the surface of, *394;* and norepinephrine, *359;* and stretch receptors, *203;* structure of, *356*

Bronchioles, and beta receptors, *407;* and cranial nerve X, *151;* dilation and epinephrine, *148;* movement of air through, *362;* and the placebo effect, *164;* and stretch receptors in, *203;* structure of, *357;* and the sympathetic NS, *136, 139*

Bronchospasm, *359*

Broomstick model, for balancing, *528–530;* and *sirsasana, 549;* and *urdhva hastasana, 537;* and *virabhadrasana III, 542;* and *vrksasana, 538*

Bruises, effect of blood flow on, *162*

Bulimia, and bright lights, *431*

Bursae, and cervical misalignment, *79;* in the gluteus maximus, *187, 263;* and the greater trochanter, *263;* in knee, *251;* structure of, *187, 263*

Bursitis, *79, 187*

C

Caduceus, *102*

Caesarian section, and stretching, *457*

Caffeine, *38*

Calcaneus, location of, *237, 252*

Calcitonin, *243;* and the thyroid, *405*

Calcium ion (Ca^{2+}), *122, 128;* in the blood, *246;* and blood clotting, *243;* and bones, *235, 242, 243;* and calcitonin, *405;* circadian excretion cycle, *397;* and detoxification, *243;* and heart contraction, *315–317, 319;* and homeostasis, *243, 246;* and muscle contraction, *173, 178;* and oscillator Y, *477;* and osteoporosis, *270;* and the parathyroid, *405;* action on troponin, *178;* and urination, *397*

Cancer, *6, 385–388;* and aging, *493;* and AIDS, *388;* and anxiety, *387;* and attitudes, *386;* and chronotherapy, *486;* death by, *501;* and depressed immunity; *387;* and depression, *387;* and estrogen, *410;* and killer T cells, *384, 385;* and lymph edema, *353;* and melatonin, *404;* and N-nitrosamines, *393, 394;* and stress, *155, 387;* and tumors, *387*

Capillaries, *329;* blood flow through, *329–331;* blood pressure in, *329;* diameter at systole, *353;* formation during stretching, *177, 184, 321;* function of, *325, 328;* and hypoxia, *367;* within the lungs, *358;* and lymph, *352;* and

red-blood-cell diameter, *330;* and type-1
  fibers, *190;* and *yogasana* practice, *321*
Carbohydrates, digestion of, *444;* as fuel for
  muscles, *184, 369;* in ground substance, *275;*
  and stress, *449;* and serotonin, *449*
Carbon dioxide (CO$_2$), in blood, *369;* chemoreceptors for, *342, 366;* and hemoglobin, *369;*
  and *kumbhaka, 382;* and panic attacks, *471*
Cardiac muscle (see also **Heart**), arrhythmia of,
  155; blood supply for, *315;* output of, *369,*
  476; pacemaker for, *20;* comparison to skeletal muscle, *314, 315;* contraction of, *313, 314;*
  synapse with acetylcholine, *123*
Cardiac notch, location of, *357, 359*
Cardiac plexus, *103, 104*
Cardiac systole, and capillary diameters, *353*
Cardiovascular system, *1, 4, 6;* and aging,
  493–495, 500; chronotherapy for, *487;* and
  exercise, *496;* and ultradian rhythms, *476;* and
  yogasana practice, *500*
Carotid artery, *327;* baroreceptors in, *220,*
  338–340; and chemoreceptors, *342, 367;*
  common, *36, 37;* and EEG changes, *341;*
  external, *36;* internal, *36;* nerve plexus, *104*
Carpal bones, location of, *237*
Carpal tunnel syndrome, *127, 459*
Carrying angle, at elbow, *259;* in *adho mukha*
  svanasana, 259
Cartilage, *275, 280, 281;* and bone formation,
  235, 239; and chondrocytes, *280;* injury to,
  281; in joints, *96;* as joint lubricant, *236, 237,*
  280, 281; and meniscus of knee, *281;* piezoelectric property of, *280*
Cataracts, *414*
Catecholamines, and adrenal medulla, *405, 406;*
  and backbending, *216–218;* and beta receptors, *406;* and bipolar disorder, *469;* and emotions, *129;* and depression, *464, 466;* and
  fight-or-flight, *407, 415;* and forced unilateral
  breathing, *378;* and gender differences, *161;*
  and glycogenolysis, *148;* in headache, *38;* and
  the heart, *148, 319;* hormonal release of, *147,*
  148; and hypertension, *335, 336;* and mania,
  469; and muscle action, *183;* as neurotransmitters, *129, 144, 145;* and pupil diameter,
  415; and stressors, *153, 154, 156;* and ultradian rhythms, *476;* and vasoconstriction, *148;*
  see also **Epinephrine** and **Norepinephrine**
Cell membrane, permeability to Na$^+$, *115–117,*
  119; permeability to K$^+$, *116, 117;* of
  organelles, *109;* structure of, *108*
Center of gravity, *56, 69, 70, 526, 527, 537;* and
  balance, *554, 555;* and extension, *554;* and

hasta padangusthasana, 537; and *malasana,*
  537
Central nervous system, *1, 13, 14, 16, 17, 63,*
  84, 107, 108, 125, 128; and the ANS, *146;*
  and the colon, *442;* habituation of, *297;* and
  the muscles, *172;* and pain, *295;* and the rectum, *442*
Central-pattern generators, *43, 87*
Central sulcus, *24, 26;* location of, *27, 173*
Central tendon, and the abdominal muscles,
  363; and the diaphragm, *360, 362, 363*
Cerebellum, *14–16, 18, 29, 172;* and balance,
  532, 533; function of, *33, 43, 177, 209;* inhibition by, *33;* location of, *24;* and tickling,
  289
Cerebral arteries, *36;* blood flow through, *26*
Cerebral cortex, *22;* and aging, *499;* and baroreceptors, *339;* hemispheres of, *4, 14, 15, 22*
Cerebral dominance, and breathing, *356;* and
  handedness, *56, 523;* and memory, *51;* and
  ultradian rhythms, *474*
Cerebral laterality, *4, 17;* in animals, *51, 52;*
  and the retinal cones, *424;* and corpus callosum, *424;* and depression, *466, 468;* and the
  EEG, *55;* and emotions, *463;* and handedness,
  425; and hearing, *433, 434;* and lesbians, *523;*
  in mammals, *52;* and nasal laterality, *54, 55,*
  381, 422; and neural crossover, *422;* oscillation of, *54, 55;* and OCD, *468;* and optical
  crossover, *422–424;* properties of, *52;* and
  pupil diameter, *424;* and shift in *savasana,*
  165; and testosterone, *50, 409;* and vision,
  422; relation to World Views, *53*
Cerebrospinal fluid, *16, 47, 84, 93–95;* composition of, *93;* flow pattern of, *95;* functions of,
  93; and *halasana, 346;* and H$^+$ ions, *367;* and
  hydrostatic pressure of, *344, 346;* and the
  hypothalamus, *93;* and B.K.S Iyengar, *95;* and
  the optic nerve, *418;* pressure of, *94, 95;* pulsations of, *94, 95, 474;* reabsorption of, *93, 94*
Cerebrum, connections to other centers, *173;*
  and kinaesthesia, *50;* location of, *24;* size in
  man and animals, *23*
Cervical flexion reflex, *218–220;* see also
  Jalandhara bandha
Cervical spine, nerves, *15, 16*
Cervical vertebrae, in extension, *82;* foramina
  in, *36, 65, 66;* and *halasana, 81;* herniated
  disc in, *74, 91;* lateral bending, *72, 73;* location of, *64, 65, 69;* misalignment of, *79;* movement of, *38;* range of motion, *67, 68, 72, 73,*
  90; rotation about, *78, 81*

Chakras, *1, 101–105;* associated colors, *103, 105;* locations of, *104;* and lymph glands, *103, 105*

Chandra bhedana, *382*

Chaturanga dandasana, *191, 230;* and co-contraction, *196;* and gravity, *556*

Chemoreceptors, *342;* for carbon dioxide, *342, 367;* for hydrogen ion, *342;* for oxygen, *342, 367;* and regulation of blood pressure, *342;* and regulation of heart rate, *342;* and regulation of respiration rate, *342*

Chewing, *19*

Chi, *105*

Child birth, *48;* and pelvis, *98, 99;* and pubic symphysis, *98;* time of, *481;* trauma of, *49*

Chloride ion, *116;* and GABA, *129*

Cholesterol, *401;* and circadian rhythm, *478, 479*

Cholinergic synapse, *407*

Chronotherapy, and anxiety, *487;* and asthma, *486, 487;* and blood pressure, *486;* and blood viscosity, *486;* and cancer, *486;* for cardiovascular problems, *486, 487;* for depression, *487;* and the heart rate, *486;* and hot flashes, *487;* for hypertension, *487;* and osteoarthritis, *487;* for rheumatoid arthritis, *487;* and the sleep/wake cycle, *488–491;* and Western medicine, *486;* and *yogasana* practice, *486, 487*

Chyme, *444, 446;* buffering of pH by, *447, 448*

Cigarette smoke/smoking, and asthma attacks, *359;* and the ANS, *147;* reaction with hemoglobin, *370;* and longevity, *498, 499;* and osteoporosis, *270;* see also **Nicotine**

Ciliary muscles, and cranial nerve III, *413, 414;* ganglia for, *423;* and lens focusing, *413;* location of, *414*

Cingulate gyrus, location of, *34*

Circadian rhythm, *476–484;* and aging, *486;* and alertness, *478, 480;* and allergies, *480–482;* and anxiety, *481;* and ANS dominance, *480, 482, 483;* and asthma, *478, 479;* and blood pressure, *478–482;* and brain hemorrhage, *481, 482;* and bronchial constriction, *479;* for Ca^{2+} excretion, *397;* and cholesterol, *478, 479;* and core temperature, *476, 478–482, 485, 486;* and cortisol, *402, 465, 476, 478–482;* and CRF, *149;* and depression, *481, 482;* and digestion, *479–481;* and entrainment, *477;* and eosinophils, *478;* and epinephrine, *478–480, 482;* and the eyes, *421;* and flexibility, *491;* and glycogen, *479;* and growth hormone, *478, 479;* and headaches, *478, 481, 482;* and T cells, *478, 479;* and heart attacks, *478–482, 484;* and hemoglobin,

479, 480; and histamine, *478, 479, 482;* and hormones, *478, 479, 481, 482;* and the hypothalamus, *483, 485;* and immune response, *481, 482;* and insulin, *478, 480;* and liver function, *478, 479;* and lung function, *478, 480, 482;* mechanism of, *484–486;* and melatonin, *479, 480, 485;* and memory, *479, 481, 482;* and menstruation, *478;* and mental acuity, *479–482;* and muscle strength, *480;* and muscle tone, *478, 479, 481;* and neutrophils, *478, 479;* and osteoarthritis, *480–482;* for Na^+ excretion, *397;* and pain, *478, 481;* and platelets, *478, 480;* for K^+ excretion, *397, 476;* and reflex sensitivity, *480;* and respiration, *480;* and rheumatoid arthritis, *479, 482;* for salivation, *393, 480;* and salt excretion, *480;* and sleep, *482, 485;* and stroke, *478–480;* and the suprachiasmatic nucleus, *422, 485;* and urinary volume, *479, 481;* and vasopressin, *47, 485;* and visual pigment, *485*

Circulation, and red color, *427;* and resting muscle tone, *205;* and *yogasana* practice, *390*

Clavicle, and the glenoid fossa, *254, 258,* location of, *237, 357, 360;* connection to manubrium, *254*

Clitoral erection, *140;* and the ANS, *462;* and REM sleep, *461, 488*

Cluster headache, *38*

Coccygeal branch, *16*

Coccygeal vertebrae, location of, *64, 65;* range of motion of, *68*

Coccyx, joint, *97;* location of, *97, 98, 237;* nerve plexus of, *104*

Cochlea, *433;* location of, *434, 438;* and *nada* sound, *436*

Co-contraction, of muscles, *188, 195, 196, 223*

Cold feet, in inversions, *349, 350*

Collagen, *242, 273, 274,* and aging, *414, 496, 497;* and amino acids, *273;* and bone, *236, 241, 242;* and bone repair, *244;* crosslinks in, *274;* fibers, *273;* fibrils, *273;* and fibroblasts, *273;* in ligaments, *262, 263;* in the sclera of eyes, *414;* in skin, *284;* as a structural member, *112*

Colon, asymmetry of, *443, 522;* and the ANS, *145;* and the central nervous system, *442;* and exercise, *446;* and fiber, *446;* and gases, *446;* and the liver, *446;* and lumbar misalignment, *80;* and microbes, *446;* and the stool, *450*

Colored lights, and alpha waves, *427;* and the ANS, *426–430;* and depression, *427, 468, 469;* and emotions, *429;* and eyeblink rate, *427;* hearing, *117;* and heart rate, *427;* and isometric contraction, *429;* and mania, *469;* and the motivational system, *429;* and muscle strength, *429;* and palmar conductance, *427;* and pink agitation, *427;* and PMS, *427;* and respiration rate, *426;* and systolic pressure, *426, 427;* as yoga props, *430;* and *yogasana* practice, *426, 428–430, 468, 469*

Color therapy, *426–428*

Coma, *32*

Compression, as a mechanical force, *76;* of nerves, *126;* of the spinal vertebrae, *91*

Compressive stress, *228, 229, 241*

Concentration gradients, *110, 111, 114, 115*

Cones, and color sensitivity, *415, 416;* and the fovea, *415, 417;* function of, *415;* neuroanatomy of, *416;* and visual laterality, *424*

Congenital weakness, and *yogasana* injury, *512, 517*

Conjunctiva, location of, *414*

Connective tissue, *273–280;* asymmetry of, *522;* and aging, *279;* and body shape, *522;* in contracting muscles, *171, 187;* contribution from bones, *238;* function of, *273;* and injury, *279, 280;* and menopause, *460;* and stretching, *189, 190, 224;* and viscoelasticity, *277*

Conrotatory twisting, *79, 91, 96;* in *maricyasana III,* *98*

Consciousness, *9–11, 17, 22, 25;* dual, *53;* and the heart, *317;* and homeostasis, *342;* mixing with subconscious, *135, 157, 172, 199, 212;* overload of, *31, 32, 107;* and receptors, *199;* regulation by reticular formation, *31*

Consolidation, *43–47;* and sleep, *47, 61*

Constipation, and depression, *464;* and inversions, *349, 397, 398, 450;* and *maricyasana III,* *450;* and peristalsis, *397;* and pregnancy, *459;* and pressure on colon walls, *450;* and relaxin, *459;* and *yogasana* practice, *397, 398, 500*

Contortion, *190*

Contractile force, *317, 320;* and baroreceptor reflex, *340, 341*

Contracture, *205*

Coracoid process, *258*

Core temperature, *137;* and bipolar disorder, *469;* and circadian rhythms, *476, 478–482;* and fever, *388;* and mania, *469;* and oscillator X, *477;* stressors and, *153*

Cornea, *18, 413;* and blinking, *414;* and blood vessels, *414;* location of, *414;* stress-strain curve for, *278*

Coronary artery, diameter of, *320;* location of, *327*

Coronary ventricles, contraction of, *325;* function of, *312–314;* location of, *310, 311*

Corpus callosum, and balancing, *543;* and cerebral laterality, *424;* function of, *29, 57;* and handedness, *523;* location of, *24, 53*

Corpus luteum, *404;* and menstruation, *453*

Cortex, *11, 14, 16, 18, 23–25, 29;* arousal of, *50;* connections with other centers, *173, 175;* location of, *24, 30;* and memory, *47;* and mental functioning, *60, 61;* size of, *25, 40*

Cortical lobes, *25*

Corticospinal tract, *176, 177;* and breathing, *366, 367*

Corticosteroids, *149, 386;* and adrenal cortex, *405;* timing of release of, *401*

Corticosterone, as steroidal hormone, *401*

Corticotropin releasing factor (CRF), and the ANS, *139, 148, 153;* and the circadian clock, *149;* and the pituitary, *403*

Cortisol, *149, 150;* and adrenal cortex, *403, 405, 406;* and ACTH, *404;* and the ANS, *139, 148, 149, 386;* chronic elevation of, *406;* and circadian rhythm, *465, 476, 478–482;* and depression, *465, 481, 482;* and digestion, *449;* diurnal rhythm of, *149;* and the EEG pattern, *59;* and the fetus, *406;* and glucose, *405, 406;* and immunity, *385, 406;* and hypertension, *406;* and memory, *44, 149;* and muscle action, *183;* oligomenorrhea, *455;* and oscillator X, *477;* and over-training, *233;* and the sarcolemma, *230;* and the sleep/wake cycle, *490;* as steroidal hormone, *401;* and stress, *40;* times of max/min concentration, *402, 406;* and time of *yogasana* practice, *405, 406;* and ulcers, *406;* and upper respiratory infection, *406*

Costal cartilage, *360;* ossification of, *362*

Costal muscles, *366*

Costovertebral joints, *359;* location of, *360*

Coughing reflex, *20;* muscles involved in, *364*

Cramps, *231, 232;* and dehydration, *231;* and lumbar misalignment, *80;* and pregnancy, *458;* and *supta virasana,* *231*

Cranial lobes, *25*

Cranial nerves, *17–20, 107;* and eye motion, *411*

Cranial nerve I, *18;* and hypothalamus, *143;* and nasal laterality, *379*

Cranial nerve II, *18, 51, 132*

Cranial nerve III, *18, 19, 31, 32;* and the cervical flexion reflex, *218;* and ciliary muscles, *151, 411, 413, 414;* target organs of, *151;* and visual relaxation, *415, 420*

Cranial nerve IV, *19, 31*

Cranial nerve V, *19, 31, 38;* and malleus excitation, *435*

Cranial nerve VI, *19, 31*

Cranial nerve VII, *19, 31;* and salivation, *393;* and stapes excitation, *436, 438;* target organs of, *151;* and tears, *151, 395*

Cranial nerve VIII, *19, 20, 31;* and hearing, *433;* and the medulla, *440;* and the vestibular organs, *440*

Cranial nerve IX, *20, 31, 342;* and salivation, *393;* and sucking, *488;* target organs of, *151*

Cranial nerve X (Vagus nerve), *20, 31, 38, 105, 150–152;* asymmetry of, *522;* and baroreceptors, *339;* and breathing, *152;* and the gall bladder, *401;* and the gastrointestinal organs, *151, 488;* and the genitals, *151;* and the heart, *151, 317;* and hunger, *441, 442;* and the liver, *151;* and the parasympathetic NS, *152, 153;* and peristalsis, *447;* and reflex arcs, *340, 341;* and the rectum, *151;* and stretch receptors in the lungs, *367;* target organs of, *151;* and the ocular-vagal heart-slowing reflex, *152, 220*

Cranial nerve XI, *20*

Cranial nerve XII, *20, 31*

Craniosacral pulse (see **Cerebrospinal fluid pulsations**)

Craniosacral therapy, *3, 95;* and stretch receptors, *95*

Craving sweets/chocolate during menstruation, *454;* and *dhanurasana*, *454;* and insulin, *454;* and *setu bandhasana*, *454*

Creatinine phosphate, in muscles, *183*

Creativity, *1, 10, 13, 24*

Cross bridges, *274;* action of, *179–181, 185, 190;* and glucose, *274;* power stroke of, *183;* structure of *178, 179*

Cross inhibition, of diaphragm and abdominals, *364*

Crosslinking, of proteins and joint stiffness, *497*

Cruciate ligaments of the knee, *251, 252;* injury of, *279*

Crutch-in-armpit reflex, *55*

Curare, *131*

Cyclic guanosine monophosphate, *131;* and Na$^+$ channels, *131;* and K$^+$ channels, *131*

D

Dandasana, *98, 260, 266*

Dead air, *364;* and the trachea, *366;* volume of, *364, 365;* and *yogasana* practice, *366*

Death, causes of, *501, 502*

Declarative learning, *42*

Decussation, *17, 18, 26, 30, 55;* of proprioception, *209;* within the spine, *85–87, 176, 177*

Deep pressure sensors, see **Pacinian corpuscles**

Defeat reaction, *161*

Defecation, *397, 398;* and the anal sphincters, *397;* and the ANS, *150, 397;* and the colon, *397;* and higher centers, *397, 447;* and the sacrum, *98;* and stool, *397;* and tachycardia, *397;* time of, *483*

Delta waves, in the EEG, *59*

Deltoid, location of, *168, 169*

Dendrites, *46, 108;* action of, *121, 125*

Depolarization waves, hopping of, in gap junctions, *119, 120, 122;* in heart, *316;* in nerves, *107, 111, 116–119;* response to Na$^+$, *123;* threshold for, *124*

Depression, *463–469;* and aging, *500;* and the ANS, *465, 467, 468;* atypical, *464;* and back-bending, *467, 468;* and beta waves, *50, 51;* and cancer, *387;* and catecholamines, *464, 466;* and cerebral laterality, *466, 468;* and chronotherapy, *487;* and colored lights, *427, 468, 469;* and constipation, *464;* and cortisol, *465, 466, 481, 482;* and dominant left frontal lobe, *523;* and dopamine, *464;* and EEG waves, *50, 51, 60, 152, 153, 466, 468;* and loss of energy, *464;* and eye position, *420;* symptoms of, *464, 465;* and fear, *468;* and the flexional reflex, *215;* and handedness, *466;* and headache, *38, 39, 49, 464, 478;* and the HPA axis, *465;* and inhalation, *467;* and immunity, *467, 470;* and inversions, *349;* and menopause, *459;* and mental pain, *464;* and nasal dominance, *466;* and lack of neurotransmitters, *130;* and norepinephrine, *464;* and the patellar knee jerk, *213;* and the placebo effect, *164, 165, 464;* and posture, *464;* and type-D PMS, *454;* and psychotherapy, *464, 467;* and SAD, *431, 469;* and serotonin, *464, 467;*and loss of sexual desire, *464, 467;* and sleep, *467;* and stress, *155;* and suppressor T cells, *467;* symptoms of, *464, 465, 470;* and time to treatment, *468;* and ultraviolet light, *469;* and visual dominance, *51;* and *yogasana* practice, *48, 464, 500*

Dermatitis, and blood flow, *162*

Dermatomes, *28, 303–307;* dorsal-root locations of, *305;* from the spinal cord, *86;* and the visceral organs, *288, 448*

Dermis, *283;* and coloration, *285;* and composition of, *284;* and Ruffini corpuscles, *208;* structure of, *284, 287;* and temperature regulation, *285*

Descending colon, location of, *443*

Descending information, *16, 32, 85, 86,*

Detached retina, and inversions, *349*

Detoxification, *444;* of emotions, *425;* and the liver, *243, 448;* and sweating, *395;* and *yogasana* practice, *243, 395*

Dhanurasana, *365;* and cravings for sweets, *454;* and type-C PMS, *455;* and type-D PMS, *454*

Dharana, *9*

Dhyana, *9*

Diabetes, and aging, *494, 501;* and insulin deficiency, *450;* and inversions, *349;* and lack of insulin response, *450;* and odor of the breath, *365;* and *yogasana* practice, *451*

Diaphragm, *63, 92;* and abdominal muscles in breathing, *363, 364, 370;* central tendon of, *360, 362, 363;* control of, *366;* cross inhibition with abdominal muscles, *363;* dermatomes for, *306;* function of, *362;* location of, *359, 360, 443;* spasm of, *450*

Diaphragmatic breathing, *371, 372;* and abdominal contraction, *371;* and asthma, *372;* and *langhana*, *374;* effect on mental clarity, *371;* and nasal laterality, *380;* and the parasympathetic NS, *371;* physiology of, *374;* and *pranayama*, *382;* and the RSA, *368;* and *yogasana* practice, *371, 372*

Diaphyses, *236, 239;* growth of, *238*

Diastolic blood pressure, *311, 312, 315, 322, 337;* and the atrial volume sensor, *341;* and isometric contraction, *368;* and vascular conditions, *326*

Diencephalon, *14, 15, 17;* function of, *33, 34;* location of, *43*

Diet, *6;* and brain aging, *501;* and the colon, *446;* and immunity, *385;* and length of digestive tract, *441;* and longevity, *498;* and the stool, *397, 398*

Diffusion, of nutrients, *281*

Digestive system/digestion, *1, 17, 20, 30;* and aging, *494;* and circadian rhythms, *479–483;* energy for, *449;* and hormones, *408;* and hydrochloric acid, *442, 445, 449;* and lymph, *352;* and lysozyme, *442;* and norepinephrine, *148;* and pancreatic enzymes, *447, 448;* and pepsin, *445;* and pressure points in feet, *450;* secretions and the ANS, *448;* tract length, *441;* and viewing yellow color, *427;* and *yogasana* practice, *443, 444, 449, 467, 468, 500;* see also **Gastrointestinal tract**

Dilator pupillae, and the ANS, *415;* and the catecholamines, *415;* function of, *415*

Disinfectants, lysozyme, *442*

Disrotatory twisting, *78, 91, 96*

Dizziness, *79, 81;* and aging, *497;* in inversions, *550, 551*

Dopamine, *39;* and aging, *499, 501;* and depression, *464;* as a neurotransmitter, *129, 407;* and Parkinson's disease, *129;* and sense of time, *473;* ultradian release of, *476*

Dorsal horn, *65, 87;* neuroreceptors in, *130*

Dorsal root, *85, 86*

Doshas, *483, 484*

Dowager's hump, see **Kyphosis**

Dreaming, *30, 59*

Drugs, abuse of, *6;* action of amphetamines, *130;* curare, *131;* LSD, *131;* mescaline, *131;* nicotine, *131;* see also **Cigarettes**

Dura mater/dural membrane, *16, 17, 93–95, 349;* and sclera, *418*

Dynamic nuclear-bag fibers, *199;* function of, *201;* innervation of, *201;* structure of, *200*

Dyslexia, and testosterone, *410*

E

Ears, *19;* and cervical misalignment, *79*

Earth, oscillations and Om, *436;* rotational period of, *473*

Edema, see **Lymph edema**

Edinger-Westphal nucleus, *31;* function of, *424;* location of, *423*

Efferent nerves, *18, 85, 86, 108, 172, 173;* types of, *120*

Ehlers Danlos syndrome, *274*

Ejaculation, *462*

Eka pada sirasana, *74*

Eka pada urdhva dhanurasana, *99*

Elastin, *229, 273–275;* aging and, *496;* in arteries and veins, *275;* in skin, *284*

Elasticity, of ligaments, *263;* of lungs, *364;* of nerves, *128*

Elbow, carrying angle at, *258;* hyperextension of, *259;* and interosseous membrane, *259*

Electrocardiogram (EKG), *318, 319*

Electroencephalogram (EEG), *341;* and aging, *500, 501;* alpha waves in, *32, 33, 58–60, 138;* and the ANS, *138;* beta waves in, *32, 59–61;* and cerebral laterality, *55;* conscious control of, *59;* and cortisol, *59;* delta waves in, *59;* and depression, *50, 51, 61, 152, 153, 466, 468;* gamma waves in, *59;* and nasal laterality, *377;* and nasal *versus* oral breathing, *374;* patterns of, *32, 40, 57–61;* and postsynaptic potentials, *57;* and *savasana*, *60, 61, 165, 490;* and sleep stages, *54, 58, 488;* synchronicity of, *138;* and theta waves, *59, 61;* and unilateral breathing, *55*

Efferent neurons, *18*

Embolism, due to injury, *324;* and *pranayama*, *518;* from thrombosis, *515, 517, 518*

Emotional center, *23;* and the hypothalamus, *135, 142*

Emotions, and aging, *499–502;* and the ANS, *463;* and the breath, *63, 374, 471, 472;* and cerebral laterality, *380, 463;* and colored lights, *429;* detoxification of, *426;* and the eyes, *426;* and gamma-motor neurons, *202;* and Golgi tendon organs, *206;* and the hypothalamus, *135, 142;* and immunity, *386, 391, 463;* and *langhana, 374;* and the limbic system, *33, 135;* and muscle tone, *463;* and forced nasal laterality, *379, 380;* and pain, *298;* and right cerebral hemisphere, *50, 426, 463;* and SAD, *431;* and *savasana, 395;* and sense of smell, *463;* and the skin, *285, 291;* and tears, *395;* and visual pathway, *426;* and *yogasana* practice, *463*

Endocrine glands, *1, 399–401;* and the ANS, *400;* hormones and the hypothalamus, *399, 400;* pacemaker for, *485;* and receptors, *399;* and solitary tract, *399;* speed of action of, *399, 400;* and visceral organs, *399*

Endogenous depression, *464, 465*

Endogenous headache, and circadian rhythms, *478, 482*

Endometriosis, and inversions, *455, 456*

Endometrium, and menstruation, *453*

Endorphins, *303;* and aging, *494;* and the ANS, *139;* and the adrenal medulla, *147;* and immunity, *385;* and pain, *130, 164, 303, 494;* and the pituitary, *131;* and runner's high, *131, 303*

Endosteum, *238*

Endothelial cells, and hormones, *335;* and injury, *324, 330*

Endurance, and *yogasana* practice, *500*

Enteric nervous system, *5, 15, 17, 108, 447;* and the gastrointestinal organs, *442;* neurotransmitters in, *137;* pacemaker in, *319, 447;* and the parasympathetic NS, *137;* and peristalsis, *447*

Entrainment, *477, 483;* and jet lag, *491*

Eosinophils, times of maximum number, *478, 479*

Epicondyles, location of, *237*

Epidermis, *283;* and *adho mukha svanasana, 283;* structure of, *284, 287;* see also **Skin**

Epiglottis, *356;* action during sneeze, *373;* location of, *357;* and swallowing, *442*

Epilepsy, *53, 60*

Epinephrine, and adrenal medulla, *403, 406, 407;* and aging, *40;* and alpha/beta receptors, *129, 406;* and backbending, *216–218;* and circadian rhythm, *478–480, 482;* and exercise, *389;* and glycogen, *406;* and headache, *38;* and the heart, *319;* and K^+ channels, *407;* as a neurotransmitter, *128, 129;* and stressors, *153–155;* and the sympathetic NS, *136, 139, 147;* and ultradian release of, *476*

Epiphyseal line, in growing bone, *236, 239*

Epiphyses, *236, 239;* and compressive stress, *260;* and epithelial cells, *394;* growth of, *238;* in the humerus, *254;* in the knee, *251*

Epithelial cells, of bronchi, *394;* of thorax, *394*

Erectile tissue, in the nose, *375;* and PMS, *375*

Erector spinae, location of *81, 82;* speed of contraction, *172*

Ergotamine, *38*

Esophagus, location of, *357, 359, 360, 443;* dermatome of, *306;* and swallowing, *442*

Estradiol, and hot flashes, *408;* and menopause, *408*

Estrogen, *149;* and adrenal cortex, *403, 405;* and amenorrhea, *455;* at birth, *406;* and breast cancer, *410;* effects of, *408–410;* and finger length, *410;* and feminine personality, *410;* and menopause, *459, 461, 494;* and menstruation, *453, 454;* and mental alertness, *461;* and oligomenorrhea, *455;* and ovaries, *408;* as a steroidal hormone, *401;* ultradian release of, *474*

Estrogen/progesterone balance; and bone density, *408, 409;* and breasts, *408;* and genitals, *408;* and FSH, *408;* and long bones, *408;* and urinary muscle tone, *408;* and water retention, *408*

Estrone, and menopause, *408*

Evaporative cooling, see **Heat**

Exercise, and brain aging, *501;* and the colon, *446;* and endurance, *499;* and epinephrine, *389;* and hormones, *403;* and immunotransmitters, *385, 389;* and leucocytes, *389;* and longevity, *498;* and lymphocytes, *389;* and mitochondria, *322;* and muscle speed, *499;* and neutrophils, *389;* and osteoporosis, *270–272;* and polio, *389, 390;*

Exhalation, and asthma, *359;* and brain movement, *364;* and forward bends and twists, *356;* and the internal costal muscles, *363;* and *langhana, 356;* and left-nostril dominance, *356;* and the parasympathetic NS, *356, 367;* and relaxation, *364;* and right-cerebral dominance, *356;* and thoracic contraction, *362;* and moving into *yogasanas, 364*

Exogenous depression, *464, 465;* and catecholamines, *466;* and circadian rhythms, *465,
481, 482;* and cortisol, *465;* and the HPA axis,
465

Extensor carpi, location of, *169*

Extensor digitorum, location of, *169*

External auditory canal, *433;* location of, *434*

External costal muscles, *359;* control of, *365;*
function of, *361;* and inhalation, *363*

External obliques, location of, *168*

Extension, *63;* and abnormal spinal curves, *71;*
and compression, *83;* of the neck, *67, 81;*
range of motion, *72*

Extracellular fluid, *111, 112;* ions in, *116, 119;*
and neurotransmitters, *118, 122*

Extrafuasal fibers, *200*

Eye(s), *19, 419–431;* and the ANS, *138, 145,
150, 151, 422;* aqueous humour and CSF, *93;*
bags and *savasana, 491;* and balance, *526,
533–535, 542, 552;* blink rate of, *413;* blood
shot, *349;* and balancing, *45, 411, 422;* arterioles of, *349;* and cataracts, *414;* and cervical
misalignment, *79;* and circadian rhythm, *421;*
and color viewing, *427;* and depression, *420;*
dilation of pupils, *19, 136, 138, 147, 150;* lateral dominance of, *426;* and emotions, *426;*
and external structure of, *411–421;* and the
fight-or-flight response, *422;* and forced unilateral breathing, *379;* and gaze of, *419–421;*
hearing colors through, *117;* and hypotension,
420; and hypothalamus, *143;* and inhalation,
368; and internal structure of, *413–415;*
intraocular pressure and the ANS, *138;* and
inversions, *349;* and *jalandhara bandha, 218;*
lens curvature and the ANS, *138, 420, 421;*
and lymph drainage, *349;* and reaction time,
422; relaxation of, *411, 419–421;* and sleep,
411; and sneezing, *373;* socket, *95, 412;* and
vestibular organs, *418;* and the visual cortex,
27, 29, 173; and *yogasana* practice, *411;* see
also **Visual aids, Visual laterality,** and
Visual stress

Eye motion, and auditory memory, *425;* and the
cranial nerves, *411, 420;* and handedness,
425; and kinaesthesia, *425;* saccadic, *413,
417, 419;* in *savasana, 420;* and thinking,
425, 426; and visual memory, *425*

Eye muscles, and cranial nerve III, *151, 411,
413;* dilator pupillae, *412;* and exercises for,
415, 419, 421; extrinsic, *19, 113;* inferior
oblique, *412;* inferior rectus, *412, 420;* intrinsic, *413–415;* lateral rectus, *412, 418, 426;*
medial rectus, *412, 418, 426;* and the stretch

reflex, *412;* superior oblique, *412;* superior
rectus, *412;* sphincter pupillae, *412*

F

Face, bones of, *96;* density of skin receptors in,
288; expression of, *19;* hair and testosterone,
408; muscles and headache, *37*

Facet joint, *66–68, 70;* structure of, *88*

Facial nerves; see **Cranial nerve VII**

Fallopian tubes, and estrogen/progesterone balance, *408;* and menstruation, *453*

Fainting, *37*

Fascia, see **Myofascia**

Fastigial nucleus, *29;* location of, *30*

Fast-twitch fibers, see **Muscle fiber, type-3**

Fat, absorption into lymph, *445, 448*

Fatigue, and immunity, *389;* and injuries, *511,
512;* and inversions, *349;* and type-C PMS,
454; and upper respiratory tract infection, *389*

Fatty acids, *321;* and aerobic oxidation, *184;* and
anaerobic oxidation, *183;* and the ANS, *139,
147;* as fuel, *369;* and stressors, *153*

Fear, *1, 11, 463;* and apocrine sweat glands, *395;*
and backbending, *215–218, 468, 471;* center,
216; and depression, *468;* of falling, *525,* and
the flexional reflex, *215;* and the hypothalamus, *142, 152, 203, 532;* of inversions, *344,
345, 351, 352, 525;* and the medulla, *345;* and
pain, *345;* and the solar plexus, *216*

Feedback, *133–135, 172, 532;* and the ANS,
134; in the muscles, *178;* supraspinal, *206*

Feedforward, *133, 135, 532, 552*

Feet, arches as shock absorbers, *69, 96;* and
digestion, *450;* joints of, *253, 254, 262;* and
myofascia, *280;* pressure sensors in, *253;*
pressing into the floor, *553, 554;* pain in, *497;*
and pregnancy, *458;* psychoanatomy of, *163;*
and sweat glands, *395;* and *tadasana, 253,
527, 553, 554;* and *trikonasana, 253, 553,
554;* and *uttanasana, 531;* and *yogasana* practice, *497*

Female sexual function, *461, 462;* clitoris and
the ANS, *461;* and gonadotropins, *461;* neuroanatomy of, *462;* and orgasm, *462;* and
ovaries, *461*

Feminine, *3,* personality and estrogen, *410*

Femoral artery, *327*

Femoral vein, and pregnancy, *458*

Femur bones, allowed motion in, *260, 261;*
condyles of, *250, 251;* joints with, *96, 97, 99,
247, 260;* location of, *237, 248;* and lordosis,
248; mass of, *242;* neck of, *247, 249;* and

pelvic motion, *100, 247, 249, 250;* rotation of, *247, 249, 250;* and *trikonasana, 249*

Fetus, and cortisol, *406;* development of, *235;* and hormones, *457;* and hyaline cartilage, *280, 281*

Fever, *388;* circadian rhythm of, *481;* and core temperature, *388;* and prostaglandins, *388*

Fibrillation, *316*

Fibroblasts, *280*

Fibrocartilage, *98, 281*

Fibula, joints of, *251–253;* location of, *237*

Fight-or-Flight response, *136, 154, 155, 156, 158, 162, 336, 483;* and catecholamines, *407, 415;* and the eyes, *422;* and the heart, *317, 320;* in inversions, *352;* and the vascular system, *335*

Finger length, and estrogen, *410;* and testosterone, *409*

Finger temperature, *293;* and autonomic balance, *159, 160*

Flexion/Flexional reflex, *63, 142, 195, 214–218;* and compression, *83;* consequences of, *215;* and depression, *215;* and fear, *215–218, 471;* and grief, *215;* of head, *63;* and impotence, *215;* and incontinence, *215;* and kyphosis, *215;* and lower-back pain, *215;* and lumbar vertebrae, *93;* and muscle tone, *214, 215;* range of motion of, *72;* see also **Forward bending**

Flexibility, and aging, *494;* and circadian rhythm, *491;* and the joints, *261;* of neurons, *159;* and protein crosslinking, *497;* and *yogasana* practice, *500*

Floating ribs, and the sternum, *72*

Follicular stimulating hormone (FSH), *143, 404;* and estrogen/progesterone balance, *408;* and gonadotropin RF, *403;* and menstruation, *453;* times of max/min concentration, *402*

Foramen magnum, *29, 84, 87, 95;* and the vertebral arteries, *515*

Forced unilateral breathing, *53;* and blood glucose, *379;* and catecholamines, *378;* and emotions, *379, 380;* and eye-blink rate, *379;* and heart rate, *379;* and intraocular pressure, *379;* and memory, *53;* and spatial tasks, *379;* and verbal tasks, *379*

Forearm, *256;* pronation/supination of, *257–260*

Forebrain, *15, 32;* development, *23;* function of, *24*

Fornix, location, *34*

Forward bending, benefits of, *83, 84;* and the cervical flexional reflex, *219;* and exhalation, *356;* and the flexional reflex, *215;* and rotation of the femurs, *249;* supported, for gastric

distress, *449;* see also **Flexion/Flexional reflex**

Fovea, and cones, *417;* fixation when moving, *418;* function of, *415;* location of, *414;* saccadic motion of, *413, 417, 419;* and visual stress, *419*

Free nerve endings, *287;* and pain, *38, 291, 296;* as temperature sensors, *290, 291*

Free radicals, and aging, *497;* and ATP, *497;* and antioxidants, *497;* and mitochondria, *497*

Free-running rhythms, *476, 477*

Frontal lobe, *15;* function, *26, 39;* and headache, *38;* location of, *24, 27, 94;* size of, *39*

Frozen joints, *261*

Fungi, *383*

G

Gall bladder*;* asymmetry of, *522;* and cranial nerve X, *401;* and dermatome for, *306, 448;* location of, *443;* and thoracic misalignment of, *80*

Gamma-aminobutyric acid, *129*

Gamma-motor neurons, effects of emotions on, *202;* effects of psychological attitudes on, *202, 214;* in muscle spindles, *113, 175, 200, 202, 205, 222;* and resting muscle tone, *202;* and stretching, *214*

Gamma waves, in the EEG, *59;* and mental functioning, *60, 61*

Ganglia, *108, 132*

Ganglion cell, in retina, *416*

Gap junctions, *122;* and the heart, *316;* and hyperpolarization, *122*

Garudasana, 38

Gas exchange, in different breathing modes, *372;* and posture, *373*

Gastrin, as a hormonal peptide, *401;* and stomach acid, *408*

Gastrocnemius, action of, *253, 280;* location of, *168, 169*

Gastrointestinal organs, *15, 441–451;* and cranial nerve X, *151;* and the enteric nervous system, *442;* nutrient absorption and the ANS, *138;* and pain, *441;* peristalsis and the ANS, *138;* secretions and the ANS, *138;* and skin, *441;* and smooth muscle, *441, 447;* and stress, *448, 449;* vascularization of, *326*

Gate theory of pain, *269, 301*

G cells, *444;* and gastrin, *445;* and histamine, *445*

General adaptation syndrome (GAS), *155*

Genitals, *1, 408–410;* and cranial nerve X, *151;* and intraocular pressure, *410*

Glands, *400–410;* types of, *401;* external secretions of, *393–396*

Glaucoma, and intraocular pressure, *421;* and inversions, *349, 421, 517;* and *urdhva dhanurasana, 421*

Glenohumeral joint, *254*

Glenoid fossa, bones of, *250, 254, 256, 257;* and the humerus, *256;* location of, *237;* opening of, *197, 198*

Glial cells, *110, 116;* and neural health, *86, 128;* and neuroglia, *112*

Globus pallidus, function of, *35;* and posture, *35*

Glossopharyngeal nerves, *20, 38*

Glucagon, and the ANS, *139, 147;* and pancreatic beta cells, *408*

Glucose, aerobic oxidation of, *184;* anaerobic oxidation of, *183, 191;* and the ANS, *138, 139, 147;* and the blood-brain barrier, *325;* and cortisol, *405, 406;* in crossbridges, *274;* and forced unilateral breathing, *379;* and hunger, *441;* insulin and absorption of, *450;* in muscles, *321;* and stressors, *153*

Glutamate ion, as a neurotransmitter, *129*

Gluteus maximus, and bursae, *187, 263;* location of, *169*

Gluteus medius, *194;* action in *vrksasana, 540*

Glycogen, and the ANS, *138, 139;* and the circadian rhythm, *479;* and epinephrine, *406;* and muscle action, *183, 184;* and vasopressin, *404*

Glycogenolysis, and the catecholamines, *148*

Golgi tendon organ, *199, 206–208, 268, 269;* and emotional factors, *207;* and inhibition, *206;* nerve type, *120;* and PNF, *204;* and proprioception, *209, 268, 269;* and stress on tendons, *206;* structure of, *206;* and the triceps brachii, *207;* and *urdhva dhanurasana, 207*

***Gomukhasana**, 38, 56;* and handedness, *520;* and neurological damage, *515*

Gonads, see **Genitals**

Gonadotropin RF, *403;* and anterior pituitary, *404;* in females, *461;* and inhibin, *408 ;* and the hypothalamus, *403;* in males, *453, 454, 461;* and menstruation, *453*

Gout, *502*

Gracilis, location of, *168, 169*

Grand mal epileptic seizure, *9*

Gray matter, *25, 33, 36;* in the brain, *93, 107;* in the spinal cord, *84–87*

Gravity/Gravitational stress, and balance, *525, 556;* and bone demineralization, *241, 242, 397;* and *malasana, 554;* and Newton's Law, *553;* and *tadasana, 555;* and *trikonasana, 555;* and *utkatasana, 555*

Greater trochanter, *194;* and bursae, *263;* location of, *237, 248;* structure of, *247, 249*

Greater tubercle, *250*

Green-color viewing, *427*

Grief, and the flexional reflex, *215*

Groins, stabilization of in *parivrtta trikonasana, 542*

Ground substance, *273;* composition of, *275;* as a lubricant, *275*

Growth hormone (GHRH), *130, 143;* and bones, *236, 244;* and circadian rhythm, *478, 479;* and oscillator Y, *477;* and over-training, *233;* and the sleep/wake cycle, *489, 490;* times of max/min concentration, *402*

Guilt, feelings of, *153*

***Gunas**, 160*

***Gyri**, 25*

H

Habituation, and the ANS, *138,* of the central nervous system, *297*

Hair, and the ANS, *308;* frequency tuning of cells, *436, 437;* and piloerection, *140, 148, 150, 308;* structure of receptors, *286;* and testosterone, *408*

***Halasana**, 345;* and anger, *226, 471;* and baroreceptors, *347, 348;* and cerebrospinal fluid, *348;* and the cervical flexional reflex, *219;* and cervical vertebrae, *81;* and constipation, *450;* and hydrostatic pressure, *348;* and neck injuries, *82, 346, 348, 516;* and spinal mobility, *497;* and thyroid circulation, *405;* and vertebral-artery lesions, *516;* as an "X-rated" pose, *513*

H2 blockers, mode of action, *445*

Hallucinations, *130*

Hallux, misalignment of, *262;* sensitivity of, *539, 551;* and *virabhadrasana III, 542;* see also **Big toe**

Hamstrings, *10, 127, 167*

***Hanumanasana**, 99*

Hand, density of skin receptors on, *288;* muscles of, *175*

Handedness, *49;* and birth trauma, *50;* and cerebral laterality, *425;* and cerebral dominance, *50, 523;* commitment to, *523;* dominance of, *520;* and eye motion, *425;* in *gomukhasana, 520;* and manual dexterity, *63, 425;* and *maricyasana III, 520;* and speech, *50, 523;* and symmetry, *520, 523*

***Hasta padangusthasana**, 204;* and the center of gravity, *537;* wall support for, *536*

Hatha yoga, *2*

Haversian channels, *238–240, 244*

Hayfever, and circadian rhythms, *479*

Head, position when balancing, *534, 540, 547, 550–552;* psychoanatomy of, *163*

Headaches, *37–39;* and anxiety, *38, 481;* and arterial constriction, *334;* and blood flow, *162;* and cervical misalignment, *79;* and circadian rhythms, *478, 481, 482;* and circulation, *162;* and depression, *38, 39, 49, 464, 478;* and epinephrine, *38;* and the frontal lobe, *38;* and green-color viewing, *427;* and inversions, *349;* and muscles, *37, 38;* and nasal laterality, *379;* and the occipital lobe, *38;* and the placebo effect, *164;* and serotonin, *38;* time of, *38;* and tonic reflex, *216;* and type-C PMS, *454;* and the ocular-vagal heart-slowing reflex, *220, 221, 334*

Health, and beauty, *519;* in man, *519;* and symmetry, *519*

Hearing, and aging, *437, 494, 495, 497;* and cerebral laterality, *51, 433, 434;* colors, *117;* and cranial nerve VIII, *433;* frequency of, *434;* loss of in inversions, *435;* nerve cells in, *109;* speech and music, *434;* and *savasana*, *435;* and the temporal lobes, *523;* and *yogasana* practice, *421, 500*

Heart, *1;* aging of cells in, *496;* and alpha receptors, *407;* anatomy of, *310, 311;* and the ANS, *137, 145, 147, 150, 364, 484;* asymmetry of, *522;* attack and circadian rhythm, *478–482, 484;* and beta receptors, *406;* and the catecholamines, *148, 315, 317, 319;* contractions of, *313, 314;* contractility of, *147;* and cranial nerve X, *151, 317;* dermatome from, *306;* enlargement of, *315, 322, 335;* depolarization wave in, *316;* and the fight-or-flight response, *317, 320;* and gap junctions, *316;* and the hypothalamus, *140, 320;* innervation of, *315, 316;* and *janu sirsasana*, *320;* location of, *443;* and lymph, *352;* and parasympathetic action, *317, 318, 320, 322;* pressure on in *savasana*, *359;* refractory period in, *316;* resting potential in, *317;* and stressors, *153, 154;* stroke volume of, *321, 369;* waist-to-hip ratio, *460, 461;* see also **Cardiac**

Heart rate, *20, 137, 312, 313, 315, 317, 320, 322;* and breathing, *53, 379;* and chemoreceptors, *342;* and chronotherapy, *486;* and circadian rhythm, *478–480, 484;* and color viewing, *427;* and cranial nerve X, *317;* and inhalation, *151, 152, 367;* pacemaker for, *309, 315–317;* and the placebo effect, *164;* in REM sleep, *488;* and *sirsasana*, *321, 337, 346;*

stopping the heart, *317, 318;* and unilateral breathing, *53, 379*

Heart and sympathetic action, *317, 318, 320;* coronary diameters, *137;* stroke volume, *137;* vascular resistance, *137*

Heart hormones, *401;* and baroreceptor reflex, *340, 341;* and inversions, *345;* and lymph leakage, *352;* and unilateral breathing, *54, 379;* and *yogasana* practice, *337, 346*

Heart function, conscious control of, *317;* and the electrocardiogram, *318;* and oxygen demand, *320, 321;* and old age, *322, 493, 494;* power stroke of, *312;* and size in old age, *495, 497;* and thoracic misalignment of, *80*

Heart valves, function of, *312, 313;* location of, *310*

Heartburn, and hydrochloric acid, *80, 443, 444, 449;* and pregnancy, *459*

Heat balance, *295;* and breathing, *375;* see also **Sweating** and **Thermoregulation**

Heels, *250*

Height, change on aging, *83*

Helicobacter pylori, in stomach, *449*

Helper T cells, *384;* and circadian rhthym, *479*

Hemispheric laterality, see **Cerebral laterality**

Hemoglobin, *369, 370;* in aerobic oxidation, *184;* and ATP, *369;* and carbon dioxide, *369;* and cigarette smoke, *369;* and circadian rhythm, *479, 481;* and cooperative binding, *369;* and hyperventilation, *373;* iron in, *369, 370, 388;* and red blood cells, *323, 369*

Hemorrhoids, *333;* and inversions, *349, 351*

Herniated intervertebral disc, *5, 74, 78, 88, 91–93, 126, 127, 302;* and the emotions, *298;* and gate-control theory, *301;* in the lumbar spine, *91–93;* and referred pain, *91, 92*

Heroin, effect on reticular formation, *33*

Herpes, *387*

Hiccups, and cranial nerve X, *450;* cure for, *450;* and spasm of diaphragm, *450*

High blood pressure, see **Hypertension**

Higher centers, and co-contraction, *195, 196;* control by, *20, 212;* and defecation, *397, 447;* and swallowing, *443, 447;* and visual laterality, *424*

High-heeled shoes, and joint misalignment, *262;* and osteoarthritis, *268*

Hindbrain, *15, 22, 29, 30;* function of, *24;* location of, *29, 30*

Hippocampus, and consolidation, *61;* function, *34, 40, 41;* location, *34;* and learning/memory, *35, 47, 149, 490;* and neurogenesis, *128, 500*

Hippocrates, *4*

Hips/Hip joint, *244, 254, 256, 260, 261;* bending at, *96;* coupling to knee joint, *265;* ligaments in, *261;* and motion of pelvis, *99;* and sacral misalignment, *80*

Histamine, and allergies, *388;* and circadian rhythm, *478, 479, 482;* and pain, *297;* sensitivity to, *479;* in stomach, *445;* and the sympathetic NS, *388*

Homeostasis, *133, 135, 297, 299;* age and, *341;* and the ANS, *150, 155;* and blood pressure, *338, 341;* of Ca^{2+} levels, *246;* and conscious control, *342;* and the hypothalamus, *135, 136;* lack of, *486;* and physiological rhythm, *476;* and T cells, *385;* following urination, *351*

Homosexuality, and testosterone, *409*

Homunculi, *28, 114;* in animals, *175;* motor, *175;* sensory, *175, 176*

Hormones, *1, 393, 399–410;* and aging, *496;* and biorhythms, *142, 403;* digestive, *408;* and endothelial cells, *335;* and the hypothalamus, *142, 401, 403, 474;* and learning, *401;* mechanism of action, *216, 217;* and memory, *401;* neurotransmitters as, *124;* peptides as, *401;* steroidal, *401*

Hormonal release, of ACTH, *476;* of dopamine, *476;* of epinephrine, *476;* of estrogen, *474;* and the hypothalamus, *401, 474;* of insulin, *474;* of luteinizing hormone, *476;* of norepinephrine, *476;* and pressure, *400, 401;* in rhythm, *401, 402;* of testosterone, *474;* and ultradian rhythm, *474;* and *yogasana* practice, *400, 401*

Hormone replacement therapy (HRT), and menopause, *459;* and osteoporosis, *272, 459, 460*

Hot flashes, and aging, *494;* and chronotherapy, *487;* and estradiol, *408;* and menopause, *459, 460*

HPA axis, *465, 467;* and exogenous depression, *465*

Human balancing tower, *537, 538*

Humerus, *197, 207, 241, 254, 255;* articulations of, *256;* epiphyses of, *254;* and glenoid fossa, *256;* location of, *171, 237, 360;* rotation of, *250, 256*

Hunger, and the ANS, *442;* and cranial nerve X, *441, 442;* drive for, *135;* and glucose, *441;* and the hypothalamus, *140, 143, 441, 442*

Hyaline cartilage, in fetus, *280, 281*

Hydrochloric acid (HCl), and digestion, *441, 448;* and dissolution of bone, *242;* and heartburn, *443, 444;* protection of stomach from, *444;* release of, *444, 445;* and stomach

enzymes, *444;* and swallowing, *444;* see also **Stomach acid**

Hydrogen ion (H$^+$), *122;* in the blood, *246, 367, 374;* buffering of, *447;* chemoreceptors for, *342;* see also **Hydrochloric acid**

Hydrostatic pressure, *343–345;* and cerebrospinal fluid, *93, 94, 344, 346;* and *halasana, 346*

Hyperextension, of the elbow, *259;* of the knee, *252*

Hyperflexibility, and injury, *203;* and loose ligaments, *263, 264;* and viscoelasticity, *203*

Hypermobility, *278;* of joints, *262–265*

Hyperpolarization, in gap junctions, *122;* of nerves, *116, 117, 120, 131, 132;* as response to K$^+$ and Cl$^-$, *123;* in the retina, *418*

Hypertension, *335, 337, 338;* and aging, *337, 494;* and atherosclerosis, *338;* baroreceptors and, *335;* and brain function, *40;* and chronotherapy, *486, 487;* and cortisol, *406;* essential, *337;* and inversions, *349, 421, 517;* and intraocular pressure, *349;* and the placebo effect, *164;* and proprioception, *338;* and speaking, *337;* and stress, *156;* and stroke, *336;* and the sympathetic NS, *337;* and listening, *337;* and *yogasana* practice, *337, 338*

Hypertensive retinopathy, *349;* inversions and, *421*

Hyperventilation, and blood chemistry, *372, 373;* and hemoglobin, *373;* and thoracic breathing, *372*

Hypnotic states, and mental dissociation, *420;* and pain, *166;* and placebo, *165;* and visual relaxation, *420;* and *yogasana, 32, 56, 156*

Hypogastric plexus, *103, 105*

Hypoglossal nerves, *20*

Hypoglycemia, *450*

Hypotension, *338, 350;* and the eyes, *420;* and the possum response, *338;* in *uttanasana, 338*

Hypothalamus, *14, 140–144, 403, 404;* and allergic reactions, *388;* and adrenal glands, *399, 403;* and anger, *142, 471;* and breathing rate, *140;* and cerebrospinal fluid, *93;* and circadian rhythm, *142, 483, 485;* connection to other centers, *173;* and control of the ANS, *135, 136;* and cranial nerve I, *143;* and emotions, *135, 142, 143, 153;* and the endocrine glands, *399, 400;* and energy resources, *140;* and the eyes, *143;* and fear, *142, 152, 203, 532;* and feeding, *140;* function of, *34, 135, 141;* and function of median eminence, *144;* and function of preoptic area, *144;* and function of supraoptic area, *144;* and gonadotropin RF, *403;* and the heart, *140, 320;* and hormones, *142, 143, 401, 474;* and hunger, *143, 441, 442;* and the limbic system, *142, 147, 165;* location of, *24, 34, 402, 403;* and memory, *143, 150;* and menstruation, *143, 453;* and metabolism, *143;* and oscillator X, *477;* and the pituitary, *34, 47, 135, 142, 143, 399, 400, 403, 404;* size of, *141;* target organs of, *403;* and temperature, *140;* and ultradian rhythm, *476;* and urination, *396;* and water retention, *140;* see also **Anterior hypothalamus** and **Posterior hypothalamus**

Hypoxia, *126, 185, 309, 367*

I

Ida nadi, *54, 101, 102, 140;* and nasal laterality, *380*

Idiot savant, *29*

Iliac, artery, *327*

Iliac crest, *194;* location of, *97;* motion of, *100*

Iliocecal valve, in gastrointestinal tract, *446*

Iliopsoas, location of, *168*

Iliotibial band, location of, *168, 169*

Ilium, *96;* fusion of, in newborn, *98;* location of, *97, 237*

Illness *versus* disease, *164*

Imagination, *13*

Immunity, and aging, *390, 391, 494, 500;* and the *anahata chakra*, *387;* and asthma, *387;* and the ANS, *140, 386, 387;* and the blood-brain barrier, *388, 389;* and blood flow, *162, 384;* and circadian rhythms, *481, 482;* and cortisol, *385, 406;* and depression, *467;* and emotions/attitudes, *386, 391, 463;* and endorphins, *385;* and fatigue, *389;* and the musculoskeletal system, *391;* and SAD, *430, 431;* and supported backbends, *389;* ultradian rhythms of, *476;* and *yogasana* practice, *384, 389, 390, 500*

Immunoglobulins, and antibodies, *384;* and trench mouth, *387*

Immunotransmitters, *385, 386;* and ACTH, *385;* and cortisol, *385;* and exercise, *385;* and stress, *385*

Impotence, and the flexional reflex, *215*

Incontinence, and the flexional reflex, *215*

Incus, *433;* location of, *434*

Indigestion, and inversions, *349;* and hydrochloric acid, *443, 444;* and pregnancy, *459;* and stress, *155*

Inebriation, in men, *482;* in women, *482*

Infants, and bones, *98, 244;* and cortisol, *406;* head size, *40;* and myelin, *119, 120;* and touching, *291;* and urination, *211*

Inferior vena cava, *329;* function of, *328, 332, 333;* location of, *310, 360;* and pregnancy, *459*

Infradian rhythms, *491;* and menstruation, *491;* and SAD, *491*

Inhalation, and abdominal muscles, *363;* and backbends, *356;* and depression, *467;* and external costal muscles, *363;* and the eyes, *368;* and the heart rate, *151, 152, 367;* and *langhana*, *356;* and left-cerebral dominance, *356;* mechanism of, *196, 197;* and motion of the brain, *364;* and right-nostril dominance, *356;* and spinal curvature, *368;* and the sympathetic NS, *356, 367;* and thoracic expansion, *362, 372*

Inhibin, and gonadotropin RF, *408*

Inhibition, by cerebellum, *33;* and the Golgi tendon organ, *206;* and interneurons, *123, 188, 195, 202;* of muscle contraction, *188;* response to K^+ and Cl^-, *123;* by synapses, *87, 108, 123, 128*

Innate immunity, *383, 384*

Innate sense of time, and dopamine, *473*

Inner ear, *20, 33, 434, 437, 438–440, 526, 533;* see also **Vestibular organs**

Injuries, *511–518;* and being too ambitious, *512;* to ankle, *540;* and congenital weakness, *512, 517;* and connective tissue, *279, 280;* to cruciate ligament, *279;* and endothelial cells, *324, 330;* and *halasana*, *82, 346, 347, 516;* to joints, *251, 252, 262;* to ligaments, *263, 279;* and *mulhabandhasana*, *281;* and neurological damage, *87, 125–128, 513–515;* and fatigue, *511, 512;* to muscle extensors, *177;* in *padmasana*, *266, 267, 279–281, 513, 514, 518;* and rest, *232, 233;* to the sciatic nerve, *127, 267, 514;* and *sirsasana*, *82, 516, 517;* and spinal extension, *91;* and spinal flexion, *9;* to teachers, *552;* and vascular damage, *324, 515–518;* and *viparita karani*, *245;* and yoga foot drop, *514*

Insomnia, and inversions, *349*

Insulin, and the ANS, *139, 150;* and circadian rhythms, *478, 480;* and glucose absorption, *450;* as a hormonal peptide, *401;* and the pancreas, *399, 407, 447;* and pancreatic beta cells, *407, 408;* and craving sweets, *454;* and ultradian rhythms, *474;* and *yogasana* practice, *408*

Intellect, *13*

Internal clock, and *yogasana*, *192, 193*

Internal costal muscles, *359;* control of, *365;* and exhalation, *363;* function of, *361;* when sneezing, *373*

Internal wall for balance, in *anantasana, 536;* in *ardha chandrasana, 536;* in *sarvangasana, 536*

Interneurons, and baroreceptor reflexes, *340;* and the breath, *366;* function of, *112, 123–125;* and muscle movement, *188, 195, 202;* and pain, *300;* and reciprocal inhibition, *194, 195;* and reflexes, *212;* in the spinal cord, *86*

Interosseus membrane, *256;* and weight-bearing on the arms, *258, 259*

Interventricular septum, location of, *310*

Intervertebral discs, *64, 66, 67, 87–93;* and aging, *88–90, 497;* changing dimensions of, *89;* dehydration of, *76, 89;* herniated, *5, 74, 78, 88, 90–93, 126, 127;* and pain, *91, 92;* prestressing of, *90;* as shock absorbers, *71, 72, 89, 90, 96;* structure of, *88, 89;* viscoelastic character of, *89;* see also **Herniated intervertebral disc**

Intervertebral foramina, *86*

Intervertebral muscles and ligaments, *68*

Intervertebral joints, *88;* degeneration of, *97*

Intestines, reflex actions of, *222*

Intracellular fluid, *111*

Intrafusal fibers, *200, 201, 205*

Intraocular pressure, *349;* and the ANS, *138;* and forced unilateral breathing, *379;* and glaucoma, *421;* and gonad removal, *410;* and hypertension, *349, 517;* in inversions, *349, 517;* in *sarvangasana, 517;* when seated, *517;* in *sirsasana, 517;* in *urdhva dhanurasana, 517;* and the ocular-vagal heart-slowing reflex, *349;* and the vitreous humour, *420*

Inverted *yogasanas*, *343–352, 544–551;* and the baroreceptors, *341, 348;* benefits of, *349, 350;* and blood pressure, *342, 349–351;* and cold feet, *349, 350;* coming down from, *545;* and constipation, *349, 397, 398, 450;* and depression, *349;* and diabetes, *349;* and dizziness in, *550, 551;* and endometriosis, *455, 456;* falling backward in, *544;* and the eyes, *349, 350, 545;* and fatigue, *349;* fear of, *157, 158, 344, 345, 351, 352;* and the fight-or-flight response, *352;* general points on, *551, 552;* and head position in, *547;* and headaches, *349;* and hearing, *435;* and the heart, *345;* and hemorrhoids, *349, 351;* and hypertension, *350, 351;* and hypertensive retinopathy, *421;* and indigestion, *349;* and injuries to the teacher, *552;* and insomnia, *349;* and intraocu-

lar pressure, *349, 517;* and loss of hearing, *435;* and the medulla, *346;* and oxygenation of the blood, *342;* and pregnancy, *456, 458;* and resistive balancing, *544;* and rheumatoid arthritis, *349;* and sinus congestion, *394, 395;* and skin, *349;* and stroke, *343;* and *svadhyaya, 456;* and the sympathetic NS, *345, 349;* and systolic blood pressure, *345;* and type-H PMS, *455;* and urination, *352, 396, 397;* and the uterus during menstruation, *349, 453, 455, 456;* and vasoconstriction, *345;* and vasodilation, *348, 350;* and venous return to the heart, *333, 348, 349;* and ventricular stroke volume, *345*

Ion channels, *109, 111*

Iris, location of, *414;* and pupillary diameter, *414*

Iron, in blood, *388;* in hemoglobin, *369, 370*

Ischemia, *126, 185;* attack of, *324;* and muscle tone, *205, 206;* neural, *513, 514;* in *padmasana, 514;* and pain, *302;* and smooth muscle, *441*

Ischial tuberosities (sitting bones), location of, *97, 98;* motion of, *100;* sitting on, *99*

Ischium, *97, 98;* and bursae, *187;* fusion in newborn, *98;* location of, *97, 237*

Isokinetic contraction, *187–189*

Isomerization, *131*

Isometric contraction, *187, 188;* and colored lights, *429;* and diastolic pressure, *368;* and PNF, *20;* and sarcomere length, *187;* and systolic pressure, *368;* and type-1 muscle fibers, *190;* and *yogasana* practice, *189*

Isotonic contraction, *188, 189;* concentric, *188, 189;* eccentric, *188, 189*

Iyengar yoga, *4, 7, 8;* as art, *7;* and body intelligence, *130;* and cerebrospinal pressure, *95;* and control of single motor unit, *114;* and pose-and-repose, *287, 288;* and Ruffini corpuscles, *208;* and skin receptors, *289;* and symmetry, *519–522*

J

Jalandhara bandha, 67, 218–220; and the baroreceptors, *220;* and chin lock, *220;* and cranial nerve III, *218;* and forward bending, *219;* and *halasana, 220;* and the parasympathetic response, *218;* and *savasana, 219*

Janu sirsasana, and the heart, *320*

Jathara parivartanasana, 78

Jet lag, *491*

Jnana nadi, 9, 105

Joint-proliferant therapy, *92*

Joints, *1, 16, 18, 260–262;* ball and socket, *247, 250;* cartilaginous, *96;* hypermobility in, *262;* and immunity, *260;* injury to, *262;* and loose ligaments, *263–265;* misalignment and high heels, *262, 268;* opening and closing of, *197, 198;* pain in, *261, 262, 267–269;* popping of, *264;* range of motion, *262, 268, 279, 494;* receptors in, *260;* and relaxin, *458;* stability of, *198, 260;* and the weather, *267;* see also **Glenohumeral, Knee**, etc.

Joint capsules, and balancing in *vrksasana, 540;* nerve type in, *120;* pain and the weather, *261;* as proprioceptive sensors, *209, 268, 269;* strain of, *231, 232*

Joint lubrication, *518;* by cartilage, *236, 237;* by synovial fluid, *237;* and warming up, *227, 518*

Jugular veins, *37*

K

Kapha, 382, 483, 484

Kapotasana, 74

Karma nadi, 9, 105

Karnapidasana, and hiccups, *450;* and lower-back pain, *215;* and premature birth, *215*

Keratin, *283;* and hair, *308*

Kidney, and aging, *500;* and backbending, *216;* hormones of, *401;* odor of the breath and disease of, *365;* in the sensory cortex, *28;* and thoracic misalignment, *80;* and vasopressin, *47;* and *yogasana* practice, *500*

Killer T cells, *384;* action of, *385;* and rheumatoid arthritis, *388*

Kinaesthesia, and the cerebral hemispheres, *50;* and eye motion, *425;* and proprioception, *209*

Kinocilium, directional sensing by, *439;* and K^+ ions, *438;* and the utricle, *438, 439*

Knee joints, coupling to hip joint, *265;* injury to, *251, 252, 279;* ligaments of, *251, 252;* meniscus of, *281;* misalignment of, *281;* allowed motions of, *252, 265, 266;* osteoarthritis of, *247, 261, 267, 268;* and rheumatoid arthritis, *265, 267, 268;* stability of, *265;* structure of, *250, 251, 260, 261, 265;* temperature of, *265;* and *ustrasana, 250*

Knock knees, *100, 247, 248*

Krounchasana, 99

Kumbhaka, 220, 381; and CO_2 levels in the blood, *382*

Kundalini, 104

Kyphosis, *67, 70, 71;* and the flexional reflex, *215;* and osteoporosis, *70, 271*

L

Lachrimal system, see **Tears**

Lactic acid, *309;* and the ANS, *139;* and soda loading, *183*

Langhana, 355, 356; and abdominal breathing, *374;* and diaphragmatic breathing, *374;* and emotional stability, *374;* and the parasympathetic NS, *374;* and *pranayama, 382;* properties of, *356*

Language, and age, *39;* function of, *25, 26, 28, 41;* site of, *25, 26;* skills, *49*

Large intestine, see **Colon**

Larynx, *356;* location of, *357*

Lateral bending, *72,* and aging, *497;* and the lumbar spine, *72, 73, 75;* and the thoracic spine, *72, 73*

Lateral geniculate nucleus, function of, *424;* location of, *423*

Latissimus dorsi, *262, 330;* location of, *168, 169;* and pull on scapulae, *196*

Laughter, and the baroreceptors, *341, 351;* and lack of muscle tone, *222, 351;* and tickling, *289;* and urination, *352*

Lead (Pb^{2+}), in bones, *243*

Learning, *19, 22, 40;* and brainwave frequencies, *60, 61;* and environmental context, *44, 45;* and hormones, *401;* and muscle memory, *233, 234;* and neural branching, *46–48;* and neurotransmitters, *45, 125;* and brain plasticity, *46, 113;* sites of, *25, 35*

Left brain/cerebral hemisphere, *3;* and the ANS, *138;* beta waves and sympathetic dominance, *140;* and depression, *523;* dominance and inhalation, *356;* effect of testosterone, *50, 409;* and language skills, *50, 380;* properties of, *50–57*

Left handedness, *49;* and longevity, *49, 50;* and speech, *50, 51;* and testosterone, *410*

Left-nostril dominance, and depression, *466;* and exhalation, *356*

Left-right preference, *49, 51;* of eye, *426;* of foot, *49*

Legs, density of skin receptors in, *288;* loss of muscle tissue in, *176;* pain and lumbar misalignment, *80;* psychoanatomy of, *163;* ranges of motion in, *253–255;* structure of, *247*

Lens, *413;* and ciliary muscle, *413*

Lesbians, and cerebral laterality, *523*

Leucocytes, *325, 383;* and bone marrow, *383;* and exercise, *389;* and lymph, *383*

Level of illumination, and balancing, *535*

Levels of consciousness, *9*

Lie detectors, and the ANS, *60, 160, 293;* and the salivary glands, *394;* and thermoregulation, *293*

Lifting of the kneecaps, *250*

Ligaments, *262–265;* and bones, *235;* and collagen, *262, 263;* composition of, *275, 276;* destabilization of, *264, 275;* in the knee, *251, 252;* in the hip joint, *261;* injury to, *263;* and mechanoreceptors, *268;* nourishment of, *263;* and pain, *263;* properties of, *262, 263, 275, 276;* stretching of, *190, 198, 263, 264*

Ligamentum flava, *275*

Ligamentum nuchea, *263, 275;* stress-strain curve for, *278*

Limbic system, *17, 18, 22, 25, 33–35;* and emotions, *33, 135, 296;* and endorphins, *303;* and the hypothalamus, *142, 147, 165;* and pain, *295, 296;* and pleasure, *297*

Lipid bilayer, *325;* structure, *108, 109, 111*

Lipolysis, and the catecholamines, *148, 183;* and triglycerides, *183*

Lithium, and bipolar disorder, *469, 470*

Liver, and aging, *500;* and the ANS, *145, 153;* asymmetry of, *522;* and bile, *448;* and the colon, *446;* and cranial nerve X, *151;* and detoxification, *243, 448;* disease and odor of the breath, *365;* function and circadian rhythms, *478, 479;* hormones of, *401;* location of, *359, 360, 443, 448;* and menstruation, *454;* portal vein of, *448;* and red-blood cells, *323, 369;* and spinal twists, *448;* and stem cells, *22;* and thoracic misalignment, *80;* and vascular system, *326;* and *yogasana* practice, *500*

Locus ceruleus, *129,* and aging, *40, 500*

Longevity, *498, 499;* and alcohol, *498;* and body weight, *498;* and diet, *498;* and exercise, *498;* and left handedness, *49, 50;* and marriage, *499;* and sleeping, *498;* and smoking, *498, 499*

Long-term memory, *43–48, 61*

Lordosis, *81, 91, 99, 101;* and rotation of the femurs, *249;* and the tonic reflex, *216*

Love, *1*

Lower-back pain, *70, 78;* and *karnapidasana, 215;* and the flexional reflex, *215;* and lumbar misalignment, *80;* and menstruation, *456;* and premature birth, *215;* psychoanatomy of, *163;* psychological cure for, *206;* and rest period, *233;* and the sacroiliac joint, *264;* and stress, *155;* and tonic reflex, *215*

Lower hinge, *96*

LSD, *131;* effect on the reticular formation, *33;* and serotonin, *130*

Lumbago, *91*

Lumbar spine, curvature of, *90, 99, 101;* nerves of, *15, 16*

Lumbar vertebrae, aging effects on, *82, 93;* and the colon, *80;* disc herniation in, *91, 93;* extension and, *75, 93, 497;* flexion of, *93;* intervertebral discs of, *88;* lateral bending of, *72, 73, 75;* loading of, *92, 93;* location of, *64, 65, 70;* lordosis of, *70, 71, 101;* range of motion, *68, 72, 73, 90;* rotation about, *78, 81;* shape of, *66, 88;* and tonic reflex, *216*

Lumen, *441;* pressure on, and release of HCl, *444*

Lungs, *311;* and aging, *494–496;* and the ANS, *145;* asymmetry of, *522;* and blood-air mixing, *358;* blood flow through, *358;* and circadian rhythm, *478, 480, 482;* and cranial nerve X, *367;* elasticity of, *364;* and exercise, *496;* function of, *312–314, 326;* location of, *443;* stretch receptors in, *203, 367;* structure of, *356–359;* and surfactants, *364;* and thoracic misalignment, *80*

Luteinizing hormone (LH), *143, 404;* and menstruation, *453;* ultradian release of, *476*

Lymph, *352–354;* circulation and *yogasana, 353;* composition of, *352;* and digestion, *352;* drainage from eyes, *349;* and emulsified fat, *445, 448;* and heart rate, *352;* and leucocytes, *383;* movement of, against gravity, *178;* system, *1;* and thoracic misalignment, *80;* and valves, *352*

Lymph edema, *230, 333, 351, 353;* and cancer, *353;* and infection, *353;* and *viparita karani, 351*

Lymph glands, relation to the *chakras, 103, 105;* shrinkage and stress, *156*

Lymph nodes, *353, 354;* and the ANS, *386;* and control of nasal laterality, *379;* function of, *353;* location of, *353;* and macrophages, *353*

Lymphocytes, *325, 353, 383–385;* action of, *384, 390;* and attitude, *385;* and the ANS, *386;* and exercise, *389*

Lysozyme, and digestion, *442;* and disinfection, *442*

M

Macrophage cells, *384;* and body temperature, *385;* and the lymph nodes, *353;* and red blood cells, *323;* and white blood cells, *324*

Malasana, and the center of gravity, *537;* and gravity, *554;* and the pubic symphysis, *458;* as a "X-rated" posture, *513*

Male sexual function, *461, 462;* and ejaculation, *462;* and gonadotropins, *461;* neuroanatomy of, *462;* penis and the ANS, *461, 462;* and temperature of sperm, *461;* testosterone and erection, *461*

Malleus, *433;* and cranial nerve V, *435;* location of, *434*

Mammillary body, location of, *34, 141*

Mandible, *94, 96;* location of, *237*

Mania, *463;* and blue-color viewing, *469;* and the catecholamines, *469;* and core temperature, *469;* and nasal laterality, *466;* and norepinephrine, *466;* relation to bipolar disorder, *469*

Manipura chakra, *103;* location of, *104;* relation to plexus, *103*

Manubrium, connection to clavicle, *254;* function of, *361;* location of, *237, 360*

Maricyasana III, *56, 72, 78, 91;* and the breath, *365;* and constipation, *450;* and handedness, *520;* and neurological damage, *513;* and sacroiliac joint, *98;* vascular compression in, *330*

Marijuana, effect on reticular formation, *33;* and formation of an embolism, *518*

Marriage, and longevity, *499*

Masculine, *3*

Masseter muscles, *19, 96;* location of, *168;* and lockjaw, *125*

Mastoid process, *94*

Matsyasana, *100*

Mechanoreceptors, *17, 125, 198–208;* in joint capsules, *268;* in ligaments, *268, 269;* in muscles, *175, 190, 198–206;* and reflex actions, *203;* see also **Baroreceptors** and **Muscle spindles**

Medial meniscus of knee, *251*

Medial suture, *94*

Meditation, *11, 59, 60, 404*

Medulla oblongata, *14–16, 24;* and baroreceptors, *339, 340;* and control of the breath, *366, 367;* and fear, *345;* function of, *30;* and hearing, *440;* location of, *30, 145;* and inversions, *346;* and nasal laterality, *378;* and spinothalamic tract, *87;* and sweating, *395;* and the vestibular organs, *440*

Meissner's corpuscles, *284, 286;* adaptation in, *290;* and light touch, *288, 289;* and proprioception, *288*

Melanocytes, *285*

Melatonin, and cancer, *404;* and circadian rhythm, *479, 480, 485;* and meditation, *404;* and the pineal gland, *404, 485;* and SAD, *431*

Memory, *22, 40, 42, 43;* and aging, *494, 501, 502;* cells for, *384;* and cerebral dominance, *51;* and circadian rhythm, *479, 481, 482;* and the cortex, *47;* and cortisol, *149;* erasure of, *44;* menopause and loss of, *461;* and handedness, *425;* and hormones, *401;* location of, *25;* and oxytocin, *48, 404;* and proteins, *45, 47;* recall, *43;* and sleep, *490;* and *savasana*, *490;* and time, *42, 43;* and vaccination, *384, 385;* and vasopressin, *47, 404, 485;* and visual laterality, *424–426*

Meninges, *37*

Meniscus of the knee, *5, 251, 281;* as shock absorber, *251, 252*

Menopause, *459–461;* and aging, *494;* and the ANS, *460;* and anxiety, *461;* and backbending, *459, 460;* and connective tissue, *460;* and depression, *459;* and estradiol, *408;* and estrogen, *459–461;* and estrone, *408;* and hot flashes, *459, 460;* and HRT, *459;* and memory, *461;* and night sweats, *459, 460;* and *niralamba sarvangasana*, *460;* and progesterone, *459;* and spinal twists, *459*

Menstruation, *453–456;* and *apana* energy, *455;* and body fat, *454;* and corpus luteum, *453;* and endometrium, *453;* and effects of estrogen, *453, 454;* and the fallopian tubes, *453;* and gonadotropins, *453;* and the hypothalamus, *143, 453;* as an infradian rhythm, *491;* and the liver, *454;* and lower-back pain, *456;* and lumbar misalignment, *80;* onset and circadian rhythm, *478;* and ovum, *453;* and pain, *456;* and the pineal gland as pacemaker, *453;* and postural weakness, *512;* and prostaglandins, *456;* and the pubic symphysis, *98;* and the sacroiliac joint, *98;* and *sirsasana*, *455;* and sperm, *453*

Menstrual cramps, *231;* and *baddha konasana*, *231;* and *supta virasana*, *231;* and *upavistha konasana*, *231*

Menstruation and inversions, *455, 456;* and *apana* energy, *455;* and blood flow in uterus, *349, 453, 455*

Mental alertness, and aging, *494;* and circadian rhythm, *479–482;* and the diaphragmatic breath, *371;* and estrogen in menopause, *461;* and the sympathetic NS, *136;* and *yogasana* practice, *500–502;* see also **Reticular formation**

Mental dissociation, and hypnotism, *420;* and the pineal gland, *420*

Merkel receptors, *286;* adaptation in, *291;* structure of, *287*

Merudanda, *101*

Mescaline, *131*

Metabolism, and the hypothalamus, *143;* and the thyroid, *404, 405*

Methane, generation in the gut, *446*

Microbes, and the colon, *446*

Microglial cells, *389*

Microsaccades, *418*

Midbrain, *14–16;* location of, *24, 30, 145*

Middle ear, *17–20, 378, 433–437;* location of, *434;* muscles of, *435;* reflex of, *435;* relaxation of, *435, 437;* and REM sleep, *436;* and the reticular formation, *437;* and *savasana, 435;* and the sneeze, *373, 435*

Migraine headache, *38, 39, 60, 79*

Mineralocorticoids, *386*

Minute volume, *364*

Mitochondria, and exercise, *322;* and free radicals, *497;* in muscles, *174, 182, 184, 496;* and oxidation of fuels, *369;* and stomach acid, *445*

Monamine oxidase, *39, 129*

Monday-morning blues, *486*

Monocytes, *324, 325, 383, 384*

Morphine, *163*

Moon, rotation of, *473*

Motivational system, *17–19, 23, 135;* and color viewing, *429;* and pleasure, *297*

Motor cortex, *16, 19;* and the ANS, *145;* function of, *26;* location of, *27, 173;* map of, *28, 424*

Motor nerves, *16, 112;* and the spinal cord, *87*

Motor unit, *113, 114;* and alpha-motor neurons, *173–176;* control of single, *114, 175;* and neural dominance, *46;* and B. K. S. Iyengar, *114*

Mouth, *442*

Mucus, and the ANS, *139, 393, 394;* and epithelial cells, *394;* and the parasympathetic NS, *376, 377, 393*

Muktasana, *127,* and damage to the sciatic nerve, *514*

Mulhabandhasana, injury in, *281*

Muladhara chakra, *9, 103;* location of, *104*

Multiple sclerosis, *121*

Multipolar cells, function of, *112, 125;* structure of, *109;* and vision, *132*

Muscles, *1, 16, 18, 167–234;* action of, *186, 187;* effect of age on, *192;* and the ANS, *139;* and breech presentation, *457;* and compression of, *221, 222;* and connective tissue, *171, 187;* and contraction headache, *38;* contraction of, *169, 172, 173, 179–181, 194;* and cortisol, *183;* cross section of, *182, 187, 229;* death of, *176;* dehydration and cramps, *231;* and filament overlap, *186, 194, 195;* and glucose, *321;* inhibition of, *188, 194;* innervation of, *176,* *177;* and interneurons, *188, 194, 202;* and ischemia, *185;* and lactic acid, *183, 184;* learning, *18, 233, 234;* loss of in legs, *176;* mass and exercising, *496, 499;* memory and age, *233, 234;* and mitochondria, *174, 182, 184, 496;* as organs of constant volume, *182;* oxygen consumption, *139, 185;* power, *186;* and proprioception, *210, 211;* and range of motion, *185, 491;* tremor, *126, 175;* vascularization of, *177, 178;* viscosity of, *224–227;* work of, *185;* and *yogasana* practice, *182, 199–201*

Muscle fiber types, *189–193;* and aging, *495, 496;* characteristics of, *191;* interconversion, *184, 192, 495, 496, 555;* in poultry, *192;* twitch time of, *174;* and *yogasana* practice, *192, 193, 421*

Muscle fibers, *171;* fasciculus in, *171, 172;* proportions of, *193;* rest period for, *232;* scars in, *232;* structure of, *173, 179;* and Schwann cells, *174;* tearing of, *232*

Muscle extensors, *170, 195;* healing of injuries to, *177;* and the myotactic stretch reflex, *213*

Muscle fiber, type 1, *120, 190, 191;* and acetylcholine, *189;* and aging, *495;* and isometric contraction, *190;* and myoglobin, *189;* and postural muscles, *190;* properties of, *191, 193;* speed of contraction of, *189, 190*

Muscle fiber, type 2, *120, 189, 191;* and acetylcholine, *189;* and aging, *495;* properties, of, *191*

Muscle fiber, type 3, *120, 183, 189–191;* and acetylcholine, *189;* and aging, *495;* and anaerobic oxidation, *191;* and injury of, *191;* properties of, *191;* speed of contraction of, *190;* and *yogasana* practice, *192, 193, 421*

Muscle movement, abductors, *170, 171; 195;* action, *186, 187;* adductors, *170, 171;* isometric action, *187;* and isotonic movement, *187;* rotators, *170;* and warming up, *227*

Muscle soreness, *184, 230, 231;* and hypertension, *337*

Muscle spindle, *190;* adaptation of receptors in, *202;* and extrafusal fibers, *200;* function of, *201–203, 205, 207;* and gamma-motor neurons, *113, 175, 200–202, 205;* and hyperflexibility, *203;* intrafusal fibers within, *200, 201, 205;* neural output during stretching, *115, 202;* and proprioceptive sense, *203, 209;* structure of, *199;* viscous flow in, *202*

Muscle strength, *173–175, 185, 186;* and aging, *494, 495, 499;* and cerebral dominance, *56;* and circadian rhythm, *480;* and emotions, *226, 227;* and muscle length, *186;* power of, *186;*

and protein crosslinking, *497;* when viewing color, *226, 429;* and weakness, *126, 127, 279;* and *yogasana* practice, *500*

Muscle stretching, *190, 223–227;* and connective tissue, *189, 190, 224;* and eccentric contractions, *230;* and delayed soreness, *230;* and mental stretching, *226, 227;* and prompt soreness, *230, 231;* and the stretch reflex, *202, 212;* and time, *224–226;* viscoelastic character of, *224–226;* see also the **Myotactic stretch reflex**

Muscle tone, *33, 48, 203–206, 224, 378;* and anxiety, *206, 471;* and the ANS, *139, 143, 147, 150, 176, 205;* and the bones, *240, 246;* and circadian rhythm, *478, 479, 481;* and circulation, *205;* and the emotions, *206, 463;* excessive, *92, 202;* and the flexional reflex, *214, 215;* and gamma-motor neurons, *201, 202, 205, 214;* and ischemia, *205, 206;* lack of, *49;* and laughter, *222, 351;* loss of, *33, 156, 222;* and postural muscles, *206;* and psychological problems, *92, 159, 206, 471;* rest length of, *186, 205;* and shivering, *143;* and stressors, *153, 154, 156, 158;* and *yogasana* practice, *205, 206, 227*

Musculoskeletal system, *391*

Music, and anaesthesia, *437;* and hearing, *434;* and the saccule, *439;* and testosterone, *410*

Myelin, in muscle fibers, *174;* and nerves, *513, 514;* neural wrapping in infants, *39, 119, 120;* and reflexive actions, *120;* in spinal cord, *84*

Myofascia, *276–280;* and muscle action, *276, 277;* price of, *277;* and range of motion, *276;* stress-strain curve for, *278;* and temperature, *279*

Myofibrils, *171, 172;* contraction of, *173;* structure of, *179*

Myoglobin, *184, 191;* and muscle fiber type 1, *189*

Myopia, *419, 420;* and retinal detachment, *419*

Myosin, *172, 180;* and ATP, *183;* overlap with actin, *181, 185, 190, 194;* structure of, *178, 179, 190*

Myotactic stretch reflex, *205, 212–214*

N

Nada **sound**, and the *anahata chakra*, *436;* source of, *436, 439*

Nadis, *9, 54, 101–105;* and nasal laterality, *105;* relation to nerves, *119, 140*

Nadi shodana, and nasal laterality, *380, 382*

Nasal allergies, and circadian rhythms, *480*

Nasal apparatus/nose, and breathing, *96;* and cervical misalignment, *79;* conchae and cooling the brain, *36, 357, 375;* and the EEG, *374;* erectile tissue in, *375;* erection and the ANS, *139;* function of, *375;* and heat dissipation, *356, 375;* mucus in, *356, 377;* and PMS, *375;* runny and circadian rhythm, *478, 480;* septum of, *375;* structure of, *357, 375;* sympathetic nerve plexi in, *375*

Nasal laterality, *55, 374–381;* and the ANS, *139, 159, 377;* and connection to cerebral laterality, *55, 381, 422;* control of, *378, 379, 381;* and cranial nerve I, *379;* and depression, *466;* and diaphragmatic breathing, *380;* and EEG activity, *377;* and emotions, *378, 380;* and good health, *378;* and lymph nodes, *379;* and mania, *466;* mechanism of, *375, 378;* and the medulla, *378;* and *nadis*, *105, 380;* and OCD, *471;* and *padadirasana*, *379;* periodicity of, *375, 377;* and orgasm, *376;* and sneeze, *376;* and *samadhi*, *376;* and ultradian rhythm, *474, 476;* and *yogasana* practice, *380;* and *yogadandasana*, *379*

Nasal/sexual interplay, *375*

Nausea, and the semicircular canals, *438, 440*

Navasana, *99, 100;* balancing in, *525;* and pregnancy, *458;* wall support for, *536*

Neck, extension of, *67; halasana* and injury to, *82, 346, 347;* muscles and headache, *37;* pain and tonic reflex, *215;* psychoanatomy of, *163*

Nerve fiber types, A_{alpha}, *120, 121, 176, 191;* A_{beta}, *120, 121, 176;* A_{gamma}, *120, 176;* B, *120;* C, *120, 121, 191;* Ia, *120, 121, 176, 188, 201, 209;* Ib, *120, 121, 176, 201;* II, *120, 121;* III, *120;* IV, *120, 121*

Nerves, *13;* damage to, *125–128, 513–515;* death of, *126, 128;* demyelination of, *513;* depolarization of, *107, 111, 116–118;* diameters of, *120, 128;* effects of pressure on, *125, 126, 217;* elasticity of, *128;* excitation of, *123–125;* hyperpolarization of, *116, 117, 120;* and inhibition, *123, 125;* and ischemia, *185, 513, 514;* and muscle types, *120;* and myelin, *84;* and reciprocal inhibition, *194;* and Schwann cells, *112, 119, 287;* strength of, *177;* tensile stress on, *126, 127*

Nervousness, and dominant right frontal lobe, *523;* and exhaustion, *124*

Nervous systems, *13–18*

Neural, adaptation, *116;* information signal, *132;* integration, *115, 117, 119;* membrane, *111;* noise, *203, 204;* plexi, *104;* receptor (postsynaptic), *121;* sensitivity, *116;* transduction, *114, 116;* transmitter (presynaptic), *121*

Neural conduction, *114–121;* compression and, *126;* refractory period in, *117, 119, 120, 123;* velocity of, *84, 117–121, 128*

Neural connections, conduction velocity in, *84, 117–121;* and learning, *46, 47;* patterns of, *42, 43;* plasticity of, *112, 113;* relation to *chakras, 105;* tracts, *107;* see also **Synapses**

Neural crossover, and balancing, *542–544;* and *parivrtta trikonasana, 543*

Neuroendocrine function, *399, 400;* and ultradian rhythms, *476*

Neurogenesis, *22, 40;* and the hippocampus, *500*

Neurolinguistic programming (NLP), *424, 425*

Neuromuscular junction, end plate structure, *173, 174;* function of, *178*

Neurotransmitters, *116, 118, 119, 122, 128–130;* and aging, *497;* binding of, *123;* degradation of, *123;* and dopamine, *129, 407;* and the enteric nervous system, *137;* and epinephrine, *128, 129;* hormones as, *124;* and learning, *45, 125;* neuropeptides, *128, 130;* reabsorption of, *123*

Neutrophils, *324, 325, 383;* action of, *384;* and exercise, *389;* and time of maximum number, *478, 479*

Newton's Law of Gravitation, *553;* and balance, *556*

Nicotine, *131, 147*

Night sweats, and menopause, *459, 460;* and sleep, *460*

Niralamba sarvangasana, 531, 536; and menopause, *460*

N-nitrosamines, and cancer, *393, 394*

Niyama, 9

Nociceptors, *195, 203,* and dermatomes, *303–307;* and pain, *296–298*

Noncyclical body clocks, *473, 500, 501*

Norepinephrine, *39;* and adrenal medulla, *403;* and aging, *500;* and alpha/beta receptors, *129, 407;* and backbending, *217;* and bipolar disorder, *469;* and blue lights, *469;* in bronchi, *359;* and depression, *464;* and exercise, *469;* and digestion, *148;* in the heart, *315, 317;* and mania, *466;* and mescaline, *130, 131;* as neurotransmitter, *117, 128, 129;* and *savasana, 490, 491;* and smooth muscles, *129;* and the sympathetic NS, *136, 139, 146;* ultradian release of, *476*

Nuclear-chain fibers, *199, 200;* functions of, *201;* innervation of, *201;* structure of, *200*

Nucleus ambiguus, and baroreceptors, *341*

Nucleus pulposus, dimensions of, *90, 92, 93;* function, *90;* herniation of, *91;* structure of, *82, 87, 88;* transformation of, *82*

Numbness, sensation of, *91, 125–127*

Nutrients, absorption and the ANS, *13;* in the brain, *93;* diffusion of, *82, 83;* in the spine, *88*

O

Obesity, *6, 270, 271*

Obsessive-compulsive disorder (OCD), *60, 468, 471;* and cerebral laterality, *468;* and nasal laterality, *471*

Occipital bone, *30*

Occipital lobe, *15, 18;* function of, *26, 28;* and headaches, *38;* location of, *24, 27, 94;* and vision, *415, 424, 533*

Occlusion, *81, 82*

Ocular-vagal heart-slowing reflex, *39, 152, 307;* and the cervical flexion reflex, *219;* and cranial nerve X, *220;* and headache relief, *220, 334;* and intraocular pressure, *349;* and inversions, *549*

Ocular-vestibular connection, *418*

Oculomotor complex, *413;* and balance, *418;* nerves for, *19, 423*

Olfactory nerve; see **Cranial nerve I**

Olfaction, *28, 463;* olfactory bulb, *34*

Oligomenorrhea, *455;* and bone loss, *455;* and high cortisol, *455;* and low estrogen, *455*

Om, and earth's oscillations, *436;* and toning, *437*

Optic chiasm, location of, *24, 141, 423, 424*

Optic crossover, and cerebral laterality, *422–424*

Optic nerves, *349, 421;* and cerebrospinal fluid, *418;* crossover of, *422–424;* function of, *416;* location of, *412, 414;* see also **Cranial nerve II**

Oral breathing, and the EEG, *374;* and heat dissipation, *375*

Orange-color viewing, *427*

Orgasm, *462;* and nasal laterality, *376;* and oxytocin, *404*

Oscillator X, and core temperature, *477;* and cortisol release, *477;* and the hypothalamus, *477;* and K^+ ion excretion, *477;* and Na^+ ion excretion, *477;* and urinary volume, *477*

Oscillator Y, and Ca^{2+} ion excretion, *477;* and growth hormone, *477;* and the rest-activity cycle, *475, 477;* and skin temperature, *477;* and slow-wave sleep, *477;* and the suprachiasmatic nucleus, *477*

Ossification, *235*

Osteoarthritis, and circadian rhythm, *480–482;* and chronotherapy, *487;* and high-heeled shoes, *268;* of the knees, *247, 261, 268;* and being overweight, *268;* of the spine, *91*

Osteoblasts, *280;* and the ANS, *246;* function of, *238, 239, 242–244;* and remodeling, *245, 246*

Osteoclasts, and the ANS, *246;* function of, *238, 239, 242–244;* and remodeling, *245, 246*

Osteoporosis, *269–272;* and aging, *270, 494, 495;* and bone density, *241, 269, 272;* and estrogen in women, *270, 272;* and HRT, *272, 460;* and kyphosis, *70, 271;* and loading, *90, 271;* and lead poisoning, *243;* and menopause, *270, 460;* and the pelvis, *269;* risk factors for, *270;* and T cells, *385;* and testosterone in men, *272;* and *yogasana* practice, *271, 272, 351*

Otolith organs, *438*

Outer ear, *433*

Oval window, *433;* location of, *434*

Ovaries, *461;* relation to *chakras*, *105;* and estrogen, *408;* location of, *402;* and progesterone, *408;* and relaxin, *408;* and sex drive, *408*

Overbalancing, *544*

Over-training, and amenorrhea, *455;* and asthma attacks, *359;* and growth hormone, *233;* and *yogasana* practice, *359*

Oxygen concentration, in arteries, *368;* chemoreceptors for, *342, 367;* and inversions, *342;* in plasma, *369*

Oxygen consumption, and aging, *496;* and the heart, *320–322;* and muscles, *139, 185;* in REM sleep, *488;* in the spinal cord, *84;* and stressors, *153;* in unilateral breathing, *53*

Oxyhemoglobin, *227*

Oxytocin, and the ANS, *139, 143;* and autism, *404;* and social memory, *47 , 404;* as a neuropeptide, *130;* and orgasm, *404;* and the posterior pituitary, *48, 404;* and pregnancy, *404, 457*

P

Pacemaker, for breathing, *365;* for endocrine glands, *485;* for the enteric nervous system, *319, 447;* for the heart, *309, 315–317;* for menstruation, *453*

Pacinian corpuscles, *132, 286;* adaptation in, *289, 290;* and balance, *526, 530;* and the big toe, *540;* and heavy pressure, *290;* and proprioception, *290;* and standing poses, *530;* structure of, *287;* and the thalamus, *290;* and balancing in *vrksasana*, *539, 540*

Padadirasana, and switching nasal laterality, *379*

Padmasana, *36, 100, 127;* and blood circulation, *334;* injury in, *251, 279–281, 513, 514, 518;* and ischemia, *514;* and knee motion,

265–267; a safe way to teach, *266, 267;* and varicosities, *266, 518*

Pain, *28, 294–307,463;* and the ANS, *295, 298, 301, 303;* and the anterior hypothalamus, *203;* and arachidonic acid, *126, 302;* and the breath, *472;* and circadian rhythms, *478, 481;* and cultural factors, *299;* and dermatomes, *303–307;* and emotions, *298;* and endorphins, *130, 164, 303;* and fear, *298, 345;* in foot, *497;* and free nerve endings, *38, 291;* and gastrointestinal organs, *441;* gate theory of, *269, 300, 301;* and habituation, *297;* of herniated disc, *91, 92;* and histamine, *297;* and ischemia, *302;* in joints, *261, 262, 268, 269;* and learning, *297;* and menstruation, *456;* mental, *464;* and muscle contraction, *295, 463;* and nociceptors, *296;* and the placebo effect, *164, 165;* and prostaglandins, *296, 297, 301, 302;* and psychological factors, *92, 295, 296, 298, 299;* radiating, *125;* receptor nerve type, *120;* referred pain, *92, 303–307;* effect on reticular formation, *33, 86, 298;* sensitization of, *297;* in *sirsasana*, *456;* and skin irritation, *302;* visceral, *150, 296, 306, 441, 448;* as a warning signal, *294;* and the weather, *261;* and *yogasana* practice, *296, 298, 299, 301–303*

Palmar conductance, *159;* and color viewing, *427*

Palms, and sweating, *395*

Pancreas, *1, 407, 408;* and alpha cells, *407;* and relation to the ANS, *145, 407, 408, 451;* and beta cells, *407;* buffering of small intestine, *445;* relation to the *chakras*, *103, 105;* and digestive enzymes, *447;* and glucagon, *407;* and insulin supply, *407, 447;* location of, *402, 443;* and thoracic misalignment, *80*

Panic attacks, and CO_2, *471*

Papilla, *415, 417*

Parasites, *325, 383;* and killer T cells, *385*

Parasympathetic nervous system, *5, 15–20, 53–55, 128, 136, 150–153;* and allergies, *388;* and alpha waves, *60;* and cerebral laterality, *52, 55;* relation to the *chakras*, *103, 105;* and the cranial nerves, *137, 146, 151, 152;* and darker colors, *356;* and defecation, *397;* and diaphragmatic breathing, *372;* and the EEG, *150;* and its effect on the enteric nervous system, *137, 397;* and exhalation, *356, 367;* and the heart, *150, 317, 318, 320, 322;* and immunity, *386, 387;* and *langhana*, *374;* and mucus, *150, 376, 377, 393;* and nasal laterality, *56;* and neurotransmitters, *137;* and saliva,

393, 394; and *sirsasana*, 337; response to stress, 336; and spinal flexion, 84; target organs for, 137, 145; and tears, 393; and urination, 351

Parathyroid gland, and Ca^{2+}, 405; location of, 402; and PTH, 405; relation to the *chakras*, 103; and vitamin D, 405

Parathyroid hormone (PTH), 243, 405

Paraventricular nucleus, function of, 144; location of, 141

Paravertebral ganglia, 128, 144–146

Parietal cells, and generation of stomach acid, 445; and the prostaglandins, 445; of the stomach, 444, 445

Parietal lobe, 15; function of, 26, 27, 39; location of, 24, 27, 94; size of, 39

Parietal-occipital sulcus, 24

Parighasana, and the knee joint, 250

Parivrtta ardha chandrasana, balancing in, 535; internal wall for, 536

Parivrtta janu sirsasana, 77; and the psoas, 248, 250

Parivrtta parsvakonasana, 56

Parivrtta trikonasana, 77, 207; balancing in, 525; internal wall for, 536; and neural crossover, 541–543; and referred pain, 307; and resistive balancing, 545; and stabilizing the groins, 542; symmetry in, 521; wall support for, 536

Parkinson's disease, 35, 39, 60; and loss of dopamine, 129

Parotid glands, see **Saliva**

Parsva halasana, 550

Parsva karnapidasana, 550

Parsvakonasana, 221; and nasal laterality, 380; and rotation of the femurs, 249

Parsva sirsasana, 78

Parsvottanasana, 263; and the calf, 264

Pasasana, 56, 291

Paschimottanasana, 10, 210, 241, 347; best time for, 491

Passion, 13

Patanjali, 2, 4, 6, 24

Patella, location of, 237, 251; structure of, 250

Patellar knee-jerk reflex, 194, 212–214, 223, 532; and the biceps femoris, 212, 213; and depression, 213; and phasic reflex, 212–214; and the quadruceps, 212, 213

Pavan muktasana, 291

Pectoralis major, action of, 255; location of, 168

Pelvis, 63; in childbirth, 99; counter-rotation of, 78; diaphragm of, 276; and the femur bones, 100; gender differences in, 98; joints of, 98; ligaments of, 98; motion of, 100; nerve plexus

of, 104; and osteoporosis, 269; in pregnancy, 99; psychoanatomy of, 163; and red blood cells, 323; and the vascular system, 326

Penile erection, 140; and the ANS, 461, 462; and REM sleep, 461, 462, 488

Pepsin, and microbes, 445; and protein digestion, 445; and ulcers, 448

Pepsinogen, and ulcers, 387

Peptides, as hormones, 401

Periaqueductal gray area, and endorphins, 303

Peripheral nervous system, 13–15, 17–20

Perineum, 326; muscles of, 16

Periodicity of body rhythms, 473–491; and blood pressure, 474; and the celestial oscillator, 474; definition of, 473; and heart rate, 474; and the pulse of cerebrospinal fluid, 474, 475; and set points, 474, 475; and the sleep/wake cycle, 474; see also **Circadian rhythms**, **Ultradian rhythms**, and **Infradian rhythms**

Periodontal bone loss, on aging, 494, 500

Periosteum, 171, 235, 238, 239, 262

Peripheral nervous system, 1, 13, 14, 17, 107, 127, 128

Peristalsis, and the abdominal breath, 371; and the ANS, 147, 150; and cranial nerve X, 447; and the enteric nervous system, 447; as a reflex, 222, 447; and the small intestine, 446

Personality, relation to breathing, 163; and visual stress, 419

Pessimism, and dominant right frontal lobe, 523; see also **Attitudes**

Phages, 383

Phalanges, of foot, 252; location of, 237

Pharyngeal plexus, 103

Pharynx, 356; location of, 357; plexus, 103; and the spine, 79

Phasic reflex, 211, 212; and patellar knee-jerk reflex, 212–214

Phospholipids, 109

Phosphorus, and bones, 235, 242

Photopigments, and circadian rhythm, 422; in the retina, 131

Piezoelectricity, and bone, 245, 246; and cartilage, 280

Piloerection, 307, 308; and the ANS, 140, 148, 150

Pincha mayurasana, balancing in, 545, 549; and filament overlap, 186; and gravity, 553, 554; internal wall for, 536; and redistributing the mass, 554

Pindasana, and constipation, 398

Pineal gland, 1, 404; and the ANS, 139; relation to the *chakras*, 103; and hormonal bio-

rhythms, *142;* location of, *402;* and mela-
    tonin, *404, 485;* and the menstrual pacemaker,
    453; and mental dissociation, *420*
Pingala nadi, *54, 102, 140;* and nasal laterality,
    380
Pink agitation, *427, 429*
Pins-and-needles sensation, *125;* relation to the
    chakras, 103
Piriformis muscle, *5, 92;* and the sacroiliac joint,
    98; and sciatica during pregnancy, *459;* and
    sciatica, *514*
Pitta, 382, 483, 484
Pituitary gland, *1, 404;* and the ANS, *147;* rela-
    tion to the *chakras, 103;* and CRF, *403;* and
    endorphins, *131;* hypothalamic control of, *34,
    47, 135, 142, 143, 399, 400, 403;* location of,
    24, 141, 402
Placebo effect, *48, 56, 163–166;* and anxiety,
    164, 165; and color, *165;* and depression, *164,
    165, 464;* examples of, *164;* and headaches,
    164; and healing, *166;* and the heart, *164;* and
    hypertension, *164;* and pain, *164, 165, 302;*
    target organs for, *403;* and surgery, *165;* and
    ulcers, *164*
Plantar fasciitis, *280;* and obesity, *280*
Platelets, *238, 324;* and blood clotting, *324;* and
    circadian rhythm, *478, 480;* and collagen,
    324; function of, *324;* and thromboses, *515;*
    and *yogasana* practice, *324*
Pleasure center, *23, 24, 35, 297, 463;* and
    amphetamines, *130;* and the hypothalamus,
    142, 297
Pleural membranes, *362*
PMS symptoms, and erectile nasal tissue, *375*
Polio, and exercise pattern, *389, 390*
Pons, *14–16, 24;* and control of the breath, *366;*
    function of, *30, 31, 437;* location of, *30, 145*
Portal vein, *448*
Pose and repose, in vision, *418*
Possum response, *336;* and hypotension, *338*
Postcentral gyrus, *15, 209, 289*
Posterior hypothalamus, *138;* and ANS control,
    140; function of, *144, 203;* location of, *141;*
    and temperature sensors, *334*
Posterior pituitary, release of oxytocin, *408;*
    release of vasopressin, *47, 404*
Postsynaptic potentials, and the EEG, *57*
Posture, and depression, *464;* and pressure at the
    ankle, *332, 333;* and ventricular stroke vol-
    ume, *369;* and the thymus, *70;* and weakness
    during menstruation, *512*
Postural muscles, and motor units, *113, 175;* and
    muscle tone, *206;* and poor posture, *309;*

properties of, *191;* strength of, *175;* and type-
    1 fibers, *190*
Postural reflexes, and the cerebellum, *33*
Potassium ion (K$^+$), *116;* in body fluids, *149;*
    channels and epinephrine, *407;* circadian
    cycle of excretion, *397, 476;* and hyperpolar-
    ization, *123;* and inhibition, *123;* and kinocili-
    um, *438;* and oscillator X, *477;* and urination,
    397
Power, *1;* definition of, *186;* stroke of heart, *312*
Prana, *9, 101–105;* energy of, *241;* relation to
    transmembrane voltage, *119*
Pranayama, *6, 9;* and the ANS, *161, 381;* and
    asthma, *359;* best time for, *484;* and breath
    control, *367;* and *brmhana, 382;* and the
    diaphragmatic breath, *382;* and formation of
    an embolism, *518;* and immunity, *389;* and
    langhana, 382
Prasarita padottanasana, 263
Pratyahara, 6, 9
Precentral gyrus, *15*
Prefrontal cortex, *142;* and alpha waves, *153;*
    and depression, *152, 153*
Pregnancy, and biorhythms, *457;* and collagen,
    457; and connexin, *457;* and constipation,
    459; and cramps, *458;* and estrogen, *406;* and
    estrogen/progesterone balance, *456, 457;* and
    fallen arches, *458;* and the femoral vein, *458;*
    and fetal hormones, *457;* and heartburn, *459;*
    and the inferior vena cava, *459;* and inver-
    sions, *456, 458;* and joint stability, *98, 264,
    265;* and leg cramps, *458;* and *navasana, 458;*
    and oxytocin, *404, 457;* and progesterone,
    406; and the prostaglandins, *457;* and respira-
    tion, *458;* and sciatica, *459;* and first-trimester
    yogasana practice, *456;* and the uterus, *457*
Premature birth, and *karnapidasana, 215;* and
    lower-back pain, *215*
Premenstrual syndrome (PMS), and color ther-
    apy, *427;* and erectile tissue in nose, *375;* and
    estrogen/progesterone balance, *454;* and REM
    sleep, *489;* and SAD phototherapy, *454*
PMS, type-A, and anxiety, *454;* and the ANS,
    454; and *balasana, 454;* and *savasana, 454*
PMS, type-C, cravings, *454;* fatigue, headache,
    454; and SAD phototherapy, *454*
PMS, type-D, and depression, *454;* and *dha-
    nurasana, 454;* and *setu bandhasana, 454;*
    and sympathetic stimulation, *454;* and *urdhva
    mukha svansana, 454*
PMS, type-H, and inversions, *455;* and water
    retention, *454*
Preoptic area, function of, *144, 202;* location of,
    141

Pressure sensors, see **Skin**

Pretectal region, *423*

Pretend knee surgery, *164*

Primary visual cortex, *9, 19*

Progesterone, and birth, *406*; and menopause, *459, 494*; and menstruation, *453*; and the ovaries, *408*; as a steroidal hormone, *401*

Projection fibers, *29*

Prolactin, *143*; and the anterior pituitary, *404*; times of max/min concentrations, *402*

Proliferants, *264, 280*

Prolotherapy, *38*

Proprioception, *8, 18, 29, 208–211, 268, 269*; and aging, *497*; and balance, *33, 526, 533*; and the cerebellum, *33, 533*; and the cerebral hemispheres, *50*; and the Golgi tendon organs, *206, 209, 268, 269*; and gravity, *556*; and hypertension, *338*; and joint capsules, *268, 269*; and kinaesthesia, *209*; and ligaments, *268, 269*; and Meissner's corpuscles, *288*; and muscle spindles, *203, 206, 210, 211*; and neural paths, *120, 209, 210*; and Pacinian corpuscles, *290*; and Ruffini corpuscles, *290*; spinal connections to sensors, *87, 114*; and left-right asymmetry, *520*; and the vestibular organs, *210*; and *yogasana* practice, *208–211*

Proprioceptive maps, *27, 28, 32, 35, 209–211, 268*

Proprioceptive neuromuscular facilitation (PNF), *203, 204, 228*; and isometric contraction, *20*

Proprioceptors, and balance, *526, 530, 532, 533*; and balancing in *vrksasana*, *539, 540*; decussation of, *209*; and joint capsules, *209*; and kinaesthesia, *209*; location of, *208*; response time of, *530*; and the sensory cortex, *209*; and static limb position, *209*

Prostaglandins, and aspirin, *296, 456*; from endothelial cells, *335*; and fever, *388*; and menstruation, *456*; and pain, *296, 297, 301, 302*; and parietal cells, *445*; and pregnancy, *457*; and temperature control, *335*

Proteins, and blood-brain barrier, *325*; channels for, *108, 109*; foreign, *383*; joint stiffness and crosslinking of, *497*; and memory, *45, 47*

Prozac, *164*

Pseudo-unipolar cells, function of, *112*; structure of, *110*

Psoas, *77*; and leg/pelvic action, *100, 248–250*; location of, *360*; and myofascia, *277*; and *parivrtta janu sirsasana*, *250*; and *upavistha konasana*, *248*

Psychoanatomy, *163*

Psychoimmunology, *390*

Psychosis, *61*

Psychotherapy, and depression, *464, 467*

Pubic bones, fusion in newborn, *98*; location of, *97, 237*

Pubic symphysis, and childbirth, *99*; as a joint, *96, 98*; location of, *97*; and *malasana*, *458*; and menopause, *98*; and menstruation, *98*; and pregnancy, *98*; and relaxin, *458*

Pulmonary, artery, *310, 326*; capillaries, *311*; function of, *314*; location of, *310, 326*

Pupils, diameters of, *378, 415, 424*; dilation of, *19, 136, 138, 147, 148, 150*; and edema, *421*; and the limbic system, *415*; and the placebo effect, *164*

Puraka, *381*

Purkinje cells, *33, 34, 109, 316*; structure of, *110*

Purvottanasana, *127, 257*

Pyloric valve, *442, 444*; and neutralization of chyme pH, *448*

Pyramidal tract, *173*

Pyrogens, *134, 383*

Q

Quadratus lumborum, *188, 360*

Quadruceps, *11, 25, 127, 167, 204*; and muscle type, *191–193*; and patella, *250, 251*; and patellar knee jerk, *212, 213*; and withdrawal reflex, *195*

R

Radius, *255, 256*; action on scapulae, *196*; artery of, *327*; articulations of, *256*; *location of, 171, 237*; reflex arc in, *212*; rotation of, *257*

Raphe nucleus, and sleep, *488*

Rapid-eye movement (REM) sleep, *54, 58, 488*; and the ANS, *138*; and atonia, *488*; beta waves in, *33*; blood pressure in, *488*; and consolidation, *47*; and genital erection, *462*; heart rate in, *488*, and the middle ear, *436*; and oscillator X, *477*; and PMS, *489*; and the rest-activity cycle, *489*; and *savasana*, *420*; and ultradian rhythm, *474*

Reason, *13*; site of, *25*

Rebound headache, *38*

Receptive fields, *417, 534*; and balancing, *417, 534, 540*

Receptor potential, *115–117*

Receptors, and consciousness, *199*; for hormones, *399*; in joints, *260*

Rechaka, *381*

Reciprocal inhibition, *10, 193–196, 202;* and interneurons, *194, 195–202;* and *uttanasana, 194*

Rectum, and the central nervous system, *442;* and cranial nerve X, *151;* and defecation, *397;* location of, *443;* stretch receptors in, *397*

Rectus abdominus, location of, *168*

Rectus femoris, location of, *168;* strength of, *253*

Red-color viewing, *427;* and the emotions, *429;* and depression, *469;* and muscle strength, *429*

Red corpuscles/Red blood cells, *22, 93;* and bone marrow, *323;* and capillary diameter, *330;* and gravity, *555;* and hemoglobin, *323, 369;* and the liver, *323, 369;* and macrophages, *323;* and the spleen, *323, 324, 353, 369;* and the sternum, *323, 369;* and the sympathetic NS, *323;* and *yogasana* practice, *324, 390*

Redistributing the mass, to balance, *536, 537;* in *adho mukha svanasana, 554;* in *virabhadrasana III, 537;* in *vrksasana, 537*

Reflex arcs, *173, 209, 211;* and cranial nerve X, *340, 341;* and interneurons, *124, 212*

Reflexive action, *10, 11, 16, 17;* conscious control of, *211, 212, 222;* and the emotions, *222;* hypothalamic control of, *34, 143;* and higher centers, *212;* intestinal, *222;* learning, *42;* and the middle ear, *435;* sensitivity and circadian rhythm, *480;* and the spinal cord, *84, 86, 87;* and *supta padangusthasana, 222;* of urination in infants, *211*

Refractory period, in the heart, *316;* in nerves, *117–119, 120, 123*

Relaxation, *17;* and anxiety, *471;* and the ANS, *420;* and beta waves, *33, 44, 488;* and the breath, *202;* and blue color, *427;* and exhalation, *364;* and hypnotism, *420;* of visual stress, *419, 420, 534;* and *yogasana* practice, *491;* see also **Savasana** and **Sarvangasana**

Relaxation response, *150, 156*

Relaxin, and constipation, *459;* and indigestion, *459;* and joints during pregnancy, *458;* and the ovaries, *408;* and the pubic symphysis, *458*

Renal artery, *327*

Renin, and the ANS, *149, 150, 407;* and angiotensin, *150;* and angiotensinogen, *335, 338;* and blood pressure, *335*

Reproductive system, *1, 23, 453–462;* and the ANS, *145*

Resistive balancing, *544, 545*

Respiratory rate, and the nucleus ambiguus, *475;* and chemoreceptors, *342;* and circadian rhythm, *480;* and color viewing, *427;* pacemaker for, *475;* and the sympathetic NS, *136, 147;* and *yogasana* practice, *337*

Respiratory system, *1;* and the breath, *355–382;* efficiency and posture, *295, 358, 359;* and pregnancy, *458;* regulation by the reticular formation, *31;* and the spine, *355;* and stressors, *154;* and venous blood flow, *333*

Respiratory sinus arhythmia (RSA), *152, 159;* mechanism of, *367, 368;* and diaphragmatic breathing, *368;* as symptomatic of health, *368*

Rest, and lower-back pain, *232;* and sleep, *491;* for injuries, *232, 233*

Rest-activity cycle, *475, 485;* and oscillator Y, *477;* and REM sleep, *489*

Reticular formation, *10, 22, 31–33;* and the ANS, *138;* arousal of, *32, 33, 57, 147, 490;* and consciousness, *31;* and the eyes, *421;* functions of, *31, 59, 60, 86, 135;* and inhibition of pain, *86, 298;* and light touch, *289;* location of, *24, 30;* and LSD, *33;* and marijuana, *33;* and mental dissociation, *420;* and the middle ear, *437;* and migraine, *39;* nuclei within, *31;* and the sleep/wake cycle, *490;* and vascular control, *31*

Retina, *18, 28, 413;* adaptation of, *417, 421;* detachment and myopia, *419;* relation to the brain, *418;* hemifields of, *422–424;* hyperpolarization in, *418;* location of, *414;* and neural convergence, *416, 417;* pigments in, *417, 485;* and stimulation of the reticular formation, *421;* stress and detachment of, *419*

Reverse breathing, *373*

Rheumatism/Rheumatoid arthritis, *261, 267;* and autoimmunity, *388;* and B and T cells, *388;* and chronotherapy, *487;* circadian rhythm of, *479, 482;* and inversions, *349;* and negative emotions, *388;* and stress, *155;* and thoracic misalignment, *80;* time of highest intensity, *268;* and the weather, *267*

Ribs/Ribcage, *359–362;* action of scapulae on, *196, 256;* attachments to, *67, 75;* clamping of motion, *72;* connection to sternum, *361;* connection to vertebrae, *361;* floating, *369;* use in inhalation, *196;* location of, *237;* motion during breathing, *363;* psychoanatomy of, *163;* and red blood cells, *323*

Right brain/Cerebral hemisphere, *3;* alpha waves and parasympathetic dominance, *140;* and the ANS, *138;* and emotions, *50, 426, 463;* and exhalation, *356;* and nervousness, *523;* and pessimism, *523;* properties of, *50, 54, 380;* and proprioception, *209;* sensory cortex in, *86*

Right frontal cortex, *41*

Right-handedness, *49;* and longevity, *49, 50;* and speech, *50, 51*

Right-nostril dominance, and inhalation, *356*

Rigor mortis, *183, 184*

Rods, function of, *415;* neuroanatomy of, *424;* and reflexive actions, *415;* spectral sensitivity of, *416;* and visual laterality, *424*

Rotator cuff, *254, 255*

Ruchikasana, *74*

Ruffini corpuscles, *199;* adaptation of, *208;* and the dermis, *208;* and B. K. S. Iyengar, *208*

Ruffini receptors, *286;* directional properties of, *290;* and proprioception, *290;* structure of, *287;* as temperature sensors, *291*

S

Saccadic motions, *413, 417, 419*

Saccharides, absorption of, *445*

Saccule, function of, *437;* location of, *434, 438;* action in *virabhadrasana III, 542;* in *sirsasana I, 550*

Sacroiliac joint, and childbirth, *98;* location of, *97;* and *maricyasana III, 99;* and menopause, *98;* and menstruation, *98;* misalignment problems of, *80;* motion of, *96, 97;* pain in, *264;* and the piriformis, *98;* and pregnancy, *98;* as a shock absorber, *97;* stability of, *98;* structure of, *96;* torque of, *78*

Sacral nerves, *15, 16, 103;* target organs of, *151*

Sacral vertebrae, *15;* location of, *64, 65, 97, 98, 237;* range of motion of, *68*

Sacrum, *1;* joints with, *96;* motion of, *100*

Sahasrara chakra, *9, 103;* location of, *104*

Salabhasana, *74;* and glaucoma, *517;* and the vertebral arteries, *516*

Saliva, and bacteria, *393, 394;* and circadian rhythm, *393, 480;* and cranial nerve VII, *19, 393;* and cranial nerve IX, *393;* as a lubricant, *393;* and *savasana, 393*

Salivary glands, *20, 393–395;* and the ANS, *139, 145, 150, 393;* and brainstem nuclei, *393;* as lie detectors, *394;* and sexual arousal, *393*

Salt excretion, and circadian rhythm, *480;* and the sleep/wake cycle, *490;* see also **Calcium ion, Potassium ion,** and **Sodium ion**

Samadhi, *6, 9;* and nasal laterality, *376*

Sarcolemma, *178;* and cortisol, *230;* structure of, *179*

Sarcomere, *178,* action within, *180, 181, 185;* in isometric contraction, *187;* permeability of, *190;* structure of, *179*

Sartorius, location of, *168*

Sarvangasana, *150, 152, 157, 158, 346, 531;* and autonomic balance, *157, 158;* and balance, *531;* and the baroreceptors, *220;* and the basilar-artery syndrome, *512, 516;* and the cervical flexion reflex, *219;* cervical vertebrae and, *74, 75, 81;* and colored lights, *430;* and constipation, *450;* and cranial blood flow, *37, 74;* and eye rolling, *420;* and glaucoma, *421, 517;* and the heart, *320;* and hiccups, *450;* and the internal wall, *536;* and intraocular pressure, *517;* and inversions, *346;* and ligaments in the neck, *229, 263;* and menopause, *460;* and menstruation, *455;* and the parasympathetic NS, *337, 346;* turning red in, *350;* and sinus congestion, *394;* and spinal mobility, *497;* and swallowing, *442;* and thyroid circulation, *405;* vision and balance in, *534;* as an "X-rated" pose, *513*

Savasana, *32, 150, 198;* and abdominal breathing, *370, 371;* and body temperature, *294;* and the center of gravity, *554;* and cerebral laterality, *55;* and the cervical flexion reflex, *218;* duration of, *407;* and the EEG, *59–61, 165, 421, 490;* and emotions, *395;* and eyebags, *491;* falling asleep in, *483;* and the flexional reflex, *215;* and gastric distress, *449;* and gravity, *525, 554;* and the heart, *359;* as hypertension treatment, *337, 338;* and hypnosis, *165;* and hypotension, *338;* and the immune system, *386;* and *jalandhara bandha, 219;* and learning, *44;* and memory, *490;* and movement of the brain, *364;* and muscles of the middle ear, *435;* and night sweats, *460;* and norepinephrine, *490, 491;* numbness in, *127;* and the parasympathetic NS, *337;* and pressure on the heart, *359;* and relaxation, *69, 321, 322;* and sleep, *420, 460;* and the reticular formation, *32, 33, 47, 165, 421, 491;* and saliva, *393;* and skin sensations, *288, 290;* and tears, *395;* and the tongue, *189;* and type-A PMS, *454*

Scapulae, *81, 195;* action and arm rotation, *257;* in *dandasana, 260;* location of, *360;* muscle attachments to, *171, 196;* and pressure on the ribs, *256, 257, 260;* and the radius, *196;* and the shoulder joint, *254, 255;* stabilizers for, *170;* structure of, *237, 238;* and the trapezius, *196, 256*

Scars, *280;* and muscle fibers, *232;* and stretching, *285*

Schizophrenia, *60*

Schwann cells, *112, 119;* in muscle fiber, *174;* in the skin, *287*

Sciatic nerve, in the aged, *540;* compression of, *514, 515;* injury of, *127, 267, 514;* length of, *118, 119;* and *muktasana, 514;* and *pad-masana, 514;* effect of the piriformis on, *514;* effect of pressure on, *126;* and *vrksasana, 541*

Sciatica, *5;* and herniated discs, *91;* and lower-back pain, *91, 92;* and lumbar misalignment, *80;* and *muktasana, 514;* and the piriformis, *514;* and pregnancy, *459;* and the tonic reflex, *216;* and *yogasana* practice, *302*

Sclera, and cataracts, *414;* and collagen, *414;* and the dura mater, *418;* location of, *414;* stress-strain curve of, *278*

Scleroderma, *274*

Scoliosis, *70, 71, 77*

Seasonal affective disorder (SAD), *430, 431;* and bipolar disorder, *470;* and depression, *469;* and the emotions, *431;* as an infradian rhythm, *491;* and melatonin, *431;* and PMS, *454;* and women, *430*

Sebaceous glands, *307, 308, 396, 401*

Semicircular canals, *439, 440;* function of, *437, 439;* location of, *434, 438;* and nausea, *438, 440*

Sense of smell, *442;* and aging, *494;* and the amygdala, *463;* and the emotions, *463;* and *yogasana* practice, *500*

Sense of taste, *20, 442;* and aging, *494;* and *yogasana* practice, *500*

Sense of time, and aging, *473, 500, 501;* and dopamine, *473*

Sensorimotor integration, *7*

Sensors, for balance, *437–440, 533, 534;* in bones, *268, 269;* in the cardiovascular system, *338–342;* in joint capsules, *208;* in ligaments, *206–208;* in muscles, *198–208;* in proprioception, *208–211;* in skin, *285–291;* in skull, *94, 95;* see also **Stretch receptors**

Sensory cortex, *18, 19, 172, 173;* location of, *27;* map of, *27, 28;* and proprioception, *209*

Sensory homunculus, *288, 424*

Sensory signals, and aging, *494;* and neurons, *112;* transduction of, *198*

Sensory systems, *17–19*

Serotonin, and the ANS, *137;* and depression, *464, 467;* and exercise, *469;* and headache, *38;* and LSD, *130;* as a neurotransmitter, *129, 137;* and platelets, *324;* and sleep, *488;* stress and carbohydrates, *449*

Serratus anterior, action during breathing, *196;* location of, *168*

Setpoint, and feedback, *134, 135, 474–476;* resetting of, *135*

Setu bandhasana, *38, 59, 61, 99, 100;* and the cervical flexional reflex, *219;* and cravings for sweets, *454;* and lower-back pain, *92;* and the parasympathetic NS, *337;* and type-C PMS, *455;* and type-D PMS, *454*

Sexuality, *1, 135, 463, 488;* and the adrenal cortex, *405;* and the ANS, *140;* and backbending, *216;* and depression, *464;* and ejaculation, *140;* and hormones, *149, 404;* and the hypothalamus, *142;* malfunction and inversions, *349;* and muscle tension, *463;* and the ovaries, *408;* and orange-color viewing, *427;* and pain, *298;* and SAD, *431;* and violet-color viewing, *427*

Shear, as a mechanical force, *76*

Shivering, *133;* and the ANS, *140, 143;* and muscle tone, *143;* and temperature regulation, *294*

Shock absorbers; cranial sutures as, *96;* in feet, *69, 96;* in the knee, *251, 252;* in the spine, *71, 72, 88, 90, 96;* and synovial joints, *63*

Short-term memory, *28, 43–45*

Shoulder joint, see **Glenoid fossa** and **Glenohumeral joint**

Shoulders, muscles and headache, *38;* psychoanatomy of, *163*

Sigmoid colon, location of, *443*

Sinoatrial (SA) node, *315, 316*

Sinus, infection and odor of the breath, *365;* and inversions, *394, 395;* and *sarvangasana, 394;* and *sirsasana, 394, 395;* and the spine, *79*

Sirsasana I, *34, 290, 348;* balancing in, *525, 532, 544, 545, 550;* and the baroreceptors, *220;* and blood in the lungs, *358;* and the broom-stick action, *549;* and constipation, *450;* and cranial sutures, *95;* and bloodshot eyes, *349;* and feedback, *532;* and feedforward, *532;* and glaucoma, *421;* and the heart rate, *321, 337, 346;* and hypertension, *350;* and intraocular pressure, *517;* and isotonic movements, *188;* and menstruation, *455;* and neck injuries, *82;* and pain, *456;* and the parasympathetic NS, *337;* and perceived sounds, *436;* and sinus congestion, *394, 395;* and swallowing, *442;* and tears, *395;* and thromboses, *516, 517;* and twisting, *81;* and the vascular system, *348;* and vision, *534, 549, 550;* and the vertebral arteries, *515, 516*

Skeletal muscles, see **Muscles**

Skin, *1, 16, 18, 19, 22, 283–308;* and aging, *289, 494;* and the ANS, *140;* as connective tissue, *284, 285;* and dermatomes, *303–307;* stress and disorders of, *291;* elastin in, *284;* electrical resistance, *140;* and emotions, *285, 291;*

and the feet, *253;* and the gastrointestinal tract, *441;* glabrous, *287;* hairy, *287;* irritation and pain relief, *302, 307;* and pain, *285;* problems and inversions, *349;* resistance to stretching, *285;* and self-comforting, *291;* spinal connections to, *87;* stress-strain curve of, *278;* structure of, *283–285;* and temperature, *140, 294;* temperature and oscillator Y, *477*

Skin receptors, *285–291;* adaptation of, *285–291;* density in body, *288;* and B.K.S. Iyengar, *289;* for pain, *285;* for temperature, *285, 334;* for tension, *285*

Skull, *30, 63, 95, 96;* bones of, *96, 237, 238;* location of, *237;* and red blood cells, *323*

Sleep, apnea, *491;* and beta waves, *33, 44, 488;* and circadian rhythm, *482;* and consolidation of memory, *47, 61;* and depression, *467;* and the eyes, *411;* latency and circadian rhythm, *480;* and longevity, *498;* and memory, *490;* and night sweats, *460;* oscillation of EEG stages, *54, 58, 488;* and the Raphe nuclei, *488;* regulation of, *31;* and *savasana*, *420, 460, 483;* oscillator Y and slow-wave, *477;* and sneezing, *373;* stages and the ANS, *138;* and urination, *397*

Sleep/wake cycle, *474, 488–491;* and alertness, *489, 490;* and the ANS, *488;* and cortisol, *490;* and the EEG, *488;* and growth hormone, *489, 490;* and learning/memory, *490;* and Raphe nucleus, *488;* and REM sleep, *488;* and the reticular formation, *490;* and salt excretion, *490;* and serotonin, *488;* and temperature, *489, 490*

Slow-twitch fibers, see **muscle fiber, type 1**

Small intestine, *445, 446;* and the ANS, *145;* area of, *446;* and bacteria, *447;* pH buffering by the pancreas, *445;* and chyme, *445;* functions of, *446;* location of, *443;* and peristalsis, *446;* and thoracic misalignment, *80*

Smile, *35*

Smooth muscles, *23, 112;* and the ANS, *139;* and arteries, *139;* and the gastrointestinal tract, *441, 447;* and ischemia, *441;* and norepinephrine, *129*

Sneezing, mechanism of, *373;* and the middle ear, *373, 435;* and nasal laterality, *376;* and sleep, *373*

Social memory, and oxytocin, *404*

Soda loading, *183*

Sodium ion (Na$^+$), *108, 111, 116, 119;* in body fluids, *149;* circadian cycle of excretion, *397;* and depolarization waves, *123;* in heart con-

traction, *316;* and oscillator X, *477;* and the pain axon, *130;* and urination, *397*

Solar plexus, *1, 103, 104, 482;* and fear, *216*

Soleus, location of, *169*

Solitary nucleus, and baroreceptors, *340, 341;* function of, *144*

Solitary tract, and the ANS, *138;* and endocrine glands, *399*

Somatostatin, and stomach acid, *408*

Speech, *20;* and handedness, *523;* hearing of, *434;* muscles of, *175*

Sperm, and menstruation, *453;* temperature of, *461;* and testosterone, *408*

Sphincter pupillae, and ANS, *414;* and ciliary ganglion, *423;* function of, *414*

Spinal column, *16, 63–84;* canal, *65, 66, 84, 91;* development of curves, *69;* dimensions of, *68, 89, 90;* health of, *82, 83;* mobility of, *67, 71–91;* muscles of, *81–83;* and osteoarthritis, *91;* as shock absorber, *69;* stenosis of, *91*

Spinal cord, *14–17, 24, 25, 84–87;* blood flow to, *36, 84, 88;* connections to other centers, *173;* and dermatomes, *86;* gray matter in, *84–87;* function of, *84;* and interneurons, *87;* and nutrients, *88;* structure of, *84, 86, 104*

Spinal curvature, *69–90;* and inhalation, *368;* and scoliosis, *70, 71, 77*

Spinal extension, and injury, *91;* and intervertebral discs, *83, 88, 90;* and relief of pain, *91*

Spinal muscles, ligaments, and tendons, erector spinae, *81, 82;* latissimus, *81;* ligamentum nuchae *81, 83, 89, 90;* and over-stretched ligaments, *92;* prestressing of, *89;* rhomboids, *81;* trapezius, *81, 92;* and tension in trapezius, *81*

Spinal flexibility, *88*

Spinal flexion, and injury, *9;* and intervertebral discs, *89, 90;* and relief of pain, *91*

Spinal nerves, *107;* impingement on, *91–93;* injuries to, *87*

Spinal reflex, and urination, *396;* see also **Patellar knee-jerk reflex**

Spinal rotation, *71, 72, 75–77, 262;* coupling to lateral bending, *75, 77;* and liver detoxification, *444, 448;* and the lumbar spine, *78, 81;* and menopause, *459;* and the upper/lower hinges, *96*

Spinal vertebrae, *63–82;* compression of, *91;* and osteoporosis, *269, 271*

Spinothalamic tract, and the medulla, *87*

Spitting, muscles involved in, *364*

Spleen, and the ANS, *386;* asymmetry of, *522;* location of, *359, 360, 443;* and red blood cells, *323, 324, 354, 369;* representation of in sensory cortex, *28*

Stage-2 sleep, and consolidation, *47*

Stagnation in practice, *8*

Standing postures, *99, 100, 537–542;* see also individual postures such as ***Trikonasana***, etc.

Stapes, *433;* and cranial nerve VII, *436, 438;* location of, *434*

Static nuclear-bag fibers, *199, 200;* function of, *200;* innervation of, *201;* structure of, *200*

Stem cells; and the liver, *22;* and T lymphocytes, *384*

Sternocleidomastoid, location of, *168, 169*

Sternocostal joints, *359;* location of, *360*

Sternum, connection to ribs, *360, 361;* and floating ribs, *72;* location of, *237, 359;* and red blood cells, *323, 369;* structure of, *361*

Steroids, as hormones, *401*

Stomach, and the ANS, *145;* asymmetry of, *522;* and cranial nerve X, *151;* dermatome for, *306;* function of, *444;* and histamine, *445;* hormones of, *401;* location of, *360, 443*

Stomach acid, *444, 445;* and energy, *445;* and mitochondria, *445;* and stress, *449;* and ulcers, *445*

Stomach enzymes, and hydrochloric acid, *444;* pepsin, *444, 449;* pepsinogen, *444*

Stomach distress, and heartburn, *80, 443, 444, 449;* and helicobacter pylori, *449;* and indigestion, *449;* and thoracic misalignment, *80*

Stool, *446;* pressure on colon walls, *450*

Strength, see **Muscle strength**

Stress/Stressors, *11;* and the ANS, *157, 205;* and the adrenal cortex, *156;* and the apocrine glands, *395;* and anxiety, *154–156;* and blink rate, *413;* and cancer, *387;* and carbohydrates, *449;* seen as challenge, *160;* and core temperature, *153;* and cortisol, *40;* and depression, *155;* and supported forward bends, *449;* fracture, *244;* and gastrointestinal tract, *448, 449;* and the heart, *153–155;* hormonal response to, *153, 154;* and hypertension, *156;* and immunotransmitters, *155, 385;* and indigestion, *155;* and longevity, *499;* and lower-back pain, *155;* and the lymph glands, *103, 105;* mental, *230;* neural response to, *154;* and overwork, *161, 162;* and parasympathetic rebalancing, *449;* and the placebo effect, *164;* and *pranayama, 381;* with *savasana, 449;* and serotonin, *449;* and skin disorders, *291;* and stomach acid, *449;* and strain, *228–230, 277–279;* and the sympathetic NS, *335, 336, 449;* seen as threat, *160;* and trench mouth, *387;* and ulcers, *156, 387;* and vision, *419–421;* and *yogasana* practice, *157–160, 500*

Stretching, *4;* ballistic, *226;* and Caesarian section, *457;* and connective tissue, *189, 190, 224;* and creep, *279;* and gamma-motor neurons, *113, 175, 200, 202, 205, 214, 222;* and muscle spindles, *198–208;* and pain, *278;* reflex and the extensors, *212;* and scars, *285;* and skin, *285;* and temperature, *202, 203, 279;* time factor in, *279*

Stretch receptors, and craniosacral therapy, *95;* in the lungs, *203, 367;* in muscles, *199–206, 211;* in the rectum, *397;* in the sutures, *95;* in the urinary bladder, *396;* in the viscera, *203*

Striate body, function of, *35*

Striate cortex, and binocular vision, *424;* function of, *424;* location of, *423;* and the visual map, *424*

Stroke, *37;* and aging, *494;* and circadian rhythm, *478–480;* and hypertension, *336;* and inversions, *343;* timing of, *37*

Subconscious, *9–11, 17, 29, 35;* mixing with conscious, *49, 208;* time sense of, *473;* transformation to consciousness, *9*

Subcutaneous layer, *283;* structure of, *284*

Substantia nigra, *35;* and memory, *35*

Sugars, as fuel, *369*

Sulci, *25*

Superconscious, *9*

Superior temporal gyrus, *433*

Superior vena cava, *329;* function of, *312, 314, 328, 332, 333;* location of, *310*

Suppressor T cells, *384;* and depression, *467*

Suprachiasmatic nucleus, and circadian rhythms, *422, 485, 491;* function of, *144, 403, 423, 485;* and hormones, *403;* location of, *141;* and oscillator Y, *477*

Supta padangusthasana, *91;* and gravity, *556;* and reflex actions, *222*

Supta virasana, *126, 213;* and menstrual cramping, *231;* as an "X-rated" pose, *513*

Surgical deaths, times for, *478*

Surya bhedana, *382*

Surya namaskar, *184, 227*

Sushumna, *104, 140;* and *yogasana* practice, *380*

Sutures, coronal, *94;* cranial, *96;* as shock absorbers, *96*

Svadhyaya, *167;* and inversions, *456*

Swadisthana chakra, *75, 102, 103;* location of, *104*

Swallowing, *20, 34, 442;* and the epiglottis, *442;* and the esophagus, *442;* and higher centers, *443, 447;* and inversion, *442;* and release of hydrochloric acid, *444*

Swara yogis, *54;* and nasal laterality, *374, 375, 378, 379*

Swastikasana, 69, 266

Sweat glands, 307, 399; apocrine and anxiety, 395; apocrine and fear, 395; apocrine and stress, 395; and detoxification, 307, 395; eccrine, 395, 401; and the feet, 395; locations of, 395; and medulla oblongata, 395

Sweating, 133, 307, 393; and the ANS, 140, 143, 150; and the medulla, 395; and the palms, 395; and stressors, 154, 155; and thermoregulation, 293, 295, 395; and warming up, 227

Symmetry, and beauty, 519; and breathing, 519; and handedness, 520; and health, 519; and lack of, 519; in man, 519; and proprioception, 520; in *yogasanas*, 519, 521

Sympathetic nervous system, 5, 15, 18, 53, 55, 144–150; and acetylcholine, 144, 145; activation of, 83, 136; and lighter colors, 350; and arterial diameters, 327; and baroreceptor reflex arc, 340, 341; and beta waves, 60; and *brmhana*, 374; and the catecholamines, 147–149; and cerebral laterality, 55; and cervical misalignment, 79; and relations to the *chakras*, 103, 105; and cortisol, 149, 150; and depression, 464, 500; and epinephrine, 136, 139, 147; and heart action, 137, 317–320; and histamine, 388; and hormones, 47, 136; and hypertension, 337; and hyperventilation, 372; and hypoxia, 309; and inhalation, 356, 367; and innervation, 144–146; and inversions, 345, 349; and mental alertness, 136; and nasal laterality, 56; nerves of, 144–147, 375; neurotransmitters in, 137; and norepinephrine, 136, 139, 146; and pain, 298; and red blood cells, 323; response to stress, 335, 336; and spinal extension, 84; target organs of, 137, 145; and thoracic breathing, 372; and type-D PMS, 454

Synapses, 14, 108, 119, 121–125; adrenergic, 407; chemical, 122; cholinergic, 128, 407; cleft of, 128, 174; electrical, 122; inhibition of, 87, 108, 123, 128; potential, 117; strength of, 46; terminal, 115; see also **Neural connections**

Synovial fluid, and bursae, 263; in knee, 251, 260; and joint lubrication, 237

Synovial joints, 63, 66, 260–262; ball and socket, 96; capsule of, 252, 261; of the jaw, 96; as shock absorbers, 63; and warming up, 518

Systolic blood pressure, 311, 312, 315, 337; and color viewing, 427; and heart condition, 336; and inversion, 345; and isometric contraction, 368; and unilateral breathing, 53

T

Tachycardia, and defecation, 397

Tadasana, 69, 77, 99–101, 127, 135; arm action in, 257; asymmetry in, 522; and blood within lungs, 358; center of gravity in, 526, 527, 554; and colored lights, 430; foot action in, 253; and gravitational stress, 555; and gravity, 553; leg rotation in, 258; stability of, 550; symmetry in, 519–521; and redistributing the mass, 554

Talus, joints with legs, 252, 253; location of, 237, 252

Tarsal bones, location of, 237

T cells, and aging, 494; circadian rhythm and numbers of, 478, 479; and homeostasis, 385; storage of, 405; and the thymus, 384, 405

Teachers, 45; injury to, 552

Teaching, and cerebral laterality, 53; and neural plasticity, 113; *yogasana*, 44, 48, 49, 291

Tears, 393, 395; and the ANS, 139, 150, 393; and bacteria, 395; and blinking, 395; composition of, 395; and cranial nerve VII, 151, 395; ducts, 401; and emotional stress, 395; and *savasana*, 395

Temperature, of core, 137, 335; of finger, 158; and the hypothalamus, 140; of the knee, 265; and macrophages, 385; sensors for, 290, 291; of skin, 140, 294; and the sleep/wake cycle, 489, 490; of sperm, 461; see also **Fever** and **Cold feet**

Temporal lobe, 15, 27; function of, 26, 28, 43; and hearing, 523

Temporomandibular joint (TMJ), 94; and *yogasana* practice, 500

Tendon, 171, 262–265; and bone, 235; composition and properties of, 275–277; elongation of 229; and Golgi tendon organs, 206; injury of, 263; and joint stabilization, 265; nourishment of, 263; stress-strain curve of, 229, 230, 278; tensile strength of, 190, 229

Tensile stress, 201, 206, 229, 241; on nerves, 126, 127; on tendons, 190

Tension, as a mechanical force, 76

Tensor fasciae latae, location of, 168

Teres major, location of, 169

Teres minor, location of, 169

Testes, and androgens, 408; relation to the *chakras*, 103; location of, 402

Testosterone, and autism, 409; and bone growth, 408; and dyslexia, 409; effects of, 408, 409; and erection, 461; and facial hair, 408; and finger length, 409; and homosexuality, 409; and left handedness, 409; effect on left hemisphere, *49, 409;* levels as one ages, *409;* and musical ability, *409;* and osteoporosis, *272;* and sperm, *408;* as a steroidal hormone, *401;* and the testes, *408;* times of max/min concentration, *402;* ultradian rhythm of release of, *474;* in vegetarians, *408;* and the voice, *408;* in women, *408;* and *yogasana* practice, *408*

Tetanus, *125*

Thalamus, *11, 14, 172;* connections to other centers, *173;* and the EEG, *60;* frequencies of, *60, 61;* functions of, *25, 29, 34, 60;* and heavy pressure, *290;* location of, *24, 30, 173;* role in proprioception, *209*

Thermoregulation, via blood vessels, *292–294, 334;* and lie detection, *293;* via sweating, *293, 395*

Theta waves, in the EEG, *59, 60;* and *savasana, 166*

Thinking, about colors, effects of, *427;* and eye motion, *425, 426;* about food, *445, 449;* and immunity, *385, 386*

"The zone", for athletes, *146*

Thirst, *135*

Thoracic breathing, and abdominal contraction, *372;* and anxiety, *372;* and *brmhana, 374;* and hyperventilation, *372;* and inefficiency of, *372;* and inhalation, *372;* physiology of, *374;* and the sympathetic NS, *372*

Thoracic spine, curvature of, *90;* nerves of, *15, 1*

Thoracic vertebrae, connection to ribs, *360, 361;* and flexion, *74;* herniation of disc in, *91;* and lateral bending of, *72, 73;* location of, *64, 65, 69, 70;* misalignment of, *80;* range of motion of, *68, 72, 73, 90;* rotation about, *78, 81;* shape of, *66;* spinal extension, *74*

Thorax, *69, 70, 359, 360;* and the aorta, *327;* expansion of, *362;* and the diaphragm, *276;* outlet syndrome, *127*

Threat *versus* challenge, *160, 161;* and the adrenal medulla, *466–468*

Throat, *1;* and cervical misalignment, *79*

Thrombosis, and embolisms, *515, 517;* and platelets, *515;* and *sirsasana, 516, 517*

Thymus gland, *1, 354;* and the ANS, *386;* degeneration of, *385, 389, 405;* and hormones of, *401;* location of, *402;* and posture, *70;* relation to the *chakras, 103, 405;* and T cells, *384, 405*

Thyroid gland, *1;* and the bones, *243;* and cervical misalignment, *79;* relation to the *chakras, 103;* and *halasana, 405;* and the hypothalamus, *143;* location of, *357, 402;* and metabolism, *404, 405;* and *sarvangasana, 405*

Thyroid hormones, and the ANS, *139;* and calcitonin, *405;* and thyroxine, *404;* and triiodothyronine, *404*

Thyroid stimulating hormone (TSH), *143;* and the anterior pituitary, *404*

Thyrotropin, times of max/min concentrations, *402;* and TSH, *404*

Thyroxine, *405;* and the ANS, *139*

Tibia, joints involving, *248, 250–253;* location of, *237*

Tibial artery, *327*

Tibialis anterior, location of, *168*

Tickling, and the cerebellum, *289;* and laughter, *289*

Tidal volume, *365, 368;* and abdominal contraction, *366*

Tingling, sensation of, *91, 125–127*

Tinnitus, *60*

T lymphocytes, *384;* and AIDS, *385–388;* efficiency and temperature of, *388;* and osteoporosis, *385;* and rheumatoid arthritis, *388;* and stem cells, *384;* and the thymus gland, *384*

Tomato effect, *4, 5, 95*

Tongue, relaxation of, *189*

Tonic reflex, *99, 205, 206, 211, 215;* and headache, *215;* and lordosis, *215*

Top brain, *24*

Top hinge, *249*

Torque/countertorque, *20;* in *adho mukha vrksasana, 546;* and balancing, *528–530;* in *sirsasana* I, *546;* in *uttanasana, 531;* in *vrksasana, 538, 539*

Touch sensors, spinal connections to, *87*

Touching, *165;* deep pressure, *289, 290;* effects on infants, *291;* light touch, *287–289;* of women by men, *292;* and *yogasana, 291, 292*

Tourniquet effect, *126*

Trachea, *356;* and the dead volume, *365;* location of, *311, 357, 443;* when sneezing, *373;* mucus and the surface of, *394*

Transmembrane voltage, *111, 113, 116, 118;* relation to *prana, 119*

Transverse colon, *443*

Trapezius, *167;* location of, *168, 169;* pull on scapulae, *196, 256;* and tension, *81*

Trench mouth, and immunoglobulin, *387;* and stress, *387*

Triangamukhaikapada paschimottanasana, 513

Triceps brachii, and filament overlap, *186;* and Golgi tendon organ, *207;* inhibition by, *196;* location of, *168, 169;* reflex arc in, *212;* use of in opening shoulders, *197*

Trigeminal nerve; see **Cranial nerve V**

Triglycerides, as muscle fuel, *183, 184*

Triiodothyronine, *405*

Trikonasana, *11, 42, 77, 212, 221, 227;* and the arches of the feet, *253;* asymmetry in, *522;* balancing in, *541, 542;* best time for, *491;* and cerebral laterality, *56;* and exhalation, *364;* and gravity, *553;* hanging on the joints in, *252, 263;* left-right symmetry in, *519, 521;* and nasal laterality, *380;* and the reticular formation, *421;* and rotation of the femurs, *249;* and the ventilation-to-perfusion ratio, *358;* and the vestibular-ocular motor reflex, *541;* and redistributing the mass, *554*

Trochlear nerves; see **Cranial nerve IV**

Troponin, *178;* action of Ca^{2+} ion on, *178;* role in muscle action, *180*

Tumors, *383;* and cancer, *387;* and killer T cells, *385*

Two-World Views, *2–4;* and cerebral laterality, *53*

Tympanic membrane, *433;* location of, *434*

U

Uddiyana bandha, and anal pressure, *447*

Ulcers, and the ANS, *160;* and cortisol, *406;* and odor of the breath, *365;* and pepsin, *448;* and pepsinogen, *387;* and the placebo effect, *165;* and stomach acid, *445;* and stress, *156, 387*

Ulna, *255, 256;* articulations of, *256;* location of, *237;* rotation of, *257;* action on the scapulae, *196*

Ulnar nerve, *126, 127;* and artery, *327;* and the cubital tunnel, *126*

Ultradian rhythms, *54, 474–476;* and the ANS, *476;* and arterial pressure, *476;* and the breathing cycle, *475, 476;* and cardiac output, *476;* and the cardiovascular system, *476;* and the catecholamines, *476;* and cerebral dominance, *474;* and cerebrospinal fluid, *475;* and diastolic pressure, *476;* and heart rate, *476;* and hormonal release, *474, 476;* and the hypothalamus, *476;* and immunity, *476;* and nasal laterality, *474, 476;* and the neuroendocrine system, *476;* and REM sleep, *489;* and stroke volume, *476;* and systolic pressure, *476*

Ultraviolet light, and depression, *469;* and good health, *426*

Unconscious, *9, 10;* and *yogasanas*, *157*

Underbalancing, *544*

Unilateral breathing, and the EEG, *55;* and the heart, *54, 379;* relation to cerebral laterality, *54;* forced, *54*

Unipolar cells, function of, *110;* structure of, *109*

Upavistha konasana, and menstrual cramps, *231;* and the psoas, *248*

Upper hinge, *96*

Upper respiratory tract infections, and cortisol, *406;* and fatigue, *389*

Urdhva dhanurasana, *61, 70, 72, 79, 100;* and the ANS, *142, 162, 216–218;* and the breath, *365;* and the center of gravity, *527;* and colored lights, *430;* and eye rolling, *420;* and fear, *216;* and filament overlap, *186;* and glaucoma, *421;* and the Golgi tendon organs, *207;* and the heart, *320;* and intraocular pressure, *517;* and joint popping, *264;* and the vertebral arteries, *516, 517;* as an "X-rated" pose, *513*

Urdhva hastasana, *186;* and becoming a broomstick, *537;* center of gravity of, *537, 554;* and redistributing the mass, *537, 540;* and rotation of the humerus, *250*

Urdhva mukha svanasana, and type-D PMS, *454;* as an "X-rated" pose, *513*

Urdhva prasarita padasana, *247*

Uric acid, *502*

Urinary system, *1;* and the ANS, *140;* and the baroreceptors, *341;* and the bladder, *396;* and circadian rhythm, *479, 481;* incontinence and aging, *494;* and muscle tone in, *408;* and the parasympathetic NS, *351;* and the sphincter, *351, 396;* and stretch receptors, *396*

Urination, *396, 397;* and acidity of, *397;* and aging, *494;* and homeostasis, *351;* and the hypothalamus, *396;* and inversions, *342, 396, 397;* and laughter, *351;* mechanism of, *396;* and the parasympathetic NS, *351;* and sleep, *397;* and spinal reflex, *396;* and vasopressin, *396;* volume and circadian rhythm, *481;* volume and oscillator X, *477;* in women, *396;* and *yogasana* practice, *396*

Use-it-or-lose-it, bone, *242, 245;* brain, *21;* nerves, *112*

Ustrasana, and blood flow to brain, *37, 67, 81, 330;* and the knee joint, *250;* and opening the spine, *262*

Uterus, *349;* and collagen during pregnancy, *457;* and connexin during pregnancy, *457;* and the estrogen/progesterone balance, *408;* and urination, *396*

Utkatasana, *251;* and gravitational stress in, *555*

Utricle, and balancing in *trikonasana*, *541;* and balancing in *sirsasana I*, *550;* and balancing in *vrksasana*, *540;* function of, *437–439;* and kinocilia, *438, 439;* location of, *434, 438*

Uttana padasana, *98*

Uttanasana, *92*, *127*, *344;* and balance, *530*, *531;* best time for, *491;* and blood circulation, *348*, *349;* and exhalation, *368;* and fainting, *348;* and hypotension, *338;* and pain, *302;* reciprocal inhibition in, *194;* and rotation of the femurs in, *249;* as an "X-rated" pose, *513*

Uvula, *442*

V

Vaccination, *384*, *385*

Vagal heart-slowing reflex, *220*

Vagus nerve, see **Cranial nerve X**

Vagina, and estrogen/progesterone balance, *408*

Vajrasana, *78*, *379;* and cramping, *231;* and neurological damage, *513;* and the parasympathetic NS, *337;* and yoga foot drop, *514*

Valsalva maneuver, *517*

Valves, in the heart, *312–314;* in the lymphatic system, *352;* in veins, *330*, *332*, *333*, *342*

Varicose veins, *333;* and inversions, *349*, *351;* and *padmasana*, *518*

Vascular damage, *324*, *515–518*

Vascular system, *325*, *326;* and diastolic blood pressure, *326;* and the fight-or-flight response, *335;* and the gastrointestinal tract, *326;* injury to, *324*, *515–518;* and the muscles, *177*, *178*

Vascular functions, diameters and their control, *133*, *177*, *334*, *341;* flow rates, *177;* regulation by reticular formation, *31*

Vascular headaches, *38*, *39*

Vasisthasana, *422;* balancing in, *525*, *534*, *541;* and vision, *534*

Vasoconstriction, and angiotensin II, *335;* and the ANS, *138;* and the catecholamines, *148;* and hypertension, *335*, *336;* and inversions, *345;* and stroke, *336*

Vasodilation, and the ANS, *138;* and the catecholamines, *148;* and inversion, *348*, *350;* in muscles, *178;* and nitric oxide, *335*

Vasopressin, mode of action, *400;* and the ANS, *139*, *143;* and blood pressure, *404;* and circadian rhythm, *485;* and glycogen, *404;* regulates kidney, *47;* effect on memory, *47*, *404*, *485;* as a neurotransmitter, *404;* and the posterior pituitary, *404;* and rest-activity cycle, *485;* and urination, *396;* and water retention, *396*, *404*

Vastus lateralis, location of, *168*

Vastus medialis, location of, *168*

Vata, *382*, *484*

Vegetarians, and testosterone, *408*

Veins, blood of, *313;* blood pressure in, *329;* collapse of, *185;* and elastin, *275;* function of, *325;* postures and pressure in ankle vein, *332*, *333;* and valves, *330*, *332*, *333*, *342;* wall structure of, *330*

Venous blood flow, *329*, *331;* against gravity, *178*, *332–334*, *342*, *555;* and circulation during the breath, *367;* in inversions, *333*, *348*, *349;* and respiration, *333;* return to heart, *178*

Ventilation-to-perfusion ratio, *358;* in the thoracic breath, *372;* and *trikonasana*, *358*

Ventral horn, *65;* and motor neurons, *200*

Ventral root, *85*, *86*

Ventricular stroke volume, *317*, *368;* during exercise, *322;* and inversions, *345;* and posture, *369;* sensor for, *342*

Venule, *311*, *329;* blood flow through, *329–331;* blood pressure in, *329*

Vertebral arteries, *36*, *37*, *327;* to the brain, *81;* and the foramen magnum, *515;* lesions and *halasana*, *516*, *550;* and *sarvangasana*, *550;* and *sirsasana*, *515*, *516;* and thromboses, *515;* and *urdhva dhandasana*, *516;* and *ustrasana*, *330*

Vertebrae, articular facets of, *67*, *83*, *88;* facet joints of, *65–67*, *88;* and red blood cells, *323;* spinous processes of, *65–67*, *72*, *81*, *82*, *88;* subluxation of, *70*, *92;* transverse processes of, *65*, *66*, *81*, *82*, *88;* wedging, *70*, *77*, *90*

Vertebral foramen, see **Spinal canal**

Vesicles, *46;* endocrine, *401;* for neurotransmitters, *122*, *123*, *128*, *174*

Vestibular-oculomotor reflex, in balancing, *418*, *526*, *535;* in *trikonasana*, *541*

Vestibular organs, *437–440;* and aging, *497*, *526;* and balance, *67*, *223*, *438–440*, *526*, *533;* connection to the eyes, *418;* innervation of, *440;* and the medulla, *440;* nerves of, *109*, *438*, *440;* in proprioception, *210;* response times of, *530*, *532;* and semicircular canals, *418;* and structure of the inner ear, *434*, *437*, *438*

V̇O$_{2max}$, *184*, *193;* and aging, *496*

Violence, *153*

Violet-color viewing, *427*

Viparita karani, *38*, *61;* and abdominal breathing, *370*, *371;* and blood distribution, *349;* and lymph edema, *351;* for leg injury, *245;* and menopause, *460;* and the parasympathetic NS, *337;* and pregnancy, *458;* and relaxation, *219*

Virabhadrasana I, *18*, *19*, *25*, *35;* and balance, *418*, *533*, *535;* and the breath, *365*

Virabhadrasana II, *72*

Virabhadrasana III, and balance, *418, 525, 535;* broomstick action in, *542;* using the eyes for balance in, *535, 542;* redistributing the mass in, *542*

Virasana, *126, 127, 187;* and cramping, *231*

Virus, *383;* attack by, *155, 325;* herpes, *387;* infection and circadian rhythm, *481;* and killer T cells, *385*

Visceral organs, asymmetry of, *522;* and dermatomes, *448;* and endocrine glands, *399;* massage by abdominal breath, *370, 371;* nervous system of, *5, 15, 17, 108, 137, 319, 442, 447;* and pain, *150, 441, 448;* pleura of, *357;* and smooth muscles, *441;* stretch receptors in, *203*

Viscoelasticity, *224, 225;* and hyperflexibility, *203;* and intervertebral discs, *89;* and muscles, *227;* and muscle spindles, *202;* and myofascia, *277*

Vision/visual aids, *17;* adaptation and pigments, *417, 418;* aging and, *494, 497;* to balance, *422, 526, 533–535, 542, 552;* and the emotions, *52;* and dominance, *52;* mechanism of, *533;* and multipolar cells, *132;* nerve cells in, *109;* and the occipital lobe, *415, 424, 533;* response time of, *530, 532;* and *virabhadrasana III*, *533, 535;* and *yogasana* practice, *500*

Vishuddha chakra, *103;* location of, *104*

Visual cortex, *28;* location of, *27, 173*

Visual laterality, *422–424;* and depression, *51;* and dominance, *52, 56, 57, 426;* and higher centers, *424;* and memory, *424;* and *yogasana* practice, *426*

Visual memory, and eye motion, *425*

Visual pigment, and circadian rhythm, *485*

Visual stress, *419, 534;* while balancing, *534;* and the gaze, *411, 419, 420;* and hypnotic states, *420;* and personality, *419;* and relaxation of, *411, 415, 419–421*

Vitamin D, and the bones, *247;* and the parathyroid, *405;* and the skin, *283*

Vitreous humour, and intraocular pressure, *420;* location of, *414*

Voice, and testosterone, *408;* and vocal-cord tension, *20*

Volition, *13, 17*

Vomiting, *20;* muscles involved in, *364, 447*

Voodoo death, *161*

Vrksasana, *135, 245, 246;* and the aged, *540;* balancing in, *525, 537, 538–541, 550;* becoming a broomstick in, *538;* and the center of gravity, *537;* and circulation in a sprained ankle, *541;* and head position, *534, 540;* and

joint capsules, *540;* redistributing the mass, *537;* and torque/countertorque, *537, 538;* wall support for, *536, 540*

Vrscikasana, *549*

W

Wall support to balance, *535, 536, 540*

Warm up, *185, 223, 227, 228, 518;* and joint lubrication, *518;* for *padmasana*, *267;* and sweating, *227;* and *surya namaskar*, *228;* and tissue damage, *230, 231*

Waist-to-hip ratio, for heart health, *460, 461*

Wall *padasana*, and type-H PMS, *455*

Water retention, and the estrogen/progesterone balance, *408;* and the hypothalamus, *140, 143;* and type-H PMS, *454;* and vasopressin, *396, 404*

Weightlessness, *555, 556;* and old age, *556*

Western medicine, *1, 2, 4–6;* and chronotherapy, *486;* and the eyes, *415;* history of, and nasal laterality, *375;* and *yogasana* injuries, *511–518*

White corpuscles/white blood cells, *22, 93;* acquired response of, *324;* and the blood-brain barrier, *325;* and circadian rhythm, *478, 479;* and defense of the body, *324;* innate response of, *324;* and macrophages, *324;* production of, *325;* and *yogasana* practice, *390*

White matter, *25, 33, 35;* in the brain, *107;* in the spinal cord, *84–87*

World views, *2–7, 52*

Wrist, and osteoporosis, *269, 271*

X

"X-rated" postures; and *halasana*, *513;* and *malasana*, *513;* and *supta virasana*, *513;* and *triangamukhaikapada paschimottanasana*, *513;* and *uttanasana*, *513;* and *urdhva dhanurasana*, *513;* and *urdhva mukha svanasana*, *513*

Xyphoid process, location of, *237, 360;* structure of, *361*

Y

Yama, *9*

Yellow-color viewing, *427*

Yin/Yang, *105*

Yogadandasana, *56;* and nasal laterality, *379*

Yoga foot drop, and *vajrasana*, *514*

Yoganidrasana, *161, 162*

Yogasana, and asthma, *359;* and bone density, *271, 272;* and boredom, *161;* detraining, *233;* goals and practice, *6, 7, 11, 17, 20, 57;* and osteoporosis, *271;* over-training, *233, 234;* pose and repose, *333;* teaching, *43, 48, 49;* and therapy, *2;* touching, *165, 291, 292*

Yogasana **practice**, and aerobic work, *320, 321;* and aging, *279, 496, 497, 499, 501;* and AIDS, *390;* and alpha waves, *337, 468;* and anxiety, *471;* and attitude, *468;* and autonomic control, *135;* and balancing, *525–552;* and beta waves in colored light, *430;* and bipolar disorder, *470;* and blink rate, *413;* and the bones, *241, 245, 246, 500;* from a book, *511;* the breath and moving into *yogasana, 364;* and capillary formation, *184, 321;* and cardio-vascular conditioning, *496, 500;* and center of gravity, *554;* lifting the chest in, *255;* and childbirth, *457;* and chronotherapy, *486, 487;* and circulation, *245, 309;* and color therapy, *426, 428–430, 468, 469;* and constipation, *397, 398, 500;* and the control of nasal laterality, *378, 379;* and cortisol, *149, 150, 406;* and the dead volume, *366;* delight in, *208;* and delta waves in colored light, *430;* and depression, *467, 468, 500;* and dermatomes, *307;* and detoxification, *243;* and diabetes, *408, 451;* and digestion, *443, 444, 449, 500;* and diaphragmatic breathing, *371, 372;* effects of, *500–502;* and the emotions, *163, 206, 463;* and endorphins, *303;* and endurance, *184, 500;* and exhalation, *364;* and the eyes, *411;* and flexibility, *500;* and foot pain, *497;* and the Golgi tendon organs, *207;* and gravity, *555;* and hearing, *500;* and the heart, *337, 346;* and hormonal release, *400, 401;* and hypertension, *337, 338;* and hypnotic states, *32, 56, 156;* when ill, *390;* and immunity, *389, 390, 500;* and injuries, *511–518;* and insulin production, *408;* and isometric con-traction, *189;* and the kidneys, *500;* and the liver, *500;* and lymph, *353;* and mental acuity, *500–502;* and muscles, *168, 199–201;* and muscle fiber types, *192, 193, 421;* and muscle mass, *496;* and muscle strength, *500;* and muscle tone, *205, 206;* and nasal laterality, *380;* and neural crossover, *543;* and neural pathways, *18, 19, 177;* and optic-nerve crossover, *422;* and osteoarthritis, *268;* and osteoporosis, *271, 272, 351;* and over-train-ing, *359;* and pain, *295, 298, 299;* and platelets, *324;* and *pranayama, 381;* precipi-tating asthma attack, *372;* and proprioception, *208–211;* and the first trimester of pregnancy, *456;* and red blood cells, *324, 390;* and redis-tributing the mass, *536, 537;* and relaxation, *491;* and reflexes, *211, 212;* and respiration, *368, 496;* and response times, *421;* and rest-ing muscle tone, *199;* and sciatica, *302;* and the sense of smell, *500;* and the sense of taste, *500;* and skin receptors, *208, 289;* and sore-ness, *184;* and stagnation, *8;* and stress, *500;* and the *sushumna nadi, 380;* and symmetry, *519, 520;* and sympathetic de-excitation, *368;* and testosterone, *408;* and thermoregulation, *294;* best time for, *483, 484, 487;* time of, and cortisol, *406;* and TMJ, *500;* and touching by the teacher, *291;* under water, *556;* when not feeling well, *390;* and white blood cells, *390;* and urination, *396;* and visual laterality, *426;* and vision, *500, 534*

Yogasana **props**, colored lights as, *430*

Z

Z discs, *178, 179;* motion of, *180, 181, 187*

Zero gravity, and anemia, *555;* and bone dem-ineralization, *555;* and muscle fiber conver-sion, *555*

9 781587 360